Maternity & Pediatric Nursing

made Incredibly Easy!

Clinical Editor
Mikki Meadows-Oliver, PHD, RN, FAAN, FAANP
Assistant Dean for Pre-Licensure Programs;
Clinical Professor
Rory Meyers College of Nursing
New York University
New York, New York

Wolters Kluwer

Philadelphia · Baltimore · New York · London
Buenos Aires · Hong Kong · Sydney · Tokyo

Vice President and Publisher: Julie K. Stegman
Director of Nursing Education and Practice Content: Jamie Blum
Acquisitions Editors: Joyce Berendes and Heather Bays-Petrovic
Development Editor: Emily Schlapp
Editorial Coordinator: Remington Fernando
Editorial Assistant: Sara Thul
Production Project Manager: Frances Gunning
Manager, Graphic Arts & Design: Stephen Druding
Art Director, Illustration: Jennifer Clements
Manufacturing Coordinator: Margie Orzech
Marketing Manager: Amy Whitaker
Prepress Vendor: S4Carlisle Publishing Services

9 8 7 6 5 4 3 2 1

Printed in Mexico

Library of Congress Cataloging-in-Publication Data

ISBN-13: 978-1-975247-72-0

Library of Congress Control Number: 2025933217

shop.lww.com

QUADM0525

Contributors

Nancy C. Banasiak, DNP, PPCNP-BC, APRN
Wendy U. and Thomas C. Naratil Professor of Nursing
Pediatric Nurse Practitioner Specialty
Yale University School of Nursing
Orange, Connecticut

Vera C. Brancato, EdD, MSN, BSN, RN, CNE
Professor Emerita
Department of Nursing
Alvernia University
Reading, Pennsylvania

Angela Chlebowski, DNP, RN, C-EFM
Clinical Assistant Professor
Rory Meyers College of Nursing
New York University
New York, New York

Cheryl Degraw, EdS, MSN, RN, CRNP
Simulation Assistant
Department of Nursing
Central Carolina Technical College
Sumter, South Carolina

Amanda C. Filippelli, MSN, MPH, APRN, PPCNP-BC
Pediatric Nurse Practitioner
Department of Pulmonology
Connecticut Children's Medical Center
Hartford, Connecticut

Mary Agnes Gallagher, DNP, MPH, CPNP-PC
Assistant Clinical Professor
Betty Irene Moore School of Nursing at UC Davis
UCSF School of Nursing
San Francisco, California

Allison Grady, MSN, PPCNP-BC
Pediatric Nurse Practitioner
Department of Pediatrics, Oncology Section
Medical College of Wisconsin
Milwaukee, Wisconsin

Kirstin Guinn, MSN-NE, RNC-OB, C-ONQS, C-EFM
Assistant Professor of Nursing Practice
Harris College of Nursing & Health Sciences
Texas Christian University
Fort Worth, Texas

Mikki Meadows-Oliver, PhD, RN, FAAN, FAANP
Assistant Dean for Pre-Licensure Programs;
Clinical Professor
Rory Meyers College of Nursing
New York University
New York, New York

Mary K. Peterson, DNP, APRN, PPCNP-BC
Senior Lecturer
Pediatric Nurse Practitioner Specialty
Yale University School of Nursing
Orange, Connecticut

Lisette Saleh, PhD, MSN, RNC-OB
Assistant Professor
Department of Nursing
Texas Christian University
Fort Worth, Texas

Patricia E. Thomas, PhD, NNP-BC, CNE
Clinical Associate Professor
College of Nursing and Health Innovation
University of Texas at Arlington
Arlington, Texas

Foreword

The primary goal of the first edition of *Maternity & Pediatric Nursing Made Incredibly Easy!* is to provide nurses interested in maternity and pediatric health with increased knowledge regarding population-specific health care conditions as they relate to nursing practice. Writing the first edition of *Maternity & Pediatric Nursing Made Incredibly Easy!* required a team of dedicated nurse experts from different regions of the country who worked to ensure that this book contained relevant information that is useful in everyday practice. While recognizing that cultural, global, and regional differences in how words are used, this first edition of *Maternity & Pediatric Nursing Made Incredibly Easy!* endeavored to use inclusive language and gender-neutral terms where possible.

Maternity & Pediatric Nursing Made Incredibly Easy! provides an introduction to essential topics for nurses with limited maternity and pediatric experience and serves as a refresher for nurses already caring for these patients. This book is also a valuable resource for students during their maternity and pediatric clinical rotations. Students will appreciate the easy-to-read format and the "Advice from the experts." Even the most experienced nurses will find a means to enhance their knowledge.

Maternity & Pediatric Nursing Made Incredibly Easy! begins with a chapter introducing the reader to maternity and pediatric nursing. This chapter defines the role of the nurse in each setting and the philosophy of family-centered care. The next few chapters review family planning, conception, physiologic adaptations to pregnancy, and prenatal care. Care of the pregnant person through labor, birth, and the postpartum period is then examined. Potential complications within the postpartum and neonatal periods are delineated, along with assessment and care of the normal neonate.

In the pediatric portion of the book, the developmental aspects of care related to infants, early/middle childhood, and adolescence are reviewed. Chapters 14 to 23 cover commonly encountered pediatric conditions relevant to various body systems—for example, cardiovascular, respiratory, and gastrointestinal. Each chapter provides the reader with an abundance of practical, useful information.

Maternity & Pediatric Nursing Made Incredibly Easy! has several icons to draw your attention to important issues. An easy-to-read format is presented to aid and engage the reader. Illustrations are presented to help you visualize the pathophysiology of the condition.

"Memory joggers" provide useful tips to help you remember important information.

Advice from the experts—presents information from skilled practitioners

It's all relative—provides topics for education for patients and their families

Growing pains—offers age and stage description, expectations, and dangers

After reading each chapter, you can test how much you've learned with the "Quick quiz" at the end of each chapter. You will then realize how valuable a resource this book is and how much this material applies to your maternity and pediatric nursing practice!

Mikki Meadows-Oliver, PHD, RN, FAAN, FAANP
Clinical Professor
Rory Meyers College of Nursing
New York University
New York, New York

Acknowledgments

I would like to thank all the nurses and nurse practitioners who made this first edition of *Maternity & Pediatric Nursing Made Incredibly Easy!* possible. Their input and suggestions helped to make this edition useful and relevant to nursing students as well as novice and experienced nurses working with pregnant people, children, and their families.

Contents

1 Introduction to maternity/pediatric nursing   1
Mikki Meadows-Oliver, PhD, RN, FAAN, FAANP

2 Conception and fetal development   9
Mikki Meadows-Oliver, PhD, RN, FAAN, FAANP

3 Family planning and contraception   40
Lisette Saleh, PhD, MSN, RNC-OB

4 Physiologic and psychosocial adaptations to pregnancy   73
Mikki Meadows-Oliver, PhD, RN, FAAN, FAANP

5 Prenatal care   107
Mikki Meadows-Oliver, PhD, RN, FAAN, FAANP

6 High-risk pregnancy   147
Mikki Meadows-Oliver, PhD, RN, FAAN, FAANP

7 Labor and birth   199
Angela Chlebowski, DNP, RN, C-EFM

8 Postpartum care   244
Kirstin Guinn, MSN-NE, RNC-OB, C-ONQS, C-EFM

9 Complications of the postpartum period   277
Kirstin Guinn, MSN-NE, RNC-OB, C-ONQS, C-EFM

10 Neonatal assessment and care   309
Mikki Meadows-Oliver, PhD, RN, FAAN, FAANP

11 High-risk neonatal conditions   346
Patricia E. Thomas, PhD, NNP-BC, CNE

12 Infancy and early childhood   379
Mikki Meadows-Oliver, PhD, RN, FAAN, FAANP

13 Middle childhood and adolescence   417
Allison Grady, MSN, PPCNP-BC

14 Infectious diseases   451
Nancy C. Banasiak, DNP, PPCNP-BC, APRN

15 Neurologic problems   480
Mikki Meadows-Oliver, PhD, RN, FAAN, FAANP

16 Cardiovascular problems   526
Mikki Meadows-Oliver, PhD, RN, FAAN, FAANP

17   **Respiratory problems**   **579**
Amanda C. Filippelli, MSN, MPH, APRN, PPCNP-BC

18   **Urinary problems**   **614**
Mary Agnes Gallagher, DNP, MPH, CPNP-PC

19   **Musculoskeletal problems**   **645**
Mary Agnes Gallagher, DNP, MPH, CPNP-PC

20   **Gastrointestinal problems**   **683**
Cheryl Degraw, EdS, MSN, RN, CRNP

21   **Endocrine and metabolic problems**   **711**
Mary K. Peterson, DNP, APRN, PPCNP-BC

22   **Hematologic and immunologic problems**   **747**
Allison Grady, MSN, PPCNP-BC

23   **Dermatologic problems**   **785**
Vera C. Brancato, EdD, MSN, BSN, RN, CNE

Index   **819**

Chapter 1

Introduction to maternity/ pediatric nursing

Just the facts

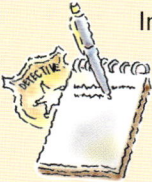

In this chapter, you'll learn:

◆ the role of maternity and pediatric nurses

◆ the philosophy of family-centered care

◆ types of family structures

◆ social determinants of health that potentially affect maternal and pediatric health.

Role of the nurse in maternity and pediatric settings

Maternity and pediatric nurses provide specialized care to patients along their health care journeys. Maternity nurses have two (or more) patients at a time: the pregnant person and the fetus or newborn. They provide specialized health care to a pregnant person during pregnancy, delivery, and postpartum. Additionally, they provide care to the neonate during the immediate postpartum period. Pediatric nurses have specialized knowledge and skills to care for neonates and children through adolescence on a continuum from health to illness.

Nurses involved in maternity and pediatric nursing assume many roles. These may include health care provider, educator, advocate, and counselor. The functions involved for each of these roles depend on the nurse's level of training and education. Nurses involved in maternity pediatric nursing may be registered nurses or advanced practice nurses such as certified nurse-midwives (CNMs), nurse practitioners (NPs), or clinical nurse specialists (CNSs).

Family–centered care

Maternity nurses are responsible for providing comprehensive care to the pregnant person, their fetus, and family members. Pediatric nurses incorporate parents, caregivers, and other family members into the child's or adolescent's care. This is known as *family-centered care or patient-family-centered care*. In some areas, it is also known as *relationship-based care*. Family-centered care encourages collaborations between health care providers and family members at all levels of care and in all health care settings. In family-centered care, patients and families define their "family" and determine how each member will participate in care and decision making.

Within pediatrics, family-centered care acknowledges the caregivers as the constant in the child's life and as experts in the care of their child. The family's input is a major force behind the development of the child's care plan.

Benefits of family-centered care

Family-centered care benefits the pregnant person, child, and family as well as the health care professional.

Benefits to families
• Less stress and heightened feelings of confidence and competence in caring for their neonates, infants, and children
• Less dependence on professional caregivers
• Empowerment to develop new skills and expertise in the care of their neonates, infants, and children

Benefits to health care professionals
• Greater job satisfaction
• Empowerment to develop new skills and expertise in maternity and pediatric nursing

A closer look at the family

Understanding different types of family structures is helpful for the nurse when providing family-centered care.

There are often four family types that are described later; however, this is not a comprehensive list as many different family types exist.

• In *two-parent families*, both parents have the same parental relationships with the child. These parents can be biological or adoptive. In a two-parent family, the parents may be married or cohabitating.
• In a *stepfamily*, the family unit is composed of one parent related to the child biologically or by adoption and one parent who is the partner or spouse of the biological/adoptive parent (i.e., stepparent).

- In a *single-parent family*, there is only one biological/adoptive parent residing with the child.
- Finally, *nonparent families* are those in which no biological/adoptive/stepparent is living in the household with the child. Examples of nonparent families would be if a child lives with a grandparent, other relative, or a nonrelative. Children in foster care would be considered part of nonparent family units.

A look at maternity and pediatric health

Maternal, infant, and childhood mortality rates are key indicators of the health of a population. These figures can provide the nurse with essential information about how and where to direct care for individual patients and the community at large.

Maternal mortality

In recent years, maternal mortality and morbidity have been a focus of clinicians and policymakers. People in the United States are more likely to die from childbirth than people living in other resource-abundant countries. Recognizing that health before, during, and after pregnancy can have a major impact on infants' health and well-being, a "Healthy People 2030" goal is to "Prevent pregnancy complications and maternal deaths and improve women's health before, during, and after pregnancy." "Healthy People" is our nation's plan to improve the health and well-being of people residing in the United States. This 10-year plan provides measurable public health objectives and tools to help track progress toward achieving them.

Regarding maternal mortality, data indicate that there were 17.4 deaths per 100,000 live births in 2018. That number increased significantly to 32.9 per 100,000 in 2021—likely due to factors related to the COVID-19 pandemic. The level of maternal mortality during the COVID-19 pandemic may have been impacted by two factors: deaths where the pregnant patient died due to the interaction between their pregnant state and COVID-19 or deaths where pregnancy complications were not prevented or managed due to disruption of health services. The most recent data indicate that the maternal mortality rate began to decrease in 2022 to 22.32 deaths per 100,000 live births. The target rate is 15.7 maternal deaths per 100,000 live births. These current rates and the target rate are contrasted with the current maternal mortality rates in resource-abundant countries such as the United Kingdom (10 deaths per 100,000 live births) and Canada which has 11 deaths per 100,000 live births.

Significant racial and ethnic disparities in maternal mortality exist in the United States. Disparities are defined as preventable differences in the burden of disease that are experienced by socially disadvantaged populations. In 2020, the mortality rate for non-Hispanic Black females was 55.3 deaths per 100,000 live births, 2.9 times higher than the rate for non-Hispanic White females (19.1) and over three times higher than the rate for Hispanic females (18.2).

Infant and childhood mortality

Infant mortality rates are the number of infant deaths during the first year of life per 1,000 live births. The infant mortality rate for the United States is 5.1 infant deaths/1,000 live births compared with 3.8 infant deaths/1,000 live births in the United Kingdom. Within the United States, the infant mortality rate varies widely by state with Massachusetts being the state with the lowest infant mortality rate (3.32/1,000 live births) and Mississippi being the state with the highest infant mortality rate (9.11/1,000 live births). The leading three causes of death during infancy are (1) congenital defects, (2) prematurity/low birthweight, and (3) sudden infant death syndrome (SIDS)/sudden unexplained infant deaths (SUID).

In 2021, the leading cause of death for children in the United States, aged 1 to 17 years, was firearm-related injuries. Of note, death by suicide is the second leading cause of death in children aged 10 to 14 years and the third leading cause of death in adolescents aged 15 to 19 years. Other leading causes of death in childhood include unintentional injuries (such as motor vehicle crashes) and childhood cancer.

Maternal and childhood morbidity

Morbidity is defined as the number of people in a population who are faced with a specific health condition at a particular point in time.

The World Health Organization (WHO) defines maternal morbidity as "any health condition attributed to and/or aggravated by pregnancy and childbirth that has a negative impact on the woman's wellbeing." The Centers for Disease Control and Prevention (CDC) defines severe maternal morbidity (SMM) as including "unexpected outcomes of labor and delivery that result in significant short- or long-term consequences to a woman's health." SMM is a key risk factor for maternal death. Examples of SMM include eclampsia, acute kidney failure, sepsis, and hemorrhage requiring a blood transfusion. The majority of SMM cases (73.5%) occur within the first 2 postpartum weeks.

For children in the United States aged 1 year and older, the most common causes of childhood morbidity include health conditions related to injuries, asthma, diabetes, obesity and overweight, developmental disabilities and differences, and mental health disorders. Congenital anomalies are the most common cause of morbidity in infants younger than 1 year.

Room for improvement

In 2023, there were 74 million children younger than 18 years old living in the United States. Of those, approximately 11 million children were living in poverty. Children remain the poorest age group in America, with children of color, children under 5 years of age, children of single birthing parent, and children in the southern United States suffering from the highest poverty rates. The COVID-19 pandemic forced children already in poverty even deeper into poverty. Four million children live without health insurance. Living in poverty or lacking health insurance has wide-ranging effects on children, putting them at a much higher risk of experiencing adverse health outcomes.

Social determinants of health

Social determinants of health (SDOH) are conditions in the environments where families live, learn, work, and play that affect their overall health and health care outcomes. SDOH can contribute to health disparities and inequities. SDOH can significantly affect care for pregnant and postpartum patients and their families. For example, families who do not have access to grocery stores with healthy foods are less likely to have good nutrition. Lack of access to healthy foods can increase the risk of health conditions like heart disease, diabetes, and obesity—which can lower life expectancy when compared to people who do have access to healthy foods.

The Healthy People 2030 document lists five domains of SDOH:

- Economic stability: In the United States, many families live in poverty and cannot afford healthy foods, health care, and adequate housing. People with steady employment are less likely to live in poverty and more likely to have employer-provided health insurance (potentially increasing access to health care).
- Education access and quality: People with higher levels of education are more likely to be healthy. Children from low-income families, children with disabilities, and children who routinely experience forms of social discrimination are less likely to graduate from high school. This, in turn, means that they may be less likely to have stable well-paying employment (with employer-provided

insurance) and be at increased risk for economic instability and being under- or uninsured.

- Health care access and quality: Nearly 10% of the population in the United States does not have health insurance coverage. Those without insurance are less likely to have a primary care provider and may not be able to afford the recommended health care services (such as cancer screenings) and needed medications.
- Neighborhood and built environment: Neighborhoods where families live can have a large impact on their health and well-being. Families may live in neighborhoods with high rates of violence, unsafe air or water, and exposure to other health and safety risks. Additionally, some people have occupational exposures that can harm their health, such as secondhand smoke or loud noises.
- Social and community context: Relationships and interactions among family, friends, and community members can have a major impact on health and well-being. Positive relationships can help reduce the negative impacts of adverse life conditions.

Health-related beliefs and practices

Health-related beliefs and practices of the family have a strong influence on how often they will seek health care. If family members hesitate to seek health care for themselves, they commonly will not seek regular care for their child until the child becomes seriously ill.

Once bitten

A family's health-related beliefs and practices are often based on previous experiences with health care. Negative experiences can make family members reluctant to seek care for themselves and for their children.

These experiences may include:
- real or perceived poor quality of care
- real or perceived insensitivity of health care professionals
- real or perceived discrimination by health care professionals
- physical or emotional pain or trauma
- death of a family member in a health care facility.

The maternity or pediatric nurse can help to make a family's health encounter positive by:
- asking family members about their past health care experiences and acknowledging their concerns
- stressing the ways the current situation may differ from past situations
- encouraging family members to participate actively in their child's health care and praising them for the care they are already providing.

Quick quiz

1. The phrase *infant mortality rates* refers to the:
   A. number of children faced with any given health problem.
   B. number of infant deaths in any given year.
   C. nutritional health of a population of infants.
   D. socioeconomic status of a population of infants.

Answer: B. Infant mortality rates refer to the number of infant deaths per 1,000 live births in any given year.

2. Children in foster care are a part of which of the following family types?
   A. Two-parent family
   B. Stepfamily
   C. Single-parent family
   D. Nonparent family

Answer: D. Children in foster care are considered to be part of non-parent families—where no biological/adoptive/stepparent lives in the household with the child.

3. A 5-year-old is in the hospital after having an appendectomy. A full liquid diet is ordered for the child. A carbonated soda, chicken broth, milk, and ice cream are on the food tray. The caregiver does not want the child to have soda or ice cream because they do not allow the child to have foods containing sugar. When considering family-centered care, which of the following actions is the nurse's best response?
   A. Explain to the caregiver that these are the only foods allowed after surgery.
   B. Consult the primary provider to determine the best foods to have postoperatively.
   C. Discuss the nutritional value of these foods after surgery.
   D. Review with the caregiver what foods are allowed and include them in the menu selection.

Answer: D. By allowing the caregiver to participate in making decisions about the child's care, the nurse is fostering family-centered care.

4. Which of the following is a condition associated with SMM among pregnant people in the United States?
   A. Preterm labor
   B. History of early pregnancy loss
   C. Acute kidney failure
   D. Gestational diabetes

Answer: C. Acute kidney failure, eclampsia, sepsis, and hemorrhage requiring a blood transfusion are all examples of SMM.

Scoring

★★★   If you answered all four items correctly, congratulations! Your introduction to maternity and pediatric nursing is empowering.

★★   If you answered three items correctly, good work! Tell your peers you have a well-centered grasp of maternity and pediatric nursing.

★   If you answered fewer than three items correctly, don't get discouraged! You have more chapters to create a positive maternity and pediatric nursing experience.

Selected References

Centers for Disease Control and Prevention. (2023). *Infant mortality rates by state*. https://www.cdc.gov/nchs/pressroom/sosmap/infant_mortality_rates/infant_mortality.htm

Central Intelligence Agency. (n.d.-a). *Infant mortality rate*. https://www.cia.gov/the-world-factbook/field/infant-mortality-rate/country-comparison/

Central Intelligence Agency. (n.d.-b). *Maternal mortality ratio*. https://www.cia.gov/the-world-factbook/field/maternal-mortality-ratio/country-comparison/

Children's Defense Fund. (2023). *Child poverty*. https://www.childrensdefense.org/tools-and-resources/the-state-of-americas-children/soac-child-poverty/

Healthy People 2030. (n.d.). *Pregnancy and childbirth*. https://health.gov/healthypeople/objectives-and-data/browse-objectives/pregnancy-and-childbirth

Institute for Patient and Family Centered Care. (2024). *Patient- and family-centered care*. https://www.ipfcc.org/about/pfcc.html

Kaiser Family Foundation. (2023). *Child and teen firearm mortality in the U.S. and peer countries*. https://www.kff.org/mental-health/issue-brief/child-and-teen-firearm-mortality-in-the-u-s-and-peer-countries/

World Health Organization. (2024). *Maternal mortality*. https://www.who.int/news-room/fact-sheets/detail/maternal-mortality

Chapter 2

Conception and fetal development

Just the facts

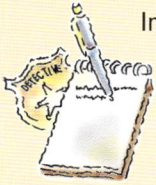

In this chapter, you'll learn:

♦ anatomic structures and functions of the male and female reproductive systems
♦ effects of hormone production on sexual development
♦ the process of fertilization
♦ stages of fetal development
♦ structural changes that result from pregnancy.

A look at conception and fetal development

Development of a functioning human being from a fertilized ovum involves a complex process of cell division, differentiation, and organization. Development begins with the union of spermatozoon and ovum (conception) to form a composite cell containing chromosomes from both caregivers. This composite cell (called a *zygote*) divides repeatedly. Finally, groups of differentiated cells organize into complex structures, such as the brain, spinal cord, liver, kidneys, and other organs that function as integrated units.

To fully understand the dramatic physical changes that occur during pregnancy, the nurse must be familiar with reproductive anatomy and physiology and the stages of fetal development.

Male reproductive system

Anatomically, the main distinction between a male and a female is the presence of conspicuous external genitalia in the male. In contrast, the major reproductive organs of the female lie within the pelvic cavity.

Making introductions

The male reproductive system consists of the organs that produce, transfer, and introduce mature sperm into the female reproductive tract where fertilization occurs. (See *Structures of the male reproductive system.*)

Structures of the male reproductive system

The male reproductive system consists of the penis, the scrotum and its contents, the prostate gland, and the inguinal structures.

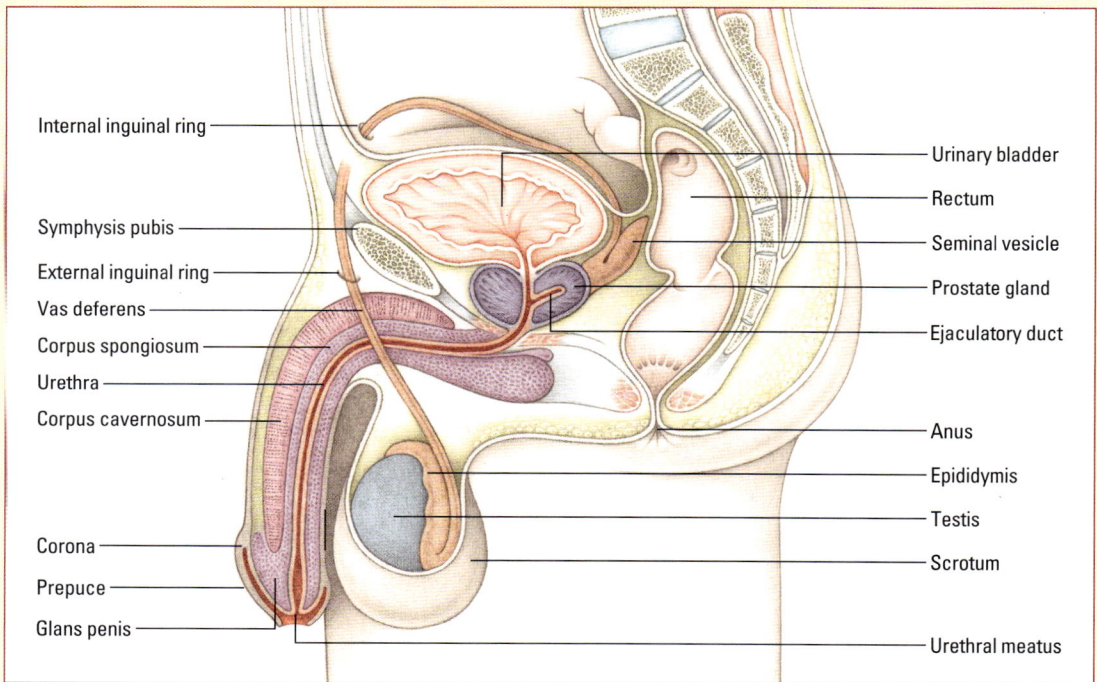

Internal inguinal ring

Symphysis pubis

External inguinal ring

Vas deferens

Corpus spongiosum

Urethra

Corpus cavernosum

Corona

Prepuce

Glans penis

Urinary bladder

Rectum

Seminal vesicle

Prostate gland

Ejaculatory duct

Anus

Epididymis

Testis

Scrotum

Urethral meatus

Multitasking

In addition to supplying male sex cells (spermatogenesis), the male reproductive system plays a part in the secretion of male sex hormones.

Penis

The organ of copulation, the penis, deposits sperm in the female reproductive tract and acts as the terminal duct for the urinary tract. The penis also serves as the means for urine elimination. It consists of an attached root, a free shaft, and an enlarged tip.

What's inside

Internally, the cylinder-shaped penile shaft consists of three columns of erectile tissue bound together by heavy fibrous tissue. Two corpora cavernosa form the major part of the penis. On the underside, the corpus spongiosum encases the urethra. Its enlarged proximal end forms the bulb of the penis.

The glans penis, at the distal end of the shaft, is a cone-shaped structure formed from the corpus spongiosum. Its lateral margin forms a ridge of tissue known as the *corona*. The glans penis is highly sensitive to sexual stimulation.

What's outside

Thin, loose skin covers the penile shaft. The urethral meatus opens through the glans to allow urination and ejaculation.

In a different vein

The penis receives blood through the internal pudendal artery. Blood then flows into the corpora cavernosa through the penile artery. Venous blood returns through the internal iliac vein to the vena cava.

Scrotum

The penis meets the scrotum, or scrotal sac, at the penoscrotal junction. Located posterior to the penis and anterior to the anus, the scrotum is an extraabdominal pouch that consists of a thin layer of skin overlying a tighter, musclelike layer. This musclelike layer, in turn, overlies the tunica vaginalis, a serous membrane that covers the internal scrotal cavity.

Canals and rings

Internally, a septum divides the scrotum into two sacs, which each contains a testis, an epididymis, and a spermatic cord. The spermatic cord is a connective tissue sheath that encases autonomic nerve fibers, blood vessels, lymph vessels, and the vas deferens (also called the *ductus deferens*).

The spermatic cord travels from the testis through the inguinal canal, exiting the scrotum through the external inguinal ring and entering the abdominal cavity through the internal inguinal ring. The inguinal canal lies between the two rings.

Loads of nodes

Lymph nodes from the penis, scrotal surface, and anus drain into the inguinal lymph nodes. Lymph nodes from the testes drain into the lateral aortic and preaortic lymph nodes in the abdomen.

Testes

The testes are enveloped in two layers of connective tissue called the *tunica vaginalis* (outer layer) and the *tunica albuginea* (inner layer). Extensions of the tunica albuginea separate the testes into lobules. Each lobule contains one to four seminiferous tubules, small tubes where spermatogenesis takes place.

Climate control

Spermatozoa development requires a temperature lower than that of the rest of the body. The dartos muscle, a smooth muscle in the superficial fasciae, causes scrotal skin to wrinkle, which helps regulate temperature. The cremaster muscle, rising from the internal oblique muscle, helps to govern temperature by elevating the testes.

Duct system

The male reproductive duct system, consisting of the epididymis, vas deferens, and urethra, conveys sperm from the testes to the ejaculatory ducts near the bladder.

Swimmers, take your mark!

The epididymis is a coiled tube that's located superior to and along the posterior border of the testis. During ejaculation, smooth muscle in the epididymis contracts, ejecting spermatozoa into the vas deferens.

Descending tunnel

The vas deferens leads from the testes to the abdominal cavity, extends upward through the inguinal canal, arches over the urethra, and descends behind the bladder. Its enlarged portion, called the *ampulla*, merges with the duct of the seminal vesicle to form the short ejaculatory duct. After passing through the prostate gland, the vas deferens joins with the urethra.

Tube to the outside

A small tube leading from the floor of the bladder to the exterior, the urethra, consists of three parts:

1. Prostatic urethra, which is surrounded by the prostate gland and drains the bladder
2. Membranous urethra, which passes through the urogenital diaphragm
3. Spongy urethra, which makes up about 75% of the entire urethra

Accessory reproductive glands

The accessory reproductive glands, which produce most of the semen, include the seminal vesicles, bulbourethral glands (Cowper glands), and prostate gland.

A pair of pairs

The seminal vesicles are paired sacs at the base of the bladder. The bulbourethral glands, also paired, are located inferior to the prostate.

Improving the odds

The walnut-size prostate gland lies under the bladder and surrounds the urethra. It consists of three lobes: the left and right lateral lobes and the median lobe.

The prostate gland continuously secretes prostatic fluid, a thin, milky, alkaline fluid. During sexual activity, prostatic fluid adds volume to semen. It also enhances sperm motility and improves the odds of conception by neutralizing the acidity of the man's urethra and the woman's vagina.

Basically basic

Semen is a viscous, white secretion with a slightly alkaline pH (7.8 to 8) that consists of spermatozoa and accessory gland secretions. The seminal vesicles produce roughly 60% of the fluid portion of semen, whereas the prostate gland produces about 30%. A viscid fluid secreted by the bulbourethral glands also becomes part of semen.

Spermatogenesis

Sperm formation (also called *spermatogenesis*) begins when a male reaches puberty and usually continues throughout life.

Divide and conquer

Spermatogenesis occurs in four stages:

1. In the first stage, the primary germinal epithelial cells, called *spermatogonia*, grow and develop into primary spermatocytes. Both spermatogonia and primary spermatocytes contain 46 chromosomes, consisting of 44 autosomes and the two sex chromosomes, X and Y.
2. Next, primary spermatocytes divide to form secondary spermatocytes. No new chromosomes are formed in this stage; the pairs only divide. Each secondary spermatocyte contains one half of the number of autosomes, 22; one secondary spermatocyte contains an X chromosome; the other, a Y chromosome.
3. In the third stage, each secondary spermatocyte divides again to form spermatids (also called *spermatoblasts*).
4. Finally, the spermatids undergo a series of structural changes that transform them into mature spermatozoa or sperm. Each spermatozoa has a head, neck, body, and tail. The head contains the nucleus; the tail, a large amount of adenosine triphosphate, which provides energy for sperm motility.

Queuing up

Newly mature sperm pass from the seminiferous tubules through the vasa recta into the epididymis. Only a small number of sperm can be stored in the epididymis. Most of them move into the vas deferens, where they're stored until sexual stimulation triggers emission.

Check the expiration date?

After ejaculation, sperm can survive for 24 to 72 hours at body temperature. Sperm cells retain their potency and can survive for up to 4 days in the female reproductive tract.

Hormonal control and sexual development

Androgens (male sex hormones) are produced in the testes and adrenal glands. Androgens are responsible for the development of male sex organs and secondary sex characteristics. One major androgen is testosterone.

Team captain

Leydig cells, located in the testes between the seminiferous tubules, secrete testosterone, the most significant male sex hormone. Testosterone is responsible for the development and maintenance of male sex organs and secondary sex characteristics, such as facial hair and vocal cord thickness. Testosterone is also required for spermatogenesis.

Calling the plays

Testosterone secretion begins approximately 2 months after conception, when the release of chorionic gonadotropins from the placenta stimulates Leydig cells in the male fetus. The presence of testosterone directly affects sexual differentiation in the fetus. With testosterone, fetal genitalia develop into a penis, scrotum, and testes; without testosterone, genitalia develop into a clitoris, vagina, and other female organs.

During the last 2 months of gestation, testosterone usually causes the testes to descend into the scrotum. If the testes don't descend after birth, exogenous testosterone may correct the problem.

Other key players

Other hormones also affect male sexuality. Two of these, luteinizing hormone (LH)—also called *interstitial cell–stimulating hormone*—and follicle-stimulating hormone (FSH), directly affect secretion of testosterone.

Waiting on the bench

During early childhood, a male child does not secrete gonadotropins and thus has little circulating testosterone. Secretion of gonadotropins from the pituitary gland, which usually occurs between ages 11 and 14 years, marks the onset of puberty. These pituitary gonadotropins stimulate testis functioning as well as testosterone secretion.

Put me in, coach!

During puberty, the penis and testes enlarge and the male reaches full adult sexual and reproductive capability. Puberty also marks the development of male secondary sexual characteristics, including:
- distinct body hair distribution
- skin changes (such as increased secretion by sweat and sebaceous glands)
- deepening of the voice (from laryngeal enlargement)
- increased musculoskeletal development
- other intracellular and extracellular changes.

Star player

After a male achieves full physical maturity, usually by age 20 years, sexual and reproductive function remain fairly consistent throughout life.

Subtle changes

With aging, adult males may experience subtle changes in sexual function, but they do not lose the ability to reproduce. For example, an older adult male may require more time to achieve an erection, experience less firm erections, and have reduced ejaculatory volume. After ejaculation, it may take longer to regain an erection.

Female reproductive system

Unlike the male reproductive system, the female system is largely internal, housed within the pelvic cavity.

External genitalia

The external female genitalia, or vulva, include the mons pubis, labia majora, labia minora, clitoris, and adjacent structures. These structures are visible on inspection. (See *Structures of the female reproductive system.*)

Structures of the female reproductive system

The female reproductive system consists of external and internal genitalia. These structures include the vagina, cervix, uterus, fallopian tubes, ovaries, and other structures. Reproductive, urinary, and gastrointestinal (GI) structures are housed in the female pelvis. These include the bladder, anus, and rectum.

View of external genitalia in lithotomy position

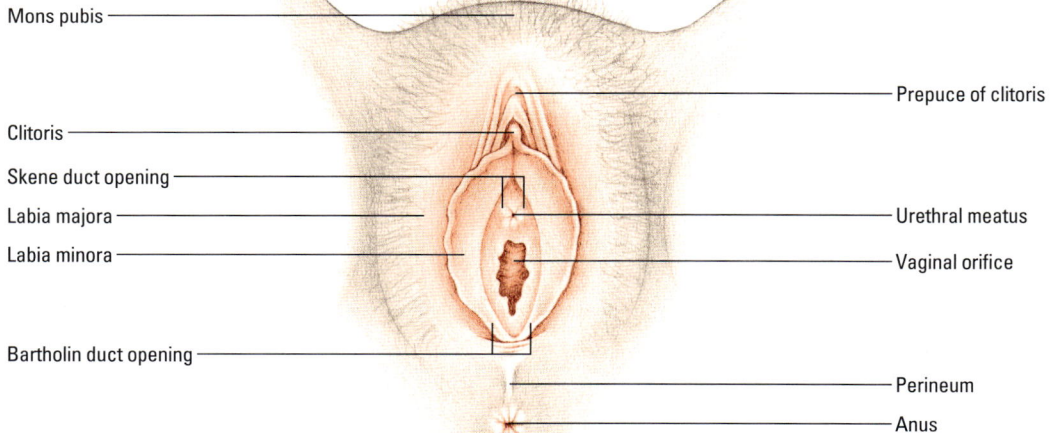

Mons pubis
Clitoris
Skene duct opening
Labia majora
Labia minora
Bartholin duct opening

Prepuce of clitoris
Urethral meatus
Vaginal orifice
Perineum
Anus

Structures of the female reproductive system (*continued*)

Lateral view of internal genitalia

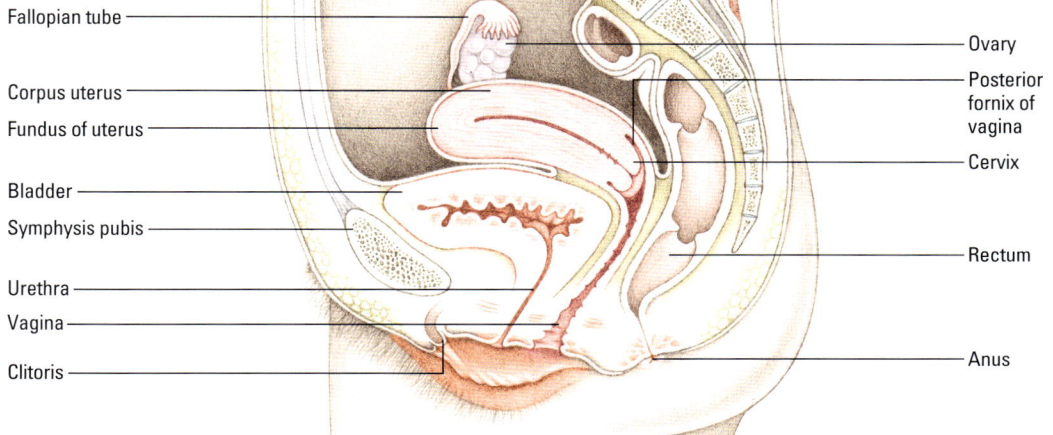

Fallopian tube

Corpus uterus

Fundus of uterus

Bladder

Symphysis pubis

Urethra

Vagina

Clitoris

Ovary

Posterior fornix of vagina

Cervix

Rectum

Anus

Anterior cross-sectional view of internal genitalia

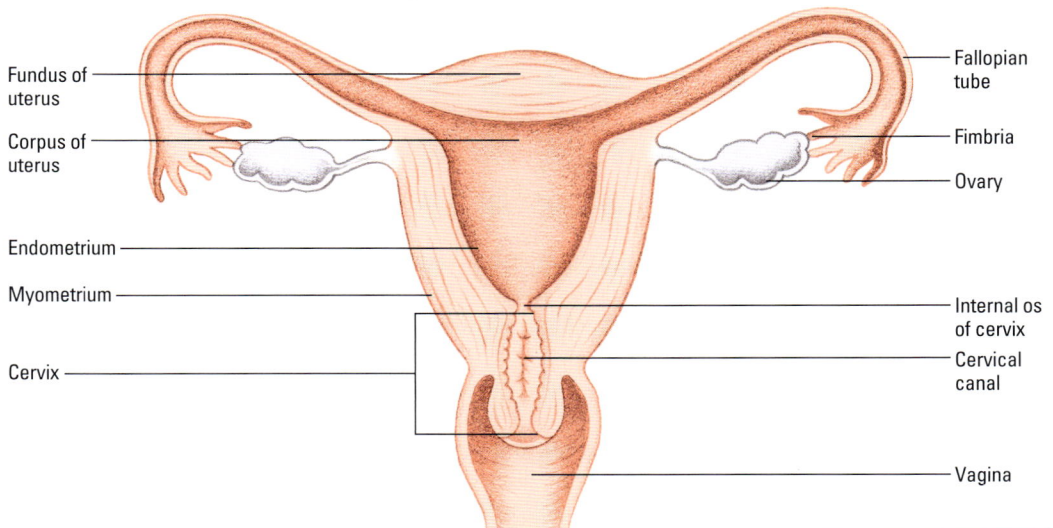

Fundus of uterus

Corpus of uterus

Endometrium

Myometrium

Cervix

Fallopian tube

Fimbria

Ovary

Internal os of cervix

Cervical canal

Vagina

Mons pubis

The mons pubis is a rounded cushion of fatty and connective tissue covered by skin and coarse, curly hair in a triangular pattern over the symphysis pubis (the joint formed by the union of the pubic bones anteriorly).

Labia majora

The labia majora are two raised folds of adipose and connective tissue that border the vulva on either side, extending from the mons pubis to the perineum. After onset of the puberty (called *pubarche*), the outer surface of the labia is covered with pubic hair.

Labia minora

The labia minora are two moist folds of mucosal tissue that lie within and alongside the labia majora. Each upper section divides into an upper and lower lamella. The two upper lamellae join to form the prepuce, a hoodlike covering over the clitoris. The two lower lamellae form the frenulum, the posterior portion of the clitoris.

The lower labial sections taper down and back from the clitoris to the perineum, where they join to form the fourchette, a thin tissue fold along the anterior edge of the perineum.

Minor in name only

The labia minora contain sebaceous glands, which secrete a lubricant that also acts as a bactericide. Like the labia majora, they are rich in blood vessels and nerve endings, making them sensitive to pain, pressure, touch, sexual stimulation, and temperature extremes. They swell in response to sexual stimulation, a reaction that triggers other changes that prepare the genitalia for coitus.

Clitoris

The clitoris is the small, protuberant organ just beneath the arch of the mons pubis. It contains erectile tissue, venous cavernous spaces, and specialized sensory corpuscles, which are stimulated during sexual activity.

Adjacent structures

The vestibule is an oval area bounded anteriorly by the clitoris, laterally by the labia minora, and posteriorly by the fourchette.

Featuring glands

The mucous-producing Skene glands are found on both sides of the urethral opening. Openings of the two mucous-producing Bartholin glands are located laterally and posteriorly on either side of the inner vaginal orifice.

The urethral meatus is the slitlike opening below the clitoris through which urine leaves the body. In the center of the vestibule is the vaginal orifice. It may be completely or partially covered by the hymen, a tissue membrane.

Not too simple

Located between the lower vagina and the anal canal, the perineum is a complex structure of muscles, blood vessels, fasciae, nerves, and lymphatics.

Internal genitalia

The female internal genitalia include the vagina, cervix, uterus, fallopian tubes, ovaries, and mammary glands. The main function of these specialized organs is reproduction.

Vagina

The vagina, a highly elastic muscular tube, is located between the urethra and the rectum.

Three layers . . .

The vaginal wall has three tissue layers: epithelial tissue, loose connective tissue, and muscle tissue. The uterine cervix connects the uterus to the vaginal vault. Four fornices (the anterior fornix, posterior fornix, and left lateral and right lateral fornix), recesses in the vaginal wall, surround the cervix.

. . . three functions

The vagina has three main functions:
1. To accommodate the penis during coitus
2. To channel blood discharged from the uterus during menstruation
3. To serve as the birth canal during childbirth

Separate but equal

The upper, middle, and lower vaginal sections have separate blood supplies. Branches of the uterine arteries supply blood to the upper vagina, the inferior vesical arteries supply blood to the middle vagina, and the hemorrhoidal and internal pudendal arteries feed into the lower vagina.

Blood returns through a vast venous plexus to the hemorrhoidal, pudendal, and uterine veins and then to the hypogastric veins. This plexus merges with the vertebral venous plexus.

Cervix

The cervix is the lowest portion of the uterus. It projects into the upper portion of the vagina. The end that opens into the vagina is called the *external os*; the end that opens into the uterus, the *internal os*. The cervix is sealed with thick mucus. This prevents sperm from entering except for a few days around ovulation when the mucus becomes thinner.

Childbirth permanently alters the cervix. In a female who hasn't delivered a child, the external os is a round opening about 3 mm in diameter; after the first childbirth, it becomes a small transverse slit with irregular edges.

Uterus

The uterus is a small, firm, pear-shaped, muscular organ situated between the bladder and rectum. It typically lies at almost a 90-degree angle to the vagina. The mucous membrane lining of the uterus is called the *endometrium*, and the muscular layer of the uterus is called the *myometrium*.

Fundamental fundus

During pregnancy, the elastic, upper portion of the uterus, called the *fundus*, accommodates most of the growing fetus until term. The uterine neck joins the fundus to the cervix, the uterine part extending into the vagina. The fundus and neck make up the main uterine body, called the *corpus*.

Fallopian tubes

Two fallopian tubes attach to the uterus at the upper angles of the fundus. These narrow cylinders of muscle fibers are where fertilization occurs.

Riding the wave

The curved portion of the fallopian tube, called the *ampulla*, ends in the funnel-shaped infundibulum. Fingerlike projections in the infundibulum, called *fimbriae*, move in waves that sweep the mature ovum (female gamete or sex cell) from the ovary into the fallopian tube.

Ovaries

The ovaries are located on either side of the uterus. The size, shape, and position of the ovaries vary with age. Round, smooth, and pink at birth, they grow larger, flatten, and turn grayish by puberty. During the childbearing years, they take on an almond shape and a rough, pitted surface; after menopause, they shrink and turn white.

Swept away

The ovaries' main function is to produce mature ova. At birth, each ovary contains approximately 400,000 graafian follicles. During the childbearing years, one graafian follicle produces a mature ovum during the first half of each menstrual cycle. Each ovum contains 22 autosomes and an X chromosome for a total of 23 chromosomes. As the ovum matures, the follicle ruptures and the ovum is swept into the fallopian tube.

The ovaries also produce estrogen and progesterone as well as a small amount of androgens.

Mammary glands

The mammary glands, located in the breast, are specialized accessory glands that secrete milk. Although present in both sexes, they typically function only in the female. Each mammary gland contains 15 to 20 lobes that are separated by fibrous connective tissue and fat. Within the lobes are clustered acini—tiny, saclike duct terminals that secrete milk during lactation.

The ducts draining the lobules converge to form excretory (*lactiferous*) ducts and sinuses (*ampullae*), which store milk during lactation. These ducts drain onto the nipple surface through 15 to 20 openings. (See *The female breast*.)

The female breast

The breasts are located on either side of the anterior chest wall over the greater pectoral and the anterior serratus muscles. Within the areola, the pigmented area in the center of the breast, lies the nipple. Erectile tissue in the nipple responds to cold, friction, and sexual stimulation.

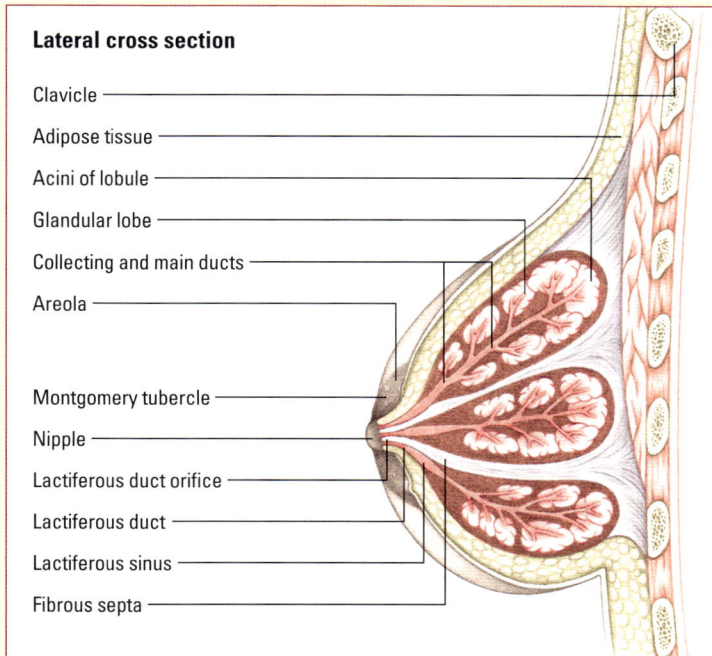

Lateral cross section

Clavicle

Adipose tissue

Acini of lobule

Glandular lobe

Collecting and main ducts

Areola

Montgomery tubercle

Nipple

Lactiferous duct orifice

Lactiferous duct

Lactiferous sinus

Fibrous septa

(*continued*)

The female breast (*continued*)

Support and separate
Each breast is composed of glandular, fibrous, and adipose tissue. Glandular tissue contains 15 to 20 lobes made up of clustered acini, tiny saclike duct terminals that secrete milk. Fibrous Cooper ligaments support the breasts; adipose tissue separates the two breasts.

Produce and drain
Milk glands in each breast produce milk by acini cells and then deliver it to the nipple by a lactiferous duct.

   Sebaceous glands on the areolar surface, called *Montgomery tubercles*, produce sebum, which lubricates the areola and nipple during breastfeeding.

Hormonal function and the menstrual cycle

Like the male body, the female body changes as it ages in response to hormonal control. When a female reaches the age of menstruation, the hypothalamus, ovaries, and pituitary gland secrete hormones—estrogen, progesterone, FSH, and LH—that affect the buildup and shedding of the endometrium during the menstrual cycle. (See *Events in the female reproductive cycle.*)

Events in the female reproductive cycle

The female reproductive cycle usually lasts 28 days. During this cycle, three major types of changes occur simultaneously: ovulatory, hormonal, and endometrial (involving the lining [endometrium] of the uterus).

Ovulatory
• Ovulatory changes, which usually last 5 days, begin on day 1 of the menstrual cycle.
• As the cycle begins, low estrogen and progesterone levels in the bloodstream stimulate the hypothalamus to secrete gonadotropin-releasing hormone (GnRH). In turn, GnRH stimulates the anterior pituitary gland to secrete FSH and LH.
• Follicle development within the ovary (in the follicular phase) is spurred by increased levels of FSH and, to a lesser extent, LH.

• When the follicle matures, a spike in the LH level occurs, causing the follicle to rupture and release the ovum, thus initiating ovulation.
• After ovulation (in the luteal phase), the collapsed follicle forms the corpus luteum, which degenerates if fertilization doesn't occur.

Hormonal
• During the follicular phase of the ovarian cycle, the increasing FSH and LH levels that stimulate follicle growth also stimulate increased secretion of the hormone estrogen.
• Estrogen secretion peaks just before ovulation. This peak sets in motion the spike in LH levels, which causes ovulation.

Events in the female reproductive cycle (*continued*)

• After ovulation (about day 14), estrogen levels decline rapidly. In the luteal phase of the ovarian cycle, the corpus luteum is formed and begins to release progesterone and estrogen.

• As the corpus luteum degenerates, levels of both of these ovarian hormones decline.

Endometrial

• The endometrium is receptive to implantation of an embryo for only a short time in the reproductive cycle. Thus, it's not intentional that its most receptive phase occurs about 7 days after the ovarian cycle's release of an ovum—just in time to receive a fertilized ovum.

• In the first 5 days of the reproductive cycle, the endometrium sheds its functional layer, leaving the basal layer (the deepest layer) intact. Menstrual flow consists of this detached layer and accompanying blood from the detachment process.

• The endometrium begins regenerating its functional layer at about day 6 (the proliferative phase), spurred by rising estrogen levels.

• After ovulation, increased progesterone secretion stimulates conversion of the functional layer into a secretory mucosa (secretory phase), which is more receptive to implantation of the fertilized ovum.

• If implantation doesn't occur, the corpus luteum degenerates, progesterone levels drop, and the endometrium again sheds its functional layer.

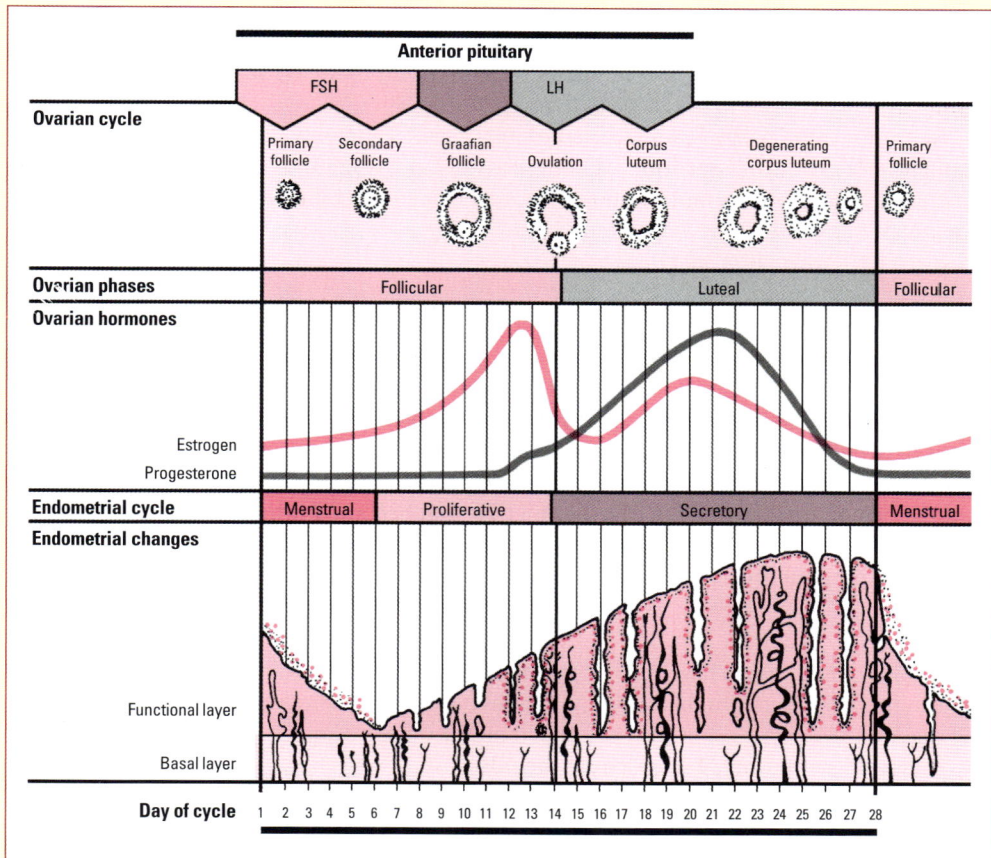

A spurt of growth

During adolescence, the release of hormones causes a rapid increase in physical growth and spurs the development of secondary sex characteristics. This growth spurt begins at approximately 11 years of age and continues until early adolescence or about 3 years later.

Irregularity of the menstrual cycle is common during this time because of inconsistent ovulation. With menarche (the first menstruation), the uterine body flexes on the cervix and the ovaries are situated in the pelvic cavity.

A monthly thing

The menstrual cycle is a complex process that involves both the reproductive and endocrine systems. The cycle averages 28 days.

Supply exhausted

In contrast to the slowly declining hormones of the aging male, the aging female's hormones decline rapidly in a process called *menopause*. Although the pituitary gland still releases FSH and LH, the body has exhausted its supply of ovarian follicles that respond to these hormones and menstruation no longer occurs.

Cessation of menses usually occurs between ages 45 and 55 years. Some people experience menopause early, possibly as a result of genetics, ovarian damage, autoimmune disorders, or surgical interventions such as hysterectomy. When menopause occurs before age 45 years, it's known as *premature menopause*.

Menopause can be broken down into three stages: perimenopause, menopause, and postmenopause.

Climactic climacteric

Perimenopause consists of the 8 to 10 years (called the *climacteric years*) of declining ovarian function that occurs before menopause. During this time, the ovaries gradually begin to produce less estrogen and the person may experience irregular menses that become further apart with a lighter flow. As menopause progresses, the ovaries stop producing progesterone and estrogen altogether.

Out of eggs

A person is considered to have reached the menopause stage after menses are absent for 1 year. At this stage, the ovaries have stopped producing eggs and have almost completely stopped producing estrogen.

Signs and symptoms of menopause include:
- hot flashes (sudden feelings of warmth that spread throughout the upper body and may be accompanied by blushing or sweating)
- irregular or skipped menses
- mood swings and irritability
- fatigue

- insomnia
- headaches
- changes in sex drive
- vaginal dryness.

Menopause can be confirmed through analysis of FSH levels or a Paplike test that assesses for vaginal atrophy.

One thing leads to another

Postmenopause refers to the years after menopause. During this stage, the symptoms of menopause cease. However, the risk of other health problems increases as a result of declining estrogen levels. These problems include:

- osteoporosis
- heart disease
- decreased skin elasticity
- vision deterioration.

Fertilization

Production of a new human being begins with *fertilization*, the union of a spermatozoon and an ovum to form a single new cell. After fertilization occurs, dramatic changes begin inside the female's body. The cells of the fertilized ovum begin dividing as the ovum travels to the uterine cavity, where it implants itself in the uterine lining. (See *How fertilization occurs*.)

How fertilization occurs

Fertilization begins when the spermatozoon is activated upon contact with the ovum. Here's what happens.

The spermatozoon, which has a covering called the *acrosome*, approaches the ovum.

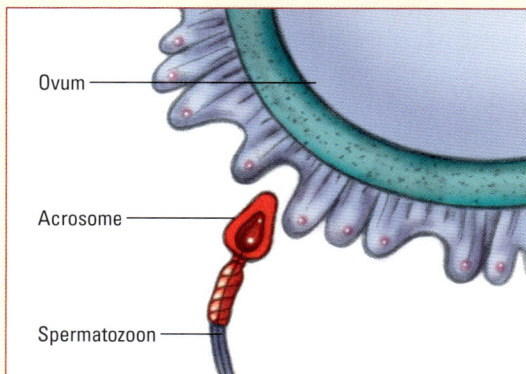

Ovum

Acrosome

Spermatozoon

(continued)

How fertilization occurs (*continued*)

The acrosome develops small perforations through which it releases enzymes necessary for the sperm to penetrate the protective layers of the ovum before fertilization.

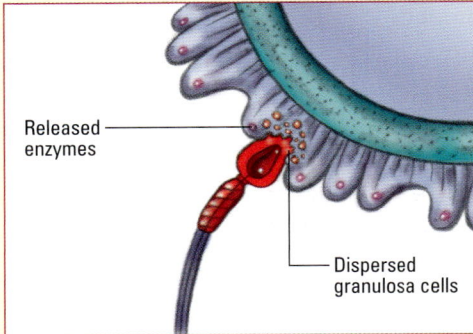

Released enzymes

Dispersed granulosa cells

The spermatozoon then penetrates the zona pellucida (the inner membrane of the ovum). This triggers the ovum's second meiotic division (following meiosis), making the zona pellucida impenetrable to other spermatozoa.

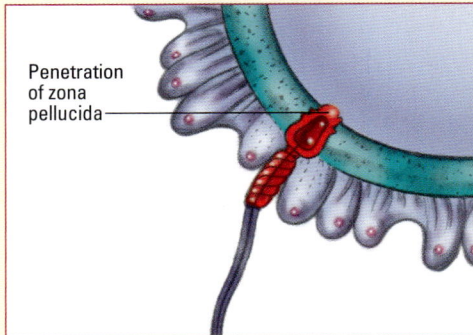

Penetration of zona pellucida

After the spermatozoon penetrates the ovum, its nucleus is released into the ovum, its tail degenerates, and its head enlarges and fuses with the ovum's nucleus. This fusion provides the fertilized ovum, called a *zygote*, with 46 chromosomes.

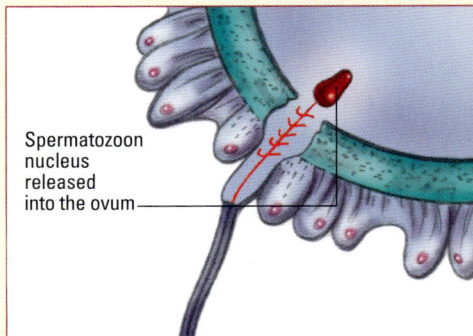

Spermatozoon nucleus released into the ovum

Survival of the fittest

For fertilization to take place, however, the spermatozoon must first reach the ovum. Although a single ejaculation deposits several hundred million spermatozoa, many are destroyed by acidic vaginal secretions. The only spermatozoa that survive are those that enter the cervical canal, where cervical mucus protects them.

Timing is everything

The ability of spermatozoa to penetrate the cervical mucus depends on the phase of the menstrual cycle at the time of transit:

- Early in the cycle, estrogen and progesterone levels cause the mucus to thicken, making it more difficult for spermatozoa to pass through the cervix.
- During midcycle, however, when the mucus is relatively thin, spermatozoa can pass readily through the cervix.
- Later in the cycle, the cervical mucus thickens again, hindering spermatozoa passage.

Help along the way

Spermatozoa travel through the female reproductive tract by means of flagellar movements (whiplike movements of the tail). After spermatozoa pass through the cervical mucus, however, the female reproductive system assists them on their journey with rhythmic contractions of the uterus that help the spermatozoa to penetrate the fallopian tubes. Spermatozoa are typically viable (able to fertilize the ovum) for up to 2 days after ejaculation; however, they can survive in the reproductive tract for up to 4 days.

Disperse and penetrate

Before a spermatozoon can penetrate the ovum, it must disperse the granulosa cells and penetrate the zona pellucida, the thick, transparent layer surrounding the incompletely developed ovum. Enzymes in the acrosome (head cap) of the spermatozoon permit this penetration. After penetration, the ovum completes its second meiotic division and the zona pellucida prevents penetration by other spermatozoa.

The spermatozoon's head then fuses with the ovum nucleus, creating a cell nucleus with 46 chromosomes. The fertilized ovum is called a *zygote*.

If the egg and sperm do not each have 23 chromosomes, genetic complications may arise and could lead to early pregnancy loss or a live birth of an infant with more or less chromosomes than is normal. An extra copy of a chromosome results in a condition referred to as trisomy. A commonly known trisomy condition is trisomy 21 otherwise known as *Down syndrome*. This condition is called trisomy 21 because there are three copies of chromosome 21 in each cell. When only one copy of a chromosome is in each cell, the condition is referred to as monosomy. An example of a monosomy condition is Turner syndrome where a female has only one sex chromosome, a single X chromosome instead of two resulting in a total of 45 chromosomes rather than the normal 46.

Pregnancy

Pregnancy starts with fertilization and often ends with childbirth. On average, a full-term pregnancy is 38 to 40 weeks. During this period (called *gestation*), the zygote divides as it passes through the fallopian tube and attaches to the uterine lining by implantation. A complex sequence of pre-embryonic, embryonic, and fetal developments transforms the zygote into a full-term fetus.

Making predictions

Because the uterus grows throughout pregnancy, uterine size serves as a rough estimate of gestation. The fertilization date is rarely known, so the female's expected delivery date is typically calculated from the beginning of their last menses. The tool used for calculating delivery dates is known as the *Nägele rule*.

The *Nägele rule* works by counting back 3 months from the first day of the last menstrual cycle and then adding 7 days. For example, if the first day of the last menses was April 29, count back 3 months, which is January 29, and then add 7 days for an approximate due date of February 5.

Stages of fetal development

During pregnancy, the fetus undergoes three major stages of development:
1. pre-embryonic period (fertilization to week 3)
2. embryonic period (weeks 4 to 7)
3. fetal period (week 8 to birth).

It all starts here

The pre-embryonic phase starts with ovum fertilization and lasts 3 weeks. As the zygote passes through the fallopian tube, it undergoes a series of mitotic divisions or cleavage. (See *Pre-embryonic development*.)

Pre-embryonic development

The pre-embryonic phase lasts from conception to approximately the end of week 3 of development.

Zygote . . .

As the fertilized ovum advances through the fallopian tube toward the uterus, it undergoes mitotic division, forming daughter cells, initially called *blastomeres*, that each contains the same number of chromosomes as the parent cell. The first cell division ends about 30 hours after fertilization; subsequent divisions occur rapidly.

The *zygote*, as it's now called, develops into a small mass of cells called a *morula*, which reaches the uterus at about day 3 after fertilization. Fluid that amasses in the center of the morula forms a central cavity.

. . . into blastocyst

The structure is now called a *blastocyst*. The blastocyst consists of a thin trophoblast layer, which includes the blastocyst cavity, and the inner cell mass. The trophoblast develops into fetal membranes and the placenta. The inner cell mass later forms the embryo (late blastocyst).

Getting attached: Blastocyst and endometrium

During the next phase, the blastocyst stays within the zona pellucida, unattached to the uterus. The zona pellucida degenerates and, by the end of week 1 after fertilization, the blastocyst attaches to the endometrium. The part of the blastocyst adjacent to the inner cell mass is the first part to become attached.

The trophoblast, in contact with the endometrial lining, proliferates and invades the underlying endometrium by separating and dissolving endometrial cells.

Letting it all sink in

During the next week, the invading blastocyst sinks below the endometrium's surface. The penetration site seals, restoring the continuity of the endometrial surface.

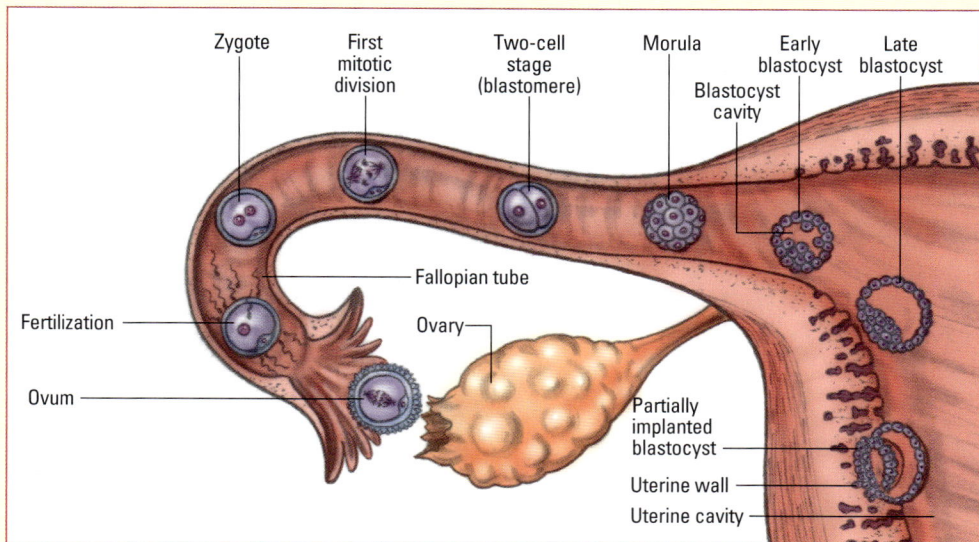

Zygote to embryo

During the embryonic period (the fourth to the seventh week of gestation), the developing zygote starts to take on a human shape and is now called an *embryo*. Each germ layer—the ectoderm, mesoderm, and endoderm—eventually forms specific tissues in the embryo. (See *Embryonic development*.)

Embryonic development

Each of the three germ layers—ectoderm, mesoderm, and endoderm—forms specific tissues and organs in the developing embryo.

Ectoderm

The ectoderm, the outermost layer, develops into the:
- epidermis
- nervous system
- pituitary gland
- tooth enamel
- salivary glands
- optic lens
- lining of the lower portion of anal canal
- hair.

Mesoderm

The mesoderm, the middle layer, develops into:
- connective and supporting tissue
- the blood and vascular system
- musculature
- teeth (except enamel)
- the mesothelial lining of pericardial, pleural, and peritoneal cavities
- the kidneys and ureters.

Endoderm

The endoderm, the innermost layer, becomes the epithelial lining of the:
- pharynx and trachea
- auditory canal
- alimentary canal
- liver
- pancreas
- bladder and urethra
- prostate.

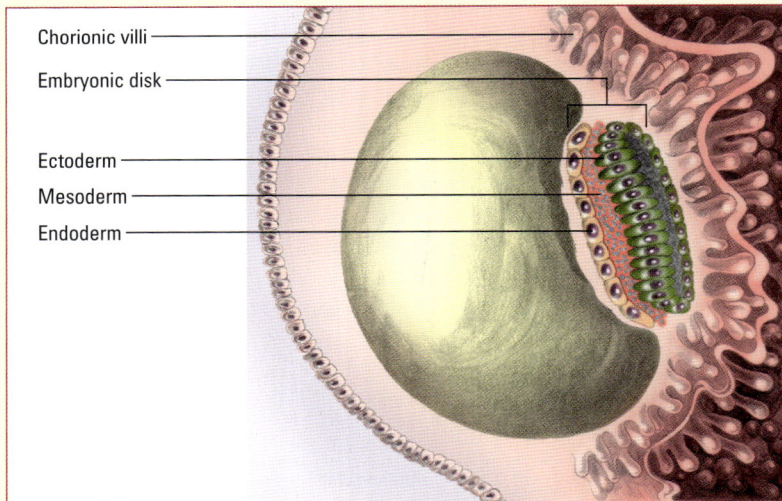

Chorionic villi
Embryonic disk
Ectoderm
Mesoderm
Endoderm

Organ systems form during the embryonic period. During this time, the embryo is particularly vulnerable to injury by maternal drug misuse, certain maternal infections, and other factors.

Baby on the way!

During the fetal stage of development, which extends from the eighth week to birth, the maturing fetus enlarges and grows heavier. (See *From embryo to fetus.*)

From embryo to fetus

Significant growth and development take place within the first 3 months following conception, as the embryo develops into a fetus that nearly resembles a full-term neonate.

Month 1

At the end of the first month, the embryo has a definite form. The head, the trunk, and the tiny buds that will become the arms and legs are discernible. The cardiovascular system has begun to function, and the umbilical cord is visible in its most primitive form.

Month 2

During the second month, the embryo—called a *fetus* from week 8—grows to 1 in (2.5 cm) and weighs 1/30 oz (1 g). The head and facial features develop as the eyes, ears, nose, lips, tongue, and tooth buds form. The arms and legs also take shape. Although the gender of the fetus is not yet discernible, all external genitalia are present. Cardiovascular function is complete, and the umbilical cord has a definite form. At the end of the second month, the fetus resembles a full-term neonate except for size.

Month 3

During the third month, the fetus grows to 3 in (7.6 cm) and weighs 1 oz (28.3 g). Teeth and bones begin to appear, and the kidneys start to function. The fetus opens its mouth to swallow, grasps with its fully developed hands, and prepares for breathing by inhaling and exhaling (although its lungs aren't functioning). At the end of the first *trimester* (the 3-month periods into which pregnancy is divided), its gender is distinguishable.

Months 4 to 9

Over the remaining 6 months, fetal growth continues as internal and external structures develop at a rapid rate. In the third trimester, the fetus stores the fats and minerals it will need to live outside the womb. At birth, the average full-term fetus measures 20 in (50.1 cm) and weighs 7 to 7½ lb (3 to 3.5 kg).

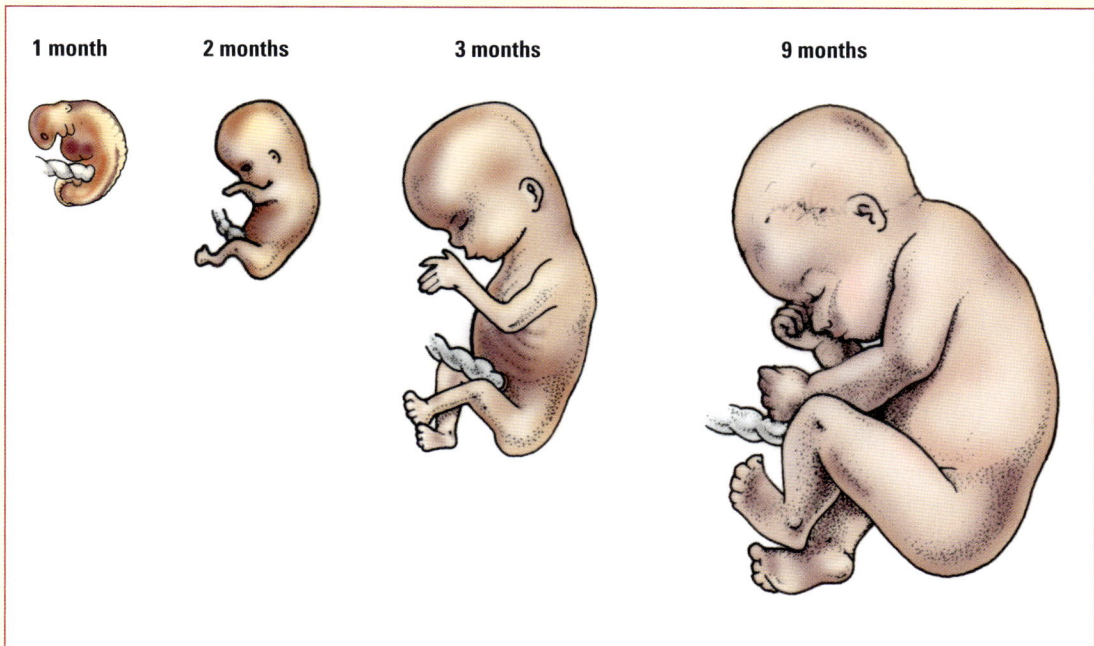

1 month   2 months   3 months   9 months

Two unusual features appear during this stage:

1. The fetus's head is disproportionately large compared to its body. (This feature changes after birth as the infant grows.)
2. The fetus lacks subcutaneous fat. (Fat starts to accumulate shortly after birth.)

Structural changes in the ovaries and uterus

During pregnancy, the reproductive system undergoes a number of changes.

Corpus luteum

Pregnancy changes the usual development of the corpus luteum and results in the development of the following structures:

- decidua
- amniotic sac and fluid
- yolk sac
- placenta.

Normal functioning of the corpus luteum requires continuous stimulation by LH. Progesterone produced by the corpus luteum suppresses LH release by the pituitary gland. If pregnancy occurs, the corpus luteum continues to produce progesterone until the placenta takes over. Otherwise, the corpus luteum atrophies 3 days before menstrual flow begins.

Hormone soup

With age, the corpus luteum grows less responsive to LH. Therefore, the mature corpus luteum degenerates unless stimulated by progressively increasing amounts of LH.

Pregnancy stimulates the placental tissue to secrete large amounts of human chorionic gonadotropin (hCG), which resembles LH and FSH. hCG prevents corpus luteum degeneration, stimulating the corpus luteum to produce large amounts of estrogen and progesterone.

Ups and downs of hCG

The corpus luteum, stimulated by the hormone hCG, produces the estrogen and progesterone needed to maintain the pregnancy during the first 3 months. hCG can be detected as early as 7 to 8 days after fertilization and can provide confirmation of pregnancy even before the first missed menses.

The hCG level gradually increases during this time, peaks at about 10 to 12 weeks' gestation, and then gradually declines.

Decidua

The decidua is the endometrial lining of the uterus that undergoes hormone-induced changes during pregnancy. Decidual cells secrete the following three substances:

- A peptide hormone, *relaxin*, which induces relaxation of the connective tissue of the symphysis pubis and pelvic ligaments and promotes cervical dilation
- Progesterone and relaxin that are secreted by the corpus luteum in early pregnancy and later in pregnancy by the placenta
- A potent (hormonelike) fatty acid, *prostaglandin*, which mediates several physiologic functions (See *Development of the decidua and fetal membranes.*)

Development of the decidua and fetal membranes

Specialized tissues support, protect, and nurture the embryo and fetus throughout its development. Among these tissues, the decidua and fetal membranes begin to develop shortly after conception.

Decidua

During pregnancy, the endometrial lining is called the *decidua*. It provides a nesting place for the developing ovum and has some endocrine functions.

Based primarily on its position relative to the embryo, the decidua may be known as the *decidua basalis*, which lies beneath the chorionic vesicle; the *decidua capsularis*, which stretches over the vesicle; or the *decidua parietalis*, which lines the remainder of the endometrial cavity.

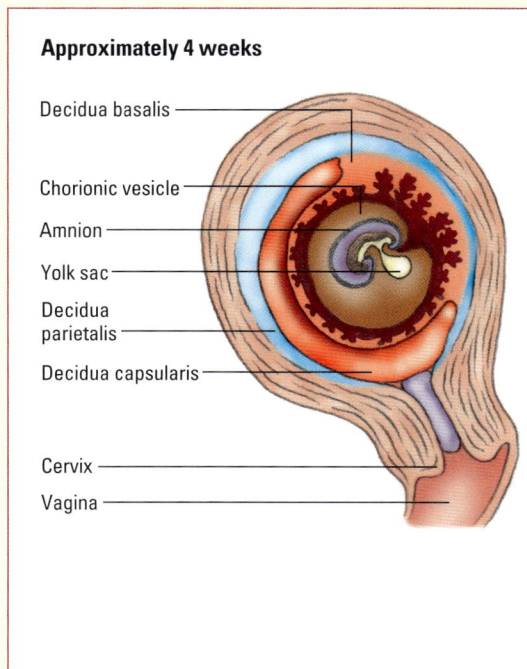

Approximately 4 weeks

Decidua basalis

Chorionic vesicle

Amnion

Yolk sac

Decidua parietalis

Decidua capsularis

Cervix

Vagina

(*continued*)

Development of the decidua and fetal membranes (*continued*)

Fetal membranes

The *chorion* is a membrane that forms the outer wall of the blastocyst. Vascular projections, called *chorionic villi*, arise from its periphery. As the chorionic vesicle enlarges, villi arising from the superficial portion of the chorion, called the *chorion laeve*, atrophy, leaving this surface smooth. Villi arising from the deeper part of the chorion, called the *chorion frondosum*, proliferate, projecting into the large blood vessels within the decidua basalis through which the maternal blood flows.

Blood vessels that form within the growing villi become connected with blood vessels that form in the chorion, in the body stalk, and within the body of the embryo. Blood begins to flow through this developing network of vessels as soon as the embryo's heart starts to beat.

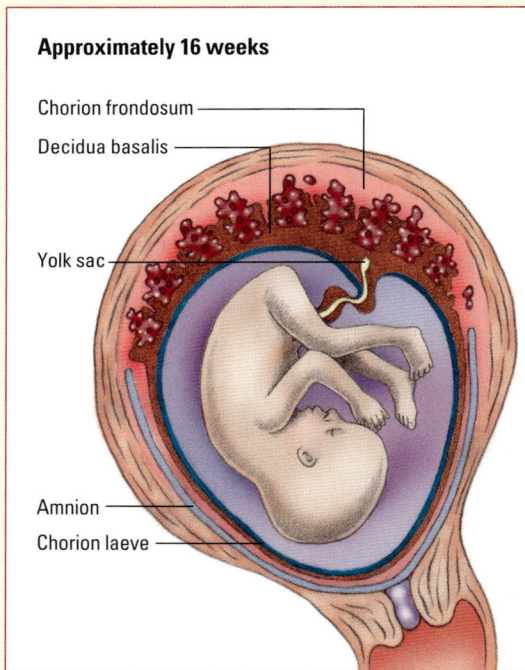

Approximately 16 weeks

Chorion frondosum

Decidua basalis

Yolk sac

Amnion

Chorion laeve

Amniotic sac and fluid

The amniotic sac, enclosed within the chorion, gradually grows and surrounds the embryo. As it enlarges, the amniotic sac expands into the chorionic cavity, eventually filling the cavity and fusing with the chorion by the eighth week of gestation.

A warm, protective sea

The amniotic sac and amniotic fluid serve the fetus in two important ways, one during gestation and the other during delivery. During gestation, the fluid gives the fetus a buoyant, temperature-controlled environment. Later, amniotic fluid serves as a fluid wedge that helps to open the cervix during birth.

Some from mom, some from baby

Early in pregnancy, amniotic fluid comes chiefly from three sources:
1. Fluid filtering into the amniotic sac from maternal blood as it passes through the uterus
2. Fluid filtering into the sac from fetal blood passing through the placenta
3. Fluid diffusing into the amniotic sac from the fetal skin and respiratory tract

Later in pregnancy, when the fetal kidneys begin to function, the fetus urinates into the amniotic fluid. Fetal urine then becomes the major source of amniotic fluid.

Every sea has its tides

Production of amniotic fluid from maternal and fetal sources balances amniotic fluid that's lost through the fetal GI tract. Typically, the fetus swallows up to several hundred milliliters of amniotic fluid each day. The fluid is absorbed into the fetal circulation from the fetal GI tract; some is transferred from the fetal circulation to the maternal circulation and excreted in maternal urine.

Yolk sac

The yolk sac forms next to the endoderm of the germ disk; a portion of it is incorporated into the developing embryo and forms the GI tract. Another portion of the sac develops into primitive germ cells, which travel to the developing gonads and eventually form *oocytes* (the precursor of the ovum) or *spermatocytes* (the precursor of the spermatozoon) after gender has been determined.

Here today, gone tomorrow

During early embryonic development, the yolk sac also forms blood cells. Eventually, it undergoes atrophy and disintegrates.

Placenta

Using the umbilical cord as its conduit, the flattened, disk-shaped placenta provides nutrients to and removes wastes from the fetus from the third month of pregnancy to birth. The placenta is formed from the chorion, its chorionic villi, and the adjacent decidua basalis.

A fetal lifeline

The normal umbilical cord contains two arteries and one vein and links the fetus to the placenta. The umbilical arteries, which transport blood from the fetus to the placenta, take a spiral course on the cord, divide on the placental surface, and branch off to the chorionic villi. (See *Picturing the placenta*.)

Picturing the placenta

At term, the placenta (the spongy structure within the uterus from which the fetus derives nourishment) is flat, cakelike, and round or oval. It measures 6 to 7¾ in (15 to 19.5 cm) in diameter and ¾ to 1¼ in (2 to 3 cm) in breadth at its thickest part. The maternal side is lobulated; the fetal side is shiny.

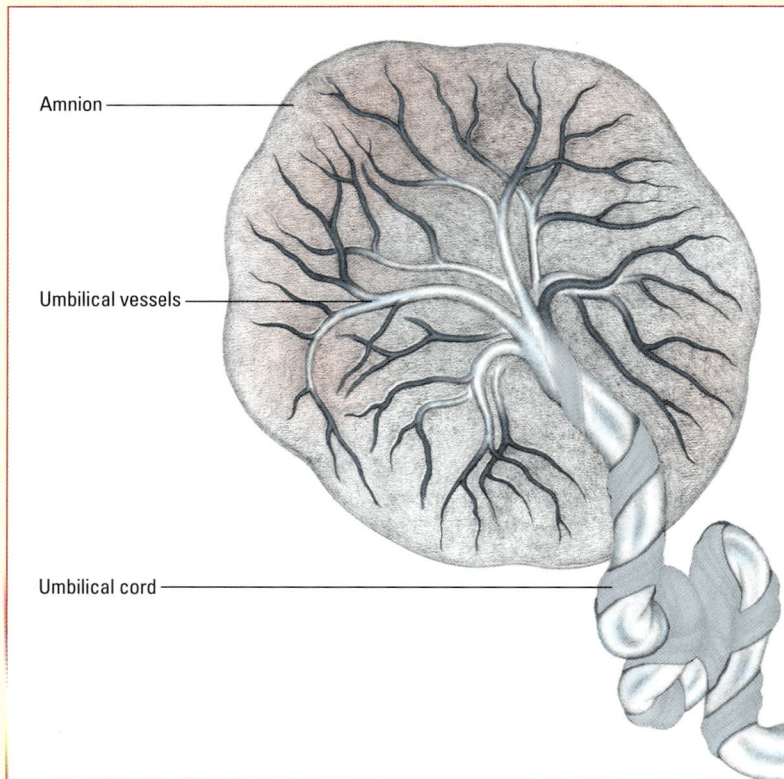

Amnion

Umbilical vessels

Umbilical cord

In a helpful vein
The placenta is a highly vascular organ. Large veins on its surface gather blood returning from the villi and join to form the single umbilical vein, which enters the cord, returning blood to the fetus.

Specialists on the job
The placenta contains two highly specialized circulatory systems:
- The *uteroplacental* circulation carries oxygenated arterial blood from the maternal circulation to the intervillous spaces—large spaces separating chorionic villi in the placenta. Blood enters the intervillous spaces from uterine arteries that penetrate the basal part of the placenta; it leaves the intervillous spaces and flows back into the maternal circulation through veins in the basal part of the placenta near the arteries.
- The *fetoplacental* circulation transports oxygen-depleted blood from the fetus to the chorionic villi by the umbilical arteries and returns oxygenated blood to the fetus through the umbilical vein.

Placenta takes charge
For the first 3 months of pregnancy, the corpus luteum is the main source of estrogen and progesterone—hormones required during pregnancy. By the end of the third month, however, the placenta produces most of the hormones; the corpus luteum persists but is no longer needed to maintain the pregnancy.

Hormones on the rise
The levels of estrogen and progesterone, two steroid hormones, increase progressively throughout pregnancy. Estrogen stimulates uterine development to provide a suitable environment for the fetus.

Progesterone, synthesized by the placenta from maternal cholesterol, reduces uterine muscle irritability and prevents spontaneous abortion of the fetus.

Keep those acids coming
The placenta also produces human placental lactogen (HPL), which resembles growth hormone. HPL stimulates maternal protein and fat metabolism to ensure a sufficient supply of amino acids and fatty acids for the parent and fetus. HPL also stimulates breast growth in preparation for lactation. Throughout pregnancy, HPL levels rise progressively.

Quick quiz

1. The term spermatogenesis refers to which of the following?
    A. The growth and development of sperm into primary spermatocytes
    B. The division of spermatocytes to form secondary spermatocytes
    C. The structural changing of spermatids
    D. The entire process of sperm formation

    Answer: D. Spermatogenesis refers to the entire process of sperm formation—from the development of primary spermatocytes to the formation of fully functional spermatozoa.

2. The primary function of the scrotum is to do which of the following?
    A. Provide storage for newly developed sperm.
    B. Maintain a cool temperature for the testes.
    C. Deposit sperm in the female reproductive tract.
    D. Provide a place for spermatogenesis to take place.

    Answer: B. The function of the scrotum is to maintain a cool temperature for the testes, which is necessary for spermatozoa formation.

3. The main function of the ovaries is to do which of the following?
    A. Secrete hormones that affect the buildup and shedding of the endometrium during the menstrual cycle.
    B. Accommodate a growing fetus during pregnancy.
    C. Produce mature ova.
    D. Channel blood discharged from the uterus during menstruation.

    Answer: C. The main function of the ovaries is to produce mature ova.

4. The corpus luteum degenerates in which phase of the female reproductive cycle?
    A. Luteal
    B. Follicular
    C. Proliferative
    D. Ovarian

    Answer: A. The corpus luteum degenerates in the luteal phase of the ovarian cycle of reproduction.

5. Which of the following are the four hormones involved in the menstrual cycle?
    A. LH, progesterone, estrogen, and testosterone
    B. Estrogen, FSH, LH, and androgens
    C. Estrogen, progesterone, LH, and FSH
    D. LH, estrogen, testosterone, and androgens

    Answer: C. The four hormones involved in the menstrual cycle are estrogen, progesterone, LH, and FSH.

6. Which of the following is the structure that guards the fetus in utero?
   A. Decidua
   B. Amniotic sac
   C. Corpus luteum
   D. Yolk sac

Answer: B. The structure that guards the fetus by producing a buoyant, temperature-controlled environment is the amniotic sac.

Scoring

⭐⭐⭐ If you answered all six questions correctly, fantastic! You're fertilization-friendly!

⭐⭐ If you answered five questions correctly, excellent! Now, reproduce that success in the chapters ahead!

⭐ If you answered fewer than five questions correctly, don't fear! Your concept of conception will improve after a little review.

Selected References

Lawson, G. W. (2020). Naegele's rule and the length of pregnancy—A review. *The Australian and New Zealand Journal of Obstetrics and Gynaecology, 61*(2), 177–182. https://doi.org/10.1111/ajo.13253

Ricci, S., Kyle, T., & Carman, S. (2021a). Anatomy and physiology of the reproductive systems. In *Maternity and pediatric nursing* (4th ed., pp. 95–112). Wolters Kluwer.

Ricci, S., Kyle, T., & Carman, S. (2021b). Fetal development and genetics. In *Maternity and pediatric nursing* (4th ed., pp. 323–349). Wolters Kluwer.

Silbert-Flagg, J. (2023a). Nursing care during normal pregnancy and care of the developing fetus. In *Maternal and child health nursing* (9th ed., pp. 177–204). Wolters Kluwer.

Silbert-Flagg, J. (2023b). Nursing care to promote fetal and maternal health. In *Maternal and child health nursing* (9th ed., pp. 262–289). Wolters Kluwer.

Chapter 3

Family planning and contraception

Just the facts

In this chapter, you'll learn:

♦ goals of family planning

♦ various methods of contraception, including the advantages and disadvantages of each

♦ surgical methods of family planning

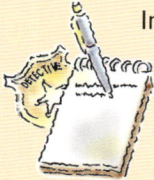

A look at family planning

Family planning involves the decisions people make regarding when (and if) they should have children, how many children to have, and how long to wait between pregnancies. Family planning also consists of choices to prevent or achieve pregnancy. Family planning is a personal decision that has many ethical, physical, emotional, religious, cultural, and legal implications. Effectiveness, cost, contraindications, and adverse effects for all family planning options should be presented to the patients and their partners so that they can make informed decisions.

A look at contraception

Contraception is the use of a delivery method to prevent conception.

Choosing a contraceptive

An appropriate contraceptive method will be safe, easily obtained, have minimal to no adverse effects, be affordable, acceptable to the patient, and minimize effects on future pregnancies. In addition, a person should use a contraceptive that is highly effective at preventing pregnancy.

Patient history

Information from the patient's menstrual and obstetric history should be used when determining which contraceptive method is best for them. The patient's history is also used to plan appropriate patient education.

An assessment for family planning involves collecting a reproductive history, including:
- beginning of menses
- interval between menses
- duration and amount of flow
- problems that occur during menses
- number of previous pregnancies
- number of previous births (and date of each)
- duration of each pregnancy
- type of each delivery
- gender and weight of children when delivered
- problems during previous pregnancies
- problems after delivery.

Scope out potential complications

The patient's health history may also identify potential risks of complications and help to determine whether hormonal contraceptives are safe for the patient to use. For example, a breastfeeding patient may desire options that have a lower chance of decreasing milk supply, such as a progesterone-only pill.

Factor in the partner

In some cases, the health of the patient's sexual partner influences which contraception method is used. For example, if the patient's sexual partner has a latex allergy, they may choose to use a latex-free condom made from polyisoprene during sex.

Implementing the chosen contraceptive

The effectiveness and safety of any contraceptive depend greatly on the patient's knowledge of and adherence to the chosen method. The patient's inability to understand proper use of the contraceptive device or an unwillingness to use it correctly or consistently may result in pregnancy. That is why patient education is such an important component of family planning. (See *Teaching tips on contraception*.)

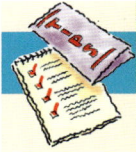

Teaching tips on contraception

Here are some points you should cover when teaching a patient about contraception:
• Teach proper use of the selected contraceptive and describe the procedure for the chosen method accurately. This may require demonstration of the method with a model to ensure proper use.
• Discuss possible adverse reactions. Direct the patient to report adverse reactions to their health care provider.
• Stress the importance of keeping follow-up appointments. During follow-up visits, contraceptive use and adverse reactions are evaluated, and it is possible that a repeat Papanicolaou test may be performed. Follow-up visits also provide an opportunity to address any questions the patient may have.
• Answer all questions in a manner that is easily understood by the patient.

With proper instruction and information, the patient should be able to:
• describe how to use the selected contraceptive correctly
• describe adverse reactions to the selected contraceptive and state the responsibility to report any that occur
• state that they will make an appointment for their next visit (if indicated)
• express that the current method of birth control is an acceptable method for them.

Methods of contraception

Contraceptive methods include abstinence, natural family planning methods, oral contraceptives, the morning-after pill (MAP) or emergency contraception (EC), the intravaginal method, transdermal contraceptive patches, intramuscular (IM) injections, intrauterine devices (IUDs), intrauterine systems, mechanical or chemical barrier methods, and permanent sterilization.

Abstinence

Abstinence, or refraining from having sexual intercourse, has a 0% failure rate. It is also the most effective way to prevent the transmission of sexually transmitted infections (STIs). However, most people—especially adolescents—do not consider it an option or a form of contraception. Abstinence should always be presented as an option to the patient in addition to information about other forms of contraception.

Natural family planning methods

Natural family planning methods are contraceptive methods that do not use chemicals, foreign materials, or devices to prevent pregnancy. Instead, it relies on the patient to monitor fertility signs throughout the menstrual cycle to determine the fertility window. Religious beliefs may prevent some people from using hormonal or internal contraceptive devices. Others just prefer a more natural method of planning or preventing pregnancy. Natural family planning methods include the rhythm (calendar) method, basal body temperature (BBT) method, cervical mucus (Billings) method, symptothermal method, ovulation awareness (cycle beads), lactational amenorrhea, and coitus interruptus.

Keeping count

For most natural family planning methods, the patient's fertile days must be calculated so that they can abstain from intercourse on those days. Various methods are used to determine the fertile period. The effectiveness of these methods depends on the patient's and partner's willingness to refrain from sex on the female partner's fertile days and accurate documentation. Failure rates vary from 10% to 20%.

Rhythm method

The rhythm, or calendar, method requires that the couple refrain from intercourse on the days that the patient is most likely to conceive based on their menstrual cycle. This fertile period usually lasts from 3 or 4 days before to 3 or 4 days after ovulation.

Dear diary

Teach the patient to keep a record of their menstrual cycle to determine when ovulation is most likely to occur. They should do this for six to eight consecutive cycles. They should begin counting day 1 as the first day of menstruation. To calculate the safe periods, tell the patient to subtract 18 from the shortest cycle and 11 from the longest cycle that they have documented. For instance, if they had six menstrual cycles that lasted 26 to 30 days, their fertile period would be from the eighth day (26 minus 18) to the 19th day (30 minus 11). To ensure that pregnancy does not occur, the patient and their partner should abstain from intercourse during days 8 to 19 of the menstrual cycle. During those fertile days, they may also choose to use contraceptive foam.

Basal body temperature

BBT is a patient's temperature when at full rest. Just before the day of ovulation, their BBT falls about one half of a degree. At the time of ovulation, the BBT rises to a full degree because of progesterone influence.

Ups and downs, highs and lows

To use the BBT method of contraception, the patient must take their temperature every morning before sitting up, getting out of bed, or beginning their morning activity. (See *Teaching a patient how to take BBT*.) By recording this daily temperature, they can see a slight dip and then an increase in body temperature. The increase in temperature indicates that they have ovulated and should refrain from intercourse for the next 3 days. Three days is significant because this is the lifespan of a discharged ovum. Because sperm can survive in the female reproductive tract for 4 days, the BBT method of contraception is typically combined with the calendar method so that the couple can abstain from intercourse a few days before ovulation as well.

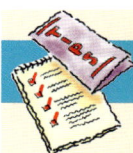

Education edge

Teaching a patient how to take BBT

Here are tips to help you teach a patient about recording BBT. Remind the patient that BBT is lower during the first 2 weeks of the menstrual cycle, before ovulation. Immediately after ovulation, the temperature begins to rise. It continues to rise until it is time for the next menses. This rise in temperature indicates that progesterone has been released into the system, which, in turn, means that the patient has ovulated.

Charting BBT does not predict the exact day of ovulation; it just indicates that ovulation has occurred. However, this can be used to help the patient to monitor their ovulatory pattern and give them a time frame during which ovulation occurs.

Getting started

Tell the patient to follow these instructions for taking BBT:
- Advise the patient to chart the days of menstrual flow by darkening the squares above the 98°F (36.7°C) mark. They should start with the first day of their menses (day 1) and then take their temperature each day after the menses ends.
- Tell the patient to use a thermometer that measures tenths of a degree.
- Instruct the patient to take their temperature as soon as they wake up. Tell them that it is important to do this at the same time each morning.
- The patient should then place a dot on the graph's line that matches the temperature reading. (Tell them not to be surprised if the waking temperature before ovulation is 96°F or 97°F [35.6°C or 36.1°C].) If they forget to take their temperature on 1 day, instruct them to leave that day blank on the graph and not to connect the dots.
- Instruct the patient to make notes on the graph if they miss taking their temperature, feel sick, cannot sleep, or wake up at a different time. Advise them that if they are taking any medicine—even over-the-counter medications such as aspirin or acetaminophen—it may affect their temperature. Remind them to mark the dates when they have sexual intercourse.

Teaching a patient how to take BBT (*continued*)

Sample chart

In the sample temperature chart, the patient used an "S" to record sexual intercourse and made notes showing they had insomnia on September 27. The patient forgot to take her temperature on September 19; notice that they didn't connect the dots on this day. Their temperature dipped on September 24 (day 15 of the cycle) and began rising afterward.

Some patient's chart will be larger and will probably include temperatures over 99.3°F (37.4°C) and under 97°F (36.1°C).

Sample temperature chart

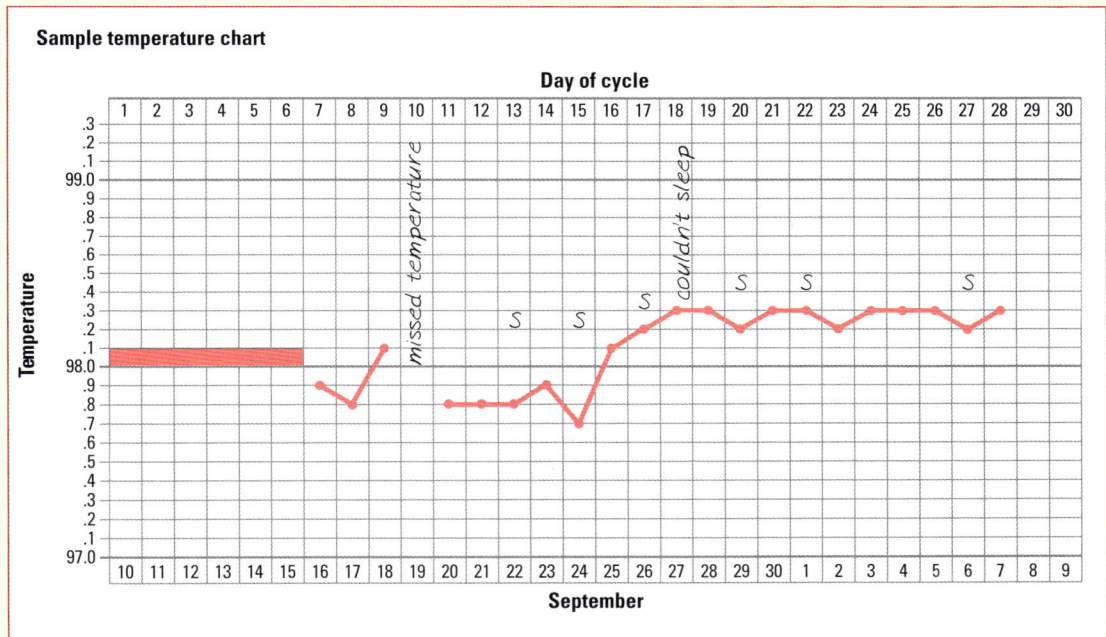

Various variables

One problem with this method is that many things can affect BBT. The patient may forget and take their temperature after rising out of bed or they may have a slight illness. These situations cause a rise in temperature. If the patient changes their daily routine, the change in activity could also affect the body temperature, which may lead them to mistakenly interpret a fertile day as a safe day and vice versa.

Cervical mucus method

The cervical mucus method (also known as the *Billings ovulation method*) predicts changes in the cervical mucus during ovulation.

During nonfertile times of the menstrual cycle, cervical mucus is thick, sticky, opaque, and impervious (inhospitable) to sperm. Just prior to ovulation, cervical mucus becomes thin, colorless, and copious in amount and is stringy and stretchy. This thin, stretchable mucus (also known as *spinnbarkeit*) is favorable to sperm and facilitates transport of sperm through the cervix into the uterus.

Slippery peaks

During the peak of ovulation, the cervical mucus becomes slippery and stretches at least 1 in (2.5 cm) before the strand breaks. Breast tenderness and anterior tilt of the cervix also occur with ovulation. The fertile period consists of all the days that the cervical mucus is copious and the 3 days after the peak date. During these days, the couple should abstain from intercourse to avoid conception.

Consistently checking consistency

Cervical mucus must be assessed every day for changes in consistency and amounts to be sure that those changes signify ovulation. Assessing cervical mucus after intercourse is unreliable because seminal fluid has a watery, postovulatory consistency, which can be confused with ovulatory mucus.

Symptothermal method

The symptothermal method combines the BBT method with the cervical mucus method. The patient takes their daily temperature and watches for the rise in temperature that signals the onset of ovulation. They also assess the cervical mucus every day. The patient abstains from intercourse until 3 days after the rise in basal temperature or the fourth day after the peak day (indicating ovulation) of cervical mucus because these signs signify the fertile period. Combining these two methods is more effective than using either method alone.

Ovulation awareness

Over-the-counter ovulation detection kits determine when ovulation occurs by measuring luteinizing hormone (LH) in the urine or a combination of LH and estrogen. Usually, during each menstrual cycle, LH levels rise suddenly (called an *LH surge*), causing an ovum to be released from the ovary 24 to 36 hours later (ovulation). This test determines the midcycle surge of LH, which can be detected in the urine as early as 12 to 24 hours after ovulation. They identify the four most fertile days. These kits are about 98% to 100% accurate, but they are fairly expensive to use as a primary means of birth control. (See *Performing a home ovulation test.*)

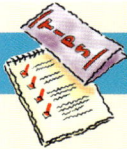

Education edge

Performing a home ovulation test

A home ovulation test helps the patient determine the best time to try to become pregnant or to prevent pregnancy by monitoring the amount of LH/estrogen found in urine. These test kits can be purchased over the counter.

Normally, during each menstrual cycle, levels of LH rise suddenly, causing an egg to be released from the ovary 24 to 36 hours later.

Getting ready

Tell the patient to follow these instructions before performing a home ovulation test:
- Read the kit's directions thoroughly before performing the test.
- Before testing, calculate the length of the menstrual cycle. Count from the beginning of one menses to the beginning of the next menses. (The patient should count the first day of bleeding as day 1. The length of their cycle will determine when to begin testing.)
- The best time to test is at the first void of the morning.
- This test can be performed at any time of the day or night, but it should be performed at the same time every day.

Taking the test

Tell the patient to follow these instructions for performing a home ovulation test:
- Remove the test stick from the packet.
- Sit on the toilet and direct the absorbent tip of the test stick downward and directly into the urine stream for at least 5 seconds or until it is thoroughly wet.
- Be careful not to urinate on the window of the stick.
- Alternatively, urinate in a clean, dry cup or container and then dip the test stick (absorbent tip only) into the urine for at least 5 seconds.
- Place the stick on a clean, flat, dry surface.

Reading the results

Explain to the patient the following instructions for reading home ovulation test results:
- Wait at least 5 minutes before reading the results. When the test is finished, a line appears in the small window (control window).
- If there is no line in the large rectangular window (test window) or if the line is lighter than the line in the small rectangular window (control window), the patient has not begun an LH surge. The patient should continue testing daily.
- If they see one line in the large rectangular window that is similar to or darker than the line in the small window, they are experiencing an LH surge. This means that ovulation should occur within the next 24 to 36 hours.
- Once the patient has determined they are about to ovulate, they will know they are at the start of the most fertile time of their cycle and should use this information to plan accordingly.

Coitus interruptus

Coitus interruptus, one of the oldest known methods of contraception, involves withdrawal of the penis from the vagina during intercourse before ejaculation. However, because pre-ejaculation fluid that is deposited outside the vagina may contain spermatozoa, fertilization can occur.

Combined oral contraceptives

Combined oral contraceptives (birth control pills) are hormonal contraceptives that consist of synthetic estrogen and progesterone. The estrogen suppresses production of follicle-stimulating hormone (FSH) and LH, which, in turn, suppresses ovulation. The progesterone complements the estrogen's action by causing a decrease in cervical mucus permeability, which limits sperm's access to the ova. Progesterone also decreases the possibility of implantation by interfering with endometrial proliferation. If a dose is late or missed (24 to more than 48 hours since the pill should have been taken), take it as soon as possible even if taking two pills in 1 day. If two or more are missed, take the most recent missed pill as soon as possible and use an additional form of contraception, such as a barrier or chemical method, for the next 7 days while continuing the pill pack.

Triple Dose

There are three types of combined oral contraceptives based on the dosing of hormones:

1. Monophasic oral contraceptives provide fixed doses of estrogen and progesterone throughout a 21-day cycle. The last 7 days are placebo pills (no active ingredient) and are often a different color than active pills. These preparations provide a steady dose of both hormones.
2. Biphasic oral contraceptives provide one dosage strength of estrogen and progesterone for the first 7 to 10 days and a second strength of the hormones for 11 to 14 days. The last 7 days are placebo pills.
3. Triphasic oral contraceptives maintain a cycle more like the natural menstrual cycle because they vary the amount of estrogen and progestin throughout the cycle with three differing levels of hormones. Triphasic oral contraceptives have a lower incidence of breakthrough bleeding than monophasic oral contraceptives.

Small but powerful

A mini pill is a progestin-only oral contraceptive available for those who cannot take estrogen-based pills because of a history of stroke, high blood pressure, or thrombophlebitis. This type of pill is taken every day—even when the patient has their menses. The progestins in the pill inhibit the development of the endometrium and thicken cervical mucus, thus preventing implantation. There are no inactive or placebo pills during the month of dosing. Progestin-only pills may also be used by patients who are breastfeeding.

The mini pill must be taken at the same time each day. If a dose is missed, take it as soon as possible even if taking two pills on 1 day.

Use an additional form of contraception for the next 7 days while continuing to take the pill pack.

In addition to being available by prescription, progestin-only pills are now available over the counter in the United States. They are marketed under the brand name Opill (norgestrel is the generic name).

21- or 28-day package deals

Monophasic, biphasic, and triphasic oral contraceptives are dispensed in either 21- or 28-day packs. The first pill is usually taken on the first Sunday following the start of menses, but it is possible to start oral contraceptives on any day. For patients who have recently given birth, oral contraceptives can be taken at least 4 weeks after delivery on the first Sunday. Patients should be advised to use an additional form of contraception for the first week after starting an oral contraceptive because the medication does not take full effect for 7 days. (See *Teaching tips on oral contraceptives*.)

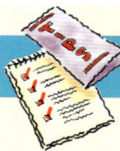

Education edge

Teaching tips on oral contraceptives

Be sure to include these tips when teaching patients about oral contraceptives:
• Inform the patient about possible adverse reactions, such as fluid retention, weight gain, breast tenderness, headache, breakthrough bleeding, chloasma, acne, yeast infection, nausea, and fatigue. It may be necessary to change the type or dosage of the contraceptive to relieve these adverse reactions.
• Instruct the patient on the dietary needs of those taking an oral contraceptive. Patients need to increase their intake of foods high in vitamin B_6 (wheat, corn, liver, meat) and folic acid (liver; green, leafy vegetables). About 20% to 30% of oral contraceptive users have dietary deficiencies of vitamin B_6 and folic acid. Moreover, health care professionals speculate that oral contraceptive users should also increase their intake of vitamins A, B_2, B_{12}, C, and niacin.
• Advise the patient to use an additional form of contraception for the first 7 days after starting the medication because it does not take full effect for 7 days.
• Advise the patient to use an additional form of contraception when taking antibiotics until the beginning of a normal menstrual period.

Birth control pills that are prescribed in a 21-day dispenser allow the patient to take a pill every day for 3 weeks. They should expect to start their menstrual flow about 4 days after taking a cycle of pills. The 28-day pills are packaged with 21 days of birth control pills and 7 days of placebos. A new pack of pills is started as soon as the previous pack finishes, eliminating the risk of forgetting to start a new pack.

It's seasonal

An additional oral contraceptive on the market is a combination of levonorgestrel and ethinyl estradiol in which one tablet is taken daily for 12 or 13 weeks. This pill extends the time between periods, allowing patients to have a period only four times a year as opposed to monthly. There is also continuous dosing with 365 active pills and no inactive pills allowing for no period to occur.

The plus side

Here are the advantages of oral contraceptives:
- Monophasic, biphasic, and triphasic oral contraceptives are 99.5% effective with "perfect use." The failure rate is about 3%; failure usually occurs because the patient forgets to take the pill or because of other individual differences in their physiology.
- They do not inhibit sexual spontaneity.
- They may reduce the risk of endometrial and ovarian cancer, ectopic pregnancy, ovarian cysts, and noncancerous breast tumors.
- They decrease the risk of pelvic inflammatory disease (PID) and dysmenorrhea.
- They regulate the menstrual cycle and may diminish or eliminate premenstrual tension.

The minus side

Here are the disadvantages of oral contraceptives:
- They do not provide protection from STIs.
- They must be taken daily at the same time every day.
- They can be expensive with a copay required every month.
- Illnesses that cause vomiting may reduce their effectiveness.
- Most combination oral contraceptives are contraindicated in those who are breastfeeding because the pills may reduce milk supply.
- Patients with a family history of stroke, coronary artery disease, thrombohemolytic disease, or liver disease should have additional testing prior to being prescribed estrogen-containing oral contraceptives. Oral contraceptives are contraindicated in patients who have a personal history of thromboembolic events such as deep vein thrombosis or pulmonary embolism.
- People who are older than age 40 years, and those who have a history of or have been diagnosed with diabetes mellitus, elevated triglyceride or cholesterol level, breast or reproductive tract malignancy, high blood pressure, obesity, seizure disorder, sickle cell disease, mental depression, and migraines or other vascular-type headaches, should be strongly cautioned about taking oral contraceptives for birth control. The possible side effects of oral contraceptives may be more severe in those who fall under these categories.

- A patient older than age 35 years is at increased risk for a fatal heart attack if they smoke and take oral contraceptives.
- Adverse effects include nausea, headache, weight gain, depression, mild hypertension, breast tenderness, breakthrough bleeding, and monilial (yeast) vaginal infections.
- When a patient wants to conceive, they may not be able to for several months after stopping oral contraceptives. The pituitary gland requires a recovery period to begin the stimulation of cyclic gonadotropins, such as FSH and LH, which help regulate ovulation. In addition, many health care providers recommend that patients not become pregnant within 2 months of stopping oral contraceptives.

Morning-after pill

Also called *emergency contraception*, the "morning-after pill" prevents pregnancy in the event of unprotected sexual intercourse or failure of a birth control method (such as a broken condom). EC is a pregnancy prevention measure, not an abortion pill. It may be obtained from various health care providers' offices and family planning clinics. Levonorgestrel EC pills may be purchased over the counter without a prescription in many pharmacies.

EC comes in three forms: progestin-only pill, a combined hormone pill, or ulipristal acetate. For the progesterone-only pill, known as "Plan B," the first dose must be taken within 72 hours of sexual intercourse. "Plan B" can be taken as one pill and contains 1.5 mg of levonorgestrel.

Another option is a patient may be prescribed a certain number of oral hormonal contraceptive pills from a birth control pack (estrogen and progesterone combination). Ella (a pill containing 30 mg ulipristal acetate) can be taken up to 5 days or 120 hours after sexual intercourse.

Medications for nausea may also be prescribed, and the patient is instructed to return to the office or clinic in 3 weeks. The patient must also be instructed to use a birth control method consistently until their menstrual period begins. The type of birth control method recommended will depend on the EC prescribed.

The plus side

Here are the advantages of the EC:
- It is 75% to 98% effective, depending on which product is used, when in the cycle intercourse occurred, and whether the patient has had unprotected intercourse within the past 72 hours or 120 hours (depending on the EC used).
- It does not inhibit sexual spontaneity.
- It is readily available when unforeseen circumstances occur.
- Ella, specifically, delays or prevents ovulation even after LHs have started to rise.

The minus side

Here are the disadvantages of the EC:
- It does not offer protection from STIs.
- It must be taken within the 72- or 120-hour period after intercourse occurs depending on what is prescribed.
- The hormone dosage is larger than that of oral hormonal contraceptives and commonly causes nausea, vomiting, and malaise.
- It can be expensive.
- It is not always readily available at a pharmacy and may have to be ordered.
- Contraindications and precautions are similar to those for other oral hormonal contraceptives.
- Ella does not work as well for those weighing more than 195 pounds.

Intravaginal method

Another method of introducing hormones (estrogen and progestin) into a patient's circulation is the intravaginal route by a cervical ring that slowly releases contraceptive hormones called the *NuvaRing* or *Annovera*. The ring is inserted into the vagina, where it stays held in by the vaginal walls, for 3 weeks. It is then removed, allowing menstruation to occur. A new ring needs to be reinserted after 1 week. If not currently using hormonal birth control and if inserted on the first day of menstrual cycle, there is no need for backup contraceptive. If changing from progestin-only, implant, injection, or IUD form, an extra barrier method of contraceptive must be used for the first 7 days. For the *Annovera*, the patient can choose to leave it in for 13 cycles or one entire year to prevent pregnancy.

The plus side

Here are the advantages of the intravaginal method:
- It is inserted only every 3 weeks.
- The patient does not have to remember to take a pill every day.
- There are fewer hormonal peaks and decreases because of the slow but steady release.
- It is 97% to 99% effective.
- It allows sexual spontaneity.
- It is discreet.
- It is easy to insert.
- *Annovera* can be used to skip cycles for an entire year.

The minus side

Here are the disadvantages of the intravaginal method:
- It does not provide protection against STIs.

- It is contraindicated in patients who are pregnant or may become pregnant; those who are breastfeeding; those who have a family history of stroke, coronary artery disease, thrombohemolytic disease, or liver disease; those who have undiagnosed vaginal bleeding; and those who are sensitive to the material in the ring.
- Patients who are older than age 35 years; those who have a history of or have been diagnosed with diabetes mellitus, elevated triglycerides or cholesterol level, breast or reproductive tract malignancy, high blood pressure, obesity, seizure disorder, sickle cell disease, depression, and migraines or other vascular-type headaches; and those who smoke should be strongly cautioned about using a hormonal contraceptive ring. The possible side effects of hormonal contraceptives may be greater in patients with a history of these disorders.

Transdermal contraceptive patches

The transdermal contraceptive patch is a highly effective, weekly hormonal birth control patch worn on the skin. The patch integrates a combination of estrogen and progestin. The hormones are absorbed into the skin and then transferred into the bloodstream.

Patchwork

The patch is very thin, beige, and smooth and measures 1¾ in (4.4 cm) square. It can be worn on the upper outer arm, buttocks, abdomen, or upper torso, and placement should be rotated each cycle. The patch is worn for 1 week and replaced on the same day of the week for 3 consecutive weeks. No patch is worn during the fourth week. Studies have shown that the patch remains attached and is effective when the patient bathes, swims, exercises, or wears it in humid weather.

The plus side

Here are the advantages of the transdermal contraceptive patch:
- It is 99% effective in preventing pregnancy if used exactly as directed.
- It is convenient. No preparation is needed before intercourse.
- It helps lessen or prevent ectopic pregnancy, and endometrial and ovarian cancers.
- It is still effective even if experiencing nausea or diarrhea.
- It is a good alternative for patients who commonly forget to take oral contraceptives.

The minus side

Here are the disadvantages of the transdermal patch:
- It does not provide protection from STIs.
- It is contraindicated in patients who are breastfeeding; those who have a family history of stroke, coronary artery disease,

thrombohemolytic disease, or liver disease; those who have undiagnosed vaginal bleeding; and those who are sensitive to the adhesive used on the patch.

- Patients who are older than age 35 years; those who have a history of or have been diagnosed with diabetes mellitus, elevated triglycerides or cholesterol level, breast or reproductive tract malignancy, high blood pressure, obesity, seizure disorder, sickle cell disease, mental depression, and migraines or other vascular-type headaches; and those who smoke should be strongly cautioned about using a transdermal contraceptive patch for birth control. The possible side effects of hormonal contraceptives may be more severe in patients who fall under these categories.
- It has been found to be slightly less effective in patients with a body mass index (BMI) of greater than 30 kg/m^2. These patients may need to consider another form of contraception.
- Some antibiotics reduce its effectiveness.

Contraceptive injections

Contraceptive injections include IM and subcutaneous (SQ) injections of medroxyprogesterone (Depo-Provera, Sayana Press, or Noristerat), which are administered every 8, 12, or 13 weeks depending on the type. Contraceptive injections release progestogen, stopping ovulation from occurring by suppressing the release of gonadotropic hormones. They also change the cervical mucosa to prevent sperm from entering the uterus and thinning the uterine lining.

The plus side

Here are the advantages of contraceptive injections:
- It is 99% effective in preventing pregnancy if used exactly as directed.
- It does not inhibit sexual response.
- It is not affected by other medication.
- It is useful for those who cannot take contraceptives containing estrogen.
- Except for abstinence, it is more effective than other birth control methods.
- It helps prevent endometrial cancer and PID.
- It can be used as a contraceptive method for patients who just gave birth if they are not breastfeeding.

The minus side

Here are the disadvantages of contraceptive injections:
- It requires an injection every 8, 12, or 13 weeks.
- If the patient wants to become pregnant, it may take 9 to 24 months after the last injection to conceive.

- It does not protect against STIs.
- Its effects cannot be reversed after it is injected.
- It may cause changes in the menstrual cycle such as irregular spotting, bleeding, or amenorrhea.
- It may cause weight gain because of an increase in appetite.
- It may cause a decrease in sex drive or desire.
- It may cause headaches, fatigue, and nervousness.
- It can cause bone density loss in some patients with continued use.
- It is contraindicated if the patient is pregnant or has liver disease, undiagnosed vaginal bleeding, breast cancer, blood clotting disorders, or cardiovascular disease.
- Patients who have a history of arterial disease, heart disease or stroke, blood clots, liver disease, diabetes, and those with a history of or current breast cancer should be advised to use another form of contraception.

Intrauterine device

The IUD is a plastic contraceptive device that is inserted into the uterus through the cervical canal and stays in place for 1 to 10 years depending on the type and brand. (See *IUD insertion*.) The IUD is inserted into and removed from the uterus most easily during menses, when the cervical canal is slightly dilated. Inserting the device during menses also reduces the likelihood of inserting an IUD into a patient who is pregnant.

IUD insertion

A bimanual examination is performed to determine uterine position, shape, and size.

Before IUD insertion, make sure that the procedure has been explained to the patient and that their questions have been addressed. Also, be sure to obtain a negative pregnancy test and informed consent.

How it's done
Here is how the device is inserted:
1. The movable flange on the inserter barrel of the IUD is set to the depth of the uterus (measured in centimeters). The loaded inserter tube is introduced through the cervical canal and into the uterus.

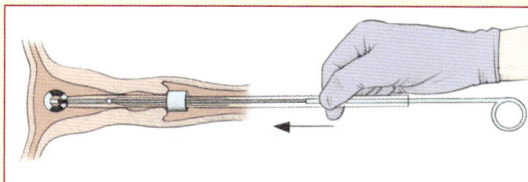

(*continued*)

IUD insertion (*continued*)

2. The IUD is inserted by retracting the inserter slowly about ½ in (1.3 cm) over the plunger while the plunger is held still. This allows the arms to open.

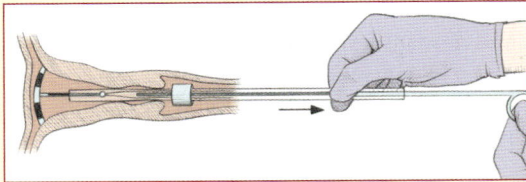

3. The plunger is gently advanced until resistance is felt. This action ensures high fundal placement of the IUD and may reduce the potential for expulsion.

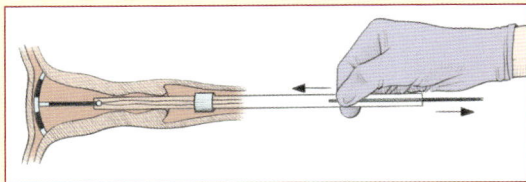

4. The solid rod is withdrawn, whereas the insertion barrel is held stationary. The insertion barrel is then withdrawn. The strings are clipped about 2 to 3 cm from the cervical os. This action leaves sufficient string for checking the placement of and removing the IUD.

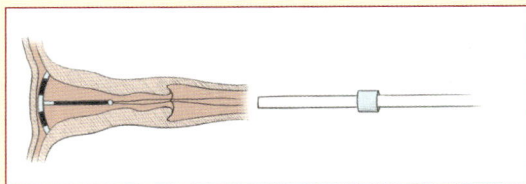

Copper interference

One type of IUD, the ParaGard-T, is a T-shaped, polyethylene device with copper wrapped around its vertical stem. The copper interferes with sperm mobility, decreasing the possibility of sperm crossing the uterine space. A knotted monofilament retrieval string is attached through a hole in the stem.

Progesterone reserve

Another type of IUD is the hormonal IUD, a T-shaped device made of soft plastic that releases small amounts of progestin over time. The hormonal method works to prevent pregnancy by causing the cervical mucus to remain thick, preventing sperm from entering, inhibiting sperm from reaching or fertilizing an egg, and inhibiting endometrial proliferation.

There are four brands of hormonal IUDs available in the United States: Mirena, Kyleena, Liletta, and Skyla. They are all hormonal IUDs used for contraceptives that release varying amounts of levonorgestrel and are approved by the U.S. Food and Drug Administration; however, they vary in the length of time they work. Mirena and Liletta last for up to 8 years, Kyleena works for up to 5 years, and Skyla works for up to 3 years. Some patients will stop having periods after about a year of continuous use of a hormonal IUD. Patients should be educated to check for strings, to be sure it is in place, once a month in between cycles.

If the patient becomes pregnant with an IUD in place, the device can be left; however, it is usually removed to reduce the risk of spontaneous abortion and infection.

The plus side

Here are the advantages of an IUD or intrauterine system:
- It is 99% effective in preventing pregnancy if used exactly as directed.
- It does not inhibit sexual spontaneity.
- It is safe to use while breastfeeding.
- It does not interact with other medications.
- Neither partner feels the device during intercourse.
- It is easily removable and patients are able to get pregnant right away.

The minus side

Here are the disadvantages of an IUD:
- It is expensive.
- It may cause uterine cramping on insertion.
- It may cause infection, especially in the initial weeks after insertion.
- It can be spontaneously expelled in the first year by 5% to 20% of patients.
- It does not protect against STIs.
- The incidence of PID increases with IUD use. Most cases of PID occur during the first 3 months after insertion. After 3 months, the risk of PID is lower unless pre-insertion screening failed to identify a person at risk for STIs. The patient should be instructed to watch for signs of PID. (See *Signs of PID*.)
- It increases the risk of ectopic pregnancy.
- Copper-containing IUDs are contraindicated in those who have Wilson disease (because of the inability to metabolize copper properly).

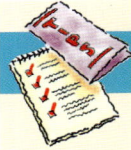

Signs of PID

If a patient has an IUD, tell them that untreated vaginal infections can progress to PID. Instruct the patient to watch for signs and symptoms of PID, such as:

- fever of 101°F (38.3°C)
- purulent vaginal discharge
- painful intercourse
- abdominal or pelvic pain
- suprapubic tenderness or guarding
- tenderness on bimanual examination.

- It is contraindicated in patients who have active, recent, or recurrent PID; infection or inflammation of the genital tract; STIs; diseases that suppress immune function, including human immunodeficiency virus (HIV); unexplained cervical or vaginal bleeding; previous problems with IUDs; cancer of the reproductive organs; or a history of ectopic pregnancy. Insertion is also contraindicated in patients who have severe vasovagal reactivity, difficulty obtaining emergency care, valvular heart disease, anatomic uterine deformities, anemia, or, in most cases, nulliparity.

Hormonal intrauterine systems are being successfully used by some family planning care providers in nulliparous patients.

Implantable methods

Etonogestrel implant (Nexplanon) is a matchstick-sized implant that is placed (and later removed) in the fat layer under the skin of the upper arm by a health care provider. Once placed, it prevents ovulation and can be more than 99% effective for up to 3 to 5 years. The implant works by stopping ovulation, thinning the lining of the uterus, and thickening cervical mucus similar to other contraceptives. Patients with an etonogestrel implant may have irregular periods, bleeding or spotting, or may stop having periods if the implant is used over a longer time period.

The plus side

Here are the advantages of implantable methods:

- It does not inhibit sexual spontaneity.
- It has long-term effectiveness without the need to take a daily pill.
- It may be used in nulliparous patients and adolescents.
- It may be used in those who cannot use estrogen-containing contraceptives.

The minus side

Here are the disadvantages of implantable methods:
- It is expensive.
- It is contraindicated if a patient has a history of thrombophlebitis, liver disease or tumor, unexplained vaginal bleeding, breast cancer, or any cancer that is sensitive to progestin.
- Patients that have a history of diabetes, high cholesterol or triglycerides, headaches, gallbladder or kidney problems, depressed mood, high blood pressure, allergies to local anesthetics or antiseptics, or smoking and are considering an etonogestrel implant should be warned that an etonogestrel implant can make these conditions worse.

Barrier methods

In the barrier methods of contraception, a chemical or mechanical barrier is inserted between the cervix and the sperm to prevent the sperm from entering the uterus, traveling to the fallopian tubes, and fertilizing the ovum. Barrier methods do not use hormones, so they're sometimes favored over hormonal contraceptives, which can cause many adverse effects. However, failure rates for barrier methods are higher than for hormonal contraceptives.

Barrier methods include spermicidal products, diaphragms, cervical caps, vaginal rings, and male and female condoms.

Spermicidal products

Before intercourse, spermicidal products are inserted into the vagina. Their goal is to kill sperm before the sperm enter the cervix. Spermicides also change the pH of the vaginal fluid to a strong acid, which is not conducive to sperm survival. Vaginally inserted spermicides are available in gels, creams, films, foams, sponges, and suppositories.

The gels, foams, and creams are inserted using an applicator and should be inserted at least 1 hour before intercourse. The patient should be instructed not to douche for 6 hours after intercourse to ensure that the agent has completed its spermicidal action in the vagina and cervix.

Spermicidal films are made of glycerin impregnated with nonoxynol-9. The film is folded and then inserted into the vagina. The film should be inserted at least 15 minutes and up to 1 hour before sexual intercourse. Once it is inserted and contacts body heat or vaginal secretions, it dissolves and releases nonoxynol-9 to protect the cervix against invading spermatozoa.

Spermicidal suppositories consist of cocoa butter and glycerin and are filled with nonoxynol-9. The suppositories are inserted into the vagina, where they dissolve to release the spermicide. Patients should be instructed to insert it 15 minutes before intercourse.

The plus side
Here are the advantages of spermicidal products:
- They are inexpensive.
- They may be purchased over the counter, which makes them easily accessible.
- They do not require a visit to a health care provider.
- Spermicidal films wash away with natural body fluids.
- Vaginally inserted spermicides may be used in combination with other birth control methods to increase their effectiveness.
- They are useful in emergency situations such as when a condom breaks.

The minus side
Here are the disadvantages of spermicidal products:
- They need to be inserted from 15 minutes to 1 hour before intercourse, so they may interfere with sexual spontaneity.
- Some spermicides may be irritating to the vagina and penile tissue.
- Spermicides with nonoxynol-9 do not protect against HIV infection and can increase the risk for contracting STIs in those with frequent use (due to mucosal wall irritation).
- Some patients are bothered by the vaginal leakage that can occur, especially after using cocoa- and glycerin-based suppositories.
- Spermicidal films are not recommended for patients who are nearing menopause because decreased vaginal secretions make the film less effective.
- Spermicidal products may be contraindicated in patients who have acute cervicitis because of the risk of further irritation.

Diaphragm

The diaphragm is another barrier-type contraceptive that mechanically blocks sperm from entering the cervix. It is composed of a soft, latex dome that is supported by a round, metal spring on the outside. A diaphragm can be inserted up to 2 hours before intercourse. Optimum effectiveness is achieved by using it in combination with spermicidal jelly that is applied to the rim of the diaphragm before it is inserted. Diaphragms are available in various sizes and must be fitted to the person. (See *Inserting a diaphragm*.)

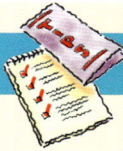

Education edge

Inserting a diaphragm

As the diaphragm is inserted, instruct the patient to prepare for inserting the diaphragm themselves. Identify structures and the feelings associated with proper insertion. Follow these steps for insertion:

1. After putting on gloves, lubricate the rim or dome of the fitting ring or diaphragm to lessen the discomfort of insertion.

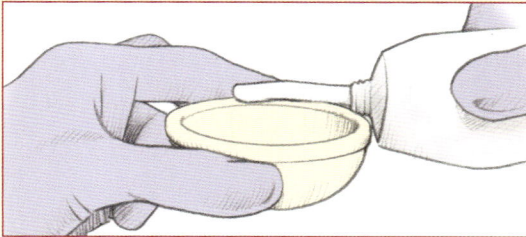

2. Fold the diaphragm in half with one hand by pressing the opposite sides together. Hold the vulva open with the other hand.

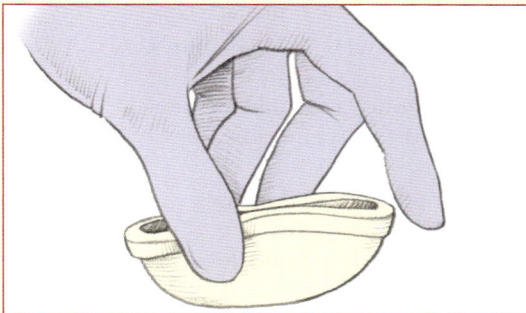

3. Slide the folded diaphragm into the vagina and toward the posterior cervicovaginal fornix.

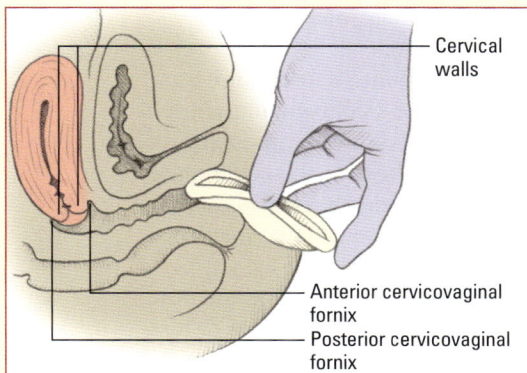

Cervical walls

Anterior cervicovaginal fornix

Posterior cervicovaginal fornix

(*continued*)

Inserting a diaphragm (*continued*)

4. The diaphragm should fit under the symphysis and cover the cervix. The proximal ring should fit behind the pubic arch with minimal pressure. Note that the cervix is palpable behind the diaphragm. The cervix feels like a "nose."

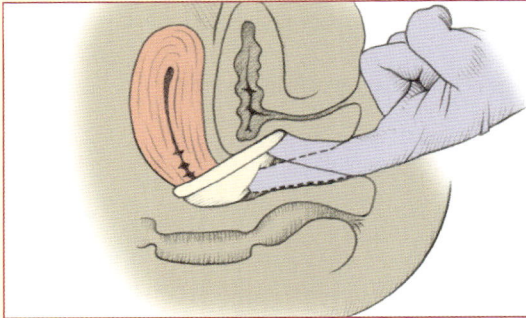

The plus side

Here are the advantages of the diaphragm:

- It is a good choice for those who choose not to use hormonal contraceptives or do not feel that they can use natural family planning methods effectively.
- Its effectiveness ranges from 80% to 93% for new users and increases to 97% for long-term users when combined with spermicidal jelly.
- It causes few adverse reactions.
- It does not alter the body's metabolic or physiologic processes.
- It can be inserted up to 2 hours before intercourse.
- Neither partner can feel it during intercourse when correctly fitted and inserted.

The minus side

Here are the disadvantages of the diaphragm:

- It must be inserted before intercourse and may interfere with spontaneity.
- Although it can be left in place for up to 24 hours, if intercourse is repeated before 6 hours (which is how long the diaphragm must be left in place after intercourse) more spermicidal gel must be inserted. The diaphragm cannot be removed and replaced because this could cause sperm to bypass the spermicidal gel and fertilization could occur.
- The pressure it creates on the urethra may cause a higher incidence of upper urinary tract infections (UTIs).
- It must be refitted after birth, cervical surgery, miscarriage, dilation and curettage (D & C), therapeutic abortion, or weight gain or loss of more than 15 lb (6.8 kg) because of cervical shape changes.

- It is contraindicated in patients who have a history of cystocele, rectocele, uterine retroversion, prolapse, retroflexion, or anteflexion because the cervix position may be displaced, making insertion and proper fit questionable.
- It is contraindicated in patients with a history of toxic shock syndrome or repeated UTIs, vaginal stenosis, pelvic abnormalities, or allergy to spermicidal jellies or rubber (latex). It is also contraindicated in patients who show an unwillingness to learn proper techniques for diaphragm care and insertion.
- It cannot be used in the first 6 weeks postpartum.

Cervical cap

The cervical cap is another barrier-type method of contraception. It is similar to the diaphragm but smaller. It is a thimble-shaped, soft rubber cup that the patient places over the cervix and is held in place by suction. The addition of a spermicide creates a chemical barrier as well. Patients who are not suited for diaphragms may use cervical caps. Failure of the cervical cap is commonly due to failure to use the device or inappropriate use of the device. (See *Recognizing a correct fit.*)

Advice from the experts

Recognizing a correct fit

With the proper fit, the gap or space between the base of the cervix and the inside of the cervical cap ring should be 1 to 2 mm (to reduce the possibility of dislodgment), and the rim should fill the cervicovaginal fornix.

To verify a good fit, leave the cervical cap in place for 1 to 2 minutes. Then, with the cap in place, pinch the dome until there is a dimple. A dimple that takes about 30 seconds to resume a domed appearance indicates good suction and a good fit. If the cap is too small, the rim leaves a gap where the cervix remains exposed. If the cap is too large, it will not fit snugly against the cervix and can be more easily dislodged.

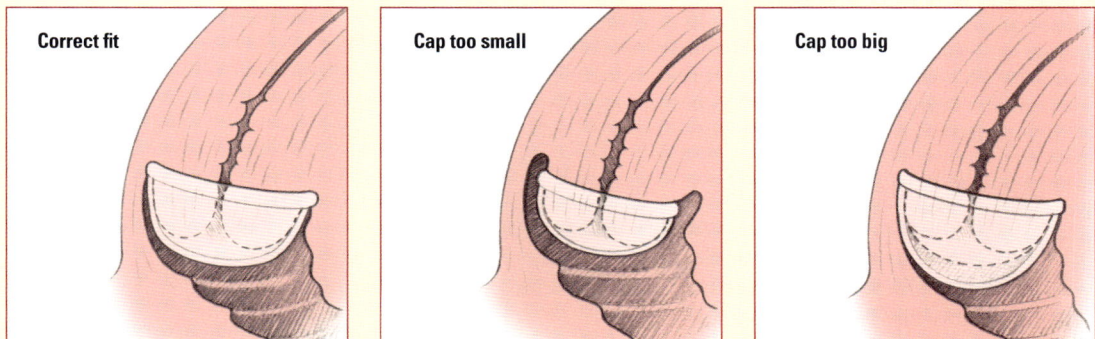

Correct fit

Cap too small

Cap too big

The plus side

Here are the advantages of the cervical cap:

- It requires less spermicide and is less likely to become dislodged during intercourse.
- It is 85% effective for nulliparous patients and 70% effective for parous patients when used correctly and consistently.
- It does not alter hormones.
- It can be inserted up to 8 hours before intercourse.
- It does not require reapplication of spermicide before repeated intercourse.
- It can remain in place longer than a diaphragm because it does not exert pressure on the vaginal walls or urethra.

The minus side

Here are the disadvantages of the cervical cap:

- It requires possible refitting after weight gain or loss of 15 lb (6.8 kg) or more, recent pregnancy, recent pelvic surgery, or cap slippage.
- It may be difficult to insert or remove.
- It may cause an allergic reaction or vaginal lacerations and thickening of the vaginal mucosa.
- It may cause a foul odor if left in place for more than 36 hours.
- It cannot be used during menstruation or during the first 6 postpartum weeks.
- It should not be left in place longer than 24 hours.
- It is contraindicated in patients with a history of toxic shock syndrome, a previously abnormal Pap test, allergy to latex or spermicide, an abnormally short or long cervix, history of PID, cervicitis, papillomavirus infection, cervical cancer, or undiagnosed vaginal bleeding.

Male condom

A male condom is a latex, synthetic sheath, or natural membrane (usually animal intestine) that is placed over the erect penis before intercourse. It prevents pregnancy by collecting spermatozoa in the tip of the condom, preventing them from entering the vagina.

The condom should be positioned so that it is loose enough at the penis tip to collect ejaculate but not so loose that it comes off the penis. The penis must be withdrawn before it becomes flaccid after ejaculation or sperm can escape from the condom into the vagina.

The plus side

Here are the advantages of the male condom:

- No health care visit is needed.
- It is available over the counter in pharmacies and grocery stores and is inexpensive.
- It is easy to carry.
- Latex and synthetic material condoms help prevent the spread of STIs.

The minus side

Here are the disadvantages of the male condom:

- It must be applied before any vulvar penile contact takes place because pre-ejaculation fluid may contain sperm.
- It is contraindicated if it contains latex in patients or partners with latex allergies.
- It needs to be stored properly and can expire, increasing the risk of failure.
- It may break during use if it is used incorrectly or is of poor quality.
- It cannot be reused.
- Natural material condoms do not offer protection from STIs due to larger pores in the material.
- Sexual pleasure may be affected.
- It may interfere with spontaneity.

Female condom

A female condom is made of latex and lubricated with nonoxynol-9. The inner ring (closed end) covers the cervix. The outer ring (open end) rests against the vaginal opening. Female condoms are intended for one-time use and should not be used in combination with male condoms. (See *Inserting a female condom.*)

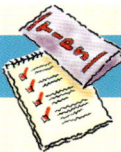

Education edge

Inserting a female condom

A female condom is made of latex and lubricated with nonoxynol-9. It has an inner ring that covers the cervix and an outer ring that rests against the vaginal opening, as shown in the image.

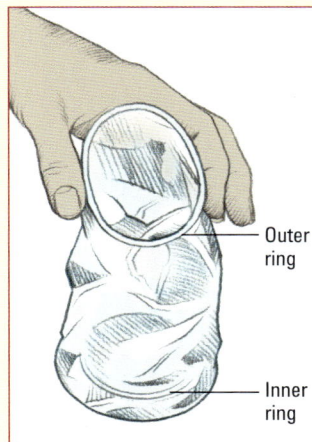

Outer ring

Inner ring

(continued)

Inserting a female condom (*continued*)

Inserting the condom

Inform the patient to take these steps when inserting the condom:

1. Fold the inner ring in half with one hand by pressing the opposite sides together, as shown in the image. When inserted, the inner ring covers the cervix.

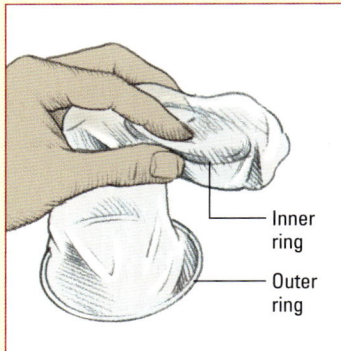

Inner ring

Outer ring

2. After the condom is inserted, the outer ring (open end) rests against the vaginal opening.

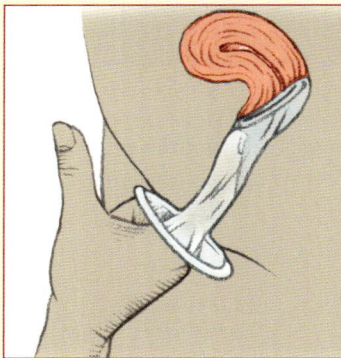

The plus side

Here are the advantages of the female condom:

- It is 95% effective.
- It helps prevent the spread of STIs.
- It can be purchased over the counter.

The minus side

Here are the disadvantages of the female condom:
- It is more expensive than the male condom.
- It is difficult to use and has not gained as much acceptance as a male condom.
- It may break or become dislodged.
- It is contraindicated in patients or partners with latex allergies.
- It may interfere with spontaneity.

Surgical methods of family planning

Surgical methods of family planning include vasectomy (for males) and tubal ligation (for females). These procedures are available to most adults (18 years of age or older) but are most commonly chosen by people over 30 years of age for those expressing a desire for child-free family planning.

Reversal reality

It is possible to reverse these procedures, but it is expensive and not always effective. Therefore, surgical sterilization should be chosen only when the patient has thoroughly discussed the options and knows that these procedures are for permanent contraception.

Vasectomy

Vasectomy is a procedure in which the pathway for spermatozoa is surgically severed. Incisions are made on each side of the scrotum, and the vas deferens is cut and tied, then plugged or cauterized. The testes continue to produce sperm as usual, but the sperm cannot pass the severed vas deferens. (See *A closer look at vasectomy.*) This procedure should be viewed as irreversible, although successful reversal is possible in 60% to 95% of cases.

The patient should be cautioned that sperm remaining in the vas deferens at the time of surgery may remain viable for as long as 6 months. An additional form of contraception should be used until two negative sperm reports have been obtained. These reports confirm that all the remaining sperm in the vas deferens has been ejaculated.

A closer look at vasectomy

In a vasectomy, the vas deferens is surgically altered to prohibit the passage of sperm. Here's how:

1. The surgeon makes two small incisions, one on each side of the scrotum.

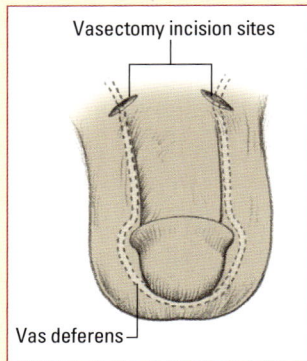

Vasectomy incision sites

Vas deferens

2. The vas deferens are cut.

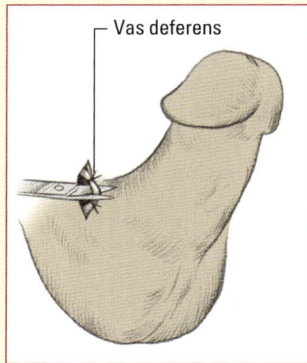

Vas deferens

3. The vas deferens is then cauterized or plugged to block the passage of sperm.

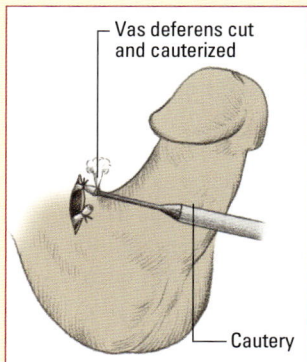

Vas deferens cut and cauterized

Cautery

The plus side

Here are the advantages of vasectomy:

- It can be done as an outpatient procedure, with little anesthesia and minimal pain.
- It is 99.99% effective.
- It does not interfere with male erection, and the male still produces seminal fluid—it just does not contain sperm.

The minus side

Here are the disadvantages of vasectomy:

- Misconceptions about the procedure may lead some patients to resist it.
- Some reports indicate that vasectomy may be associated with the development of kidney stones.
- It is contraindicated in people who aren't entirely certain of their decision to choose permanent sterilization and in those with specific surgical risks such as an anesthesia allergy.

Tubal sterilization

In tubal sterilization, a laparoscope is used to cauterize, crush, clamp, or block the fallopian tubes, thus preventing pregnancy by blocking the passage of ova and sperm. The procedure is performed after menses and before ovulation. This procedure can be performed during a caesarean section (surgical birth) or at least 4 hours (although it is more typically done within 12 to 24 hours) after the vaginal birth of a baby or after an abortion. A signed informed consent is required.

Here is how it works:

1. A small incision is made in the abdomen.
2. Carbon dioxide is pumped into the abdominal cavity to lift the abdominal wall, providing an easier view of the surgical area.
3. A lighted laparoscope is inserted, and the fallopian tubes are located.
4. An electrical current is then used to cauterize the tubes, or the tubes are clamped and cut.

After surgery, patients may notice some abdominal bloating from the carbon dioxide, but this subsides. (See *A closer look at tubal sterilization.*)

Patients should be cautioned to not have unprotected intercourse before the procedure because sperm that can become trapped in the tube could fertilize an ovum, resulting in an ectopic pregnancy.

This procedure should be viewed as irreversible. Although reversal is successful in 30% to 75% of patients, this process is difficult and could cause an ectopic pregnancy.

A closer look at tubal sterilization

In a laparoscopic tubal sterilization, the surgeon inserts a laparoscope and occludes the fallopian tube by cauterizing, crushing, clamping, or blocking. This prevents the passage of ova and sperm.

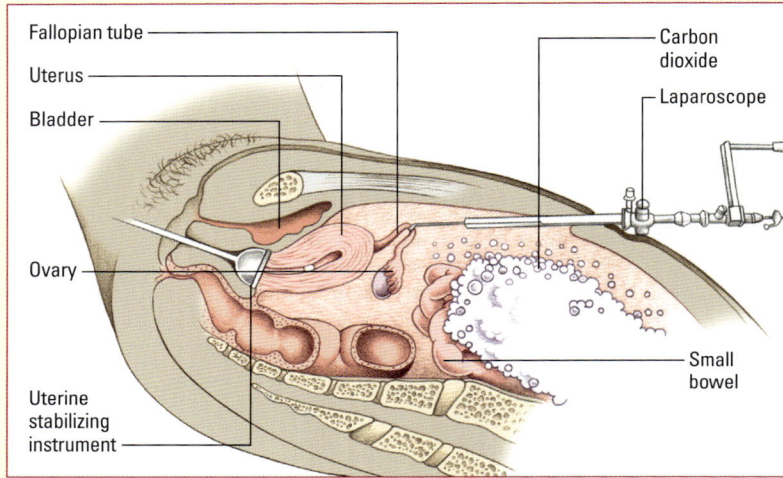

The plus side

Here are the advantages of tubal sterilization:
- It can be performed on an outpatient basis, and the patient is usually discharged within a few hours after the procedure.
- It is 99.6% effective.
- It has been associated with a decreased incidence of ovarian cancer.
- Intercourse can be resumed 2 to 3 days after having the procedure.

The minus side

Here are the disadvantages of tubal sterilization:
- Complications include a risk of bowel perforation and hemorrhage and the typical risks of general anesthesia (allergy, arrhythmia) during the procedure.
- Contraindications include umbilical hernia and obesity.
- Post-tubal ligation syndrome may occur. This includes vaginal spotting and intermittent vaginal bleeding as well as severe lower abdominal cramping.
- It is not recommended for people who are not certain of their decision to choose permanent sterilization.

Quick quiz

1. Which family planning method requires assessment of the quality of cervical mucus throughout the menstrual cycle?
- A. Rhythm method
- B. Coitus interruptus
- C. Billings method
- D. BBT

Answer: C. The Billings method requires assessment of cervical mucus, which is minimal and not stretchy until ovulation occurs. At the time of ovulation, the cervical mucus is present in greater quantity, is stretchy, and is more favorable to penetration by sperm.

2. A vasectomy is considered 100% effective after which of the following time frames?
- A. Approximately 2 weeks
- B. Approximately 4 weeks
- C. Two consecutive sperm counts show zero sperm
- D. Six consecutive sperm counts show zero sperm

Answer: C. A vasectomy is considered 100% effective after two consecutive sperm counts show zero sperm. Some sperm remain in the proximal vas deferens after vasectomy. It may take up to several months to clear the proximal ducts of sperm.

3. Which of the following patients is the best candidate for using an IUD?
- A. A patient with Wilson disease
- B. A patient with two children with no history of PID
- C. A patient with one child who has a history of severe dysmenorrhea
- D. A 35-year-old patient with recent history of PID

Answer: B. An IUD is an optimal contraceptive for a patient who has no history of PID, dysmenorrhea, or previous IUD failures.

4. A 20-year-old woman arrives at a family planning clinic seeking EC 48 hours after they had unprotected sexual intercourse. The nurse correctly responds by stating which of the following?
- A. "Come right in so we can get you started."
- B. "You must wait 72 hours before the pill will work."
- C. "You need to wait until you have missed your period."
- D. "The pills must be started the morning after intercourse."

Answer: A. The first dose of hormones must be taken within 72 hours of sexual intercourse.

Scoring

☆☆☆ If you answered all four questions correctly, super! Your conception of the material is right on target!

☆☆ If you answered three questions correctly, smile! Your planning method seems to work!

☆ If you answered fewer than three questions correctly, don't worry. Just make plans to do some extra family planning review!

Selected References

American College of Obstetricians and Gynecologists. (2019). *Sterilization by laparoscopy.* https://www.acog.org/womens-health/faqs/sterilization-by-laparoscopy

American Pregnancy Association. (2024). *How to track ovulation with irregular periods.* https://americanpregnancy.org/getting-pregnant/track-ovulation-irregular-periods/

Bayer. (2023). *Mirena.* www.mirenahcp.com

Centers for Disease Control and Prevention. (2024a). *Combined hormonal contraceptives.* https://www.cdc.gov/contraception/hcp/usspr/combined-hormonal-contraceptives.html

Centers for Disease Control and Prevention. (2024b). *Progestin-only pills.* https://www.cdc.gov/contraception/hcp/usspr/progestin-only-pills.html

Healthline. (2022). *Yes, you can order birth control online—These are the 8 services we trust.* https://www.healthline.com/health/birth-control-pills

Mayo Clinic. (2022). *Birth control.* https://www.mayoclinic.org/healthy-lifestyle/birth-control/in-depth/best-birth-control-pill/art-20044807

Mayo Clinic. (2023). *Infertility.* https://www.mayoclinic.org/diseases-conditions/infertility/diagnosis-treatment/drc-20354322

Organon. (2024). *How Nexplanon works.* https://www.nexplanon.com/how-does-nexplanon-work/

Chapter 4

Physiologic and psychosocial adaptations to pregnancy

Just the facts

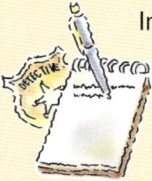

In this chapter, you'll learn:

♦ presumptive, probable, and positive signs of pregnancy
♦ ways in which the major body systems are affected by pregnancy
♦ methods of promoting acceptance of pregnancy
♦ psychosocial changes that occur during each trimester.

A look at pregnancy changes

During pregnancy, a patient undergoes many physiologic and psychosocial changes. Their body adapts in response to the demands of the growing fetus while their mind prepares for the responsibilities that come with being a caregiver. Physiologic changes occur throughout pregnancy as the fetus grows and develops. Psychosocial changes will vary from trimester to trimester.

Physiologic signs of pregnancy

Pregnancy produces several types of physiologic changes that must be evaluated before a definitive diagnosis of pregnancy is made. The changes can be:
- presumptive (subjective: what the pregnant patient feels)
- probable (objective: what the health care provider sees)
- positive: proof of pregnancy.

Neither presumptive nor probable signs confirm pregnancy because both can be caused by other medical conditions; they simply suggest pregnancy, especially when several are present at the same time. (See *Making sense out of pregnancy signs.*)

Making sense out of pregnancy signs

This chart classifies the signs of pregnancy into three categories: presumptive, probable, and positive.

Sign	Weeks from implantation	Other possible causes
Presumptive		
Breast changes, including feelings of tenderness, fullness, or tingling, and enlargement or darkening of areola	2	• Hormonal contraceptives • Hyperprolactinemia induced by tranquilizers • Infection • Prolactin-secreting pituitary tumor • Pseudocyesis • Premenstrual syndrome
Feeling of nausea or vomiting upon arising	2	• Gastric disorders • Infections • Psychological disorders, such as pseudocyesis and anorexia nervosa
Amenorrhea	2	• Anovulation • Blocked endometrial cavity • Endocrine changes • Illness • Medications (phenothiazines, medroxyprogesterone acetate [Depo-Provera]) • Metabolic changes • Stress
Frequent urination	3	• Emotional stress • Pelvic tumor • Kidney disease • Urinary tract infection (UTI)
Fatigue	12	• Anemia • Chronic illness • Depression • Stress
Uterine enlargement in which the uterus can be palpated over the symphysis pubis	12	• Ascites • Obesity • Uterine or pelvic tumor
Quickening (fetal movement felt by the patient)	18	• Excessive flatus • Increased peristalsis
Linea nigra (line of dark pigment on the abdomen)	24	• Cardiopulmonary disorders • Estrogen–progestin hormonal contraceptives • Obesity • Pelvic tumor
Melasma (dark pigment on the face)	24	• Cardiopulmonary disorders • Estrogen–progestin hormonal contraceptives • Obesity • Pelvic tumor

Making sense out of pregnancy signs (*continued*)

Sign	Weeks from implantation	Other possible causes
Striae gravidarum (red streaks on the abdomen)	24	• Cardiopulmonary disorders • Estrogen–progestin hormonal contraceptives • Obesity • Pelvic tumor
Probable		
Serum laboratory tests revealing the presence of human chorionic gonadotropin (hCG) hormone	1	• Cross-reaction of luteinizing hormone (similar to hCG) • Hydatidiform mole
Chadwick sign (vagina changes color from pink to violet)	6	• Hyperemia of cervix, vagina, or vulva
Goodell sign (cervix softens)	6	• Estrogen–progestin hormonal contraceptives
Hegar sign (lower uterine segment softens)	6	• Excessively soft uterine walls
Sonographic evidence of gestational sac in which characteristic ring is evident	6	None
Ballottement (Fetus can be felt to rise against abdominal wall when lower uterine segment is tapped on during bimanual examination.)	16	• Ascites • Uterine tumor or polyps
Braxton Hicks contractions (periodic uterine tightening)	20	• Gastrointestinal (GI) distress • Hematometra • Uterine tumor
Palpation of fetal outline through abdomen	20	• Subserous uterine myoma
Positive		
Sonographic evidence of fetal outline	8	None
Fetal heart audible by Doppler ultrasound	10–12	None
Palpation of fetal movement through abdomen	20	None

Presumptive signs of pregnancy

Presumptive signs of pregnancy are those that suggest pregnancy until more concrete signs develop. These are signs felt by and noticed by the patient. These signs include breast changes, nausea and vomiting, amenorrhea, urinary frequency, fatigue, uterine enlargement, quickening, and skin changes. A pregnant patient typically reports some presumptive signs.

Breast changes

Tingling, tender, or swollen breasts can occur as early as a few days after conception. The areola may darken and tiny glands around the nipple, called *Montgomery tubercles*, may become elevated.

Nausea and vomiting

At least 50% of pregnant patients experience nausea and vomiting early in pregnancy (commonly called *morning sickness*). Although it is called morning sickness, and most patients experience symptoms upon waking, the nausea and vomiting can last all day. These symptoms are typically the first sensations experienced during pregnancy. Nausea and vomiting usually begin at 4 to 6 weeks' gestation. These symptoms usually stop at the end of the first trimester, but they may last slightly longer in some patients. Some patients may have nausea and vomiting throughout the entire pregnancy.

Amenorrhea

Amenorrhea is the cessation of menses. For a patient who has regular menses, this may be the first indication of pregnancy.

Urinary frequency

A pregnant patient may notice an increase in urinary frequency during the first 3 months of pregnancy. This symptom continues until the uterus rises out of the pelvis and relieves pressure on the bladder.

When lightening strikes

Urinary frequency may return at the end of pregnancy as lightening occurs (the fetal head exerts renewed pressure on the bladder due to the fetus moving farther down into the pelvis to prepare for labor).

Fatigue

A pregnant patient may report feeling fatigued. During the first trimester, the body works hard to adjust to the physical demands of pregnancy while the pregnant patient mentally and emotionally prepares for parenthood. Around 16 weeks' gestation, the body has adjusted to the pregnancy, the placenta's development is complete, and the patient should start to have more energy. The second trimester of pregnancy is often referred to as the *honeymoon phase*. Energy is renewed, and most patients have relief from nausea and vomiting. Once the third trimester comes, the patient becomes more fatigued due to the increasing size of the baby.

Uterine enlargement

Softening of the uterus and fetal growth cause the uterus to enlarge and stretch the abdominal wall.

Quickening

Quickening is recognizable movements of the fetus. It can occur anywhere between the 14th and 26th weeks of pregnancy but typically is noticed between weeks 18 and 22. Patients who have been pregnant before usually notice it before those experiencing their first pregnancy. Quickening may feel like fluttering movements in the patient's lower abdomen.

Skin changes

Numerous skin changes occur during pregnancy, including those listed here:
- *Linea nigra* refers to a dark line that extends from the umbilicus or above to the mons pubis. In the primigravida patient, this line develops at approximately the third month of pregnancy. In the multigravida patient, linea nigra typically appears before the third month. (See *Skin changes during pregnancy*.)

Skin changes during pregnancy

Linea nigra and melasma are two skin changes that occur during pregnancy. Both fade after pregnancy, with striae gravidarum fading to glistening silvery lines.

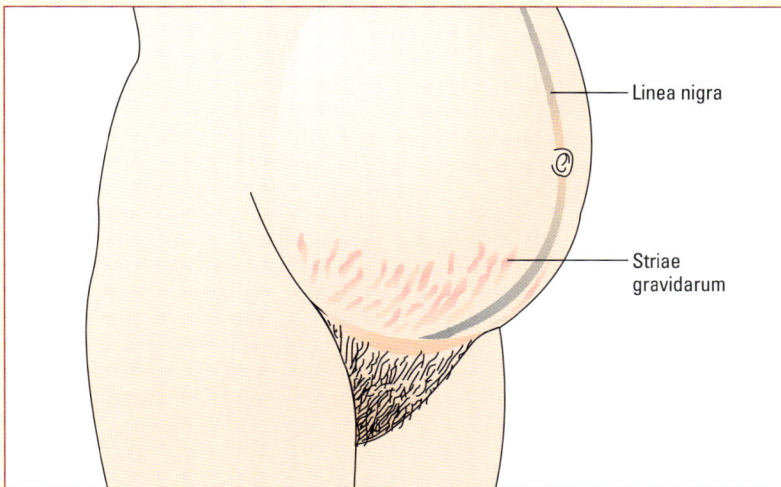

- *Melasma*, also known as *chloasma* or the "mask of pregnancy," are darkened areas that may appear on the face, especially on the cheeks and across the nose. Melasma appears after the 16th week of pregnancy and gradually becomes more pronounced. After childbirth, it typically fades.
- *Striae gravidarum* are red or pinkish streaks that appear on the sides of the abdominal wall and sometimes on the thighs.

Probable signs of pregnancy

Probable signs of pregnancy strongly suggest pregnancy. They are more reliable indicators of pregnancy than presumptive signs, but they can also be explained by other medical conditions. Probable signs include positive laboratory tests, such as serum and urine tests, positive results on a home pregnancy test, Chadwick sign, Goodell sign, Hegar sign, sonographic evidence of a gestational sac, ballottement, and Braxton Hicks contractions.

Laboratory tests

Laboratory tests for pregnancy are used to detect the presence of hCG—a hormone created by the chorionic villi of the placenta—in the urine or blood serum. Because hCG is produced by trophoblast cells—preplacental cells that would not be present in a nonpregnant person—detection of hCG is considered a sign of pregnancy.

Looking for hCG in all the right places

Tests for hCG include radioimmunoassay, enzyme-linked immunosorbent assay, and radioreceptor assay. For these tests, hCG is measured in milli-international units (mIU). Trace amounts of hCG appear in the serum as early as 24 to 48 hours after implantation of the fertilized ovum. They reach a measurable level of about 50 mIU/mL between 7 and 9 days after conception. Levels peak at about 100 mIU/mL between the 60th and 80th days of gestation. After this point, the level declines. At term, hCG is barely detectable in serum or urine. An at-home pregnancy test tests for hCG in the urine. This will either show up as a negative or positive result. Quantitative hCG is done by serum and gives a specific number that correlates with how far along the pregnancy is. In a normal pregnancy, this number will double every 48 hours.

Home pregnancy tests

Home pregnancy tests, which are available over the counter, are 97% accurate when performed correctly. They are convenient and easy to use, taking only 3 to 5 minutes to perform.

Dip stick

Here is how the home pregnancy test works:
- A reagent strip is dipped into the urine stream.
- A color change on the strip denotes pregnancy.
  Most manufacturers suggest to wait until the day of the missed menstrual period to test for pregnancy.

Chadwick sign

Chadwick sign is a bluish coloration of the mucous membranes of the cervix, vagina, and vulva. It can be observed at 6 to 8 weeks' gestation by speculum examination.

Goodell sign

Goodell sign is a softening of the cervix that occurs at 6 to 8 weeks' gestation. The cervix of a nonpregnant person typically has the same consistency as the tip of the nose. The cervix of a pregnant person feels more like an earlobe. This is felt during a bimanual examination.

Hegar sign

Hegar sign is a softening of the uterine isthmus that can be felt on bimanual examination at 6 to 8 weeks' gestation. As pregnancy advances, the isthmus becomes part of the lower uterine segment. During labor, it expands further.

Ultrasonography

Ultrasonography, or sonographic evaluation, can detect probable and positive signs of pregnancy. At 4 to 6 weeks' gestation, a characteristic ring indicating the gestational sac is visible on sonographic evaluation, making this a probable rather than a positive sign of pregnancy.

Ballottement

Ballottement is passive movement of the fetus. It can be identified at 16 to 18 weeks' gestation.

Braxton Hicks contractions

Braxton Hicks contractions are uterine contractions that begin early in pregnancy and become more frequent after 28 weeks' gestation. Typically, they result from normal uterine enlargement that occurs to accommodate the growing fetus. Sometimes, however, they may be caused by a uterine tumor.

Positive signs of pregnancy

Positive signs of pregnancy include sonographic evidence of the fetal outline, an audible fetal heart rate, and fetal movement felt by the examiner. These signs confirm pregnancy because they cannot be attributed to other conditions.

Ultrasonography

Ultrasonography can confirm pregnancy by providing an image of the fetal outline, which can typically be seen by the eighth week. The fetal outline on the ultrasound is so clear that a crown to rump measurement can be made to establish gestational age. Fetal heart movement may be visualized as early as 6.5 to 7 weeks' gestation.

Audible fetal heart rate

Fetal heart rate can be confirmed by auscultation or visualization during an ultrasound. Fetal heart sounds may be heard as early as the 10th to 12th week by Doppler ultrasonography.

Fetal movement

Even though the pregnant patients can feel fetal movement at a much earlier date (usually around 16 to 20 weeks), other people are not able to feel fetal movement until the 20th to 24th week. Patients with obesity may not feel fetal movement until later in pregnancy because of excess adipose tissue.

Physiologic changes in body systems

As the fetus grows and hormones shift during pregnancy, physiologic adaptations occur in every body system to accommodate the fetus. These changes help the patient maintain health throughout the pregnancy and physically prepare for childbirth. Physiologic changes also create a safe and nurturing environment for the fetus. Some of these changes take place even before the patient knows that they are pregnant.

Reproductive system

In addition to the physical changes that initially indicate pregnancy, such as Hegar sign and Goodell sign, the reproductive system undergoes significant changes throughout pregnancy.

Out and about

External reproductive structures affected by pregnancy include the labia majora, labia minora, clitoris, and vaginal introitus. These structures enlarge because of increased vascularity. Fat deposits also contribute to the enlargement of the labia majora and labia minora. These structures reduce in size after childbirth but may not return to their prepregnant state because of loss of muscle tone or perineal injury (such as from an episiotomy or a vaginal tear). Varices may be caused by pressure on vessels in the perineal and perianal areas.

The inside story

Internal reproductive structures, including the ovaries, uterus, and other structures, change dramatically to accommodate the developing fetus. These internal structures may not regain their prepregnant states after childbirth.

Ovaries

When fertilization occurs, ovarian follicles cease to mature, and ovulation stops. The chorionic villi, which develop from the fertilized ovum, begin to produce hCG to maintain the ovarian corpus luteum. The corpus luteum produces estrogen and progesterone until the placenta is formed and functioning. At 8 to 10 weeks' gestation, the placenta assumes production of these hormones. The corpus luteum, which is no longer needed, then involutes (becomes smaller due to a reduction in cell size).

Uterus

In a nonpregnant person, the uterus is smaller than the size of a fist, measuring approximately 3 in $\times$ 2 in $\times$ 1 in (7.5 cm $\times$ 5 cm $\times$ 2.5 cm). It can weigh 2 to 2½ oz (60 to 70 g) in a nulliparous patient (a patient who has never been pregnant) and 3½ oz (100 g) in a parous patient (a patient who has given birth). In a nonpregnant state, the uterus can hold up to 10 mL of fluid. Its walls are composed of several overlapping layers of muscle fibers that adapt to the developing fetus and help in expulsion of the fetus and placenta during labor and childbirth.

More strength, more stretch

After conception, the uterus retains the developing fetus for approximately 280 days or 9 calendar months. During this time, the uterus undergoes progressive changes in size, shape, and position in the abdominal cavity. In the first trimester, the pear-shaped uterus lengthens and enlarges in response to elevated levels of estrogen and progesterone. This hormonal stimulation primarily increases the size of myometrial cells (hypertrophy), although a small increase in cell number (hyperplasia) also occurs. These changes increase the amount of fibrous and elastic tissue to more than 20 times that of the nonpregnant uterus. Uterine walls become stronger and more elastic.

During the first few weeks of pregnancy, the uterine walls remain thick and the fundus rests low in the abdomen. The uterus cannot be palpated through the abdominal wall. After 12 weeks of pregnancy, however, the uterus typically reaches the level of the symphysis pubis (the joint at the pubic bone) and then may be palpated through the abdominal wall.

Shape shifters

In the second trimester, the corpus and fundus become globe shaped. As pregnancy progresses, the uterus lengthens and becomes oval in shape. The uterine walls thin as the muscles stretch. The uterus rises out of the pelvis, shifts to the right, and rests against the anterior abdominal wall. At 20 weeks' gestation, the uterus is palpable just below the umbilicus and reaches the umbilicus at 22 weeks' gestation. As uterine muscles stretch, Braxton Hicks contractions may occur, helping to move blood more quickly through the intervillous spaces of the placenta.

Reach and descend

In the third trimester, the fundus reaches nearly to the xiphoid process (the lower tip of the breast bone). Between weeks 38 and 40, the fetus begins to descend into the pelvis (lightening), which causes fundal height to gradually drop. The uterus remains oval. Its muscular walls become progressively thinner as it enlarges, finally reaching a muscle wall thickness of ¼ in (5 mm) or less. At term (40 weeks), the uterus typically weighs approximately 2 lb (1,100 g), holds 5 to 10 L of fluid, and has stretched to approximately 11 in × 9½ in × 8¼ in (28 cm × 24 cm × 21 cm). (See *Fundal height throughout pregnancy*.)

Fundal height throughout pregnancy

This illustration shows approximate fundal heights at various times during pregnancy. Note that between weeks 38 and 40, the fetus begins to descend into the pelvis.

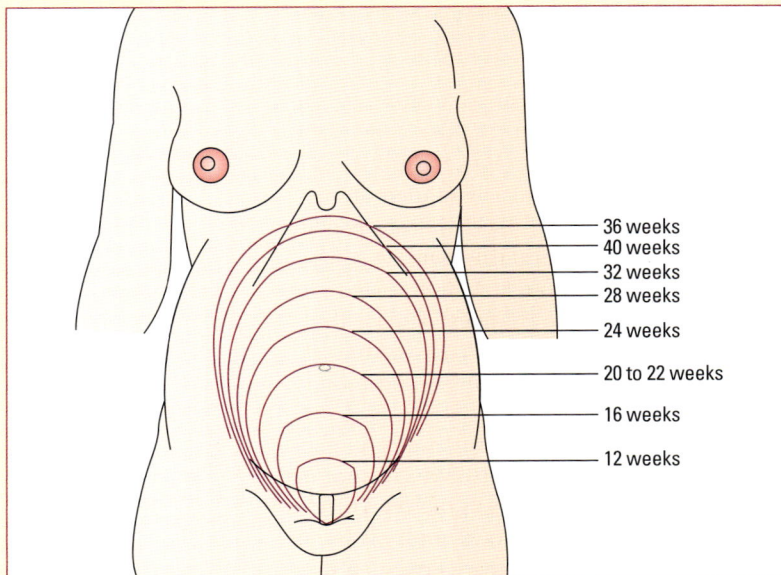

- 36 weeks
- 40 weeks
- 32 weeks
- 28 weeks
- 24 weeks
- 20 to 22 weeks
- 16 weeks
- 12 weeks

Endometrial development

During the menstrual cycle, progesterone stimulates increased thickening and vascularity of the endometrium, preparing the uterine lining for implantation and nourishment of a fertilized ovum. After implantation, menstruation stops.

The endometrium then becomes the decidua, which is divided into three layers:

1. Decidua capsularis, which covers the blastocyst (fertilized ovum)
2. Decidua basalis, which lies directly under the blastocyst and forms part of the placenta
3. Decidua vera, which lines the rest of the uterus

Vascular growth

As the fetus grows and the placenta develops, uterine blood vessels and lymphatics increase in number and size. Vessels must enlarge to accommodate the increased blood flow to the uterus and placenta. By the end of pregnancy, an average of 500 mL of blood may flow through the maternal side of the placenta each minute. Maternal arterial pressure, uterine contractions, and maternal position affect uterine blood flow throughout pregnancy.

Because one sixth of the body's blood supply is circulating through the uterus at any given time, uterine bleeding during pregnancy is always potentially serious and can result in major blood loss. (See *Uterine bleeding*.)

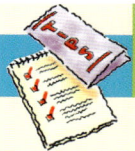

Education edge

Uterine bleeding

Uterine bleeding in a pregnant patient is potentially serious because it can result in major blood loss. A pregnant patient should be warned that such blood loss poses a major health risk. The pregnant patient should be advised to contact their health care provider if uterine bleeding occurs. Blood loss in the pregnant patient means blood loss in the fetus. This can result in altered development or even death of the fetus. Heavy vaginal bleeding in a pregnant patient is an emergency!

Cervical changes

The cervix consists of connective tissue, elastic fibers, and endocervical folds. This composition allows it to stretch during childbirth. During pregnancy, the cervix softens. It also takes on a bluish color during the second month due to increased vasculature. It becomes edematous and may bleed easily on examination or sexual activity.

Bacteria blocker

During pregnancy, hormonal stimulation causes the glandular cervical tissue to increase in cell number and become hyperactive, secreting thick, tenacious mucus. This mucus thickens into a mucoid weblike structure, eventually forming the mucus plug that blocks the cervical canal. This creates a protective barrier against bacteria and other substances attempting to enter the uterus. Patients may "lose" their mucus plug a few weeks before going into labor. This does not mean labor is imminent. Losing of the mucus plug is just one of the ways the body prepares for labor.

Vagina

During pregnancy, estrogen stimulates vascularity, tissue growth, and hypertrophy in the vaginal epithelial tissue. White, thick, odorless, and acidic vaginal secretions increase. This normal, harmless discharge is called *leukorrhea*. The acidity of these secretions helps prevent bacterial infections but, unfortunately, also fosters yeast infections, a common occurrence during pregnancy. (See *Fighting* Candida *infection*.)

Advice from the experts

Fighting *Candida* infection

Changes in the pH of vaginal secretions during pregnancy favor the growth of *Candida albicans*, a species of yeastlike fungi.

Medication is prescribed to treat and prevent transmission of *Candida* infection if it is properly diagnosed beforehand. To keep on top of possible infections, the patient should be asked if they have experienced signs and symptoms such as itching, burning, and a cottage cheese–like discharge.

Other vaginal changes include:
- development of a bluish color due to increased vascularity
- hypertrophy of the smooth muscles and relaxation of connective tissues, which allow the vagina to stretch during childbirth
- lengthening of the vaginal vault
- possible heightened sexual sensitivity.

Breasts

In addition to the presumptive signs that occur in the breasts during pregnancy (such as tenderness, tingling, darkening of the areola, and appearance of Montgomery tubercles), the nipples enlarge, become more erectile, and darken in color. The areolae widen from a diameter of less than 1½ in (3 cm) to 2 in or 3 in (5 cm or 6 cm) in the primigravida patient.

Lactation preparation

The breasts also undergo several changes in preparation for lactation. As blood vessels enlarge, veins beneath the skin of the breasts become more visible and may appear as intertwining patterns over the anterior chest wall. The breasts increase in size and weight, and there is a proliferation of ductular sprouting, branching and lobular formation, which forms the glandular system under the influence of human placental lactogen (hPL), estrogen, and progesterone.

Increasing hormone levels cause the secretion of colostrum (a yellowish, viscous fluid) from the nipples. High in protein, antibodies, and minerals—but low in fat and sugar relative to mature human milk—colostrum may be secreted as early as week 16 of pregnancy (lactogenesis stage 1), but it is most common during the last trimester. It continues secreting until 2 to 4 days after delivery and is followed by lactogenesis stage 2, which is triggered by the rapid drop in patient's progesterone levels causing the onset of copious secretion of the milk. (See *Comparing the nonpregnant and pregnant breast.*)

Comparing the nonpregnant and pregnant breast

Dramatic changes appear in the breasts of a pregnant patient because of increased estrogen and progestin production.

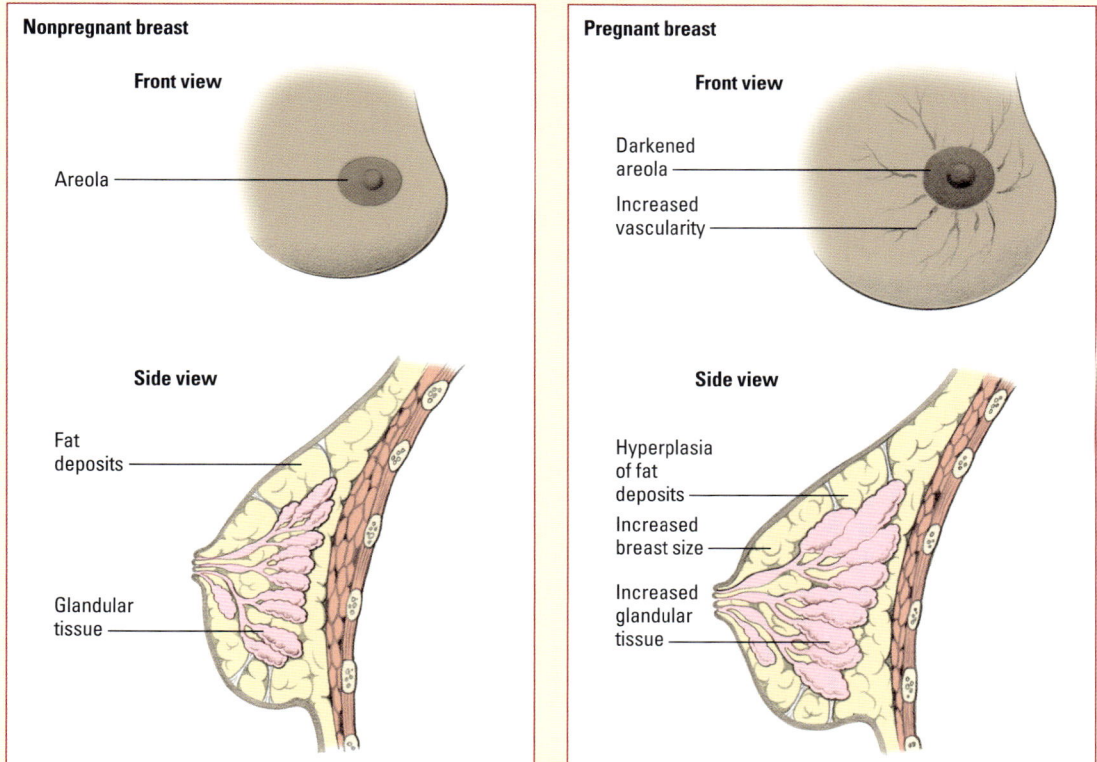

Nonpregnant breast

Front view

Areola

Side view

Fat deposits

Glandular tissue

Pregnant breast

Front view

Darkened areola

Increased vascularity

Side view

Hyperplasia of fat deposits

Increased breast size

Increased glandular tissue

Endocrine system

The endocrine system undergoes many fluctuations during pregnancy. Changes in hormone levels and protein production help support fetal growth and maintain body functions.

Placenta

The most striking change in the endocrine system during pregnancy is the addition of the placenta. The placenta is a finite, endocrine organ that produces large amounts of estrogen, progesterone, hCG, hPL, relaxin, and prostaglandins.

The estrogen produced by the placenta causes breast and uterine enlargement as well as palmar erythema (redness in the palm of the hand). Progesterone helps maintain the endometrium by inhibiting uterine contractility. It also prepares the breasts for lactation by stimulating breast tissue development.

Maxin' and relaxin

Relaxin is secreted primarily by the corpus luteum to help inhibit uterine activity. It also helps to soften the cervix, which allows for dilation at delivery, and soften the collagen in body joints, which allows for laxness in the lower spine and helps enlarge the birth canal.

How stimulating!

hCG is secreted by the placenta's trophoblast cells in early pregnancy. It stimulates progesterone and estrogen synthesis until the placenta assumes this role.

Alternate energy source

The hormone hPL is secreted by the placenta. It promotes fat breakdown (lipolysis), providing the patient with an alternate source of energy so that glucose is available for fetal growth. hPL inhibits the action of insulin and as a result, increasing insulin resistance during pregnancy can occur.

Prostaglandins

Prostaglandins are found in high concentration in the reproductive tract and the decidua during pregnancy. They affect smooth muscle contractility to such an extent that they may trigger labor at the pregnancy's term.

Pituitary gland

The pituitary gland undergoes various changes during pregnancy. High estrogen and progesterone levels in the placenta stop the pituitary gland from producing follicle-stimulating hormone and luteinizing hormone. Increased production of growth hormone and melanocyte-stimulating hormone causes skin pigment changes.

Late-breaking developments

Late in pregnancy, the posterior pituitary gland begins to produce oxytocin, which stimulates uterine contractions during labor. Prolactin production also starts late in pregnancy as the breasts prepare for lactation after birth.

Thyroid gland

As early as the second month of pregnancy, the thyroid gland's production of thyroxine (T_4)-binding protein increases, causing total T_4 levels to rise. Because the amount of unbound T_4 does not increase, these thyroid changes do not cause hyperthyroidism. However, they increase basal metabolic rate (BMR), cardiac output, pulse rate, vasodilation, and heat intolerance. BMR increases by about 20% during the second and third trimesters as the growing fetus places additional demands for energy on the pregnant patient's system. By term, the patient's BMR may increase by 25%. It returns to the prepregnant level within 1 week after childbirth.

In addition to T_4 level changes, increased estrogen levels augment the circulating amounts of triiodothyronine (T_3). Like the elevation of T_4, the elevation of T_3 levels does not lead to a hyperthyroid condition during pregnancy because much of this hormone is bound to proteins and is therefore nonfunctional.

Parathyroid gland

As pregnancy progresses, fetal demands for calcium and phosphorus increase. The parathyroid gland responds by increasing hormone production during the third trimester to as much as twice the prepregnancy level.

Adrenal gland

Adrenal gland activity increases during pregnancy as production of corticosteroids and aldosterone escalates.

Corticosteroids deployed

Some researchers believe that increased corticosteroid levels suppress inflammatory reactions and help reduce the possibility of the patient's body rejecting the foreign protein of the fetus. Corticosteroids also help to regulate glucose metabolism in the pregnant patient.

Aldosterone zone

Increased aldosterone levels help to promote sodium reabsorption and maintain the osmolarity of retained fluid, indirectly helping to safeguard the blood volume and provide adequate perfusion pressure across the placenta.

Pancreas

Although the pancreas itself does not change during pregnancy, maternal insulin, glucose, and glucagon production do. In response to the additional glucocorticoids produced by the adrenal glands, the pancreas increases insulin production. Insulin is less effective than normal, however, because estrogen, progesterone, and hPL all act as insulin antagonists. Despite insulin's diminished action and increased fetal demands for glucose, the pregnant patient's glucose levels remain fairly stable because their fat stores are used for energy. However, these changes can lead to gestational diabetes, which is why it is recommended that all pregnant patients be screened for gestational diabetes at 24 weeks' gestation (or after).

Respiratory system

Throughout pregnancy, changes occur in the respiratory system in response to hormonal changes. These changes can be anatomic (biochemical) or functional (mechanical) and help promote gas exchange, providing the patient with more oxygen.

Anatomic changes

The diaphragm rises by approximately 1 3/8 in (4 cm) during pregnancy, which prevents the lungs from normally expanding inspiration. The diaphragm compensates for this by increasing its excursion (outward expansion) ability, allowing more normal lung expansion. In addition, the anteroposterior and transverse diameters of the rib cage increase by approximately 3/4 in (2 cm), and the circumference increases by 2 to 2¾ in (5 to 7 cm). This expansion is possible because increased progesterone relaxes the ligaments that join the rib cage. As the uterus enlarges, thoracic breathing replaces abdominal breathing.

All that vascularization

Increased estrogen production leads to increased vascularization of the upper respiratory tract. As a result, the patient may develop respiratory congestion, voice changes, and epistaxis as capillaries become engorged in the nose, pharynx, larynx, trachea, bronchi, and vocal cords. Increased vascularization may also cause the eustachian tubes to swell, leading to problems such as impaired hearing, earaches, and a sense of fullness in the ears. This increased stuffiness in the nose, pharynx, and larynx—combined with the pressure the enlarged uterus places on the patient's diaphragm—may make the patient feel as if they are short of breath.

Functional changes

Changes in pulmonary function improve gas exchange in the alveoli and facilitate oxygenation of blood flowing through the lungs. Respiratory rate typically remains unaffected in early pregnancy. By the third trimester, however, increased progesterone may increase the rate by approximately 2 breaths/min.

Rising tide

Tidal volume (the amount of air inhaled and exhaled) rises throughout pregnancy because of increased progesterone and increased diaphragmatic excursion. In fact, a pregnant patient breathes 30% to 40% more air during pregnancy. Minute volume (the amount of air expired per minute) increases by approximately 50% by term.

The difference between changes in tidal volume and minute volume creates a slight hyperventilation, which decreases carbon dioxide in the alveoli. The resulting lowered partial pressure of arterial carbon dioxide in maternal blood leads to a greater partial pressure difference of carbon dioxide between fetal and maternal blood, which facilitates diffusion of carbon dioxide from the fetus.

Hyperprotective

An elevated diaphragm decreases functional residual capacity (the volume of air remaining in the lungs after exhalation), which contributes to hyperventilation. Hyperventilation in the pregnant patient is considered a protective measure that prevents the fetus from being exposed to excessive levels of carbon dioxide. Vital capacity (the largest volume of air that can be expelled voluntarily after maximum inspiration) increases slightly during pregnancy. These changes, along with increased cardiac output and blood volume, provide adequate blood flow to the placenta.

Assorted aberrations

During the third month of pregnancy, increased progesterone sensitizes respiratory receptors and increases ventilation, leading to a drop in carbon dioxide levels. This increases pH, potentially causing mild respiratory alkalosis. However, the decreased level of bicarbonate present in a pregnant patient partially or completely compensates for this increase in pH.

Cardiovascular system

Pregnancy alters the cardiovascular system so profoundly that its changes would be considered pathologic, and even life threatening, in a person who is not pregnant. However, during pregnancy, these changes are vital.

Anatomic changes

The heart enlarges slightly during pregnancy, likely because of increased blood volume and cardiac output, and reverses after childbirth. As pregnancy advances, the uterus moves up and presses on the diaphragm, displacing the heart upward and rotating it on its long axis. The amount of displacement varies depending on the position and size of the uterus, the firmness of the abdominal muscles, the shape of the abdomen, and other factors.

Auscultatory changes

Heart sounds alter during pregnancy because of changes in blood volume, cardiac output, and the size and position of the heart.

S_1 tends to exhibit a pronounced splitting, and each component tends to be louder. An occasional S_3 sound may occur after 20 weeks' gestation. Many pregnant patients exhibit a systolic ejection murmur over the pulmonic area. This is considered a physiologic murmur that does not need treatment and will resolve after the baby is delivered.

Break in rhythm

Cardiac rhythm disturbances, such as sinus arrhythmia, premature atrial contractions, and premature ventricular contractions, may occur. In pregnant patients with no underlying heart disease, these arrhythmias do not require therapy and do not indicate the development of cardiac disease.

Hemodynamic changes

Hemodynamically, pregnancy affects heart rate and cardiac output, venous and arterial blood pressures, circulation and coagulation, and blood volume.

Heart rate and cardiac output

During the second trimester, heart rate gradually increases. It may reach 10 to 15 beats/min above the patient's prepregnancy heart rate. During the third trimester, heart rate may increase by 15 to 20 beats/min above the patient's prepregnancy heart rate. The patient may feel palpitations occasionally throughout pregnancy.

All about output

Increased tissue demands for oxygen and increased stroke volume raise cardiac output by up to 50% by the 32nd week of pregnancy. The increase is highest when the patient is lying on their side and lowest when they are lying on their back. The side-lying position reduces pressure on the great vessels, which increases venous return to the heart. Cardiac output peaks during labor, when tissue demands are greatest.

Venous and arterial blood pressure

When the patient is supine, femoral venous pressure increases threefold from early pregnancy to term because the uterus exerts pressure on the inferior vena cava and pelvic veins, slowing venous return from the legs and feet. The patient may feel lightheaded if they rise abruptly after lying flat—which may lead them to become faint or pass out. Edema in the legs and varicosities in the legs, rectum, and vulva may occur.

Progesterone to smooth muscles: relax!

Early in pregnancy, increased progesterone levels relax smooth muscles and dilate arterioles, resulting in vasodilation. Despite the hypervolemia that occurs during pregnancy, the blood pressure does not normally rise because the increased action of the heart enables the body to handle the increased amount of circulating blood. In most patients, blood pressure decreases slightly during the second trimester because of lowered peripheral resistance to circulation that occurs as the placenta rapidly expands. The pregnant patient's blood pressure is at its lowest during the second half of the second trimester, and it gradually returns to first trimester levels during the third trimester. By term, arterial blood pressure approaches prepregnancy levels.

Position, position, position

Brachial artery pressure is lowest when the pregnant patient lies on their left side because this relieves uterine pressure on the vena cava. Brachial artery pressure is highest when the patient lies on their back (supine). The weight of the growing uterus presses the vena cava against the vertebrae, obstructing blood flow from the lower extremities. This results in a decrease in blood return to the heart and, consequently, immediate decreased cardiac output and hypotension. (See *A look at supine hypotension*.)

A look at supine hypotension

When a pregnant person lies on their back, the weight of the uterus presses on the vena cava and aorta, as shown in the image (left). This obstructs blood flow to and from the legs, resulting in supine hypotension. In a side-lying position, shown in the image (right), pressure on the vessels is relieved, allowing blood to flow freely.

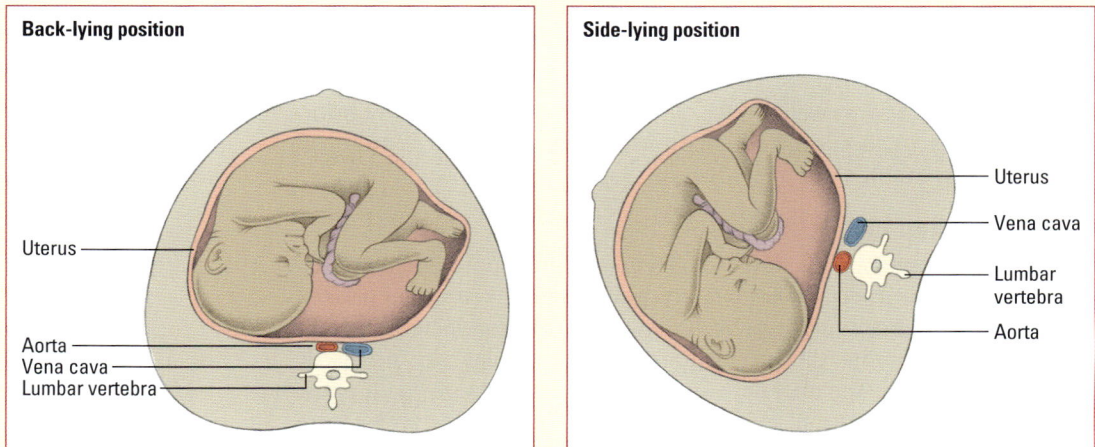

Back-lying position

Uterus
Aorta
Vena cava
Lumbar vertebra

Side-lying position

Uterus
Vena cava
Lumbar vertebra
Aorta

Circulation and coagulation

Venous return decreases slightly during the eighth month of pregnancy and, at term, increases to normal levels. Blood can clot more easily during pregnancy and the postpartum period because of increased levels of clotting factors VII, IX, and X. Pregnant patients and those in the immediate postpartum period are at a high risk for blood clots, even if they have no other risk factors.

Blood volume

Total intravascular volume increases beginning between 10 and 12 weeks' gestation and peaks with an increase of approximately 40% between weeks 32 and 34. This increase can total 5,250 mL in a pregnant patient compared with 4,000 mL in a nonpregnant patient. Volume decreases slightly in the 40th week and returns to normal several weeks after delivery.

The ABCs of red blood cells

Increased blood volume, which consists of two-thirds plasma and one-third red blood cells (RBCs), performs several functions:
- It supplies the hypertrophied vascular system of the enlarging uterus.
- It provides nutrition for fetal and maternal tissues.
- It serves as a reserve for blood loss during childbirth and puerperium.

As the plasma volume first increases, the concentration of hemoglobin and erythrocytes may decline, leading to physiologic anemia or pseudoanemia. The body compensates for this change by producing more RBCs. The body can create nearly normal levels of RBCs by the second trimester.

Hematologic changes

Hematologic changes occur during pregnancy, such as iron demands and absorption, as well as RBC, white blood cell (WBC), and fibrinogen levels. In addition, bone marrow becomes more active, producing an excess of RBCs of up to 30%.

Ironing out deficiencies

During pregnancy, the developing fetus requires approximately 350 to 400 mg of iron per day for healthy growth, and the pregnant patient's iron requirement increases by 400 mg/day. This iron increase is necessary to promote RBC production and accommodate the increased blood volume. The total daily iron requirements of a pregnant patient and their fetus amount to roughly 800 mg. Because the average store of iron is only about 500 mg for pregnant patients, they should take iron supplements.

Iron supplements may also be necessary to accommodate for impaired iron absorption, potentially caused by decreased gastric acidity (iron is absorbed best from an acid medium). In addition, increased plasma volume (from 2,600 mL in a nonpregnant person to 3,600 mL in a pregnant person) is disproportionately greater than the increase in RBCs, which lowers the patient's hematocrit (the percentage of RBCs in whole blood) and may cause anemia. Hemoglobin level also decreases. Hematocrit below 35% and hemoglobin level below 11.5 g/dL indicate pregnancy-related anemia. Iron supplements are commonly prescribed during pregnancy to reduce the risk of this complication.

WBC mystery

Pregnancy is associated with leukocytosis (increased WBC count). A pregnant patient's WBC count increases in the second month of pregnancy and levels out in the second to third trimester with a count usually between 9,000 and 15,000. WBC count will also slightly rise when the patient is in labor.

Fibrin factor

Fibrinogen (a protein in blood plasma) is converted to fibrin by thrombin and is known as *coagulation factor I*. In a nonpregnant person, levels average 250 mg/dL. In a pregnant patient, levels average 450 mg/dL, increasing as much as 50% by term. This increase in the coagulation factor plays an important role in preventing hemorrhage in the pregnant patient during childbirth.

Urinary system

The kidneys, ureters, and bladder undergo profound changes in structure and function during pregnancy.

Anatomic changes

Significant dilation of the kidney pelves, calyces, and ureters begins as early as 10 weeks' gestation, likely due to increased estrogen and progesterone levels. As pregnancy advances and the uterus undergoes dextroversion (movement toward the right), the ureters and kidney pelves become more dilated above the pelvic brim, particularly on the right side. In addition, the smooth muscle of the ureters undergoes hypertrophy and hyperplasia, and muscle tone decreases, primarily because of the muscle-relaxing effects of progesterone. These changes slow the flow of urine through the ureters and may result in hydronephrosis and hydroureter (distention of the kidney pelves and ureters with urine), predisposing the pregnant patient to UTIs. In addition, because of the delay between the formation of urine in the kidneys and its arrival in the bladder, inaccuracies may occur during urine clearance tests.

Maximal capacity, minimal comfort

Hormonal changes cause the bladder to relax during pregnancy, permitting it to distend to hold approximately 1,500 mL of urine. However, pressure from the growing uterus causes bladder irritation, manifested as urinary frequency and urgency, even if the bladder contains little urine. Bladder vascularity increases and the mucosa bleeds easily.

When the uterus rises out of the pelvis, urinary symptoms reduce. As term approaches, symptoms can return because the presenting part of the fetus engages in the pelvis exerting pressure on the bladder again.

Functional changes

Pregnancy affects fluid retention; kidney, ureter, and bladder function; renal tubular resorption; and nutrient and glucose excretion.

Fluid retention

Fluid accumulates during pregnancy because the adrenal glands produce more aldosterone and cortisol, which causes the patient's body to retain fluids. The enlarging uterus interferes with blood flow from the legs to the heart, also causing fluid to accumulate and be retained. As a result, fluid backs up in the veins of the legs and seeps out into the surrounding tissues.

A running theme

To provide sufficient fluid volume for effective placental exchange, a pregnant patient's total body water increases by about 7.5 L from prepregnancy levels of 30 to 40 L. To maintain osmolarity, the body must increase sodium reabsorption in the tubules. To accomplish this, the body's increased progesterone levels stimulate the angiotensin–renin system in the kidneys to increase aldosterone production. Aldosterone helps with sodium reabsorption. Potassium levels, however, remain adequate despite the increased urine output during pregnancy because progesterone is potassium-sparing and does not allow excess potassium to be excreted in the urine.

Kidney function

During pregnancy, the kidneys must excrete the waste products of the patient's body as well as those of the growing fetus. Also, the kidneys must be able to break down and excrete additional protein and manage the demands of increased kidney blood flow. The kidneys may increase in size, which changes their structure and ultimately affects their function.

During pregnancy, urine output gradually increases from 60% to 80% more than prepregnancy output (1,500 mL/day). In addition, urine specific gravity decreases. The glomerular filtration rate (GFR) and renal plasma flow (RPF) begin to increase in early pregnancy to meet the increased needs of the circulatory system. By the second trimester, the GFR and RPF have increased by 30% to 50% and remain at this level for the duration of the pregnancy. This rise is consistent with that of the circulatory system increase, peaking at about 24 weeks' gestation. This efficient GFR level leads to lowered blood urea nitrogen and lowered creatinine levels in the patient's plasma.

Ureter and bladder function

During pregnancy, the uterus is pushed slightly toward the right side of the abdomen by the increased bulk of the sigmoid colon. The pressure on the right ureter caused by this movement may lead to urinary stasis and pyelonephritis (inflammation of the kidney caused by bacterial infection). Pressure on the urethra may lead to poor bladder emptying and possible bladder and kidney infections. Infection in the kidneys, which serve as the filtering system for toxins in the blood, can be dangerous for the pregnant patient. UTIs are also potentially dangerous to the fetus because they are associated with preterm labor.

Renal tubular resorption

To maintain sodium and fluid balance, renal tubular resorption increases by as much as 50% during pregnancy. The patient's sodium requirement increases because they need more intravascular and extracellular fluid. Patients may accumulate 6.2 to 8.5 L of water to meet their needs and those of the fetus and placenta.

Posture of elimination

Late in pregnancy, changes in the patient's posture affect sodium and water excretion. The patient excretes less when lying on their back because the enlarged uterus compresses the vena cava and aorta, causing decreased cardiac output. This decreased cardiac output reduces kidney blood flow, which in turn decreases kidney function. The patient excretes more when lying on the left side because, in this position, the uterus does not compress the great vessels, and cardiac output and kidney function remain unchanged.

Nutrient and glucose excretion

A pregnant patient loses increased amounts of some nutrients, such as amino acids, water-soluble vitamins, folic acid, and iodine. Proteinuria (protein in the urine) can occur during pregnancy because the filtered load of amino acids may exceed the tubular reabsorptive capacity. When the kidney tubules cannot reabsorb the amino acids, protein may be excreted in small amounts in the patient's urine. Values of +1 protein on a urine dipstick are not considered abnormal until the levels exceed 300 mg/24 h. Glycosuria (glucose in the urine) may also occur as GFR increases without a corresponding increase in tubular resorptive capacity.

GI system

Changes during pregnancy affect anatomic elements in the GI system and alter certain GI functions. These changes are associated with many of the most commonly discussed discomforts of pregnancy.

Anatomic changes

The mouth, stomach, intestines, gallbladder, and liver are affected during pregnancy. (See *Crowding of abdominal contents.*)

Crowding of abdominal contents

As the uterus enlarges because of the growing fetus, the intestinal contents are pushed upward and to the side. The uterus usually remains midline, although it may shift slightly to the right because of the increased bulk of the sigmoid colon on the left.

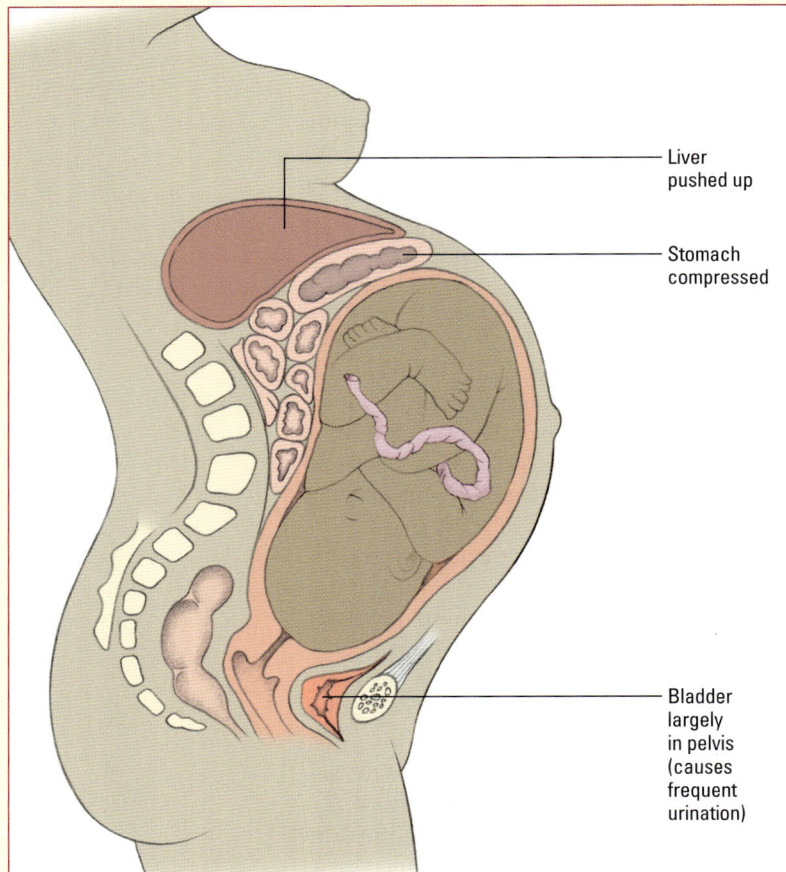

Liver
pushed up

Stomach
compressed

Bladder
largely
in pelvis
(causes
frequent
urination)

Mouth

The salivary glands become more active in the pregnant patient, especially in the latter half of pregnancy. The gums become edematous and bleed easily because of increased vascularity. Due to the hormonal shifts, this can cause the gingiva to become inflamed and overgrown. Taking care of teeth during pregnancy is very important to prevent infection.

Stomach and intestines

As progesterone increases during pregnancy, gastric tone and motility decrease, thus slowing the stomach's emptying time and possibly causing regurgitation and reflux of stomach contents. This may cause the patient to complain of reflux or heartburn.

Make room for the uterus

As the uterus enlarges, it tends to displace the stomach and intestines toward the back and sides of the abdomen. About halfway through the pregnancy, the pressure may be sufficient to slow intestinal peristalsis and the emptying time of the stomach, leading to heartburn, constipation, and flatulence. Relaxin may contribute to decreased gastric motility, which may cause a decrease in blood supply to the GI tract as blood is drawn to the uterus.

The enlarged uterus also displaces the large intestine and puts increased pressure on veins below the uterus. This may predispose the patient to hemorrhoids.

Gallbladder and liver

As smooth muscles relax, the gallbladder empties sluggishly. This can lead to reabsorption of bilirubin into the maternal bloodstream, causing subclinical jaundice (generalized itching). A patient who has had previous gallstone formation may have an increased tendency for stone formation during pregnancy because of the increased plasma cholesterol level and additional cholesterol incorporated in bile. A patient with a peptic ulcer generally finds their condition improved during pregnancy because the acidity of the stomach decreases.

Biliary overtime

The liver does not enlarge or undergo major changes during pregnancy. However, hepatic blood flow may increase slightly, causing the liver's workload to increase as BMR increases. Factors within the liver as well as increased estrogen and progesterone decrease bile flow.

Some liver function studies show changes during pregnancy, possibly caused by increased estrogen levels. Test results may show:

- increased alkaline phosphatase levels, caused in part by increased alkaline phosphatase isoenzymes from the placenta
- decreased serum albumin

- increased plasma globulin levels, causing decreases in albumin–globulin ratios
- decreased plasma cholinesterase levels.

These changes would suggest hepatic disease in a nonpregnant patient but are considered normal in the pregnant patient.

Functional changes

Nausea and vomiting during pregnancy may affect appetite and food consumption, even when the patient's energy demand increases.

Appetite and food consumption

A pregnant patient's appetite and food consumption fluctuate due to several things. For example, the patient may experience nausea and vomiting that decrease their appetite and food consumption. These symptoms are more noticeable in the morning when the patient first arises, hence the term *morning sickness*. However, some patients will experience nausea and vomiting at any time of the day. Nausea and vomiting can also occur when the patient experiences fatigue and may be more frequent if the patient smokes. Nausea and vomiting tend to be noticeable when hCG and progesterone levels begin to rise. These conditions may also be a reaction to decreased glucose levels (because glucose is used in significant quantities by the growing fetus) or increased estrogen levels.

In addition to the reduced appetite caused by nausea and vomiting, increased hCG levels and changes in carbohydrate metabolism may reduce the patient's appetite. The patient's appetite and metabolic needs increase when nausea and vomiting stop.

Carbohydrate, lipid, and protein metabolism

The pregnant patient's carbohydrate needs rise to meet increasing energy demands. They need more glucose, especially during the second half of pregnancy. Plasma lipid levels increase starting in the first trimester. Cholesterol, triglyceride, and lipoprotein levels increase as well. The total concentration of serum protein decreases, mainly serum albumin and, perhaps, gamma-globulin. The primary immunoglobulin lowers in the patient's serum as it is transferred to the fetus.

Musculoskeletal system

The patient's musculoskeletal system changes in response to hormones, weight gain, and the growing fetus. Musculoskeletal changes during pregnancy include changes to the skeleton, muscles, and nerves. These changes may affect the patient's gait, posture, and comfort. In addition, the patient's increased metabolism creates the need for greater calcium intake. If the patient ingests insufficient calcium, hypocalcemia and muscle cramps may occur.

Skeleton

The enlarging uterus tilts the pelvis forward, shifting the patient's center of gravity. The lumbosacral curve increases accompanied by a compensatory curvature in the cervicodorsal region. The lumbar and dorsal curves become even more pronounced as breasts enlarge and their weight pulls the shoulders forward, producing a stoop-shouldered stance. Increasing hormones relax the sacroiliac, sacrococcygeal, and pelvic joints. These changes cause marked alterations in posture and gait. Relaxation of the pelvic joints may also cause the patient's gait to change. Shoe and ring sizes tend to increase because of weight gain, hormonal changes, and dependent edema. Although these changes may persist after childbirth, in most cases, they return to prepregnancy states.

Muscles

In the third trimester, the prominent rectus abdominis muscles (rectus muscles of the abdomen) separate, allowing the abdominal contents to protrude at the midline. Occasionally, the abdominal wall may not be able to stretch enough, and the rectus muscles may actually separate, a condition known as *diastasis*. If this happens, a bluish groove appears at the site of separation after pregnancy.

Nerves

In the third trimester, carpal tunnel syndrome may occur when the median nerve of the carpal tunnel of the wrist is compressed by edematous surrounding tissue. The patient may notice tingling and burning in the dominant hand, possibly radiating to the elbow and upper arm. Numbness or tingling in the hands may also result from pregnancy-related postural changes such as slumped shoulders that pull on the brachial plexus.

Integumentary system

Skin changes vary greatly among pregnant patients. Because some skin changes may remain after childbirth, they are not considered important signs of pregnancy in a patient who has given birth before. The patient may need the nurse's help to integrate these skin changes into their self-concept. Skin changes associated with pregnancy include striae gravidarum, pigment changes, and vascular markings.

Striae gravidarum

The patient's weight gain and enlarging uterus, combined with the action of adrenocorticosteroids, lead to stretching of the underlying connective tissue of the skin, creating striae gravidarum in the second and third trimesters. Better known as *stretch marks*, striae on patients with lighter skin appear as pink or slightly reddish streaks with slight depressions. On patients with darker skin, they appear darker than the surrounding skin tone. They develop most commonly on the skin covering the breasts, abdomen, buttocks, and thighs. After labor, they typically grow lighter until they appear silvery white on patients with light skin tones and light brown on patients with dark skin tones.

Pigment changes

Pigmentation begins to change at approximately 8 weeks' gestation partly because of melanocyte-stimulating and adrenocorticotropic hormones and partly because of estrogen and progesterone. These changes are more pronounced in hyperpigmented areas, such as the breasts (especially nipples), axillae, abdomen, anal region, inner thighs, and vulva. Specific changes may include linea nigra and melasma.

Vascular markings

Tiny, bright-red angiomas may appear during pregnancy due to estrogen release, which increases subcutaneous blood flow. They are called vascular spiders or spider angiomas because of the branching pattern that extends from each spot. They occur mostly on the chest, neck, arms, face, and legs and disappear after childbirth.

Pink-handed

Palmar erythema, commonly seen along with vascular spiders, refers to well-delineated, pinkish areas over the palmar surface of the hands. This condition reverses when pregnancy ends and estrogen levels decrease.

Bubbled gums

Epulides, also known as *gingival granuloma gravidarum*, are raised, red, fleshy areas that appear on the gums as a result of increased estrogen. They may enlarge, cause severe pain, and bleed profusely. An epulis that grows rapidly may require excision.

Other integumentary changes

Nevi (also called moles) are circumscribed, benign proliferations of pigment-producing cells in the skin that may develop on the face, neck, upper chest, or arms during pregnancy. Oily skin and acne from increased estrogen may also occur. Hirsutism (excessive hair growth) may occur but reverses when pregnancy ends. By the sixth week of pregnancy, fingernails may soften and break easily—a problem that may be exacerbated by gel nails and artificial nails.

Immune system

Immunologic competency naturally decreases during pregnancy, most likely to prevent the patient's body from rejecting the fetus. Immunoglobulin G (IgG) production is decreased, which increases the risk of infection during pregnancy. A simultaneous increase in the WBC count may help to counteract the decrease in IgG response.

Neurologic system

Functional disturbances called *entrapment neuropathies* occur in the peripheral nervous system as a result of mechanical pressure. Nerves become trapped and pinched by the enlarging uterus and enlarged edematous vessels, making them less functional. For example, the patient may experience meralgia paresthetica, tingling, and numbness in the anterolateral portion of the thigh that results when the lateral femoral cutaneous nerve becomes entrapped in the area of the inguinal ligaments. This feeling is more pronounced in late pregnancy, as the gravid uterus presses on the nerves and as vascular stasis occurs. Additionally, some patients report becoming forgetful and having "pregnancy brain," but this is not proven.

Psychosocial changes

Pregnancy and childbirth are events that deeply affect the lives of caregivers, partners, and family members. Psychological, social, economic, and cultural factors as well as family and individual influences toward parental and family roles affect responses to pregnancy and childbirth. A nurse faces many responsibilities regarding the expectant family's psychosocial care.

First trimester

During the first trimester, the family's main psychosocial challenge is to resolve any ambivalence. The pregnant patient copes with the physical changes and common discomforts of the first trimester. The partner or other support people begin to accept the reality of the pregnancy.

Ambivalence

The first trimester is known as the *trimester of ambivalence* because patients may experience mixed feelings. Many patients have unrealistic ideas about parental instincts, expecting to feel only loving, happy thoughts about the fetus and parenthood. However, most patients feel some ambivalence about pregnancy and parenthood.

Sharing the joy (and the doubt)

Feelings of ambivalence are inevitable and normal. Encourage partners to communicate these feelings to each other. Partners who discuss these feelings can usually resolve their concerns and fears and enjoy the gratifications of expecting a child. When partners share feelings, they may find they are experiencing similar conflicts.

Psychological responses to physical changes

In the early weeks of the first trimester, the patient may watch for body changes that confirm the pregnancy. Their body image and mental image of how their body looks, feels, and moves, and how others see them may change as the breasts enlarge, menses cease, and they begin to experience nausea, fatigue, waist thickening, and general weight gain. Depending on their acceptance of the pregnancy, the patient may or may not embrace these changes.

In the mood . . . or not!

A patient's response to the physical changes incurred during pregnancy, as well as other factors, can affect the sexual relationship between them and their partner.

The partner's acceptance and preparation

During the first trimester, the patient's partner may find the pregnancy intangible. The idea of the fetus may be abstract because they cannot observe physical changes in their partner. Accepting the reality of pregnancy is the main psychological task for a partner during the first trimester.

Second trimester

During the second trimester, psychosocial tasks include parental-image development, coping with body image and sexuality changes, and development of prenatal attachment.

Parental-image development

As the second trimester begins, the pregnant patient now experiences periods of introspection and has started to determine what kind of caregiver they want to be. This parental image is a composite of the patient's characteristics gleaned from role models, readings, and their imagination.

While the pregnant patient develops their parental image, the partner begins to form their image, often based on their relationship with adult figures in their lives, previous parenting experiences, and the parenting styles of friends and family members. When the patient's expectations about their partner's role do not match their partner's, conflict may develop, and the couple may need to be referred for counseling.

Prenatal bonding

A new phase begins at approximately 17 to 20 weeks' gestation, when the patient feels fetal movements for the first time. Fetal movements signify good health and may dispel the fear of early pregnancy loss. The pregnant patient becomes attentive to the type and timing of movements and fetal responses to environmental factors, such as music, abdominal strokes, and meals.

Yes, that's my baby

The pregnant patient may demonstrate bonding behaviors, such as stroking and patting their abdomen, talking to the fetus, engaging their partner in conversations with the fetus, eating a balanced diet, and engaging in other health-promoting behaviors. Bonding is influenced by the patient's health, developmental stage, and culture. Social support improves prenatal bonding, which may increase feelings of competence and effectiveness.

Third trimester

As the third trimester begins, the patient may feel sentimental about the approaching end of the pregnancy. At the same time, however, the patient may look forward to giving birth because the last months of pregnancy involve bulkiness, insomnia, childbirth anxieties, and concern about the neonate's health.

Time to address the special delivery

During the third trimester, the patient must adapt to activity changes, develop birth plans, prepare for labor, and prepare for parenting. At this time, the patient may have fears about the unknown, labor pain, loss of self-esteem, and loss of control.

Adaptation and preparation

The growing fetus makes daily activities more difficult for the patient and forces them to slow down. As the patient's body grows, so does the anticipation of parenthood. To prepare for parenting, the patient may now focus on concrete tasks, such as preparing the nursery, making decisions about childcare, and planning postpartum events.

Support and nurture

A patient's support system through the childbearing cycle is paramount. With adequate support, there may be greater satisfaction and closeness during the pregnancy. Relationships that allow flexibility and growth may ease the transition into parenthood.

Acceptance of body image and sexuality changes

A patient's body image can change as the pregnancy progresses and more weight is gained. Poor body image may cause interest in sex to drop off. Patients that desire sexual intimacy in the third trimester must be creative, using new positions and techniques.

Quick quiz

1. Nausea and vomiting are common during pregnancy because of changes in which of the following hormone levels?
   A. Increased progesterone levels
   B. Decreased progesterone levels
   C. Increased estrogen levels
   D. Decreased estrogen levels

Answer: C. Nausea and vomiting may occur as a systemic reaction to increased estrogen levels.

2. Which of the following changes in respiratory function during pregnancy is considered normal?
   A. Increased tidal volume
   B. Increased expiratory volume
   C. Decreased inspiratory capacity
   D. Decreased oxygen consumption

Answer: A. A pregnant person breathes more deeply, which increases the tidal volume of gas moving in and out of the respiratory tract with each breath.

3. Which of the following may cause decreased gastric mobility around midpregnancy?
   A. Estrogen
   B. Progesterone
   C. Relaxin
   D. Folic acid

Answer: C. Relaxin (a hormone produced by the ovaries) can contribute to decreased gastric motility, which may cause a decrease in blood supply to the GI tract as blood is drawn into the uterus.

4. Which of the following conditions is common in the second trimester of pregnancy?

    A. Mastitis
    B. Metabolic acidosis
    C. Physiologic anemia
    D. Respiratory acidosis

Answer: C. Physiologic anemia. Hemoglobin and hematocrit values decrease during pregnancy and the increase in plasma volume exceeds the increase in RBC production.

5. Which of the following cardiac conditions is considered normal during pregnancy?

    A. Cardiac tamponade
    B. Heart failure
    C. Endocarditis
    D. Systolic murmur

Answer: D. Systolic murmurs are heard in up to 90% of pregnant patients, and the murmur disappears soon after birth.

6. Which of the following are presumptive signs of pregnancy? Select all that apply.

    A. Breast tenderness
    B. Chadwick sign
    C. Amenorrhea
    D. Fatigue

Answer: A, C, and D are all presumptive signs of pregnancy that the pregnant person feels. Chadwick sign is a probable sign of pregnancy.

7. Which of the following hormones causes insulin to become less effective during pregnancy?

    A. hCG, estrogen, progesterone
    B. Relaxin, progesterone, inhibin
    C. Estrogen, progesterone, hPL
    D. Estrogen, progesterone, aldosterone

Answer: C. Estrogen, progesterone, and hPL are responsible for insulin being less effective in pregnancy. These hormones act as an insulin antagonist.

Scoring

☆☆☆ If you answered all seven questions correctly, bravo! You're a pregnancy adaptations star!

☆☆ If you answered five or six questions correctly, take a bow! Your brain has adapted to all your new knowledge!

☆ If you answered fewer than four questions correctly, the show must go on! Do a quick review, then get ready for the next act!

Selected References

Abu-Raya, B., Michalski, C., Sadarangani, M., & Lavoie, P. (2020). Maternal immunological adaptation during normal pregnancy. *Frontiers in Immunology, 11*, 575197. https://doi.org/10.3389/fimmu.2020.575197

Alves, C., Jenkins, S., & Rapp, A. (2023). Early pregnancy loss (spontaneous abortion). In *StatPearls* [Internet]. StatPearls Publishing. https://www.ncbi.nlm.nih.gov/books/NBK560521/

Centers for Disease Control and Prevention. (2021). *Vulvovaginal candidiasis (VVC)*. https://www.cdc.gov/std/treatment-guidelines/candidiasis.htm

Iftikhar, S., & Biswas, M. (2023). Cardiac disease in pregnancy. In *StatPearls* [Internet]. StatPearls Publishing. https://www.ncbi.nlm.nih.gov/books/NBK537261/

Kampmann, U., Knorr, S., Fuglsang, J., & Ovesen, P. (2019). Determinants of maternal insulin resistance during pregnancy: An updated overview. *Journal of Diabetes Research, 2019*, 5320156. https://doi.org/10.1155/2019/5320156

Pillay, J., & Davis, T. (2023). Physiology-lactation. In *StatPearls* [Internet]. StatPearls Publishing. https://www.ncbi.nlm.nih.gov/books/NBK499981/

Ricci, S., Kyle, T., & Carman, S. (2021). Maternal adaptation during pregnancy. In *Maternity and pediatric nursing* (4th ed., pp. 350–379). Wolters Kluwer.

Chapter 5

Prenatal care

Just the facts

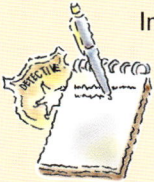

In this chapter, you'll learn:

♦ components of a prenatal patient history and physical assessment
♦ different types of prenatal testing
♦ nutritional needs of the pregnant patient
♦ common discomforts of pregnancy and ways to minimize them.

A look at prenatal care

Prenatal care is essential to the overall health of the neonate and the pregnant patient. Traditional elements of prenatal care include assessing the patient, performing prenatal testing, providing nutritional care, and minimizing the discomforts of pregnancy.

After the fact

Prenatal care after the patient has conceived consists of a thorough assessment, including a health history and physical examination, prenatal testing, nutrition, lifestyle, and psychosocial health. Each of these factors should be addressed at the first prenatal visit.

Occasion for education

The first prenatal visit is also when the pregnant patient can receive information and counseling about what to expect during pregnancy, including necessary care. This promotes the development of healthy behaviors and helps to prevent complications. Keep in mind that the patient education provided during pregnancy will vary depending on the patient's age and parity as well as their cultural background. Warn the patient ahead of time that the first prenatal visit may be a long one.

Assessment

The first prenatal visit is the best time to establish baseline data for the pregnant patient. A thorough assessment of the reproductive system should be included. As with other body systems, this assessment depends on an accurate history and a thorough physical examination. (See *Tips for a successful interview*.)

Advice from the experts

Tips for a successful interview

Here are some tips that can help you obtain an accurate and thorough patient history.

Location
Pregnancy is too private to discuss in public areas. Make every effort to interview your patient in a private, quiet setting. Trying to talk to a pregnant patient in a crowded area, such as a busy waiting room in a clinic, is rarely effective. Remember patient confidentiality and respect the patient's privacy, especially when discussing intimate topics.

Checklist
To ensure that your history is complete, be sure to ask about:
• the patient's overall patterns of health and illness
• the patient's medical and surgical history
• the patient's history of pregnancy or abortion
• the date of the patient's last menses and whether the menses are regular or irregular
• the patient's sexual history, including the number of partners, frequency, the current method of birth control, and satisfaction with the chosen method of birth control
• the patient's family history
• the patient's support system
• any allergies the patient has
• health-related habits, such as smoking or vaping and drug or alcohol use.

Health history

Information from the patient's health history helps establish baseline data, which can be used to plan health promotion strategies for every subsequent visit and identify potential complications. (*Further discussed in Chapter 6, High-risk pregnancy.*)

The health history you conduct should be extensive. Be sure to include biographic data, information on the patient's nutritional status, a medical history, a family history, a gynecologic history, and an obstetric history.

Biographic data

When obtaining biographic data, assure the patient that the information will remain confidential. Topics to discuss include age, cultural considerations (such as race and religion), relationship status, occupation, and education.

Age

The patient's age is an important factor because reproductive risks increase among adolescents and those older than age 35 years. For example, pregnant adolescents are more likely to have preeclampsia. Pregnant patients older than age 35 years are at risk for problematic conditions, including placenta previa, preeclampsia, hydatidiform mole, and vascular, neoplastic, or degenerative diseases. (See Chapter 6, High-risk pregnancy.)

Race, ethnicity, and religion

It is essential to learn about the cultural communities in which you work and become familiar with their cultural practices. The patient's race, ethnicity, religion, and other cultural considerations may impact a pregnancy. Obtaining information from your patient about these topics can help you plan patient care. (See *Cultural considerations for assessment*.)

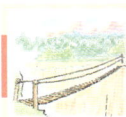

Bridging the gap

Cultural considerations for assessment

Encourage the patient to discuss their cultural beliefs regarding health, illness, and health care. Be considerate of the patient's cultural background. Also, be aware that patients may be reluctant to talk about sexual matters.

Relationship status

Knowing the patient's relationship status may help determine possible stress factors and whether support systems are available.

Occupation

Ask about the patient's occupation and work environment to assess possible risk factors. If the patient works in a high-risk environment with exposure to such hazards as chemicals, inhalants, or radiation, then inform them of the dangers of these substances as well as the possible effects on the pregnancy. Knowing the patient's occupation can also help identify such risks as working long hours, lifting heavy objects, and standing for prolonged periods.

Education

The patient's formal education, health literacy, and life experiences may influence several aspects of the pregnancy, including:
- their attitude toward the pregnancy
- their willingness to seek prenatal care
- the adequacy of their at-home prenatal care and nutritional status
- their knowledge of infant care
- their emotional response to childbirth and the responsibilities of parenting.

Obtaining information about the patient's educational level can help you to plan appropriate patient education.

Nutritional status

Adequate nutrition is especially vital during pregnancy. During the prenatal assessment, take a 24-hour diet history (recall). For more information, see the section on nutritional care later in this chapter.

Medical history

When taking a medical history, determine whether the patient is taking any prescription or over-the-counter (OTC) medications, including vitamins and herbal remedies. Also, ask about smoking or vaping practices, alcohol use, and use of illegal drugs.

Brushing up on current events

Ask the patient about previous and current medical problems that may jeopardize the pregnancy. For example:
- Diabetes can worsen during pregnancy and adversely affect the pregnant patient and fetus.
- Maternal hypertension, which is more common in patients with essential hypertension, kidney disease, or diabetes, increases the risk of preeclampsia and placental abruption.
- Rubella infection during the first trimester can cause malformation in the developing fetus.
- Genital herpes can be transmitted to the neonate during birth.

Obstacle course

Specific problems that you should ask the pregnant patient about include cardiac disorders; respiratory disorders such as tuberculosis; reproductive issues such as STIs and endometriosis; phlebitis; epilepsy; and gallbladder disorders. Also, ask the patient whether they have a history of urinary tract infections (UTIs), cancer, alcohol or substance misuse disorders, smoking or vaping, or psychiatric diagnoses.

Family history

Knowing the medical histories of the patient's family members can help you plan care and guide your assessment by identifying complications for which the patient may be at greater risk.

Gynecologic history

The gynecologic portion of your assessment should include a menstrual and contraceptive history.

Menstrual history

When obtaining a menstrual history, be sure to ask the patient:
- When did your last menstrual period (menses) begin?
- How many days are there between the start of one of your periods and the start of the next?
- Was your last period normal? Was the one before that normal?
- How many days does your flow usually last, and is it light, moderate, or heavy?
- Have you had bleeding or spotting since your last normal menstrual period?

Menarche plays a part

Age at menarche (the first menses/period) is essential when determining pregnancy risks in adolescents. When pregnancy occurs within 3 years of menarche, there is an increased risk of maternal and fetal mortality. Keep in mind that pregnancy can also occur before regular menses are established.

Contraceptive history

To obtain a contraceptive history, ask the patient:
- What form of contraception did you use before your pregnancy?
- How long did you use it?
- Were you satisfied with the method?
- Did you experience any complications while on this type of birth control?

Patients who took hormonal contraceptives before becoming pregnant should be asked how long it took to become pregnant once the contraceptives were stopped.

Obstetric history

Obstetric history is another important part of assessment because it provides helpful information about the patient's past pregnancies. Never assume this is their first pregnancy. (See *Pregnancy classification system.*)

Pregnancy classification system

When referring to the obstetric and pregnancy history of a patient, keep these terms in mind:
- A *primigravida* is a patient who is pregnant for the first time.
- A *primipara* is a patient who has delivered one child past the age of viability.
- A *multigravida* is a patient who has been pregnant before but may not necessarily have carried to term.
- A *multipara* is a patient who has carried two or more pregnancies to viability.
- A *nulligravida* is a patient who has never been and is not currently pregnant.

Getting the details

The obstetric history should include specific details about past pregnancies, including difficulty getting pregnant, difficult or long labors, and any complications.

Do it in order

Always record the patient's obstetric history chronologically. For a list of the types of information, you should include in a complete obstetric history, see *Taking an obstetric history*.

Taking an obstetric history

When taking the pregnant patient's obstetric history, be sure to ask them about:
- genital tract anomalies
- medications used during this pregnancy
- history of hepatitis, pelvic inflammatory disease, human immunodeficiency virus (HIV), blood transfusions, and herpes or other STIs
- partner's history of STIs
- previous abortions
- history of infertility.

Taking an obstetric history (*continued*)

Pregnancy particulars

Also, ask the patient about past pregnancies. Note the number of past full-term and preterm pregnancies and obtain the following information about each of the patient's past pregnancies, if applicable:

- Was the pregnancy planned?
- Did any complications—such as spotting, swelling of the hands and feet, surgery, or falls—occur?
- Did the patient receive prenatal care? If so, when did it start?
- Did the patient take any medications? If so, what were they? How long did they take them? Why?
- What was the duration of the pregnancy?
- How was the pregnancy overall for the patient?

Birth and baby specifics

Also, obtain the following information about the birth and postpartum condition of all previous pregnancies:

- What was the duration of labor?
- What type of birth was it?
- What type of anesthesia, if any, did the patient have?
- Did the patient experience any complications during pregnancy or labor?
- What were the birthplace, condition, sex, weight, and Rh factor of the neonate?
- Was the labor as expected? Better? Worse?
- Did the patient have stitches after birth?
- What was the condition of the infant after birth?
- What was the infant's Apgar score?
- Was special care needed for the infant? If so, what?
- Did the neonate experience any problems during the first several days after birth?
- What's the child's present state of health?
- Was the infant discharged from the health care facility with the caregiver(s)?
- Did the patient experience any postpartum problems?

What's your type?

In addition to asking about pregnancy history, ask whether the patient knows their blood type. If the patient's blood type is Rh-negative, then ask whether they received $Rh_o(D)$ immune globulin (RhoGAM) after miscarriages, abortions, or previous births so that you will know whether Rh sensitization occurred. If they did not receive RhoGAM after any of these situations, then the current pregnancy may be at risk for Rh sensitization.

Gravida and para

Two important components of a patient's obstetric history are the gravida and para status. *Gravida* represents the number of times the patient has been pregnant. *Para* refers to the number of children above the age of 20 weeks' gestation the patient has delivered.

GTPAL and GTPALM

To provide more detailed information about the patient's obstetric history, many facilities now use one of the following classification systems: GTPAL or GTPALM. These systems involve the assignment of numbers to various aspects of a patient's obstetric past.

How often, how many, how viable

In GTPAL, the most basic of the two systems, the patient is assigned a five-digit number as follows:

- G (Gravida) is the number of pregnancies no matter the outcome, including the current pregnancy.
- T (Term) is the number of pregnancies that ended at term (37 weeks' gestation or later).
- P (Preterm) is the number of pregnancies that ended after 20 weeks' gestation and before the end of 36.6 weeks' gestation.
- A (Abortions) is the number of pregnancies that ended in spontaneous or induced abortions before 20 weeks' gestation.
- L (Living) is the number of children who are alive at the time the history is obtained.

Note that the patient's gravida number remains the same, but the GTPAL system allows subclassification of the para status. In most cases, a health care provider includes the patient's gravida status in addition to their GTPAL number. Here are some examples:

- A patient who has had two previous pregnancies, has delivered two-term children, and is pregnant again is assigned a GTPAL of 3-2-0-0-2.
- A patient who is pregnant for the sixth time, has delivered four-term children and one preterm child, and has had one spontaneous abortion and one elective abortion is assigned a GTPAL of 6-4-1-2-5.

Details, details

In GTPALM, a number is added to the GTPAL to represent the number of multiple pregnancies the patient has experienced (M). Note that a patient who has not given birth to multiple pregnancies does not receive a number to represent M.

Here is an example:

- If a patient who is pregnant with twins delivers at 35 weeks' gestation and the neonates survive, then the patient is classified as a gravida 1, para 2 and is assigned a GTPAL of 1-0-2-0-2. Using the GTPALM system, the same patient would be identified as 1-0-2-0-2-1.

Physical assessment

Physical assessment should occur throughout pregnancy, starting with the first prenatal visit and continuing throughout labor, delivery, and the postpartum period. Physical assessment includes evaluation of maternal and fetal well-being.

Rounding the baselines

At the first prenatal visit, measurements of height and weight establish baselines for the patient and allow comparison with expected values throughout the pregnancy. Vital signs, including blood pressure, respiratory rate, and pulse rate, are also measured for baseline assessment. (See *Monitoring vital signs.*)

Advice from the experts

Monitoring vital signs

Monitoring the patient's vital signs, especially blood pressure, during each prenatal visit is an important part of ongoing assessment. A sudden increase in blood pressure is a dangerous sign of gestational hypertension. Likewise, a sudden increase in pulse or respiratory rate may suggest bleeding, such as in an early placenta previa or an abruption.

Be sure to report any of these signs or alterations in the patient's vital signs to the health care provider for further assessment and evaluation.

Scheduled surveillance

Prenatal care visits are usually scheduled every 4 weeks for the first 28 weeks of pregnancy, every 2 weeks until the 36th week, and then weekly until 40 weeks, after which they are twice a week until delivery. Patients who have known risk factors for complications and those who develop complications during pregnancy require more frequent visits.

And now back to our regularly scheduled visit

Regular prenatal visits usually consist of weight measurements, vital signs checks, palpation of the abdomen, and fundal height checks. The patient should also be assessed for preterm labor symptoms, fetal heart tones, and edema. Also, be sure to ask whether the patient has felt the baby move.

Getting started

At the start of the first prenatal visit, the patient should undress, put on a gown, and empty their bladder. Emptying the bladder makes the pelvic examination more comfortable, allows for easier identification of pelvic organs, and provides a urine specimen for laboratory testing.

Head-to-toe assessment

A thorough physical assessment should include inspection of the patient's general appearance, head and scalp, eyes, nose, ears, mouth, neck, breasts, heart, lungs, back, rectum, extremities, and skin.

General appearance

Inspect the patient's general appearance. This helps form an impression of their overall health and well-being. The way a patient dresses and speaks, in addition to their body posture, can reveal how they feel about themselves. Be sure to document all findings.

Head and scalp

Examine the head and scalp for symmetry, normal contour, and tenderness. Check the hair for distribution, thickness, dryness or oiliness, and use of hair dye. Look for chloasma, an extra pigment on the face that may accompany pregnancy. Dryness or sparseness of hair suggests poor nutrition. Lack of cleanliness may suggest fatigue.

Eyes

Be sure to perform a careful inspection of the eyes. Look for edema in the eyelids. Ask the patient whether they ever see spots before their eyes, have diplopia (double vision), or other vision problems. (See *Watching for vision changes*.) These findings may indicate gestational hypertension.

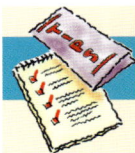

Education edge

Watching for vision changes

Poor vision can be a dangerous sign of pregnancy, possibly indicating preeclampsia. Instruct the pregnant patient to watch for symptoms of poor vision, such as spots in the eyes or double vision, and to report them as soon as possible. If the patient does close desk work on a regular basis, such as computer work or work with small numbers and lists or charts that require tedious and close attention, then advise them to take a break every hour so that work-related eyestrain is not confused with actual danger signs.

Nose

Inspect the nose for nasal congestion and nasal membrane swelling, which may result from increased estrogen levels.

Ears

During early pregnancy, nasal stuffiness may lead to blocked eustachian tubes, which can cause a feeling of "fullness" and dampening of sound. This disappears as the body adjusts to the new estrogen level.

Mouth

Examine the inside and outside of the mouth. Cracked corners may reveal a vitamin A deficiency. Pinpoint lesions with an erythematous base on the lips suggest herpes infection. Gingival (gum) hypertrophy may result from estrogen stimulation during pregnancy; the gums may be slightly swollen and tender to the touch. (See *Taking care of the teeth*.)

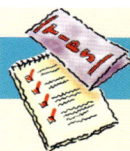

Education edge

Taking care of the teeth

Advise the patient that dental hygiene and taking care of dental caries are important during pregnancy. Dental x-rays can be taken during pregnancy if the dentist is aware of the patient's pregnancy and uses a lead apron. Extensive dental work requiring anesthesia should not be done during pregnancy without approval from the patient's health care provider.

Neck

Slight thyroid hypertrophy may occur during pregnancy because overall metabolic rate is increased. Lymph nodes normally are not palpable and, if enlarged, may indicate an infection.

Breasts

During pregnancy, the areola may darken, breast size increases, and breasts become firmer. Blue streaking of veins may occur on the breasts. Colostrum may be expressed as early as 16 weeks' gestation. Montgomery tubercles may become more prominent.

Heart

Assess the patient's heart. Heart rate should range from 70 to 80 beats/min. Occasionally, a benign functional heart murmur, caused by increased vascular volume, may be auscultated.

All about the blood pressure

Blood pressure during pregnancy is usually lower than the patient's average in the first trimester. It typically stabilizes in the second trimester. Pregnant patients are watched very carefully for high blood pressure because it impacts fetal growth and well-being in utero. Some high blood pressure issues in pregnancy can even cause organ damage to the pregnant patient. See the following for definitions of these different disorders.

Gestational hypertension

Systolic blood pressure greater than or equal to 140 mm Hg or diastolic blood pressure greater than or equal to 90 mm Hg in a previously normotensive pregnant patient who is at least 20 weeks' gestation and who does not have proteinuria or symptoms of organ disturbances

Preeclampsia

Gestational hypertension with the addition of proteinuria (more than 300 mg in a 24-hour period) or severe features

Severe preeclampsia

Preeclampsia is considered severe if one or more of the following criteria are present:
- blood pressure greater than or equal to 160/110 mm Hg on two occasions at least 6 hours apart
- proteinuria of more than 5 g in 24 hours
- thrombocytopenia
- oliguria of less than 500 mL in 24 hours
- cerebral or visual disturbances
- pulmonary edema
- epigastric pain
- impaired liver function.

Hemolysis, elevated liver enzymes, and low platelets

Hemolysis, elevated liver enzymes, and low platelets (HELLP) syndrome. HELLP syndrome is typically a severe form of preeclampsia.

Eclampsia

Grand mal seizures in a patient with preeclampsia

Lungs

Assess respiratory rate and rhythm. Late in pregnancy, diaphragmatic excursion (diaphragm movement) is reduced because the diaphragm cannot descend as fully as usual because of the distended uterus.

Back

When examining the patient's back, be sure to assess for scoliosis. Typically, the lumbar curve is accentuated when standing so that the patient can maintain body posture in the face of increasing abdominal size.

Rectum

Assess the rectum for hemorrhoidal tissue, which commonly results from pelvic pressure that prevents venous return.

Extremities and skin

Assess for palmar erythema, an itchy redness in the palms that occurs early in pregnancy because of high estrogen levels. Assess for varicose veins and check the filling time of nail beds. Observe for edema and assess the patient's gait.

Pelvic examination

A pelvic examination provides information on the health of internal and external reproductive organs and is valuable in assessment.

Shall I compare thee?

Record the patient's uterine fundal height and fetal heart sounds during the examination. Compare the new fundal height findings with the information obtained in the patient's history to ensure that the information obtained about the patient's last menstrual period and the expected date of delivery (EDD) correlate with the current fundal height.

On the move

At about 12 to 14 weeks' gestation, the uterus is palpable over the symphysis pubis as a firm globular sphere. It reaches the umbilicus at 20 to 22 weeks, the xiphoid at 36 weeks, and then, in many cases, returns to about 4 cm below the xiphoid due to lightening at 40 weeks.

If the patient is past 12 weeks of pregnancy, then palpate fundus location, measure fundal height (from the notch above the symphysis pubis to the superior aspect of the uterine fundus), and plot the height on a graph. This information helps detect variations in fetal growth.

Estimation of pelvic size

The size and shape of the patient's pelvis can affect their ability to deliver the neonate vaginally. It is impossible to predict from outward appearances whether the patient's pelvis is adequate for the passage of a fetus.

Clearly clearance counts

Internal pelvic measurements give the actual diameters of the inlet and outlet through which the fetus passes. The internal pelvis must be large enough to allow a patient to give birth vaginally without difficulty.

Now or later?

Pelvic measurements can be taken at the initial visit or at a later visit, when the pelvic muscles are more relaxed. If a routine ultrasound is scheduled, then estimations of pelvic size may be made through a combination of pelvimetry and fetal ultrasound.

Estimation of pelvic adequacy should be done by the 24th week of pregnancy. If the patient has already given birth vaginally, then the pelvis has proven to be adequate and it does not need to be remeasured, unless it has sustained trauma since the last vaginal birth.

Prenatal testing

The fetus is assessed by using direct and indirect monitoring techniques. Common tests include fetal heart rate (FHR) monitoring, ultrasonography, fetal activity determination, maternal urinalysis and serum assays, amniocentesis, chorionic villi sampling (CVS), percutaneous umbilical blood sampling (PUBS), fetoscopy, blood studies, prepartum nonstress test (NST), prepartum contraction stress test (CST), and nipple stimulation CST.

Fetal heart rate

The FHR can be obtained by placing a fetoscope or Doppler ultrasound stethoscope on the patient's abdomen and counting fetal heartbeats. Simultaneously palpating the patient's pulse helps to avoid confusion between maternal and fetal heartbeats.

Heart to heart

A fetoscope can detect fetal heartbeats as early as 20 weeks' gestation. The Doppler ultrasound stethoscope, a more sensitive instrument, can detect fetal heartbeats as early as 10 weeks' gestation and remains a useful tool throughout labor.

Because FHR usually ranges from 110 to 160 beats/min, auscultation yields only an average rate at best. It can detect gross (but commonly late) signs of fetal distress, such as tachycardia and bradycardia, and is thus recommended only for a patient with an uncomplicated pregnancy. For a patient with a high-risk pregnancy, indirect or direct electronic fetal monitoring provides more accurate information on fetal status. (See *Evaluating FHR*.)

Evaluating FHR

To evaluate FHR, position the fetoscope or Doppler ultrasound stethoscope on the patient's abdomen, midway between the umbilicus and symphysis pubis for cephalic presentation and above or at the level of the umbilicus for breech presentation. Locate the loudest heartbeats and palpate the maternal pulse. Monitor maternal pulse and count fetal heartbeats for 60 seconds. Notify the health care provider immediately of marked changes in FHR from the baseline.

Fetoscope

A fetoscope is a modified stethoscope attached to a headpiece. A fetoscope can detect fetal heartbeats as early as 20 weeks' gestation. The fetoscope is not often used in practice.

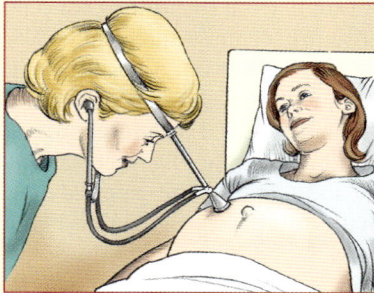

Doppler ultrasound stethoscope

A Doppler ultrasound stethoscope uses ultrasound waves that bounce off the fetal heart to produce echoes or a clicking noise that reflects the fetal heartbeat rate. It can detect fetal heartbeats as early as 10 weeks' gestation and is more sensitive than the fetoscope.

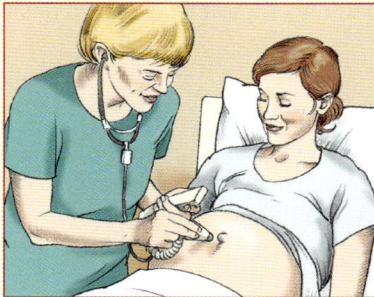

Ultrasonography

Using sound waves that bounce off internal structures, ultrasonography allows visualization of the fetus without the hazards of x-rays. Ultrasonography allows the patient to see the fetus, and it produces an image called a *sonogram*.

How ultra-useful!

Ultrasonography is used to:
- verify the due date and correlate it with fetus's size
- evaluate the condition of the fetus through observation of fetal activity, breathing movements, and amniotic fluid volume
- determine the condition of the fetus when there's a greater-than-average risk of an abnormality or a greater-than-average concern
- rule out pregnancy by week 7 if there has been a suspected false-positive pregnancy test
- determine the cause of bleeding or spotting in early pregnancy
- locate an IUD that was in place at the time of conception
- locate the fetus before amniocentesis and during CVS
- determine the condition of the fetus if no heartbeat has been detected by week 14 with a Doppler device or if no fetal movement has occurred by week 22 diagnose multiple pregnancy, especially if the patient has taken fertility medications or the uterus is larger than it should be for the expected due date
- determine if abnormally rapid uterine growth is being caused by excessive amniotic fluid
- determine the condition of the placenta when deterioration might be responsible for fetal growth restriction or distress
- verify presentation and uncommon fetal or cord position before delivery.

Screen debut

An ultrasound is performed by placing an ultrasonic transducer on the pregnant patient's abdomen. The transducer transmits high-frequency sound waves through the abdominal wall. These sound waves deflect off the fetus, bounce back to the transducer, and transform into a visual image on a monitoring screen.

A fluid fill-up

To prepare a patient for an abdominal ultrasound, have them drink 1 qt (1 L) of fluid 1 to 2 hours before the test. Instruct them not to void before the test because a full bladder serves as a landmark to define other pelvic organs.

A bladder-friendly version

Transvaginal ultrasonography is another type of imaging. It is well tolerated because it eliminates the need for a full bladder and is usually used during the first trimester of pregnancy. It allows visualization of the developing fetus at a much earlier gestation.

Fetal activity determination

The fetus's activity (kick counts) determines its condition in utero. Daily movement evaluation provides an inexpensive, noninvasive way of assessing fetal well-being. Decreased activity in a previously active fetus may reflect a disturbance in fetal well-being.

The first noticeable movement of the fetus by the pregnant patient is called *quickening*. The acknowledgment of fetal movements may be delayed if the due date is miscalculated or the patient does not recognize the sensation. A patient who has had a baby before will likely recognize movement earlier. If the patient has not felt any movements by week 22, then an ultrasound may be ordered to assess the fetus's condition.

Looking for some fetal action

To track fetal movement, have the patient mark the time and then count fetal movements, excluding hiccups, until 10 movements are felt. If the patient does not feel 10 movements within 2 hours, then they should contact their obstetric provider for further instructions. The closer the patient is to the due date, the more critical regular checking of fetal movements becomes.

Maternal urinalysis

During pregnancy, a baseline urinalysis is obtained in the first prenatal visit. Some pregnant patients may have a condition called *bacteriuria without symptoms* where they have a UTI but do not present symptoms. This needs to be treated because, without treatment, it can lead to pyelonephritis (infection of the kidneys) later in pregnancy, which can place the patient at increased risk of preterm labor.

Maternal serum assays

Serum assays—including those for estrogens, human placental lactogen (hPL), and hCG—are used in addition to urinalysis to monitor the pregnant patient for problems. hCG is typically drawn at the beginning of the pregnancy to help determine how far along a patient is. hCG is not helpful after the first trimester. Estrogen and hPL are drawn as part of genetic screens offered to all pregnant patients but are not routine prenatal care.

Fetal fibronectin

Fetal fibronectin (fFN) is a glycoprotein that acts as an adhesive between the fetal membranes and the placenta. Typically, fFN is present in cervical secretions before 20 weeks' gestation and after 37 weeks' gestation. The *fFN test* measures this glycoprotein between weeks 24 and 35 by using a swab from the posterior fornix of the cervix. This test is done on patients who present with complaints of contractions or other signs of preterm labor. A positive test indicates that the patient is at risk for premature labor. With this knowledge, precautions can be taken to decrease the risk of preterm labor and maintain fetal viability.

Human placental lactogen

Also known as *human chorionic somatomammotropin*, hPL works with prolactin to prepare the breasts for lactation. It indirectly provides energy for maternal metabolism and fetal nutrition and facilitates the protein synthesis and mobilization essential for fetal growth.

The purposes of hPL testing are to:

- assess placental function and fetal well-being (combined with measurement of estriol levels)
- aid diagnosis of hydatidiform moles and choriocarcinoma
- aid diagnosis and monitor treatment of nontrophoblastic tumors that ectopically secrete hPL.

Human chorionic gonadotropin

Although the precise function of hCG (a glycoprotein hormone produced in the placenta) is still unclear, it appears that hCG and progesterone maintain the corpus luteum during early pregnancy. Production of hCG increases steadily during the first trimester, peaking around 10 weeks' gestation. Levels then fall to less than 10% of first-trimester peak levels during the remainder of the pregnancy.

The serum test for hCG, which is more sensitive and costlier than the routine pregnancy test using a urine sample, provides a quantitative analysis. It is used to:

- detect pregnancy and can sometimes tell how far along in pregnancy a patient is
- determine adequacy of hormonal production in high-risk pregnancies
- aid diagnosis of trophoblastic tumors, such as hydatidiform moles and choriocarcinoma
- detect tumors that ectopically secrete hCG
- monitor treatment for induction of ovulation and conception.

Amniocentesis

Amniocentesis is the sterile needle aspiration of fluid from the amniotic sac for analysis. This procedure is recommended when:

- the patient is older than age 35 years

- the couple had a child with a chromosomal abnormality (such as Down syndrome) or a metabolic disorder (such as Hunter syndrome)
- the patient is a carrier of an X-linked genetic disorder, such as hemophilia, which they have a 50% chance of passing on to a male child
- a caregiver is known to have a condition, such as Huntington chorea, that is passed on by autosomal dominant inheritance, giving the baby a one in two chances of inheriting the disease
- both caregivers are carriers of an autosomal recessive inherited disorder, such as Tay-Sachs disease or sickle cell disease, and thus have a one in four chances of bearing a child with the disorder
- results of quadruple screening tests and ultrasonography are abnormal, and amniotic fluid evaluation is necessary to determine whether there is a fetal abnormality.

Generally speaking, not for general use

Complications of amniocentesis include spontaneous abortion, spontaneous rupture of membranes, trauma to the fetus or placenta, bleeding, premature labor, infection, and Rh sensitization from fetal bleeding into the maternal circulation. Because of the potential severity of possible complications, amniocentesis is contraindicated as a general screening test.

Chorionic villi sampling

Performed between 8 and 10 weeks' gestation, CVS involves aspirating chorionic villi from the placenta for prenatal diagnosis of genetic disorders. Chorionic villi are fingerlike projections that surround the embryonic membrane and eventually give rise to the placenta. Cells obtained from the sample are of fetal origin—rather than from the pregnant patient—and can be analyzed for fetal abnormalities.

Trans times two

A transcervical or transabdominal approach can be used to obtain a CVS specimen. In transcervical sampling, a sterile catheter is introduced into the cervix using direct visualization with real-time ultrasonography. A small portion of chorionic villi is aspirated through the catheter into a syringe. In transabdominal sampling, the pregnant patient's abdomen is cleaned, and an 18G to 20G needle is inserted into the chorion frondosum under ultrasound guidance. The specimen is then aspirated into a syringe. Aspirated villi are placed into a sterile medium for cytogenetic analysis.

Complicated matters

Test complications include failure to obtain tissue, ruptured membranes or leakage of amniotic fluid, bleeding, intrauterine infection, spontaneous abortion, contamination of the specimen, and possible Rh isoimmunization. If the patient is Rh-negative, then administer RhoGAM, as ordered, to cover the risk of Rh sensitization from the procedure. Also, research indicates an incidence of limb malformations in neonates who underwent CVS in utero. However, this incidence appears low when CVS is performed after 10 weeks' gestation.

Percutaneous umbilical blood sampling

PUBS, which is used to obtain blood samples directly from the fetal circulation, is indicated for prenatal diagnosis of inherited blood disorders, detection of fetal infection, and assessment of the acid–base status of a fetus with intrauterine growth restriction. PUBS can also be used to administer blood products or medications directly to the fetus. Allowing for treatment of the fetus in utero, PUBS reduces the risk of prematurity and mortality for a neonate with erythroblastosis fetalis (hemolytic disease of the newborn due to Rh incompatibility).

Fetoscopy

Fetoscopy is a procedure in which a fetoscope—a telescope-like instrument with lights and lenses—is inserted into the amniotic sac, where it can view and photograph the fetus. This procedure makes it possible to diagnose, through blood and tissue sampling, several blood and skin diseases that amniocentesis cannot detect. Fetoscopy is a relatively risky procedure, and because other safer techniques are becoming available to detect the same disorders, it is not widely used.

Biophysical profile

A biophysical profile assesses fetal well-being in the later stages of pregnancy and aids in detecting central nervous system depression in the fetus. It uses five variables: amniotic fluid volume, fetal body movements, fetal breathing movements, FHR reactivity, and fetal muscle tone. Each variable can score a maximum of 2 points. The total score is then calculated. A score of 8 to 10 indicates a potentially healthy fetus, a score of 6 is suspicious, and a score of 4 indicates that the fetus may be in jeopardy. (See *Scoring the biophysical profile.*)

Scoring the biophysical profile

Parameter	Diagnostic tool	Factor for a score of 2
Amniotic fluid volume	Ultrasound	Presence of a pocket of amniotic fluid measuring >1 cm in vertical diameter
Fetal breathing movements	Ultrasound	At least one episode of sustained fetal breathing movement for 30 seconds within 30 minutes
FHR reactivity	NST	Two or more FHR accelerations of at least 15 beats/min above baseline and 15 seconds duration occurring with fetal movement over 20 minutes
Fetal body movements	Ultrasound	At least three separate episodes of fetal limb or trunk movement within 30 minutes
Fetal muscle tone	Ultrasound	Extension and then flexing of the spine or extremities at least once in 30 minutes

Blood studies

During pregnancy, blood studies are ordered to assess the pregnant patient's health, screen for conditions that may endanger the fetus, detect genetic defects, and monitor fetal well-being. Initial studies include blood typing, antibody screening tests, and a serologic test for syphilis and gonorrhea. If indicated, then other tests may be performed to assess AFP levels, blood glucose, and other chemicals.

Blood typing

Blood typing, including Rh factor, is performed to determine the patient's blood type and detect possible incompatibilities. The patient's Rh status is also tested to determine if they are Rh-negative or Rh-positive. If the patient is Rh-negative, then they will need to receive RhoGAM at 28 weeks' gestation, within 72 hours after delivery, and anytime there is a concern that fetal and maternal blood have mixed. Patients who are Rh-negative and suffer a miscarriage will also need a dose of RhoGAM. RhoGAM is given not to protect the current pregnancy but against Rh sensitization in the next pregnancy. An Rh-negative patient will receive RhoGAM with every pregnancy.

Antibody screening tests

The blood studies performed during pregnancy also include antibody screening tests for Rh compatibility (indirect Coombs test), rubella, and hepatitis B. Antibodies for varicella (chickenpox) may also be assessed.

Indirect coombs test

The indirect Coombs test screens the pregnant patient's blood for RBC antibodies. This test should be performed on a patient who is Rh-negative. If the fetus is Rh-positive and its blood mixes with the maternal blood during pregnancy or delivery, then the pregnant patient's immune system produces antibodies against the fetus's RBCs. This antibody response is called *Rh sensitization*. Rh sensitization usually is not a problem with the first Rh-positive fetus. However, future Rh-positive fetuses are in danger of having their RBCs destroyed by the pregnant person's immune system. After sensitization, the fetus can develop mild-to-severe problems such as Rh or hemolytic disease of the newborn or hydrops fetalis, a swelling of two or more areas in the fetus.

If the patient does not show Rh sensitivity, then the test is usually repeated at 28 weeks' gestation. If the titers are not elevated, then an Rh-negative pregnant patient would receive RhoGAM at this time and after any procedure that might cause fetal and blood to mix (amniocentesis or CVS).

Rubella titer

A rubella (German measles) titer detects antibodies in pregnant patient's blood for the virus that causes rubella. If antibodies are found, then the patient is immune to rubella. Most patients have either had the virus as a child or have received a vaccination for rubella and, therefore, have antibodies in the blood.

Rubella exposure during pregnancy can lead to blindness, deafness, and heart defects in the fetus. If tests reveal that the patient is not immune, then they should avoid anyone who has the infection. They cannot receive the vaccination while pregnant, but they should receive it after giving birth to provide protection during future pregnancies.

Hepatitis B

The *hepatic antibody surface antigen* (HbsAg) test is used to determine whether a patient has hepatitis B. In many cases, the HbsAg test is the only way to tell whether a patient has hepatitis B because many people who carry the virus have no symptoms. Hepatitis B can be passed to the baby during delivery.

If the patient tests positive for hepatitis B, then the neonate must receive injections of hepatitis B immunoglobulin and hepatitis B vaccine immediately after birth to prevent liver damage. The neonate then receives additional doses of the vaccine at 2 to 4 months and again at 6 to 18 months.

HIV testing

The Centers for Disease Control and Prevention (CDC) recommends that all pregnant people be tested for HIV.

What happens next?

A patient who is antibody positive for HIV may begin therapy with zidovudine (AZT) to decrease the risk of transmitting the disease to the fetus.

Serologic tests

The Venereal Disease Research Laboratories (VDRL) test and rapid plasma reagin (RPR) test are serologic tests for syphilis. Syphilis needs to be treated early in pregnancy before fetal damage occurs.

Pregnant patients who test positive for syphilis must receive treatment before 16 weeks' gestation. Untreated syphilis infection during pregnancy can cause miscarriage, premature birth, stillbirth, or congenital anomalies. At-risk patients should be tested again for syphilis at 28 weeks.

AFP testing

AFP testing—sometimes called the *MSAFP* test or *maternal serum AFP* test—is usually used to detect neural tube defects. AFP is a protein secreted by the fetal liver and excreted in the pregnant patient's blood. When testing by immunoassay, AFP values are less than 15 ng/mL in nonpregnant patients.

Multiples of median levels

The test is considered positive for an increased risk of neural tube defect when the AFP level is greater than 2.5 times the median (midpoint of levels of a group of patients at the same gestational age) or 2.5 MOM (multiples of median).

Congenital anomalies, such as Down syndrome, may be associated with low MSAFP concentrations. Elevated MSAFP levels may suggest neural tube defects or other anomalies. Definitive diagnosis requires ultrasonography and amniocentesis. High AFP levels can also indicate intrauterine death or other anomalies, such as duodenal atresia, omphalocele, tetralogy of Fallot, and Turner syndrome.

Glucose tolerance testing

If the patient has a history of previously unexplained fetal loss, has a family history of diabetes, has previously delivered a large-for-gestational age neonate (over 9 lb [4.1 kg]), is obese, or has glycosuria, then a 50-g oral 1-hour glucose loading or glucose tolerance test should be scheduled toward the end of the first trimester. This test is performed to rule out or confirm gestational diabetes. For all other pregnant patients, it is routinely done between 24- and 28-weeks' gestation to evaluate insulin-antagonistic effects of placental hormones, but in high-risk pregnancies, testing should be performed earlier. Fasting plasma glucose levels should not be above 140 mg/dL.

Quadruple screen

The quadruple screen is a routine blood test between weeks 15 and 20. It measures four chemicals: AFP, unconjugated estriol, inhibin-A, and hCG.

Picking up on patterns

By detecting chemical patterns, the test predicts whether there is an increased risk of bearing a child with a chromosomal abnormality or a neural tube defect.

Suggestive, not definitive

Quadruple screening does not definitively answer whether a fetus has a congenital anomaly. It only suggests that there is a possibility for congenital anomalies. In some cases, results appear to be abnormal because the fetus is younger or older than initially estimated. Suspicions can be confirmed by amniocentesis.

Nonstress testing

Performed by a specially trained nurse, a prenatal NST evaluates fetal well-being by measuring the fetal heart response to fetal movements. Such movements produce transient accelerations in the heart rate of a healthy fetus. Usually ordered during the third trimester of pregnancy, this noninvasive screening test uses indirect electronic monitoring to record FHR and the duration of uterine contractions.

Getting it on the record

To perform the test, the patient is placed in a semi-Fowler or lateral-tilt position with a pillow under one hip. The patient should not be placed in the supine position because pressure on the maternal great vessels from the gravid uterus may cause hypotension and reduced uterine perfusion. Conductive gel is applied to the abdomen, and transducers are placed on the patient's abdomen to transmit and record FHR and fetal movement.

Shake it up

The patient is then instructed to depress the monitor's mark or test button when they feel the fetus move. If there are two or more FHR accelerations that exceed the baseline by at least 15 beats/min, lasting at least 15 seconds, occurring in a 20-minute window, then the test is "a reactive NST." This indicates that the fetus is well-oxygenated and has an intact autonomic nervous system at that time. If no spontaneous fetal movement occurs within 40 minutes, then the test is considered "nonreactive," and the fetus requires further evaluation.

Contraction stress test

The prepartum CST evaluates placental function and indicates whether the fetus can withstand the stress of labor. It is performed during labor and delivery and uses indirect electronic monitoring to measure fetal heart response to spontaneous or oxytocin-induced uterine contractions. The CST is indicated when the NST fails to produce reactive results.

Contraindications to the CST include the following maternal conditions:

- Preterm labor or preterm membrane rupture
- Previous vertical incision cesarean birth
- Abruptio placentae
- Placenta previa
- Incompetent cervical os
- Previous uterine rupture

If the test must be performed despite the presence of one of these conditions, then prepare for emergency delivery.

Places, everyone!

To perform the test, the patient is placed in a semi-Fowler or lateral-tilt position with a pillow beneath one hip. As with the NST, the supine position should not be used because pressure on the maternal great vessels from the gravid uterus may cause hypotension and reduced uterine perfusion. To release oxytocin naturally, the patient will be asked to perform nipple stimulation. If that fails to elicit uterine contractions, then an intravenous (IV) line will be placed to deliver an oxytocin drip. This test is rarely performed anymore.

Roll ultrasound . . . and action!

A tocotransducer and an ultrasound transducer are placed on the abdomen for 20 minutes to record baseline vital signs and measurements of uterine contractions, fetal movements, and FHR. The contractions cause a temporary decrease in blood and oxygen flow to the fetus, which most fetuses can tolerate. Three contractions, each lasting 40 seconds, must occur within 10 minutes. The test is considered normal if the fetus's heart rate stays constant.

The lowdown on a slowdown

The fetus may experience a decelerated heart rate during the test. If 50% or more of the contractions cause late decelerations, then the test is stopped, results are considered abnormal, and the test is reported as a "positive CST." If test results are abnormal, then the patient should be observed for 30 minutes after the test to ensure that contractions do not continue. FHR should not drop below baseline at the end or after the contraction. This is termed *late deceleration* and can be indicative of fetal hypoxia.

Nutritional care

Nutritional needs must also be addressed as part of prenatal care. Nutritional intake—including calories, protein, fat, vitamins, minerals, and fluid—needs to be increased to provide sufficient nutrients for the growing fetus.

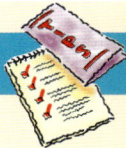

Foods to avoid during pregnancy

Although several nutritional needs increase during pregnancy, other food restrictions become necessary. Tell the patient to avoid the following food products.

Alcohol
A pregnant patient should not drink alcohol because alcohol crosses the placental barrier and can result in fetal alcohol syndrome (FAS). FAS can cause prenatal and postnatal growth failure, microcephaly, facial and musculoskeletal abnormalities, and intellectual disabilities.

Caffeine
Caffeine is a central nervous system stimulant that increases heart rate, urine production in the kidneys, and secretion of acid in the stomach. Foods and beverages with caffeine should be avoided or limited during pregnancy. Sources of caffeine include chocolate, soft drinks, tea, and coffee. Daily caffeine intake of more than 300 mg has been associated with low birth weight. If the patient continues to drink caffeine, then intake should be limited to less than 200 mg/day. To reduce caffeine intake, suggest that the patient switch to decaffeinated beverages, such as decaffeinated tea or coffee.

Artificial sweeteners
Artificial sweeteners, such as saccharin and aspartame, are not recommended during pregnancy. Although no definitive study has been performed that indicates that aspartame crosses the placental barrier, a patient should be advised to avoid ingesting food products with aspartame during pregnancy.

Additives
There are many food additives that should be avoided including various food colorings.
- **Blue no. 1**—has been known to cause inhibition of nerve cell development in vitro
- **Red no. 3**—has been known to cause cancerous thyroid tumors
- **Yellow no. 5**—has most reports of serious damage including asthma and anaphylactic shock
- **Red no. 40**—has been known to cause DNA damage to the colon, developmental toxicity and behavioral toxicity in animals, and damage to the reproductive system
- **Yellow no. 6**—increases the number of kidney and adrenal gland tumors in rats. It may also cause chromosomal damage as well as allergic reactions.
- **Nitrates**—Nitrates are used as preservatives in cured meats such as deli meats, bacon, ham, and smoked fish to prevent spoilage. Nitrates form cancer-causing compounds known as *nitrosamines* in the gastrointestinal (GI) tract.

Calories

During the first trimester, a pregnant person's energy needs are essentially the same as those of a nonpregnant person. In the second and third trimesters, however, the increased need for energy ranges from 300 to 400 calories per day. Because nutrient needs increase more than calorie needs, a pregnant patient's food choices need to be nutrient-dense. More calories (2,700 to 3,000 per day) may be needed for active, large, or nutritionally deficient patients. Inadequate calorie intake can lead to protein breakdown for energy, depriving the fetus of essential protein.

Ascertain weight gain

The easiest way to determine whether your patient's calorie intake is adequate is to assess weight gain. The patient's weight gain pattern is as important as the total weight gain. Pregnancy weight gain should be as follows based on the patient's body mass index (BMI) before pregnancy:

Underweight (BMI less than 18.5)—Gain between 28 and 40 lb
Normal (BMI 18.5 to 24.9)—Gain between 25 and 35 lb
Overweight (BMI 25 to 29)—Gain between 15 and 25 lb
Obese (BMI more than 30)—Gain between 11 and 20 lb

Protein

Recommended protein intake during pregnancy increases from 10 to 15 g/day to 60 g/day total. Many pregnant patients consume more than this already and do not need to increase protein intake.

You complete me

Good animal sources of protein include meat, poultry, fish, cheese, yogurt, eggs, and milk. Because the protein in these forms contains all nine essential amino acids, it is considered *complete protein*. However, lunch meats such as bologna and salami should not be consumed regularly because they are high in fat, contain nitrates, and are typically not good sources of protein.

Full of complements

The protein found in nonanimal sources does not contain all nine essential amino acids. Vitamin B_{12} is found exclusively in animal proteins. Therefore, a pregnant patient who excludes animal proteins from their diet may have a vitamin B_{12} deficiency. Complete protein can be obtained through nonanimal sources by cooking different protein sources together. For example, eating complementary proteins, such as beans and rice, legumes and rice, or beans and wheat together, can provide the patient with all nine essential amino acids.

Got milk?

Milk products are also rich in protein and may be consumed in various forms—buttermilk, yogurt, cheese, custards, eggnogs, and cream soups—to meet daily protein requirements. If the patient is lactose intolerant, then lactose supplements may be purchased OTC. These supplements predigest milk and make it palatable for the patient.

Fats

Linoleic acid is an essential fatty acid that is necessary for new cell growth. It is not manufactured in the body but can be found in vegetable oils such as safflower, corn, olive, peanut, and cottonseed. In addition, these vegetable oils are low in cholesterol compared with animal oils such as lard. They are also recommended for all adults to prevent hypercholesterolemia and atherosclerosis.

Vitamins

Requirements of fat- and water-soluble vitamins increase during pregnancy to support the growth of new fetal cells. A healthy, varied diet with plenty of fruits and vegetables usually allows the pregnant patient to meet these requirements. A specially designed multivitamin supplement is usually also prescribed.

Stocking the stores

Pregnant patients need to include good sources of vitamin A, vitamin B_6, and folic acid in their diet in early pregnancy. Vitamin A can be found in milk, eggs, yellow fruits and vegetables, dark-green fruits and vegetables, and liver. Vitamin B_6, is present in whole grains, organ meats, brewer's yeast, blackstrap molasses, and wheat germ. Folic acid can be found in citrus fruits, tomatoes and other vegetables, grain products, and most ready-to-eat cereals (fortified with folic acid).

Minerals

Minerals such as calcium, phosphorus, and iodine are needed for fetal cell development. They are found in many foods, so most mineral deficiencies in pregnant patients are rare. For those whose intake of minerals is below daily requirements, supplements may be necessary.

Calcium and phosphorus

Calcium and phosphorus are vital to the structure of bones and teeth. Between 1,200 and 1,500 mg of calcium and 1,200 mg of phosphorus are recommended per day during pregnancy. In the last trimester of pregnancy, fetal skeletal growth is greatest and the fetus draws calcium directly from the pregnant patient's stores.

Inadequate calcium intake can result in diminished maternal bone density. The pregnant patient should eat foods that are high in protein to ensure adequate phosphorus intake because most foods that are high in protein are also high in phosphorus.

Iodine

The recommended daily requirement of iodine during pregnancy is 175 mg. Iodine is essential for the formation of thyroxine and proper functioning of the thyroid gland. The best sources of this mineral are ocean fish, including cod, haddock, sole, and ocean perch (Atlantic redfish).

If iodine deficiency occurs, then it may result in thyroid enlargement (goiter) in the pregnant patient or fetus and, in extreme cases, can cause hypothyroidism (cretinism) in the fetus.

Iron

The recommended daily allowance (RDA) of iron for pregnant patients is 30 mg. In most cases, about one half of this intake comes from supplements because dietary intake alone cannot provide enough iron. Remember to tell the patient to take iron supplements with orange juice to enhance absorption. Inform them that the iron supplements may cause the stools to be black and that constipation may develop if enough fluids and fiber are not included in the diet.

Because the richest sources of iron are also the most expensive—organ meats, eggs, green leafy vegetables, whole grain, enriched breads, and dried fruits—a patient with a low income may have trouble taking in adequate amounts of iron in their diet. Today, many cereals are iron fortified, but even these foods may not supply the amount of iron that the patient needs.

Sodium

Sodium is a major electrolyte that regulates fluids in the body. It helps with retention of fluid in the maternal circulation to ensure a pressure gradient for optimal exchange across the placenta. It also plays a role in maintaining the acid–base balance of blood and helps nutrients cross cell membranes.

During pregnancy and lactation, the patient's sodium metabolism (utilization) is altered by hormone activity. As a result, sodium needs are slightly higher during these times. However, there is rarely a need for additional sodium intake because a typical diet usually provides adequate amounts. Unless the patient is hypertensive or has heart disease, seasoning foods as usual is recommended during pregnancy. However, extremely salty foods, such as lunch meats and potato chips, should be avoided. Excessive salt intake could result in fluid retention, which strains the heart.

Zinc

Zinc is necessary for the synthesis of DNA and RNA as well as cell division and growth. Zinc deficiency has been associated with preterm birth. The RDA of zinc during pregnancy is 15 mg daily. Meat, liver, eggs, seafood, and prenatal vitamins are good sources of zinc.

Fluid

Because the pregnant patient is excreting not only their own waste products but also those of their fetus, the patient's body requires extra water to promote kidney function.

Recommended fluid intake is 2 qt (8 cups) daily. The patient should avoid excess intake of caffeinated beverages. The pregnant patient should primarily be drinking water to stay as hydrated as possible. Dehydration can lead to contractions, which puts patients at risk for preterm labor.

Minimizing discomforts of pregnancy

Being aware of patient discomforts during pregnancy allows you to provide information on how to alleviate them. In addition, early monitoring of certain conditions can help to reduce their occurrence.

Have them share so you can provide care

A pregnant patient may not mention their concerns or discomforts, unless they are specifically asked. The patient may not be aware of the significance of their problems or they may be reluctant to take up a lot of time during a prenatal visit. Encourage the patient to discuss whatever concerns they have at their prenatal visits. Although some issues may represent minor common discomforts associated with normal pregnancy, others may be early indicators of potential problems. For example, a problem such as constipation, which the patient may consider a minor discomfort, may result in hemorrhoids, which can become a long-term problem if left to progress throughout the pregnancy.

On the other hand, a patient may see the discomforts of pregnancy as deterrents to good health. Discomforts of pregnancy may not seem minor to the patient, especially if they occur daily and make them wonder if they will ever feel like themselves again. Provide empathetic and sound advice for relieving discomforts and helping promote the overall health and well-being of a pregnant patient. (See *Dealing with pregnancy discomforts.*)

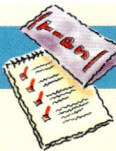

Education edge

Dealing with pregnancy discomforts

This table lists common discomforts associated with pregnancy and suggestions that you can give to the patient on how to prevent and manage them.

Discomfort	Patient education
Urinary frequency	• Void as necessary. • Avoid caffeine. • Perform Kegel exercises.
Fatigue	• Try to get a full night's sleep. • Schedule a daily rest time. • Maintain good nutrition.
Breast tenderness	• Wear a supportive bra. • Wear a bra at night if breast discomfort interferes with sleep.
Vaginal discharge	• Wear cotton underwear. • Avoid tight-fitting pantyhose. • Bathe daily.
Backache	• Avoid standing for long periods. • Keep within the recommended weight range during pregnancy. • Avoid high-heeled shoes. • Bend at the knees, not the waist.

(continued)

Dealing with pregnancy discomforts (*continued*)

Discomfort	Patient education
Round ligament pain	• Slowly rise from a sitting position. • Bend forward to relieve pain. • Avoid twisting motions. • Lie on the side opposite the discomfort. • Soak in a warm (not hot) bath. • May use acetaminophen as directed by your health care provider
Constipation	• Increase fiber intake in the diet. • Set a regular time for bowel movements. • Drink more fluids, including water and fruit juices (unless contraindicated). Avoid caffeinated drinks.
Nasal stuffiness	• Use a cool mist vaporizer. • Use saline nose drops. • Avoid medicated nasal sprays because of rebound stuffiness with repeated use.
Hemorrhoids	• Avoid constipation. • Set a regular time for bowel movements. • Take sitz baths with warm water as often as needed to relieve discomfort. • Apply ice packs for reduction of swelling, if preferred over heat.
Varicosities	• Exercise regularly. • Rest with the legs elevated daily. • Avoid standing or sitting for long periods. • Avoid crossing the legs. • Avoid wearing constrictive knee-high stockings; wear support stockings instead. • Keep within the recommended weight range during pregnancy.
Ankle edema	• Avoid standing or sitting for long periods. • Rest with the feet elevated. • Avoid wearing garments that constrict the lower extremities.
Leg cramps	• Straighten the leg and dorsiflex the ankle. • Avoid pointing the toes. • Rest frequently with legs elevated.

First trimester

Although the pregnant patient may be excited about pregnancy and childbirth, the many discomforts that occur during the first trimester can take away from those joyful feelings. Such discomforts are usually accepted as an expected part of pregnancy. However, there are ways to ease discomforts and prevent further complications. You should pass this information along to your patient as necessary.

Nausea and vomiting

Nausea and vomiting are the most common discomforts during the first trimester. Although these symptoms are commonly referred to as *morning sickness*, they can last all day for some patients. Nausea and vomiting rarely interfere with proper nutrition enough to harm the developing fetus.

Queasiness cause

Although a specific cause of nausea during pregnancy has not been determined, it has been suggested that nausea is the body's reaction to the high levels of hCG that occur during the first trimester. Other possible contributors to nausea include the rapid stretching of the uterine muscles, the relative relaxation of the muscle tissue in the digestive tract (making digestion less efficient), excess acid in the stomach, and the pregnant patient's enhanced sense of smell. (See *Reducing nausea*.)

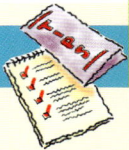

Education edge

Reducing nausea

To help the patient relieve nausea during pregnancy, provide these tips:
• Before getting out of bed in the morning, eat a high-carbohydrate food, such as saltines, melba toast, or other crackers.
• Eat small, frequent meals rather than large, infrequent ones.
• Avoid greasy and highly seasoned foods.
• Delay breakfast (or dinner, if experiencing evening nausea) until nausea passes. Make up for missed meals at another time to maintain nutrition.
• Avoid sudden movements and fatigue, which are known to increase nausea.
• If breakfast is usually eaten late in the morning, then eat a snack before bedtime to help avoid long periods between meals.
• Use a wrist acupressure band that may help to reduce motion sickness.
• Sip carbonated beverages, water, or herbal decaffeinated tea.
• Take a walk outside or take deep breaths through an open window to inhale fresh air.
• Try ginger, an alternative remedy thought to settle the stomach and help quell queasiness. Drink ginger ale made with real ginger. (Most supermarket ginger ales aren't.) Grate some fresh ginger into hot water to make ginger tea or see if ginger candies or crystallized ginger helps. Research shows that taking powdered ginger root in capsules may provide some relief. Unfortunately, there is no way to be sure how much of the active ingredient you are getting in these ginger supplements, so talk to your health care provider before taking them. (As with many other things that are helpful in small amounts, the effects of megadoses are unknown.)
• Consider seeing an acupuncturist who has experience treating nausea during pregnancy.

(continued)

Reducing nausea (*continued*)

• Experiment with aromatherapy. Some patients find scents such as lemon, mint, or orange useful. Use a diffuser to dispense an essential oil or carry a drop or two of an essential oil on a handkerchief to smell when feeling queasy. (Essential oils are very strong, so use only one or two drops.)
• Patients can talk with their obstetric provider for medications, if none of the earlier listed treatments work.

Fatigue

Fatigue is common early in pregnancy and may be caused by the body's increased metabolic requirements. Fatigue can also intensify morning sickness. For example, if the patient becomes too tired, then they may not eat properly. If they remain on their feet without minimal breaks during the day, then the risk of varicosities and thromboembolic complications increases.

Putting fatigue to rest

When in bed, a modified Sims position with the top leg forward is a good resting position. This puts the weight of the fetus on the bed, not on the patient, and allows good circulation to the lower extremities.

Second and third trimesters

Although the patient may be focused on bonding with the fetus, they must be reminded to report any discomforts they have to ensure that nothing serious is occurring. In addition, at the midpoint of pregnancy, review with the patient precautionary measures that help prevent constipation, varicosities, and hemorrhoids and discuss new symptoms that may occur.

Indigestion

Indigestion may be caused by large amounts of progesterone and estrogen, which tend to relax smooth muscle tissue throughout the body—including the GI tract. This causes food to move through the system more slowly and may result in bloating and indigestion. This slowdown is beneficial because it allows for better absorption of nutrients into the bloodstream and subsequently into the fetus's system.

Feeling the burn

Heartburn results when the cardiac sphincter relaxes, allowing food and digestive juices to back up from the stomach into the esophagus. This irritates the lining, causing a burning sensation. This problem may increase later in pregnancy because of the pressure of the fetus on the pregnant patient's internal organs. (See *Relieving heartburn and indigestion.*)

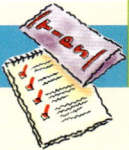

Education edge

Relieving heartburn and indigestion

To decrease the incidence of heartburn and indigestion in the pregnant patient, advise them to:

- avoid gaining too much weight (this puts excess pressure on the stomach)
- avoid wearing clothing that is tight around the abdomen and waist
- eat frequent, small meals instead of three large ones
- eat slowly and chew thoroughly
- avoid highly seasoned foods, fried and fatty foods, processed meats, chocolate, coffee, alcohol, carbonated beverages, and spearmint or peppermint
- avoid smoking and vaping
- avoid bending at the waist
- sleep with their head elevated about 60 degrees (15 cm).

If measures fail to relieve symptoms, then a low-sodium antacid or other OTC medication that is safe to use during pregnancy may be recommended. Sodium or sodium bicarbonate solutions should be avoided because they can exacerbate heartburn.

Varicose veins

Varicose veins are tortuous veins that develop during pregnancy because the weight of the distended uterus puts pressure on the veins returning blood from the lower extremities. This causes blood to pool in the vessels, and the veins become engorged, inflamed, and painful. Varicose veins are common in patients with a family history or patients who have a large fetus or multiple pregnancies. Sitting for prolonged periods with the legs dependent also promotes venous stasis.

Hemorrhoids

Hemorrhoids are varicosities of the rectal veins that can occur during pregnancy because the bulk of the growing uterus puts pressure on the veins. Measures taken early in pregnancy to prevent their occurrence are key to reducing their incidence as well as severity.

Constipation

As pregnancy progresses, the growing uterus presses against the bowel and slows peristalsis, resulting in constipation and sometimes flatulence. Prescribed oral iron supplements also contribute to constipation. Reinforce not only the need for the supplements to build fetal iron stores but also help the patient to find a method to relieve or prevent constipation.

Advise the patient not to use home remedies, such as mineral oil and enemas. Mineral oil interferes with the absorption of fat-soluble vitamins (A, D, E, and K), which are necessary for fetal growth, and enemas might initiate labor through their action. OTC laxatives are contraindicated during pregnancy, unless specifically prescribed or authorized by the patient's health care provider. (See *Preventing constipation*.)

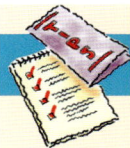

Education edge

Preventing constipation

When teaching the pregnant patient about preventing constipation, include these tips:
- Encourage them to evacuate their bowels regularly.
- Advise them to increase the amount of roughage in their diet by eating raw fruits, bran, and vegetables.
- Provide instructions to drink extra amounts of water daily.

If the patient experiences excessive flatulence, then recommend avoiding gas-forming foods, such as cabbage and beans. In addition, if dietary measures and regular bowel evacuation fail, then a stool softener (such as docusate sodium [Colace]) and evacuation suppositories (such as glycerin) may be prescribed.

Lightheadedness

Lightheadedness in the first trimester may be caused by the blood supply inadequately filling the rapidly expanding circulatory system. During the second trimester, lightheadedness may be caused by the pressure of the expanding uterus on maternal blood vessels. Faintness can occur when the patient rises from a sitting or prone position (postural hypotension) because the blood suddenly shifts away from the brain when blood pressure drops rapidly. Advise the patient to get up slowly in these situations.

Lightheadedness may also result from low glucose levels caused by skipping meals. Carrying fruit or crackers to snack on is helpful to quickly increase glucose levels.

If the patient feels faint, then advise them to lie down with their legs elevated or sit down and place their head between their knees until faintness subsides. The patient should also report any lightheadedness because it can be a sign of severe anemia or another illness and should be evaluated.

Shortness of breath

As the expanding uterus puts pressure on the diaphragm, the lungs may compress, causing dyspnea (shortness of breath). This may be more noticeable to the patient on exertion or during the night, when their body is flat.

Sitting upright and allowing the weight of the uterus to fall away from the diaphragm can help relieve the problem. As pregnancy progresses, the patient may require two or more pillows to sleep on at night to avoid dyspnea.

Always question the patient about shortness of breath at prenatal visits to be certain the sensation is not continuous. Constant shortness of breath may indicate cardiac problems or a respiratory tract infection.

Abdominal discomfort and Braxton Hicks contractions

A patient may experience uncomfortable abdominal pressure early in pregnancy. A patient with a multiple pregnancy may notice this throughout pregnancy. This pressure may be relieved by putting gentle pressure on the uterine fundus or by standing with the arms crossed in front.

Pain around the round ligaments

When standing up quickly, the patient may experience a pulling pain in the right or left lower abdomen from tension on the round ligaments. It can be very sharp and frightening and may be prevented by always rising slowly from a lying to a sitting position or from a sitting to a standing position. Keep in mind that round ligament pain may simulate the abrupt pain that occurs with ruptured ectopic pregnancy. The patient's description of the pain needs to be evaluated carefully.

As early as the 12th week of pregnancy, the uterus periodically contracts and relaxes again. These contractions, termed *Braxton Hicks contractions*, usually are not noticeable early in pregnancy. In middle and late pregnancy, the contractions become stronger, causing the patient to tense and possibly feel pain similar to a hard menstrual cramp. These feelings are normal and are not a sign of beginning labor.

Be certain the patient understands that a rhythmic pattern of contractions, characteristic of labor, should not be mistaken for Braxton Hicks contractions.

Quick quiz

1. A pregnant patient who is older than 35 years is at greater risk for having which of the following? Select all that apply.

    A. A low-birth-weight infant
    B. A preterm infant
    C. Preeclampsia
    D. Placenta previa
    E. Large-for-gestational age infant

Answer: B, C, and D. Pregnant patients who are older than 35 years are at risk for preeclampsia; placenta previa; hydatidiform mole; and vascular, neoplastic, and degenerative diseases. They are also at risk for having fraternal twins or infants with genetic abnormalities, especially Down syndrome.

2. Which of the following conditions, with familial risk factors, is most likely to cause discomfort during pregnancy?

    A. Anemia
    B. Varicose veins
    C. Cancer
    D. Colitis

Answer: B. Varicose veins are an inherited weakness in blood vessel walls that become evident during pregnancy and can cause the patient discomfort.

3. A patient has had two previous pregnancies, has had no abortions or miscarriages, delivered two full-term neonates, and is currently pregnant. Using GTPAL, you would consider this patient a:

    A. 3-2-0-2-0.
    B. 3-2-0-0-2.
    C. 2-3-0-0-2.
    D. 3-2-0-2-2.

Answer: B. This patient would be considered a 3-2-0-0-2. G is the total number of pregnancies (3). T is the number of pregnancies that end at term (38 weeks or later), which totals 2. P is for preterm, the number of pregnancies that ended after 20 weeks and before the end of 37 weeks' gestation, which is 0 for this patient. A is the number of pregnancies that ended in spontaneous or induced abortions, which is 0 for this patient. L is the number of living children.

4. Normal FHR occurs in which of the following ranges?
   A.   100 to 140 beats/min.
   B.   110 to 160 beats/min.
   C.   130 to 170 beats/min.
   D.   140 to 180 beats/min.

Answer: B. Normal FHR usually ranges from 110 to 160 beats/min.

5. A pregnant patient who is fatigued is likely to be more comfortable in which of the following positions?
   A.   Modified Sims
   B.   Supine with legs elevated
   C.   Supine with head elevated
   D.   Sitting upright with legs elevated

Answer: A. A good resting position is a modified Sims position with the top leg forward. This puts the weight of the fetus on the bed, not on the patient, and allows good circulation in the lower extremities.

Scoring

☆☆☆ If you answered all five questions correctly, wow! You've sailed through prenatal care!

☆☆ If you answered four questions correctly, great job! You have smooth seas ahead!

☆ If you answered fewer than four questions correctly, don't go overboard! Forge ahead after a quick review!

Selected References

American College of Obstetricians and Gynecologists. (2023). *Nutrition during pregnancy.* https://www.acog.org/womens-health/faqs/nutrition-during-pregnancy

American College of Obstetricians and Gynecologists. (2023). *Weight gain during pregnancy.* https://www.acog.org/clinical/clinical-guidance/committee-opinion/articles/2013/01/weight-gain-during-pregnancy

Kampmann, U., Knorr, S., Fuglsang, J., & Ovesen, P. (2019). Determinants of maternal insulin resistance during pregnancy: An updated overview. *Journal of Diabetes Research, 2019,* 5320156. https://doi.org/10.1155/2019/5320156

Lawson, G. (2020). Naegele's rule and the length of pregnancy—A review. *The Australian and New Zealand Journal of Obstetrics and Gynaecology, 61,* 177–182. https://doi.org/10.1111/ajo.13253

Smith, J. A., Fox, K. A., & Clark, S. M. (2023). *Nausea and vomiting of pregnancy: Treatment and outcome.* https://www.uptodate.com/contents/nausea-and-vomiting-of-pregnancy-treatment-and-outcome/print

U.S. Department of Agriculture. (2020). Women who are pregnant or lactating. In *Dietary guidelines for Americans 2020-2025*. https://www.dietaryguidelines.gov/resources/2020-2025-dietary-guidelines-online-materials

Who Health Organization. (2023). *Restricting caffeine intake during pregnancy*. https://www.who.int/tools/elena/interventions/caffeine-pregnancy

Yount, S., Fay, R., & Kissler, K. (2021). Prenatal and postpartum experience, knowledge and engagement with Kegels: A longitudinal, prospective, multisite study. *Journal of Women's Health, 30*, 891–901. https://doi.org/10.1089/jwh.2019.8185

Chapter 6

High-risk pregnancy

Just the facts

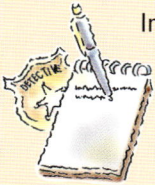

In this chapter, you'll learn:

♦ pathologic factors that contribute to a high-risk pregnancy

♦ how to identify high-risk situations based on signs and symptoms and key assessment findings

♦ appropriate treatment regimens for each complication of high-risk pregnancies

♦ relevant nursing interventions associated with each complication of high-risk pregnancies

♦ the care and needs of the childbearing patient with a high-risk pregnancy.

A look at high-risk pregnancy

Pregnancy can be a relatively normal process, but for patients who have a preexisting condition, it can have many implications. In addition, complications may occur throughout the pregnancy, from fertilization to delivery, regardless of the patient's self-care. Complications may also occur with an external factor that can impact the health and well-being of the pregnant patient or the fetus.

Keep in mind that the health of a pregnant patient and their fetus is interdependent. Changes in the patient's health may affect fetal health, and changes in fetal health may affect the pregnant patient's physical and emotional health.

Age

Reproductive risks increase among adolescents younger than 15 years and patients older than 35 years. Adolescent patients are at risk for increased incidence of intrauterine growth restriction (IUGR), preterm labor, anemia, labor dysfunction, cephalopelvic disproportion, cesarean birth, preeclampsia, and gestational hypertension. Pregnant patients older than 35 years are at risk for placenta previa, cesarean birth, stillbirth, preterm birth, or gestational hypertension and diabetes. Additionally, they are at risk for having fraternal twins or infants with genetic abnormalities, especially Down syndrome.

Current obstetric status

Current obstetric status can also place a patient at high risk for complications. The following factors may place the patient at high risk:

- Inadequate prenatal care
- Intrauterine growth–restricted fetus
- Large-for-gestational-age fetus
- Gestational hypertension, preeclampsia, eclampsia, HELLP (hemolysis, elevated liver enzyme, and low platelets)
- Abnormal fetal surveillance tests
- Hydramnios
- Placenta previa
- Abnormal presentation
- Maternal anemia
- Weight gain of less than 10 lb (4.5 kg)
- Weight loss of more than 5 lb (2.3 kg)
- Overweight or underweight status
- Fetal or placental malformation
- Rh sensitization
- Preterm labor
- Multiple gestation
- Premature rupture of membranes (PROM)
- Abruptio placentae (placental abruption)
- Postdate pregnancy
- Fibroid tumors
- Fetal manipulation
- Cervical cerclage (purse-string suture placed around incompetent cervix to prevent premature opening and subsequent spontaneous abortion)
- Sexually transmitted infections (STIs)
- Maternal infection
- Poor immunization status

Obstetric and gynecologic history

Many factors in the pregnant patient's obstetric and gynecologic history can place a pregnancy at high risk. These factors may include:

- grand multiparity (five or more births after 20 weeks' gestation)
- previous preterm labor or preterm birth
- previous low-birth-weight infant
- one or more stillbirths at term
- one or more neonates born with gross anomalies, neurologic deficit, or birth injury
- pelvic inadequacy or abnormal shaping
- last delivery less than 1 year before conception
- uterine or cervical incompetency, position, or structural anomalies
- history of infertility
- history of multiple pregnancy, placental anomalies, amniotic fluid abnormalities, or poor weight gain
- history of gestational diabetes, gestational hypertension, or infection
- history of delivering a postterm or macrosomic infant
- history of dystocia or prolonged labor, precipitous delivery, cervical or vaginal lacerations caused by labor and delivery, previous forceps delivery, cephalopelvic disproportion, hemorrhage during labor and delivery, retained placenta, or previous cesarean birth
- lack of previous prenatal care
- previous ectopic pregnancy
- previous multiple gestation
- previous hydatidiform mole or choriocarcinoma.

In addition, a pregnancy that occurs within 3 years of menarche indicates an increased risk of maternal mortality and morbidity and places the patient at risk for delivering a neonate who is small for gestational age.

Medical history

Carefully assessing the patient's medical, gynecologic, and obstetric history is necessary to determine any risk factors associated with the current pregnancy. A medical history of the following may pose a threat to the patient or fetal well-being:
- Cardiac disease
- Metabolic disease
- Kidney disease
- Recent urinary tract infection (UTI) or bacteriuria
- Gastrointestinal (GI) disorders
- Seizure disorders
- Family history of severe inherited disorders
- Surgery during current pregnancy
- Psychiatric/emotional disorders or intellectual disability

- Previous surgeries, particularly those involving the reproductive organs
- Pulmonary disease
- Endocrine disorders
- Hemoglobinopathies
- STI
- Chronic hypertension or history of gestational hypertension
- History of abnormal Papanicolaou smear
- Malignancy
- Reproductive tract anomalies.

Insulin influx

Diabetes can worsen during pregnancy and harm the pregnant patient and fetus. Pregnant patients typically develop insulin resistance and those with diabetes need increased amounts of insulin during pregnancy. The fetus of a patient with diabetes tends to be large, or macrosomic, because insulin production increases to counteract the overload of glucose and stimulates fetal growth. This, in turn, can lead to problems of cephalopelvic disproportion and dystocia and puts the pregnant patient at risk for postpartum hemorrhage. The newborn is also at risk for traumatic injuries, such as shoulder dystocia, which can lead to brachial plexus injury or a broken clavicle.

Gravida aggravations

Stomach displacement by the gravid uterus, along with cardiac sphincter relaxation and decreased GI motility caused by increased progesterone, may aggravate symptoms of peptic ulcer disease, such as gastric reflux. Also, the increase in blood volume and cardiac output associated with pregnancy can exhaust a patient with underlying cardiac disease.

Lifestyle

Psychosocial and lifestyle factors also need to be considered and can have a negative effect on the current pregnancy. Some psychosocial factors are:

- social factors (e.g., low socioeconomic status; low formal education level)
- inadequate nutrition or food insecurity
- more than two children at home with no additional support
- lack of acceptance of pregnancy

- substandard housing or unstable housing
- race, ethnicity, and cultural background (Black or Native American people have increased risk of maternal mortality, sickle cell anemia occurs primarily in people of African and Mediterranean descent, and Tay-Sachs disease is about 100 times more common in people of Eastern European Jewish [Ashkenazi] ancestry than in the general population.)
- occupation (may give an idea of environmental exposure hazards and insurance coverage)
- inadequate support systems.

Meanwhile, some lifestyle factors that can negatively affect a patient's pregnancy are:

- smoking or vaping
- long commute to work
- refusal to use seat belts
- high-risk exposure at work environment
- heavy lifting or long periods of standing
- lack of smoke and carbon monoxide detectors in the home.

Make the patient aware that what they consume and are exposed to can seriously affect their pregnancy. For example, taking some over-the-counter (OTC) and prescription medications can be detrimental to the fetus. In addition, smoking cigarettes is associated with IUGR and low-birth-weight neonates. Exposure to toxic substances, such as lead, organic solvents, radiation, and carbon monoxide, can also lead to fetal malformations.

Substance misuse

Alcohol and substance misuse is another cause of fetal anomalies. Substance misuse may interfere with the pregnant patient's ability to obtain adequate nutrition, which can adversely affect fetal growth. After birth, the neonate may experience withdrawal. Additionally, if the substance misuse involves injection, the pregnant patient is at risk for infection with hepatitis B and human immunodeficiency virus (HIV).

Nourish to flourish

Adequate nutrition is vital during pregnancy. Inadequate nutrition can lead to a deficiency of iron, folic acid, or protein. Iron-deficiency anemia during pregnancy is associated with low fetal birth weight and preterm birth. Folic acid deficiency is associated with neural tube defects. Protein deficiency can lead to poor fetal development and growth restriction.

Family history

Certain conditions and disorders that contribute to high-risk pregnancy are familial. For example, a family history of multiple births, congenital diseases or deformities, or mental disability may place a pregnancy at higher risk.

Don't forget!

Some fetal congenital anomalies may be traced to the non-birthing parent's exposure to environmental hazards. Blood type and Rh status are also important because isoimmunization in the fetus may occur if the non-birthing parent is Rh-positive, the birthing parent is Rh-negative, and the fetus is Rh-positive.

On the home front

The family environment is also important in determining whether a pregnancy is high risk. A history of domestic violence, a lack of support people, inadequate housing, social issues, single parenting, minority status, psychiatric history, or lack of adequate finances can increase risk during pregnancy.

Abruptio placentae (placental abruption)

Placental abruption, or premature separation of the placenta, occurs when a normally implanted placenta detaches from the uterine wall prematurely, typically seen after 20 weeks' gestation. Placental abruption is an obstetric emergency as it can result in severe hemorrhage or maternal or fetal death. Hemorrhage is a leading cause of perinatal mortality in the world.

What causes it

The cause of placental abruption is unknown. Predisposing factors include:
- traumatic injury such as a direct blow to the uterus (domestic violence or injury)
- placental site bleeding caused by a needle puncture during amniocentesis
- chronic hypertension or gestational hypertension, which raises pressure on the patient's side of the placenta
- multiparity (more than five)
- short umbilical cord
- dietary deficiency

- smoking
- cocaine use
- preterm premature rupture of membranes (PPROM)
- pressure on the vena cava from an enlarged uterus. (See *Understanding placental abruption.*)

Understanding placental abruption

With placental abruption, lack of resiliency or abnormal changes in the uterine vasculature cause blood vessels at the placental bed to rupture spontaneously. Hypertension and an enlarged uterus that cannot contract sufficiently to seal off the torn blood vessels further complicate the situation. As a result, bleeding continues unchecked, potentially shearing off part of or the entire placenta.

External versus internal

About 80% of bleeding is external (marginal), meaning that a peripheral portion of the placenta separates from the uterine wall. The bleeding is internal (concealed) if the central portion of the placenta becomes detached and the still intact peripheral portions trap the blood. This occurs in about 20% of cases.

Effects of bleeding

As blood enters the muscle fibers, detached and still intact peripheral portions of the placenta trap the blood. Complete relaxation of the uterus becomes impossible. Uterine tone and irritability increase. If bleeding into the muscle fibers is profuse, the uterus turns blue or purple and the accumulated blood prevents its normal contractions after delivery (known as *Couvelaire uterus* or *uteroplacental apoplexy*).

What to look for

Placental abruption produces a wide range of signs and symptoms, such as sudden and forceful severe and steady pain; hard, board-like abdomen; and external or concealed dark red blood. Fetal heart tones may be present with or without abnormalities, or absent; and cervical dilation may occur very rapidly. In addition to the major complications of placental abruption—hemorrhage and hemorrhagic shock—it may also cause kidney failure, postpartum pituitary necrosis (Sheehan syndrome), disseminated intravascular coagulation (DIC), and death of the pregnant patient or fetus.

Three degrees of separation

Three degrees of separation can occur with placental abruption:
1. *Mild* placental abruption (marginal separation) develops gradually and produces mild to moderate bleeding, vague lower abdominal

discomfort, mild to moderate abdominal tenderness, and uterine irritability. Fetal heart tones often remain strong and regular.

2. *Moderate* placental abruption (about 50% placental separation) may develop gradually or abruptly and produces continuous abdominal pain, moderate dark red vaginal bleeding, a tender uterus that remains firm between contractions, barely audible or irregular and bradycardic fetal heart tones, and, possibly, signs of shock. Labor typically starts within 2 hours and usually proceeds rapidly.

3. *Severe* placental abruption (70% placental separation) develops abruptly and causes agonizing, unremitting uterine pain (described as tearing or knifelike); a boardlike, tender uterus; moderate vaginal bleeding; rapidly progressive shock; and absence of fetal heart tones (related to fetal cardiac distress). (See *Placental separation in placental abruption.*)

Placental separation in placental abruption

Here are descriptions and illustrations of the three degrees of placental separation in placental abruption.

Mild separation

Mild separation begins with small areas of separation and internal bleeding (concealed hemorrhage) between the placenta and uterine wall.

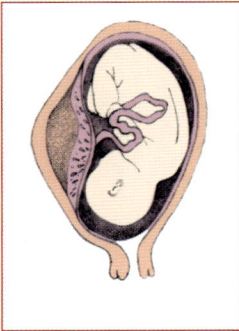

Moderate separation

Moderate separation may develop abruptly or progress from mild to extensive separation with external hemorrhage.

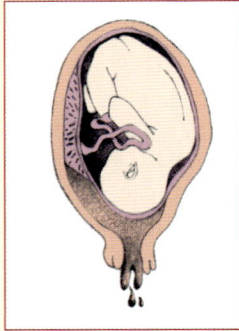

Severe separation

With severe separation, external hemorrhage occurs, along with shock and, possibly, fetal cardiac distress.

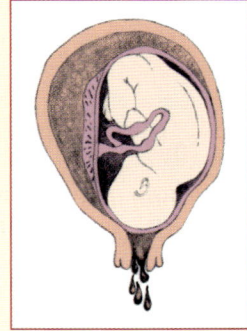

What tests tell you

Vaginal examination (in preparation for emergency cesarean birth) and ultrasonography are performed to rule out placenta previa. Decreased hemoglobin levels and platelet counts support the diagnosis. Periodic assays for fibrin split products aid in monitoring the progression of placental abruption and in detecting DIC. Differential diagnosis excludes placenta previa, ovarian cysts, appendicitis, and degeneration of leiomyomas.

How it's treated

Treatment of placental abruption focuses on assessing, controlling, and restoring the amount of blood lost, delivering a viable neonate, and preventing coagulation disorders.

First things first!

Immediate measures for treatment of placental abruption include:

- starting an intravenous (IV) infusion (through a large-bore catheter) of lactated Ringer solution to combat hypovolemia
- placing a central venous pressure (CVP) line and urinary catheter to monitor fluid status
- drawing blood for hemoglobin level, hematocrit, coagulation studies, and typing and cross-matching
- performing external electronic fetal monitoring and monitoring of patient's vital signs and vaginal bleeding
- administering blood replacement as necessary.

Delivery details

After the severity of placental abruption has been determined and fluid and blood have been replaced, prompt cesarean birth is necessary if the fetus is in distress or if heavy bleeding continues. If the fetus is not in distress, monitoring continues.

Because of possible fetal blood loss through the placenta, a neonatal team should be ready at delivery to assess and treat the neonate for shock, blood loss, and hypoxia. If placental separation is severe and no signs of fetal life are present, vaginal delivery may be performed unless it is contraindicated by uncontrolled hemorrhage or other complications.

What to do

- Assess the patient's extent of bleeding and monitor fundal height every 30 minutes for changes. Count the number of perineal pads used, weighing them as needed to determine the amount of blood loss.
- Monitor the patient's blood pressure, pulse rate, respirations, CVP, intake and output every 10 to 15 minutes.
- Begin electronic fetal monitoring to assess fetal heart rate (FHR) continuously.
- Have equipment for emergency cesarean birth readily available.

- If vaginal delivery is elected, provide emotional support during labor. Because of the neonate's prematurity, the pregnant patient may not receive analgesic agents during labor and may experience intense pain. Reassure the patient of their progress through labor and keep them informed of the fetus' condition.
- Prepare the patient and their family for the possibility of an emergency cesarean birth and the changes to expect in the postpartum period. Offer emotional support and an honest assessment of the situation.
- Tactfully discuss the possibility of neonatal death. Tell the pregnant patient that the neonate's survival depends primarily on gestational age, the amount of blood lost, and associated hypertensive disorders. Assure them that frequent monitoring and prompt management greatly reduce the risk of death.
- Encourage the patient and their family to verbalize their feelings.
- Help the patient and their family develop effective coping strategies. Refer them for counseling if necessary.

Cardiac disease

A pregnant patient with preexisting cardiac disease is considered high risk. Despite improvements in early identification and management of cardiac problems, these disorders contribute to complications in approximately 1% to 4% of pregnancies.

Rating the risk

The World Health Organization (WHO) has developed a modified risk classification of cardiovascular risk in pregnant patients.
- I: No identifiable elevated risk of morbidity or mortality in the pregnant patient
- II: Mildly elevated mortality and moderate elevation of morbidity for the pregnant patient
- III: Substantially elevated risk in mortality and severe elevation of morbidity for the pregnant patient. It is recommended that close follow-up be initiated with cardiac specialists. Cardiac monitoring should continue regularly throughout (and also after) pregnancy.
- IV: Extremely elevated risk of mortality and severe elevation of morbidity for the pregnant patient. Pregnancy is contraindicated. If the patient chooses to pursue pregnancy, they should be monitored closely as class III people.

What causes it

Some common cardiovascular diseases are cardiomyopathy, coronary artery disease, pregnancy-associated myocardial infarction, and valvular disease.

What to look for

Signs and symptoms of cardiac disease in a pregnant patient depend on the type and severity of the underlying disease. Primarily, these signs and symptoms are those associated with heart failure. (See *The weaker weeks*.) Fetal signs of maternal cardiac disease are nonspecific—such as abnormally low FHR and fetal growth retardation—so diagnosis depends mainly on the patient's signs and symptoms.

The weaker weeks

The most dangerous time for a pregnant patient with cardiac disease and their fetus is between weeks 28 and 32 of gestation. During this time, blood volume peaks and the patient's heart may be unable to compensate adequately for the increase. As a result, cardiac decompensation can occur, causing the patient's cardiac output to drop, possibly to such an extent that perfusion to vital organs, including the placenta, is significantly affected. Consequently, oxygen and nutrients are not delivered in adequate amounts to the cells, including those of the fetus.

What tests tell you

An electrocardiogram (ECG) may show cardiac changes in the patient but may be less accurate later in pregnancy as the enlarged uterus pushes the diaphragm upward and displaces the heart. Echocardiography can show cardiomegaly, hemodynamic changes, biventricular function, valve function, and the presence or absence of pulmonary hypertension. If the patient's cardiac decompensation has reached the point of placental insufficiency and incompetency, late decelerations during fetal monitoring may indicate fetal distress. Ultrasonography of the fetus may show growth retardation.

How it's treated

Treatment focuses on ensuring the health and safety of the pregnant patient and fetus. Commonly, more frequent prenatal visits are scheduled, such as every 2 weeks and then every week during the last month. Additionally, the pregnant patient may also see a maternal–fetal medicine specialist who specializes in closer management and monitoring of patients with complicated pregnancies.

Minor adjustments

If the patient was taking cardiac medications before becoming pregnant, the medications are typically continued during pregnancy. However, maintenance doses may need to be increased to aid in compensating for the increased blood volume associated with pregnancy.

The deal with other drugs

If the patient required digoxin (Lanoxin) before pregnancy, they can continue to use it during pregnancy with minimal risk. Even if the patient was not taking digoxin before pregnancy, they may require it to help increase or strengthen cardiac output as the pregnancy advances. The effects on pregnancy of propranolol (Inderal), a beta-adrenergic blocker commonly used for cardiac dysrhythmia, are not known. However, the medication does not appear to cause fetal abnormalities. The effects of nitroglycerin (NitroQuick), a compound commonly prescribed for angina, are also unknown. However, the medication appears to be safe. A patient who is taking heparin for venous thromboembolic disease should not take any after labor begins. If the patient has had a valve replacement and is receiving warfarin (Coumadin) therapy, warfarin—which is associated with an increase in fetal anomalies—is discontinued and heparin is used instead.

Prophylactic tactics

For patients with valvular or congenital cardiac disease, some health care providers may begin prophylactic antibiotic therapy near to the expected due date to prevent the development of possible subacute bacterial endocarditis secondary to bacterial invasion from the placental site into the bloodstream, although the American College of Cardiology (ACC) and the American Heart Association (AHA) are not recommending prophylactic antibiotics routinely if having an uncomplicated vaginal or cesarean birth. Antibiotics are optional and should be based on specific and individual risk factors and type of delivery. If the patient was taking prophylactic antibiotics to prevent a recurrence of rheumatic fever before becoming pregnant, the antibiotics are continued during pregnancy.

Rest for the weary

Another key area of treatment is rest. A pregnant patient with cardiac disease requires more rest than the average pregnant patient. In addition, health care providers commonly recommend complete bed rest for the patient after gestational week 30 to ensure the fetus is carried to term or at least to week 36.

A weighty subject

Maintaining good nutrition is an important component of ensuring a healthy pregnant patient and fetus. For the patient with cardiac disease, it is especially important that weight gain be balanced to ensure that the nutritional needs of the patient and fetus are met while also ensuring that the patient's heart is not overburdened. As a general practice, salt intake may be limited. However, it should not be severely restricted because sodium is needed for fluid volume. Prenatal vitamins are essential to help ensure adequate iron intake and avoid anemia, which reduces the blood's capacity to carry oxygen. The pregnant patient with cardiac disease and their fetus need as much oxygen as possible, so anemia must be avoided.

What to do

- Assess the patient's vital signs and cardiopulmonary status closely for changes. Ask the patient about increased shortness of breath, palpitations, or edema. Monitor FHR for changes.
- Monitor weight gain throughout pregnancy. Assess for edema and note any pitting.
- Explain signs and symptoms of worsening disease and tell the patient to report them immediately.
- Reinforce use of prescribed medications to control cardiac disease. Explain possible adverse reactions to these medications and instruct the patient to report these reactions immediately.
- Anticipate the need for increased doses of maintenance medications. Explain to the patient the rationale for this increase.
- Assess the patient's nutritional pattern. Work with them to develop a feasible meal plan. Stress the need for prenatal vitamins.
- Assess FHR and ultrasound results to monitor fetal growth.
- Encourage frequent rest periods throughout the day. Discuss measures for pacing activities and conserving energy.
- Advise the patient to immediately report signs and symptoms of infection, such as upper respiratory infection or UTI, to prevent overtaxing the heart.
- Advise the patient to rest in the left lateral recumbent position to prevent supine hypotension and provide the best possible oxygen exchange to the fetus. If necessary, use semi-Fowler position to relieve dyspnea.

- Prepare the patient for labor, anticipating the use of epidural anesthesia to avoid overtaxing the patient's heart.
- Monitor FHR, uterine contractions, and the patient's vital signs closely for changes during labor.
- Assess vital signs closely after delivery. Anticipate anticoagulant and cardiac glycoside therapy immediately after delivery for the patient with severe heart failure.
- Encourage ambulation, as ordered, as soon as possible after delivery.
- Anticipate administration of prophylactic antibiotics, if not already ordered, after delivery to prevent subacute bacterial endocarditis.

Diabetes

Diabetes is a metabolic disorder characterized by hyperglycemia (elevated serum glucose level) resulting from lack of insulin, lack of insulin effect, or both. It is a disorder of carbohydrate, protein, and fat metabolism.

Three general classifications are recognized:

1. *Type 1 diabetes* is characterized by absolute insulin insufficiency. The patient requires exogenous insulin and dietary management to achieve control of their diabetes.
2. *Type 2 diabetes* is characterized by insulin resistance with varying degrees of insulin secretory defects. It is treated with diet and exercise in combination with various antidiabetic medications. Treatment may also include insulin therapy.
3. *Gestational diabetes* (diabetes that emerges during pregnancy) typically develops during the middle of the pregnancy when insulin resistance is most apparent.

Losing balance

Diabetes may affect up to 18% of all pregnancies in the United States. The overall challenge associated with diabetes and pregnancy is controlling the balance between glucose levels and insulin requirements. Inadequate glucose control can adversely affect the pregnant patient, the fetus, or both. Moreover, continued fetal consumption of glucose may lead to hypoglycemia in the pregnant patient, especially between meals and during the night. Additionally, polyhydramnios (increased amount of amniotic fluid) may occur because of increased fetal urine production caused by fetal hyperglycemia.

Neonates who are born to patients with poorly controlled diabetes typically are large, or macrosomic, possibly more than 10 lb (4.5 kg).

This large size may complicate labor and delivery, resulting in labor dystocia, shoulder dystocia, or necessitating a cesarean birth. The risks of spontaneous abortions and stillbirths also increase in patients with diabetes that is not well controlled.

What causes it

Evidence indicates that diabetes has various causes, including:
- heredity
- environment (infection, diet, exposure to toxins, and stress)
- lifestyle in genetically susceptible people.

It's all relative

Although the cause of type 1 diabetes is not known, scientists believe that the tendency to develop diabetes may be inherited and related to exposure to viruses. In people with a possible genetic predisposition to type 1 diabetes, a triggering event (possibly infection with a virus) spurs the production of autoantibodies that destroy the pancreas' beta cells. The destruction of beta cells causes insulin secretion to decrease or ultimately stop. When more than 90% of the beta cells have been destroyed, the subsequent insulin deficiency leads to hyperglycemia, enhanced lipolysis (decomposition of fat), and protein catabolism.

Impaired, inappropriate . . .

Type 2 diabetes is a chronic disease caused by one or more of these factors:
- Impaired insulin production
- Inappropriate hepatic glucose production
- Peripheral insulin receptor insensitivity
- History of gestational diabetes
- Stress

. . . and intolerant

Gestational diabetes occurs when a patient who has not been previously diagnosed with diabetes shows glucose intolerance during pregnancy. Of those patients who do not have diabetes when they become pregnant, approximately 2% to 10% develop gestational diabetes. It is not known whether gestational diabetes results in a combination of hormonal changes, weight gain, and insulin resistance. Identifiable risk factors include:
- having a history of gestational diabetes during a previous pregnancy
- obesity

- race and ethnicity (Black, Hispanic or Latino, American Indian, Alaska Native, Native Hawaiian, Pacific Islander)
- hypertension
- history of delivering large neonates (usually more than 9 lb), unexplained fetal or perinatal loss, or evidence of congenital anomalies in previous pregnancies
- age older than 25 years
- family history of type 2 diabetes
- personal history of polycystic ovarian syndrome (PCOS).

What to look for

The signs and symptoms noted in the pregnant patient with diabetes are the same as those for any person with diabetes. Common signs and symptoms include hyperglycemia, glycosuria, and polyuria. Dizziness and confusion may be related to hyperglycemia. In addition, the patient may experience an increased incidence of monilial infections. Hydramnios may be present along with poor FHR and variability arising from inadequate tissue (placental) perfusion.

The patient with type 1 or 2 diabetes may also exhibit signs and symptoms related to microvascular and macrovascular changes, such as peripheral vascular disease, retinopathy, nephropathy, and neuropathy.

What tests tell you

All patients are screened for gestational diabetes during pregnancy with a glucola screen. Testing typically occurs between weeks 24 and 28, when the diabetic hormones are influencing insulin performance, and may be repeated at week 32 if the patient is obese or older than 40 years. If the patient has risk factors for gestational diabetes, this screening takes place at the first prenatal visit and again between weeks 24 and 28.

The glucose challenge

The glucola screen involves an oral glucose challenge test (a test that obtains a fasting plasma glucose level) using a 50-g glucose solution (glucola). One hour after ingestion, a venous blood sample is obtained. If the glucose level is greater than 140 mg/dL, the patient is scheduled for a 3-hour fasting glucose tolerance test using a 100-g glucose load. A fasting plasma glucose as well as plasma glucose at 1-, 2-, and 3-hour intervals after ingestion of the glucose solution is measured. (See *Glucose challenge values in pregnancy*.)

Glucose challenge values in pregnancy

Here are normal values for pregnant patients taking the oral glucose challenge test to determine risk of diabetes. These values are determined after a 100-g glucose load. Normal blood glucose levels should remain between 90 and 120 mg/dL. If a pregnant person's plasma glucose value exceeds these levels, they should be treated as a potential patient with diabetes.

Test type	Pregnancy glucose level (mg/dL)
Fasting	95
1 hour	180
2 hours	155
3 hours	140

If the patient is known to have diabetes, serial blood glucose monitoring and measurement of glycosylated hemoglobin (HgbA1C) levels are used to determine the degree of glucose control.

How it's treated

Any patient with diabetes, whether preexisting or gestational, requires more frequent prenatal visits to ensure optimal control of glucose levels, minimizing the risks to the pregnant patient and the fetus. Additionally, treatment focuses on balancing rest with exercise and maintaining adequate nutrition for fetal growth and strict control of blood glucose levels.

Ideally, patients with preexisting diabetes should consult with their health care provider before becoming pregnant to ensure the best possible health for themselves and their fetus. At that time, blood glucose levels can be assessed closely, and medication adjustments can be made to ensure optimal regulation before they become pregnant.

Crucial calories

Nutritional therapy is crucial in the treatment of patients with diabetes. Typically, a 1,800- to 2,200-calorie diet is prescribed for pregnant patients with diabetes. Alternatively, caloric requirements may be calculated at 30 to 35 kcal/kg of ideal body weight. The caloric requirement is usually divided among three meals and three snacks, allowing the calories to be distributed throughout the day in an attempt to maintain constant glucose levels.

Additional dietary recommendations include reduced saturated fat and cholesterol and increased dietary fiber. Carbohydrates should make up 40% to 45% of daily caloric intake, with protein at 20% to 25%, and fat at 35% to 40% with mostly monounsaturated and polyunsaturated fats. The goal is to allow a weight gain of approximately 25 to 35 lb (11.3 to 15.9 kg) for those with a normal prepregnancy weight, 15 to 25 lb (6.8 to 11.3 kg) for patients who are overweight, 28 to 40 lb (12.7 to 18.2 kg) for patients who are underweight, and 11 to 20 lb (5 to 9.1 kg) for patients who are obese. This way, the neonate does not grow too large and vaginal delivery remains a possibility. Furthermore, patients with diabetes should engage in 30 minutes of moderate-intensity aerobic exercise 5 days a week.

Adjust, reduce, increase

For the patient with preexisting diabetes, insulin adjustments are necessary. Early in pregnancy, insulin may be reduced because of the increased use of glucose by the fetus for growth. However, later in pregnancy, an increase in insulin typically occurs because of an increase in the patient's metabolism. Insulin therapy dosages and types are highly individualized. A continuous subcutaneous insulin infusion via a pump may be ordered to maintain constant blood glucose levels. The patient with gestational diabetes may require insulin if diet therapy does not adequately control blood glucose levels.

Check 1: Glucose levels

To assist with blood glucose control, fingerstick blood glucose monitoring is important. For the patient with preexisting diabetes, typically this monitoring is performed daily, possibly as often as four times per day. For patients with gestational diabetes, however, blood glucose monitoring may be performed only weekly. Regardless of monitoring frequency, the goal is to obtain fasting blood glucose levels below 95 mg/dL and 2-hour postprandial values below 120 mg/dL and below 140 mg/dL at 1 hour.

Check 2: Eyes and urinary tract

Follow-up monitoring is performed throughout the pregnancy. A urine culture may be done each trimester to detect UTIs that produce no symptoms. Ophthalmic examination is done at each trimester for the patient with preexisting diabetes and at least once during pregnancy for the patient with gestational diabetes. Retinal changes may develop or progress during pregnancy.

Check 3: The fetus

Because the risk of fetal complications is high, fetal monitoring is crucial. A serum alpha-fetoprotein (AFP) level may be done at 15 to 17 weeks' gestation to assess for neural tube defects. Ultrasonography may be done at 18 to 20 weeks to detect gross abnormalities, and then be repeated at 28 weeks and again at 36 to 38 weeks to determine fetal growth, amniotic fluid volume, placental location, and biparietal diameter. Starting at 32 to 34 weeks of gestation (or earlier if there is a presence of other comorbidities), the patient will be under close antepartum surveillance to assess fetal well-being where they will undergo fetal nonstress tests (NSTs) and biophysical profiles (BPPs).

Preferred delivery route

Early delivery prior to 39 to 40 weeks' gestation for patients with gestational diabetes mellitus (GDM) is not indicated unless the patient's GDM is not adequately controlled. Additionally, vaginal delivery has become the preferred route of delivery. During labor, uterine contractions and FHR are monitored continuously. The patient's glucose level is regulated with IV infusions of regular insulin based on blood glucose levels that are obtained hourly.

What to do

- Carefully monitor the patient's weight gain, blood glucose levels, and nutritional intake as well as fetal growth parameters throughout pregnancy.
- Review results of fingerstick blood glucose monitoring.
- Assess for signs and symptoms of hypoglycemia and hyperglycemia.
- Assist with scheduling of follow-up laboratory studies, including HgbA1C levels and urine studies as necessary.
- Encourage the patient to maintain a consistent exercise program and explain the benefits of eating snacks consisting of protein or complex carbohydrates before exercise. This may help prevent hypoglycemia during exercise.
- Instruct the patient in all aspects of managing diabetes, including insulin administration techniques, self-monitoring, nutrition, and danger signs and symptoms. (See *Teaching topics for pregnant patients with diabetes.*)

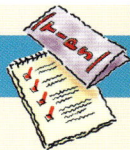

Teaching topics for pregnant patients with diabetes

Be sure to cover the following topics when teaching a pregnant patient with diabetes:
- Insulin type and dosage
- Insulin syringe preparation and injection technique or insulin pump use and care
- Sites to use (Most patients prefer not to use the abdomen as an injection site.)
- Site rotation (Insulin is absorbed more slowly from the thigh than from the upper arm.)
- Blood glucose monitoring technique, including frequency of monitoring and desired glucose levels
- Nutritional plan, including suggestions for appropriate foods to include and avoid
- Consistent exercise regimen
- Signs and symptoms of urinary tract and monilial infections, including the need to report one immediately
- Signs and symptoms of hypoglycemia and hyperglycemia
- Measures to prevent and manage hypoglycemia and hyperglycemia
- Fetal monitoring methods, including fetal movement count and follow-up testing
- Preparations for labor and delivery
- Care after delivery

- Arrange for a consult with a dietitian.
- Assist with preparations for labor, including explanations about possible labor induction and required monitoring.
- Closely assess the patient in the postpartum period for changes in blood glucose levels and insulin requirements. Typically, the patient with preexisting diabetes will require no insulin in the immediate postpartum period (because insulin resistance is gone) and will not return to the prepregnancy insulin requirements for several days. The patient with gestational diabetes usually exhibits normal blood glucose levels within 24 hours after delivery, requiring no further insulin or diet therapy.
- Encourage the patient with gestational diabetes to keep all follow-up appointments so that glucose testing can be performed to detect possible type 2 diabetes.

Gestational hypertension

Gestational hypertension, previously called *pregnancy-induced hypertension*, is a potentially life-threatening disorder that typically develops after 20 weeks' gestation in a previously normotensive pregnant patient. It occurs most commonly in nulliparous patients. Currently, gestational hypertension is one of the most common causes of maternal and fetal death in developed countries.

To seize or not to seize

Preeclampsia, the nonconvulsive form of the disorder, is marked by the onset of hypertension after 20 weeks' gestation with the presence of proteinuria or thrombocytopenia, pulmonary edema, impaired lived function, or new-onset headache that does not respond to medication. It develops in about 7% of pregnancies and may be mild or severe. The incidence is significantly higher in patients from low socioeconomic groups. Eclampsia, the convulsive form, often occurs between 24 weeks' gestation and the end of the first postpartum week. The incidence increases among nulliparous patients, patients with multiple pregnancy, and those with a history of vascular disease.

About 5% of those with preeclampsia develop eclampsia, which is the onset of seizures that can end in a coma. Of these 5%, about 15% die of eclampsia or its complications. The incidence of fetal mortality is high because of the increased incidence of premature delivery.

Complicating the situation

Generalized arteriolar vasoconstriction associated with gestational hypertension is thought to produce decreased blood flow through the placenta and the patient's organs. This can result in IUGR, placental infarcts, and placental abruption. HELLP syndrome is associated with severe preeclampsia. Other possible complications include stillbirth of the neonate, seizures, coma, premature labor, kidney failure, and hepatic damage in the patient.

What causes it

Hypertensive disorders are one of the most common complications of pregnancy. Although the exact cause of gestational hypertension is unknown, systemic peripheral vasospasm occurs and affects every organ system. (See *Changes associated with gestational hypertension.*)

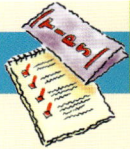

Changes associated with gestational hypertension

This flowchart illustrates the physiologic effects of gestational hypertension on the pregnant patient's body.

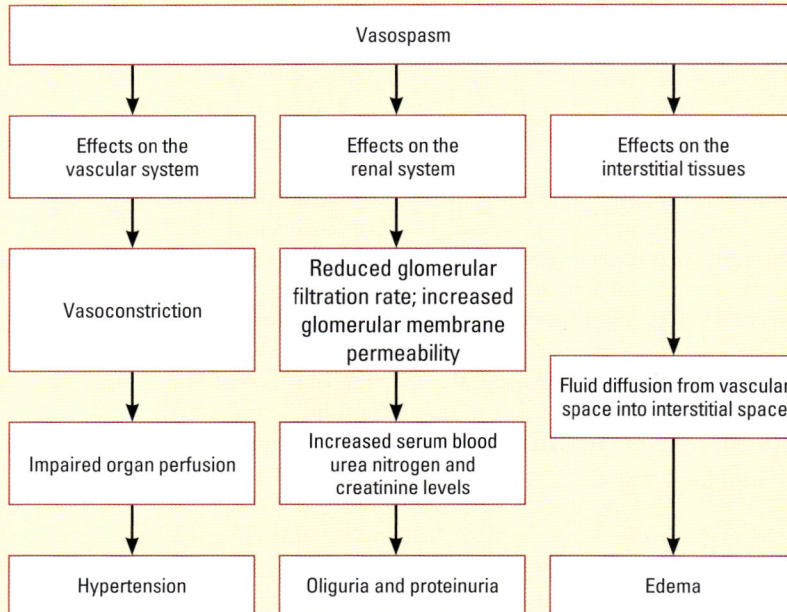

```
                              Vasospasm
        │                         │                         │
        ▼                         ▼                         ▼
  Effects on the          Effects on the            Effects on the
  vascular system         renal system              interstitial tissues
        │                         │                         │
        ▼                         ▼                         │
                         Reduced glomerular                 │
   Vasoconstriction      filtration rate; increased         │
                         glomerular membrane                │
                         permeability                       │
        │                         │                         ▼
        ▼                         │               Fluid diffusion from vascular
                                  │               space into interstitial space
 Impaired organ perfusion  Increased serum blood          │
                           urea nitrogen and               │
                           creatinine levels               │
        │                         │                         │
        ▼                         ▼                         ▼
    Hypertension        Oliguria and proteinuria          Edema
```

Geographic, ethnic, racial, nutritional, immunologic, and familial factors may contribute to preexisting vascular disease that, in turn, may contribute to the disorder's occurrence. Age is also a factor. Adolescents and primiparas older than 35 years are at higher risk for preeclampsia.

Other possible causes include potential toxic sources (such as autolysis of placental infarcts), autointoxication, uremia, sensitization to total proteins, and pyelonephritis.

What to look for

The classic triad of symptoms in preeclampsia is hypertension, proteinuria, and edema. A patient with mild preeclampsia typically reports a sudden weight gain of more than 3 lb (1.4 kg) per week in the second trimester or more than 1 lb (0.5 kg) per week during the third trimester. The patient's history reveals hypertension, as evidenced by high blood pressure readings (140 mm Hg or more systolic, or an increase of 30 mm Hg or more above the patient's normal systolic pressure, measured on two occasions, 6 hours apart; and 90 mm Hg or more diastolic, or an increase of 15 mm Hg or more above the patient's normal diastolic pressure, measured on two occasions, 6 hours apart). Further examination may reveal generalized edema, especially of the face. Palpation may reveal pitting edema of the legs and feet. Deep tendon reflexes may indicate hyperreflexia.

As preeclampsia worsens, the patient may demonstrate oliguria (urine output of 400 mL/day or less), blurred vision caused by retinal arteriolar spasms, epigastric pain or heartburn, irritability, and emotional tension. They may also complain of a severe frontal headache.

Pressure, spasm, hemorrhage—oh my!

In severe preeclampsia, blood pressure readings increase to 160/110 mm Hg or higher on two occasions, 6 hours apart, during bed rest. Ophthalmoscopic examination may reveal vascular spasm, papilledema, retinal edema or detachment, and arteriovenous nicking or hemorrhage.

Enter eclampsia

The onset of seizures signifies eclampsia. The patient with eclampsia may appear to cease breathing, then suddenly take a deep, gasping breath and resume breathing. The patient may then lapse into a coma, lasting a few minutes to several hours. When waking from the coma, the patient may have no memory of the seizure. Mild eclampsia may involve more than one seizure; severe eclampsia, up to 20 seizures.

Kicked up a notch

In eclampsia, physical examination findings are similar to those in preeclampsia but more severe. Systolic blood pressure may increase to 180 mm Hg or even to 200 mm Hg. Marked edema may be present. Some patients, however, do not show visible signs of edema.

What tests tell you

A differential diagnosis is used to distinguish the disorder from viral hepatitis, idiopathic thrombocytopenia, cholecystitis, hemolytic uremic syndrome, peptic ulcer, appendicitis, renal calculi, pyelonephritis, and gastroenteritis. Laboratory test findings reveal proteinuria (more than 300 mg/24 hours [1+] with preeclampsia and 5 g/24 hours [5+] or more with severe eclampsia). Test results may also suggest HELLP syndrome. Additionally, ultrasonography, stress tests and NSTs, and BPPs are used to evaluate fetal well-being.

How it's treated

Prevention strategies such as adequate nutrition, good prenatal care, and control of preexisting hypertension during pregnancy help decrease the incidence and severity of preeclampsia. However, if preeclampsia does develop, early recognition and prompt treatment can prevent progression to eclampsia.

Suppress the progress

The treatment priority for preeclampsia is to stop the disorder's progression and ensure fetal survival. Some health care providers advocate the prompt inducement of labor, especially if the patient is near term. Others follow a more conservative approach. Therapy may include:

- complete bed rest in the preferred left lateral recumbent position to enhance venous return
- administration of antihypertensive medications, such as methyldopa (Aldomet) and hydralazine (Apresoline)
- administration of magnesium sulfate to prevent seizures, provide neurologic protection for the fetus, promote diuresis, reduce blood pressure, and prevent seizures if blood pressure fails to respond to bed rest and antihypertensive agents (persistently rising above 160/100 mm Hg) or central nervous system (CNS) irritability increases.

Plan B

If these measures fail to improve the patient's condition or if fetal life is endangered (as determined by stress tests or NSTs and BPPs), cesarean birth may be required. If the patient develops seizures, emergency treatment consists of immediate IV administration of magnesium, oxygen therapy, IV administration of antihypertension medications (labetalol, hydralazine), along with electronic fetal monitoring. After the patient's condition stabilizes, cesarean birth may be indicated.

What to do

- Monitor the patient regularly for changes in blood pressure, pulse rate, respiratory rate, FHR, vision, level of consciousness, and deep tendon reflexes as well as headache unrelieved by medication. Report changes immediately. Assess these signs and symptoms before administering medications. (See *Emergency interventions for gestational hypertension.*)

Emergency interventions for gestational hypertension

When caring for a patient with gestational hypertension, be prepared to perform these nursing interventions:
- Observe for signs of fetal distress by closely monitoring the results of stress tests, NSTs, and electronic fetal monitoring.
- Keep emergency resuscitative equipment and anticonvulsant medications readily available in case of seizures and cardiac or respiratory arrest.
- Maintain a patent airway and have oxygen readily available.
- Carefully monitor the IV infusion of magnesium sulfate, observing for signs and symptoms of toxicity, such as diminished or absence of deep tendon reflexes, flushing, muscle flaccidity, decreased urine output, a significant drop in blood pressure (more than 15 mm Hg), and respiratory rate less than 12 breaths/min.
- Keep calcium gluconate readily available at the bedside to counteract the toxic effects of magnesium sulfate.
- Prepare for emergency cesarean birth if indicated.
- Maintain seizure precautions to protect the patient from injury. Never leave an unstable patient unattended.

- If the patient is receiving IV magnesium sulfate, administer the loading dose over 15 to 30 minutes and then maintain the infusion at a rate of 1 to 2 g/h. (See *Administering magnesium sulfate safely.*)

Administering magnesium sulfate safely

If your patient requires IV magnesium therapy, use caution when administering the medication because magnesium toxicity may occur. Follow these guidelines to ensure the patient's safety during administration.
- Always administer the medication as a piggyback infusion so that it can be discontinued immediately if the patient develops signs and symptoms of toxicity.

Administering magnesium sulfate safely (*continued*)

• Obtain a baseline serum magnesium level before initiating therapy and monitor levels frequently thereafter.
• Keep in mind that for IV magnesium to be effective as an anticonvulsant agent, serum magnesium levels should be between 5 and 8 mg/dL. Levels above 8 mg/dL indicate toxicity and place the patient at risk for respiratory depression, cardiac dysrhythmia, and cardiac arrest.
• Assess the patient's deep tendon reflexes. If the patient has received epidural anesthesia, test the biceps or triceps reflex. Diminished or hypoactive reflexes suggest magnesium toxicity.
• Have calcium gluconate readily available at the patient's bedside. Anticipate administering this antidote for IV magnesium.

- Monitor the extent and location of edema. Elevate affected extremities to promote venous return. Avoid constricting pantyhose, slippers, and bed linens.
- Assess fluid balance by measuring intake and output and checking daily weight. Insert an indwelling urinary catheter, if necessary, to provide a more accurate measurement of output and assess hourly urine output.
- Provide a quiet, darkened room. Limit visitation by friends and family members until the patient's condition stabilizes. Enforce complete bed rest.
- Provide emotional support for the patient and their family. Encourage them to verbalize their feelings.
- Encourage the patient to eat a well-balanced, high-protein diet. Limit high-sodium foods and include high-fiber foods. Drink at least eight 8-oz glasses of noncaffeinated beverages each day.
- Teach the patient to report signs and symptoms that indicate worsening gestational hypertension, which include headache, vision disturbances (blurring, flashes of light, "spots" before the eyes), GI symptoms (nausea, pain especially in the right upper quadrant of the abdomen), worsening edema (especially of the face and fingers), and a noticeable decrease in urine output.
- Teach the patient the importance of keeping prenatal appointments, which will be more frequent because they have gestational hypertension.
- Help the patient and their family develop effective coping strategies.
- Prepare to administer betamethasone IM as indicated to promote fetal lung maturity if the patient is between 24 and 34 weeks' gestation and at risk for delivery in the next 7 days.

HELLP syndrome

HELLP is an acronym that stands for **h**emolysis, **e**levated **l**iver enzymes, and **l**ow **p**latelets. HELLP syndrome is a category of gestational hypertension that involves changes in blood components and liver function. It is a form of severe preeclampsia and a disease involving multisystems. The patient exhibits a variety of complaints along with specific laboratory markers.

Temporary HELLP

HELLP syndrome develops in 12% of patients with gestational hypertension. It can occur in primigravidas and multigravidas. When it occurs, the mortality is high for both the patient and their infant. Approximately one fourth of patients and one third of infants die from this disorder. However, after birth, laboratory results return to normal—usually within 1 week—and the postpartum patient experiences no further problems.

What causes it

The exact cause of HELLP is unknown. Hemolysis is believed to result because RBCs are damaged by their travel through small, impaired blood vessels. Elevated liver enzymes are believed to result from obstruction in liver flow by fibrin deposits. Low platelets are believed to be the result of vascular damage secondary to vasospasm. Patients with severe preeclampsia are at high risk for developing HELLP syndrome.

What to look for

Typically, the patient complains of pain most commonly in the right upper quadrant, epigastric area, or lower chest. Additional signs and symptoms include nausea, vomiting, general malaise, and severe edema. The right upper quadrant may be tender on palpation because of a distended liver. In addition, the patient may show few signs of preeclampsia and may receive a non-obstetric diagnosis due to the vagueness of the symptoms. This may ultimately lead to a delay in treatment and an increase in morbidity and mortality for the patient and the fetus.

What tests tell you

Laboratory studies reveal:
- hemolysis of RBCs (appearing fragmented and irregular on a peripheral blood smear)

- thrombocytopenia (a platelet count below 100,000/mm^3)
- elevated levels of alanine aminotransferase and serum aspartate aminotransferase.

How it's treated

Treatment involves intensive care management for the patient and their fetus. Medication therapy, such as with magnesium sulfate, is instituted to reduce blood pressure and prevent seizures. Transfusions of fresh-frozen plasma or platelets may be used to reverse thrombocytopenia. Delivery of the fetus may occur vaginally or by cesarean birth and generally resolves the condition.

What to do

- Assess the patient's vital signs and FHR frequently. Be alert for signs and symptoms of complications, including hemorrhage, hypoglycemia, hyponatremia, subcapsular liver hematoma, and kidney failure.
- Maintain a quiet, calm, dimly lit environment to reduce the risk of seizures. Limit visitation.
- Avoid palpating the abdomen because this increases intra-abdominal pressure, which could lead to rupture of a subcapsular liver hematoma.
- Institute bleeding precautions and monitor the patient for signs and symptoms of bleeding. Administer blood transfusions and medications as ordered.
- If the patient develops hypoglycemia, expect to administer IV dextrose solutions.
- Prepare the patient for delivery, explain all events and procedures, and assist with evaluations for fetal maturity.
- Be aware that because of the increased risk of bleeding due to thrombocytopenia, the patient may not be a candidate for epidural or spinal anesthesia.
- Assess the patient carefully throughout labor and delivery for possible hemorrhage.

Hyperemesis gravidarum

Unlike the transient nausea and vomiting that is normally experienced until about the 12th week of pregnancy, hyperemesis gravidarum is severe and unremitting nausea and vomiting that persists after the first trimester. It usually occurs with the first pregnancy and commonly affects pregnant patients with conditions that produce high levels of hCG, such as gestational trophoblastic disease or multiple pregnancy. It might be mild symptoms initially; however, eventually, true hyperemesis may progress to the point where the patient vomits everything consumed.

The prognosis is usually good. However, if untreated, hyperemesis gravidarum produces substantial weight loss, starvation with ketosis and acetonuria, dehydration with subsequent fluid and electrolyte imbalance (hypokalemia), and acid–base disturbances (acidosis and alkalosis). Retinal, neurologic, and kidney damage may also occur.

What causes it

The specific cause of hyperemesis gravidarum is unknown. Possible causes include pancreatitis (elevated serum amylase levels are common), biliary tract disease, decreased secretion of free hydrochloric acid in the stomach, decreased gastric motility, drug toxicity, inflammatory obstructive bowel disease, and vitamin deficiency (especially vitamin B_6). Increased levels of hCG may also be a cause. In some patients, this disorder may be related to psychological factors.

What to look for

The patient typically complains of unremitting nausea and vomiting. The vomitus initially contains undigested food, mucus, and small amounts of bile. Later, it contains only bile and mucus. Finally, the vomitus includes blood and material that resembles coffee grounds.

Enough is enough!

The patient may report thirst, hiccups, oliguria, vertigo, and headache as well as substantial weight loss and eventual emaciation caused by persistent vomiting. They may appear confused or delirious. Lassitude, stupor, and, possibly, coma may occur. Additional findings may include:
- pale, dry, waxy, and, possibly, jaundiced skin with decreased skin turgor
- dry, coated tongue
- subnormal or elevated temperature
- rapid pulse
- fetid, fruity breath (from acidosis).

What tests tell you

Diagnostic tests are used to rule out other disorders, such as gastroenteritis, cholecystitis, peptic ulcer, and pancreatic or liver disorders, which produce similar clinical effects. Differential diagnosis also rules out gestational trophoblastic disease, hepatitis, inner ear infection, food poisoning, emotional problems, and eating disorders.

Urine test results show ketonuria and slight proteinuria. The following results of serum analysis support a diagnosis of hyperemesis gravidarum:

- Decreased protein, chloride, sodium, and potassium levels
- Increased blood urea nitrogen levels
- Elevated hemoglobin levels
- Elevated WBC count

How it's treated

The patient with hyperemesis gravidarum may require hospitalization to correct electrolyte imbalances and prevent starvation. IV infusions are used to maintain nutrition until the patient can tolerate oral feedings.

Infuse while you snooze—and snack

An infusion of 3,000 mL of IV fluid over 24 hours will usually cause a reduction in symptoms. Potassium chloride is typically added to the IV in order to prevent hypokalemia. Oral fluids and food are usually withheld until there is no vomiting for 24 hours, after which clear liquids can be initiated. Antiemetic medications may be administered to control vomiting. The patient progresses slowly to a clear liquid diet; then a full liquid diet; and finally small, frequent meals of high-protein solid foods. A midnight snack helps stabilize blood glucose levels. Parenteral vitamin supplements and potassium replacements are used to help correct deficiencies.

Easy does it

If persistent vomiting jeopardizes the patient's health, antiemetic medications may be prescribed. Note, however, that no medication has been approved by the U.S. Food and Drug Administration (FDA) for the treatment of nausea and vomiting during pregnancy. Therefore, any antiemetic agent must be prescribed with caution and the benefits must outweigh the risks to the patient and the fetus. Meclizine (Antivert) and diphenhydramine (Benadryl) may be prescribed. More commonly, however, a continuous IV infusion of an antiemetic agent is administered through a portable IV pump worn under the patient's clothes. The latter treatment is highly successful.

After vomiting stops and the patient's electrolyte balance has been restored, the pregnancy usually continues without recurrence of hyperemesis gravidarum. Most patients feel better as they begin to regain normal weight, but some continue to vomit throughout the pregnancy, requiring extended treatment and total parenteral nutrition. If appropriate, some patients may benefit from consultations with clinical nurse specialists, psychologists, or psychiatrists.

What to do

- Administer IV fluids as ordered until the patient can tolerate oral feedings.
- Monitor fluid intake and output, vital signs, skin turgor, daily weight, serum electrolyte levels, and urine for ketones. Anticipate the need for electrolyte replacement therapy.
- Provide frequent mouth care.
- Consult a dietitian to provide a diet high in dry, complex carbohydrates. Suggest decreased liquid intake during meals. Provide company and encourage diversionary conversation at mealtime.
- Instruct the patient to remain upright for 45 minutes after eating to decrease reflux.
- Suggest that the patient eat two or three dry crackers before getting out of bed in the morning to alleviate nausea.
- Provide reassurance and a calm, restful atmosphere. Encourage the patient to discuss their feelings about pregnancy and the disorder.
- Help the patient develop effective coping strategies. Refer to a mental health professional for additional counseling if necessary (hyperemesis may be an extreme response to psychosocial problems). Refer the patient to the social service department for help in caring for other children at home, if appropriate.
- Teach the patient protective measures to conserve energy and promote rest. Include relaxation techniques, fresh air and moderate exercise (if tolerated), and activities scheduled appropriately to prevent fatigue.

Isoimmunization

Isoimmunization, also called *Rh incompatibility*, refers to a condition in which the pregnant patient is Rh-negative but their fetus is Rh-positive. This condition, if left untreated, can lead to hemolytic disease in the neonate. Isoimmunization develops in about 7% of all pregnancies in the United States. Before the development of RhoGAM, this condition was a major cause of kernicterus (bilirubin-induced neurologic damage) and neonatal death.

What causes it

During the first pregnancy, a patient who is Rh-negative may become sensitized to Rh antigens by:
- being exposed to Rh-positive fetal blood antigens inherited from the non-birthing parent
- receiving alien Rh antigens from a blood transfusion, causing agglutinins (antibodies in the patient's blood) to develop

- receiving inadequate doses of Rho(D) or failing to receive Rho(D) after significant fetal–maternal leakage from placental abruption.

   Subsequent pregnancy with an Rh-positive fetus provokes increasing amounts of the patient's agglutinating antibodies to cross the placental barrier, attach to Rh-positive cells in the fetus, and cause hemolysis and anemia. To compensate for this, the fetus steps up the production of RBCs, and erythroblasts (immature RBCs) appear in the fetal circulation. Extensive hemolysis results in the release of large amounts of unconjugated bilirubin, which the liver cannot conjugate and excrete, causing hyperbilirubinemia and hemolytic anemia. (See *Pathogenesis of Rh isoimmunization*.)

Pathogenesis of Rh isoimmunization

Rh isoimmunization progresses throughout pregnancies in Rh-negative patients who give birth to Rh-positive neonates. The following illustrations outline the process of isoimmunization.

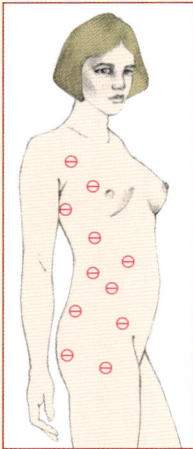

| A nonpregnant patient has Rh-negative blood. | They become pregnant with an Rh-positive fetus. Normal antibodies appear. | Placental separation occurs. | After delivery, the postpartum patient develops anti–Rh-positive antibodies. | With the next Rh-positive fetus, antibodies enter fetal circulation, causing hemolysis. |

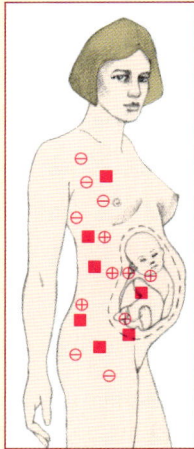

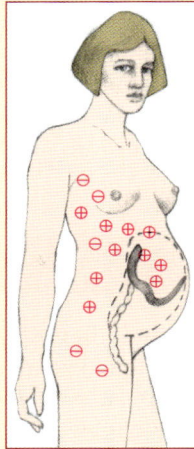

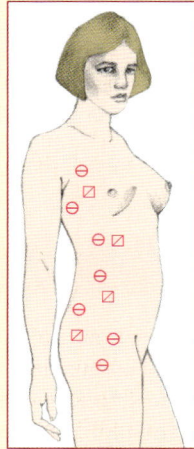

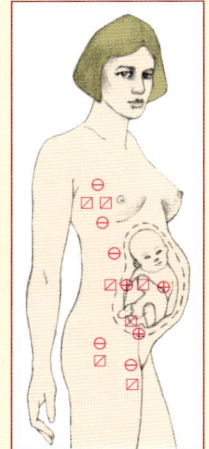

What to look for

Typically, the pregnant patient does not exhibit signs or symptoms of this disorder. The fetus—and subsequently the neonate—is affected.

What tests tell you

At the first prenatal visit, an anti-D antibody titer should be performed on all pregnant patients with Rh-negative blood. If the results are normal (titer is 0) or the titer is minimal (a ratio below 1:8), the test will be repeated at week 28. No therapy is needed at this time.

A sensitive situation

An anti-D antibody titer of 1:16 or greater indicates Rh sensitization. Titer monitoring continues every 2 weeks for the remainder of the pregnancy.

Amniocentesis may be performed to evaluate the status of the fetus. During amniocentesis, the fluid density of the amniotic fluid is determined using spectrophotometry. The results are plotted on a graph and correlated with gestational age to determine the extent of involvement and the amount of bilirubin present. Amniotic fluid analysis may show increased bilirubin levels (indicating possible hemolysis) and increased anti-Rh titers.

Radiologic studies may show edema and, in those with hydrops fetalis (edema of the fetus), the halo sign (edematous, elevated subcutaneous fat layers).

How it's treated

Treatment focuses on preventing Rh isoimmunization by administering RhoGAM to any unsensitized Rh-negative patient as soon as possible after the birth of an Rh-positive neonate or after spontaneous or elective abortion. In addition, screening for Rh isoimmunization or irregular antibodies is indicated for:

- Rh-negative patients during their first prenatal visit and at 28 weeks and sometimes more often if needed
- Rh-positive patients with a history of transfusion, a neonate with jaundice, stillbirth, cesarean birth, induced abortion, placenta previa, or placental abruption.

Towering titer

If the pregnant patient's Rh antibody titer is high, they may be given high doses of gamma-globulin to help reduce fetal involvement. The goal is to interfere with the rapid destruction of fetal RBCs. The fetus may receive a blood transfusion in utero via an injection of RBCs directly into a vessel in the fetal cord or instillation in the fetal abdomen via amniocentesis. After birth, the neonate may receive an exchange transfusion to remove hemolyzed RBCs and replace them with healthy blood cells.

Bilirubin levels in amniotic fluid are monitored for early delivery intervention or intrauterine fetal transfusion if needed. Repeated transfusions may be needed in the neonate.

What to do

- Assess all pregnant patients for possible Rh incompatibility.
- Expect to administer RhoGAM IM, as ordered, to Rh-negative patients at 28 weeks' gestation and after transfusion reaction, ectopic pregnancy, spontaneous or induced abortion, or during the second and third trimesters to patients with placental abruption, placenta previa, or amniocentesis. (See *Administering RhoGAM*.)

Advice from the experts

Administering RhoGAM

Rho(D) immune globulin (human), also known as *RhoGAM*, is a concentrated solution of immune globulin containing Rho(D) antibodies. IM injection of RhoGAM keeps the Rh-negative patient from producing active antibody responses and forming anti-Rho(D) to Rh-positive fetal blood cells and endangering future Rh-positive fetuses.

RhoGAM is administered to an Rh-negative patient after abortion, ectopic pregnancy, delivery of a neonate with Rho(D)-positive blood and cord blood that is direct Coombs negative, inadvertent transfusion of Rh-positive blood, amniocentesis, placental abruption, or abdominal trauma. It is given within 72 hours to prevent future maternal sensitization. Administration at approximately 28 weeks' gestation can also protect the fetus of an Rh-negative patient.

RhoGAM is given IM into the gluteal site. When administering RhoGAM, the same steps are followed as for any IM injection. However, be sure to include these steps:

- Check the vial's identification numbers with another nurse and sign the triplicate form that comes with the RhoGAM.
- Attach the top copy to the patient's chart.
- Send the remaining two copies, along with the empty RhoGAM vial, to the laboratory or blood bank.
- Give the patient a card indicating their Rh-negative status and instruct them to carry it with them or keep it in a convenient location.

- Assist with intrauterine transfusion as indicated. Before intra-uterine transfusion, obtain a baseline FHR through electronic monitoring and explain the procedure and its purpose. Afterward, carefully observe the patient for uterine contractions and fluid leakage from the puncture site. Monitor FHR for tachycardia or bradycardia.
- Prepare the patient for a planned delivery, usually 2 to 4 weeks before term date depending on the health history, serologic tests, and amniocentesis.
- Assist with labor induction, if indicated, from 34 to 38 weeks' gestation. During labor, monitor the fetus electronically. Obtain capillary blood scalp sampling to determine acid–base balance. An indication of fetal distress necessitates immediate cesarean birth.
- Administer RhoGAM within 72 hours of delivery to prevent complications in subsequent pregnancies.
- Provide emotional support to the patient and their family. Encourage them to express their fears concerning possible complications of treatment.

Placenta previa

Placenta previa occurs when the placenta implants in the lower uterine segment, obstructing the internal cervical os and failing to provide as much nourishment as implantation in the fundus would supply. The placenta tends to spread out, seeking the blood supply it needs, and it becomes larger and thinner than normal. Hemorrhage occurs as the internal cervical os effaces and dilates, tearing the uterine vessels. One of the most common causes of bleeding during the second half of pregnancy, this disorder occurs in about 1 in 200 pregnancies and more commonly in multigravidas than primigravidas. If the patient has heavy bleeding and is then diagnosed with placenta previa, the pregnancy may be terminated.

It's a cover-up!

The placenta may cover all or part of the internal cervical os, or it may gradually overlap the os as the cervix dilates. Complete obstruction is known as *total, complete,* or *central placenta previa*. Partial obstruction is known as *incomplete* or *partial placenta previa*. When a small placental edge is felt through the cervical os, the placenta previa is referred to as *low marginal*. (See *Three types of placenta previa*.) Obstruction that occurs as the cervix dilates is caused by marginal implantation or a low-lying placenta.

Three types of placenta previa

There are three basic types of placenta previa: low marginal, partial, and complete.

Low marginal
In low-marginal placenta previa, a small placental edge can be felt through the cervical os.

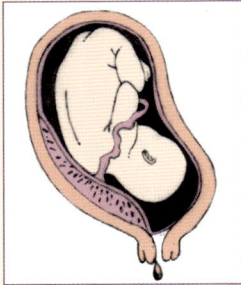

Partial
In partial placenta previa, the placenta partially caps the internal os.

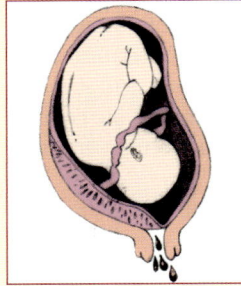

Complete
In complete placenta previa, the placenta completely covers the internal os.

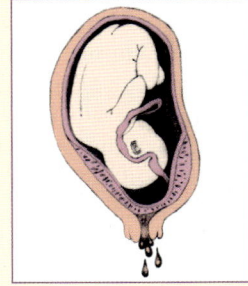

The apparent degree of placenta previa may depend largely on the extent of cervical dilation at the time of examination. The patient's prognosis is good if hemorrhage can be controlled. Fetal prognosis depends on gestational age and the amount of blood lost.

What causes it

The specific cause of placenta previa is unknown. Factors that may affect the site of the placenta's attachment to the uterine wall include:
- defective vascularization of the decidua
- multiple pregnancy (The placenta requires a larger surface for attachment.)
- previous uterine surgery or previous cesarean birth
- multiparity
- smoking
- previous placenta previa
- advanced maternal age.

What to look for

Typically, a patient with placenta previa reports the onset of painless, bright red vaginal bleeding after the 20th week of pregnancy. Such bleeding, beginning before the onset of labor, tends to be episodic; it starts without warning, stops spontaneously, and resumes later.

About 7% of patients with placenta previa are with no symptoms. In these patients, ultrasound examination reveals the disorder incidentally.

Palpation may reveal a soft, nontender uterus. Abdominal examination using Leopold maneuvers reveals various malpresentations because the placenta's abnormal location has interfered with descent of the fetal head. Minimal descent of the fetal presenting part may indicate placenta previa. The fetus remains active, however, with good heart tones audible on auscultation.

What tests tell you

A differential diagnosis is necessary to exclude genital lacerations, excessive bloody show, placental abruption, and cervical lesions. Laboratory studies may reveal decreased hemoglobin levels (due to blood loss).

Ultrasound is most sound

Transvaginal ultrasonography is used to determine placental position. Radiologic tests, such as femoral arteriography, retrograde catheterization, or radioisotope scanning or localization, may be done to locate the placenta. However, these tests have limited value, are risky, and are usually performed only when ultrasound is unavailable.

Cesarean-ready

Pelvic examination should be performed only in a surgical suite or a birthing room that is equipped for cesarean birth in the event that hemorrhage necessitates immediate delivery.

How it's treated

Treatment of placenta previa focuses on assessing, controlling, and restoring blood loss; delivering a viable neonate; and preventing coagulation disorders. Immediate therapy includes:
- starting an IV infusion using a large-bore catheter
- drawing blood for hemoglobin levels, hematocrit, typing, and cross-matching
- initiating external electronic fetal monitoring
- monitoring the patient's blood pressure, pulse rate, and respirations
- assessing the amount of vaginal bleeding.

When the bun's not done

If the fetus is premature (following determination of the degree of placenta previa and necessary fluid and blood replacement), treatment consists of careful observation to allow the fetus more time to mature. If clinical evaluation confirms complete placenta previa, the patient is usually hospitalized because of the increased risk of hemorrhage. As soon as the fetus is sufficiently mature, or in cases of severe hemorrhage, immediate cesarean birth may be necessary. Vaginal delivery is considered only when the bleeding is minimal and the placenta previa is marginal or when the labor is rapid.

Have hands on hand

Because of possible fetal blood loss through the placenta, a pediatric team should be on hand during such a delivery to immediately assess and treat neonatal shock, blood loss, and hypoxia.

What to do

- If the patient with placenta previa shows active bleeding, continuously monitor their blood pressure, pulse rate, respirations, CVP, intake and output, and amount of vaginal bleeding; continuously monitor the FHR and rhythm.
- Anticipate the need for electronic fetal monitoring and assist with application as indicated.
- Have oxygen readily available in case fetal distress occurs. Evidence of fetal distress includes bradycardia, tachycardia, or late or variable decelerations.
- If the patient is Rh-negative, administer RhoGAM after every bleeding episode.
- Institute complete bed rest.
- Prepare the patient and their family for a possible cesarean birth and the birth of a preterm neonate. Thoroughly explain postpartum care, so the patient and their family know which measures to expect.
- If the fetus is not mature, expect to administer an initial dose of betamethasone (Celestone) IM to aid in promoting fetal lung maturity. Explain that additional doses may be given again in 24 hours and, possibly, 1 to 2 weeks.
- Provide emotional support during labor. Because of the fetus's prematurity, the patient may not be given analgesic agents, so labor pain may be intense. Reassure the patient of progress throughout labor and keep them informed of the fetus's condition.
- If the patient's bleeding ceases and they return home on bed rest, anticipate the need for a referral for home care.

- Assess for signs of infection (fever, chills). The patient is at increased risk for infection because of the proximity of vaginal organisms to the placenta and the susceptibility of the placental environment to the growth of microorganisms.
- Teach the patient to identify and report signs of placenta previa (bleeding, cramping) immediately.
- During the postpartum period, monitor the patient for signs of hemorrhage and shock caused by the uterus' diminished ability to contract.
- Tactfully discuss the possibility of neonatal death. Tell the pregnant patient that the neonate's survival depends primarily on gestational age, the amount of blood lost, and associated hypertensive disorders. Assure the patient that frequent monitoring and prompt management greatly reduce the risk of death.
- Encourage the patient and their family to verbalize their feelings and help them develop effective coping strategies. Refer them for counseling if necessary.

Premature labor

Premature labor, also known as *preterm labor*, is the onset of rhythmic uterine contractions that produce cervical changes after fetal viability but before fetal maturity. It usually occurs between weeks 20 and 37 of gestation. Between 5% and 10% of pregnancies end prematurely; about 75% of neonatal deaths result from premature labor.

Weighing in

In premature labor, fetal prognosis depends on birth weight and length of gestation. Fetuses born before 26 weeks' gestation and weighing less than 1 lb, 10 oz (737 g) have a survival rate of about 10%. Fetuses born at 27 to 28 weeks' gestation and weighing between 1 lb, 10 oz (737 g) and 2 lb, 3 oz (992 g) have a survival rate of more than 50%. Those born after 28 weeks' gestation and weighing 2 lb, 3 oz (992 g) to 2 lb, 11 oz (1,219 g) have a 70% to 90% survival rate.

What causes it

Causes of premature labor include PROM (in 30% to 50% of cases), gestational hypertension, chronic hypertensive vascular disease, hydramnios, multiple pregnancy, placenta previa, placental abruption, incompetent cervix, abdominal surgery, trauma, structural anomalies of the uterus, infections (such as group B streptococci), and fetal death.

What to look for

The patient reports the onset of rhythmic uterine contractions, possible rupture of membranes (ROMs), passage of the cervical mucus plug, and a bloody discharge. The health history indicates that they are in weeks 20 to 37 of pregnancy. Vaginal examination shows cervical effacement and dilation.

What tests tell you

Premature labor is confirmed by the combined results of prenatal history, physical examination, presenting signs and symptoms, and ultrasonography (if available), showing the position of the fetus in relation to the pregnant patient's pelvis. Additionally, the health care provider may order a vaginal swab to assess for fetal fibronectin (fFN) test, which can indicate that the patient's body is preparing to go into preterm labor.

How it's treated

Treatment is designed to suppress preterm labor when tests show immature fetal pulmonary development, cervical dilation of less than 4 cm, and the absence of factors that contraindicate continuation of pregnancy. Such treatment consists of bed rest and, when necessary, corticosteroids, magnesium sulfate, and tocolytic medication therapy.

Prevention first

Taking steps to prevent premature labor is important. This requires good prenatal care, adequate nutrition, and proper rest. Inserting a purse-string suture (cerclage) to reinforce an incompetent cervix at 14 to 18 weeks' gestation may prevent premature labor in a patient with a history of incompetent cervix.

In some patients, premature labor is prevented with at-home tocolytic medication therapy (either orally or through an IV infusion pump). At-risk patients who are treated at home can have their contractions monitored remotely.

Promotion of fetal well-being

If there is a chance that preterm labor can be delayed, or avoided, certain medications can be administered to promote fetal well-being after birth. If the patient is less than 32 weeks pregnant, magnesium sulfate may be used to help reduce the risk of cerebral palsy, which is often associated with preterm birth. Additionally, if the patient is between 24 and 34 weeks' gestation, corticosteroids may be given.

Corticosteroids cross the placenta and can help promote the rapid development of the infant's lungs, brain, and digestive organs.

Slow to a stop

Several types of medication therapy may be used to stop the patient's contractions. Magnesium sulfate is typically the first medication of choice. It acts as a CNS depressant, resulting in the slowing and cessation of contractions. A beta-adrenergic agent such as terbutaline (Brethine) is used to stimulate beta-2 receptors, thus inhibiting the contractility of uterine smooth muscle. Brethine is the most widely used medication for tocolysis.

Indomethacin (Indocin), a prostaglandin synthesis inhibitor, may be given, but its use has been associated with premature closure of ductus arteriosus if given after 34 weeks' gestation.

Weighing the risks

Sometimes, preterm delivery is the lesser risk if factors such as intrauterine infection, placental abruption, placental insufficiency, and severe preeclampsia jeopardize the fetus. Fetal problems, particularly isoimmunization and congenital anomalies, can become more perilous as pregnancy nears term and may require preterm delivery.

Treatment and delivery require intensive team effort. The fetus' health requires continuous assessment through fetal monitoring.

Close at hand

Ideally, treatment of active premature labor should take place in a perinatal intensive care center, where the staff is specially trained to handle this situation. In such settings, the neonate can remain close to their caregivers.

Sedatives and narcotics, which may harm the fetus, should not be used because they may depress CNS function and may cause fetal respiratory depression. Therefore, they should be administered in the smallest doses possible when absolutely necessary.

Amniotomy (rupture of the amniotic fluid membranes) is avoided, if possible, to prevent cord prolapse or damage to the fetus's tender skull. Adequate hydration is maintained with IV fluids.

What to do

- Closely observe the patient in premature labor for signs of distress in the patient or fetus and provide comprehensive supportive care.
- Make sure the patient maintains bed rest during attempts to suppress premature labor.
- Administer medications as ordered. (See *Administering terbutaline.*)

Administering terbutaline

IV terbutaline (Brethine) may be ordered for a patient in premature labor. When administering this medication, follow these steps:

• Obtain baseline vital signs from the patient, FHR, and laboratory studies, including hematocrit, and serum glucose and electrolyte levels.

• Institute external monitoring of uterine contractions and FHR.

• Prepare the medication with lactated Ringer solution instead of dextrose in water to prevent additional glucose load and hyperglycemia.

• Administer the medication as an IV piggyback infusion into a main IV solution so that it can be discontinued immediately if adverse effects occur.

• Use microdrip tubing and an infusion pump to ensure an accurate flow rate.

• Expect to adjust the infusion flow rate every 10 minutes until contractions cease or adverse effects become problematic.

• Monitor the patient's vital signs every 15 minutes while the infusion rate is increased and every 30 minutes thereafter until contractions cease.

• Monitor FHR every 15 to 30 minutes.

• Auscultate breath sounds for evidence of crackles or changes. Be alert for complaints of dyspnea and chest pain.

• Monitor the patient for a pulse rate greater than 120 beats/min; blood pressure less than 90/60 mm Hg; or persistent tachycardia or tachypnea, chest pain, dyspnea, or abnormal breath sounds, which may indicate developing pulmonary edema. Notify the health care provider immediately.

• Watch for fetal tachycardia or late or variable decelerations in FHR pattern because these could indicate possible uterine bleeding or fetal distress necessitating emergency birth.

• Monitor intake and output closely, every hour during the infusion and every 4 hours thereafter.

• Expect to continue the infusion for 12 to 24 hours after contractions have ceased. Administer the first dose of oral therapy 30 minutes before discontinuing the IV infusion.

• Teach the patient how to take the oral Brethine and stress the importance of continuing therapy until 37 weeks' gestation or fetal lung maturity has been confirmed by amniocentesis. Alternatively, if the patient is prescribed subcutaneous terbutaline therapy via a continuous pump, teach them how to use the pump.

• Teach the patient how to measure their pulse rate before each dose of oral terbutaline or at the recommended times with subcutaneous therapy. Instruct the patient to call the health care provider if their pulse rate is over 120 beats/min or if they experience palpitations or extreme nervousness.

• Give sedatives and analgesic agents sparingly because they may be harmful to the fetus. Minimize the need for these medications by providing comfort measures, such as frequent repositioning and good perineal and back care.

• Monitor blood pressure, pulse rate, respirations, FHR, and uterine contraction pattern when administering a beta-adrenergic stimulant, sedative, or narcotic. Minimize adverse reactions by keeping the patient in a side-lying position as much as possible to ensure adequate placental perfusion.

- Administer fluids as ordered to ensure adequate hydration.
- Assess deep tendon reflexes frequently when administering magnesium sulfate. Monitor the neonate for signs of magnesium toxicity, including neuromuscular and respiratory depression.
- During active premature labor, remember that the preterm fetus has a lower tolerance for the stress of labor and is more likely to become hypoxic than a full-term fetus. If necessary, administer oxygen to the patient through a nasal cannula. Encourage the patient to lie on their left side or sit up during labor to prevent vena caval compression, which can cause supine hypotension and subsequent fetal hypoxia.
- Observe fetal response to labor through continuous monitoring. Prevent the patient from hyperventilating. Use a rebreathing bag as necessary. Continually reassure the patient throughout labor to help reduce their anxiety.
- Prepare to administer IM betamethasone as indicated (corticosteroids).
- Help the patient proceed through labor with as little analgesia and anesthesia as possible. To minimize fetal CNS depression, avoid administering an analgesic agent when delivery seems imminent. Monitor the patient's and fetus' response to local and regional anesthetics.
- Anticipate that the patient may have an extended hospitalization if the neonate is delivered before 34 weeks' gestation.

Premature rupture of membranes

PROM is a spontaneous break or tear in the amniotic sac before onset of regular contractions, resulting in progressive cervical dilation. This common abnormality of parturition occurs in nearly 10% of all pregnancies longer than 20 weeks' gestation. More than 80% of neonates are mature. Labor usually starts within 24 hours.

In labor limbo

The latent period (between membrane rupture and labor onset) is generally brief when membranes rupture near term. When the neonate is premature, the latent period is prolonged, which increases the risk of mortality from maternal infection (amnionitis, endometritis), fetal infection (pneumonia, septicemia), and prematurity.

PROM problems

Maternal complications associated with PROM include:
- endometritis
- amnionitis
- septic shock and death if amnionitis is untreated.

Baby's PROM predicament

Neonatal complications of PROM include:
- increased risk of respiratory distress syndrome
- asphyxia
- pulmonary hypoplasia
- congenital anomalies
- malpresentation
- cord prolapse
- severe fetal distress that can result in neonatal death.

What causes it

Although the cause of PROM is unknown, malpresentation and a contracted pelvis commonly accompany the rupture.

Usual suspects

Predisposing factors include:
- lack of proper prenatal care
- STIs
- previous preterm birth
- history of PROM
- second or third trimester bleeding
- poor nutrition and hygiene
- smoking
- incompetent cervix
- increased intrauterine tension from hydramnios or multiple gestations
- reduced amniotic membrane tensile strength
- uterine infection.

What to look for

Typically, PROM causes blood-tinged amniotic fluid containing vernix caseosa particles to gush or leak from the vagina. Maternal fever, fetal tachycardia, and foul-smelling vaginal discharge indicate infection.

What tests tell you

Differential diagnosis is used to exclude urinary incontinence or vaginal infection as the underlying cause. Passage of amniotic fluid confirms the rupture. Slight fundal pressure or Valsalva maneuver may expel fluid through the cervical os. Physical examination is performed to determine if multiple pregnancy is involved. Abdominal palpation (Leopold maneuvers) determines fetal presentation and size. Patient history and physical examination findings determine gestational age.

Diagnosis of PROM is confirmed by the following test results:

- Alkaline pH of fluid collected from the posterior fornix turns nitrazine paper deep blue. (The presence of blood can give a false-positive result.) Staining the fluid with Nile blue sulfate reveals two categories of cell bodies. Blue-stained bodies represent sheath fetal epithelial cells. Orange-stained bodies originate in sebaceous glands. Incidence of prematurity is low when more than 20% of cells stain orange.
- If fluid is amniotic, a smear of the fluid placed on a slide and allowed to dry takes on a fernlike pattern (because of the high sodium and protein content of amniotic fluid). Verification of amniotic fluid leakage confirms PROM.
- An AmniSure test may be performed to aid in the detection of ROM. This test is noninvasive, taken by a sterile swab inserted into the vagina, and elicits results within minutes.
- Vaginal probe ultrasonography allows visualization of the amniotic sac to detect tears or ruptures.

How it's treated

Treatment of PROM depends on fetal age and the risk of infection. In a term pregnancy, if spontaneous labor and vaginal delivery do not result within a relatively short time (usually within 24 hours after the membranes rupture), induction of labor with oxytocin usually follows. If induction fails, a cesarean birth is performed. In a preterm pregnancy, measures will be taken to prevent labor from starting as well as to prevent infection. Vaginal exams will be limited to reduce risk of infection. A magnesium sulfate infusion may be initiated as a method to slow contractions and to promote neuroprotection of the fetus, tocolytics may be administered, corticosteroids will be given, and antibiotic therapy will be initiated to prevent infection in both patient and fetus.

Heed the signs

Management of a preterm pregnancy of less than 34 weeks is controversial. Treatment of preterm pregnancy between 28 and 34 weeks includes hospitalization and observation for signs of infection (such as maternal leukocytosis or fever and fetal tachycardia) while the fetus matures.

Suspect infect? Induce to reduce

If the presence of infection is suspected, baseline cultures and sensitivity tests are appropriate. If these tests confirm infection, labor must be induced, followed by IV administration of an antibiotic. Antibiotic therapy for the neonate may be indicated as well. During such a delivery, resuscitative equipment must be readily available to manage neonatal distress.

What to do

- Prepare the patient for a vaginal examination. Before physically examining a patient who is suspected of having PROM, explain all diagnostic tests and clarify any misunderstandings.
- During the exam, stay with the patient and offer reassurance.
- Provide sterile gloves and sterile lubricating jelly. Do not use iodophor antiseptic solution because it discolors nitrazine paper and makes pH determination impossible.
- After the examination, provide proper perineal care.
- Send fluid specimens to the laboratory promptly because bacteriologic studies require immediate evaluation.
- Anticipate administering prophylactic antibiotics to the patient who is positive for streptococcal B infection to reduce the risk of this infection in the neonate.
- If labor starts, observe the contractions and monitor vital signs every 2 hours.
- Watch for signs and symptoms of infection in the pregnant patient (fever, abdominal tenderness, changes in amniotic fluid such as purulence, and foul odor) and fetal tachycardia. Fetal tachycardia may precede fever in the pregnant patient. Report such signs and symptoms immediately.
- Perform patient education. (See *Teaching about PROM.*)

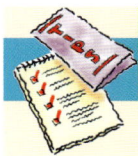

Teaching about PROM

Here are some guidelines to follow when teaching a patient about PROM.
- Inform the patient about PROM, including its signs and symptoms, during the early stages of pregnancy.
- Make sure the patient understands that amniotic fluid does not always "gush." It sometimes leaks slowly in PROM.
- Stress the importance of immediately reporting PROM (prompt treatment may prevent dangerous infection).

Teaching about PROM (*continued*)

- Warn the patient not to engage in sexual intercourse, douche, or take a tub bath after the membranes rupture.
- Advise the patient to refrain from orgasm and breast stimulation after ROMs, which can stimulate uterine contractions.
- Tell the patient to report to the health care provider a temperature above 100.4°F (38°C), which may indicate the onset of infection.

- Encourage the patient and their family to express their feelings and concerns related to the fetus' health and survival.
- Tell the patient to record fetal kick counts and to report fewer than 10 kicks in a 12-hour period. A decrease in fetal kick counts may indicate fetal distress.
- Tell the patient to report uterine contractions, reduced fetal activity, or signs of infection (fever, chills, foul-smelling discharge).

Early pregnancy loss (spontaneous abortion)

Early pregnancy loss refers to the spontaneous (occurring without medical intervention) expulsion of the products of conception from the uterus with a gestation of fewer than 20 weeks. (See *Types of early pregnancy loss*.)

Types of early pregnancy loss

Early pregnancy loss occurs without medical intervention and in various ways:

- In *complete pregnancy loss*, the uterus passes all products of conception.
- *Recurrent pregnancy loss* refers to the spontaneous loss of three or more consecutive pregnancies.
- In *incomplete pregnancy loss*, the uterus retains part or all of the products of conception.
- In *inevitable pregnancy loss*, symptoms (e.g., bleeding and cramping) are present and the cervical os is open.
- In *pregnancy loss without symptoms* (*missed abortion*), the uterus retains the products of conception after the fetus has died.
- In *septic pregnancy loss*, an early pregnancy loss is complicated by an intrauterine infection.
- In *threatened pregnancy loss*, symptoms (e.g., bleeding and cramping) of an impending early pregnancy loss occur. However, the cervical os remains closed.

What causes it

Early pregnancy loss may result from abnormal fetal, placental, or maternal factors.

Small flaws

When caused by fetal factors, early pregnancy loss usually occurs at 6 to 10 weeks' gestation. Such factors include defective embryologic development from abnormal chromosome division (the most common cause of fetal death), faulty implantation of the fertilized ovum, and failure of the endometrium to accept the fertilized ovum.

Poor placenta performance

When placental factors are involved, early pregnancy loss usually occurs around the 14th week, when the placenta takes over the hormone production needed to maintain the pregnancy. Placental factors include premature separation of the normally implanted placenta, abnormal placental implantation, and abnormal platelet function.

Maternal mechanical difficulties

When caused by maternal factors, early pregnancy loss usually occurs between weeks 11 and 19. Such factors include infection, severe malnutrition, and abnormalities of the reproductive organs (especially incompetent cervix in which the cervix dilates painlessly and without blood in the second trimester). Other factors include endocrine problems (such as thyroid dysfunction and lowered estriol secretion), trauma (including any type of surgery that requires manipulation of the pelvic organs), ABO blood group incompatibility and Rh isoimmunization, and drug ingestion.

What to look for

Prodromal symptoms of early pregnancy loss include a pink discharge for several days or a scant brown discharge for several weeks before the onset of cramps and increased vaginal bleeding. For a few hours, the cramps intensify and occur more frequently and then the cervix dilates for expulsion of uterine contents. If the entire contents are expelled, cramps and bleeding subside. However, if contents remain, cramps and bleeding continue.

What tests tell you

Diagnosis of early pregnancy loss is based on evidence of expulsion of uterine contents, vaginal examination, and laboratory studies (such as decreased hCG levels). Vaginal examination determines the size of the uterus and whether that size is consistent with the stage of the pregnancy. Expelled tissue cytology provides evidence of products of conception. Laboratory tests may also reflect decreased hemoglobin levels and hematocrit from blood loss. Ultrasonography confirms the presence or absence of fetal heartbeats or an empty amniotic sac.

How it's treated

An accurate evaluation of uterine contents is necessary before planning treatment. Early pregnancy loss cannot be stopped, except in those cases attributed to an incompetent cervix. Control of severe hemorrhage requires hospitalization. Severe bleeding requires transfusion with packed RBCs or whole blood. Initially, IV administration of oxytocin stimulates uterine contractions. If there are remnants in the uterus, the preferred treatment is dilation and vacuum extraction or dilation and curettage.

The Rh factor

After a pregnancy loss, an Rh-negative patient with a negative indirect Coombs test should receive RhoGAM to prevent future Rh isoimmunization.

Unfortunate habit

Recurrent pregnancy loss can result from an incompetent cervix. Treatment involves surgical reinforcement of the cervix (cerclage) about 14 to 16 weeks after the patient's last menses. A few weeks before the estimated delivery date, the sutures are removed and the patient waits for the onset of labor.

What to do

- Do not allow bathroom privileges because the patient may expel uterine contents without knowing it. After they use the bedpan, inspect the contents carefully for intrauterine contents.
- Note the amount, color, and odor of vaginal bleeding. Save all pads the patient uses for evaluation.

- Place the patient's bed in Trendelenburg position as ordered.
- Administer analgesic agents and oxytocin as ordered.
- Assess vital signs every 4 hours for 24 hours (or more frequently depending on the extent of bleeding).
- Monitor urine output closely.
- Provide good perineal care by keeping the area clean and dry.
- Check the patient's blood type and cross-match (in cases of severe hemorrhage) and administer RhoGAM as ordered.
- Provide emotional support and counseling during the grieving process. Refer the patient and their family to loss or grief counselors (as appropriate).
- Encourage the patient and their partner to express their feelings. Some patients may want to talk to a member of the clergy.
- Help the patient develop effective coping strategies.
- Explain all procedures and treatments to the patient and provide teaching about aftercare and follow-up. (See *After early pregnancy loss.*)

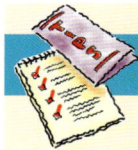

Education edge

After early pregnancy loss

If your patient experiences an early pregnancy loss, be sure to include these instructions in your teaching plan:
- Expect vaginal bleeding or spotting to continue for several days.
- Immediately report bleeding that lasts longer than 8 to 10 days or bleeding that is excessive or appears as bright red blood.
- Watch for signs of infection, such as a temperature higher than 100.4°F (38°C) and foul-smelling vaginal discharge.
- Gradually increase daily activities to include whatever tasks are comfortable to perform, as long as the activities do not increase vaginal bleeding or cause fatigue.
- Nothing in the vagina for approximately 2 weeks or until cleared by the health care provider. This means no sex, tampons, or douching.
- Abstain from sexual intercourse for approximately 2 weeks.
- Use a contraceptive when resuming intercourse.
- Avoid the use of tampons for 1 to 2 weeks.
- Schedule a follow-up visit with the health care provider in 2 to 4 weeks.

Quick quiz

1. The risks for a pregnant patient with cardiac disease and their fetus are greatest between which of the following gestational week intervals?

    A. 8 and 12
    B. 16 and 24
    C. 28 and 32
    D. 36 and 40

Answer: C. Although the risks for the pregnant patient with cardiac disease and their fetus are always present, the most dangerous time is between weeks 28 and 32, when blood volume peaks and the patient's heart may be unable to compensate adequately for this change.

2. Screening for gestational diabetes is usually performed at which of the following time intervals?

    A. 4 to 8 weeks' gestation
    B. 12 to 16 weeks' gestation
    C. 24 to 28 weeks' gestation
    D. 32 to 36 weeks' gestation

Answer: C. All pregnant patients are typically screened for gestational diabetes at 24 to 28 weeks' gestation.

3. After an early pregnancy loss, a patient who is Rh-negative would be given which of the following medications?

    A. Magnesium sulfate
    B. RhoGAM
    C. Terbutaline
    D. Betamethasone

Answer: B. A patient who is Rh-negative would receive RhoGAM after an early pregnancy loss to reduce the risk of possible isoimmunization of the fetus in a future pregnancy.

4. Assessment of a patient with placenta previa would most likely reveal:

    A. absence of fetal heart tones.
    B. boardlike abdomen.
    C. painless, bright red vaginal bleeding.
    D. signs of shock.

Answer: C. A patient with placenta previa would most likely report the onset of painless, bright red vaginal bleeding after week 20 of gestation.

Scoring

☆☆☆ If you answered all four questions correctly, congratulations! You've labored long and hard to optimize your knowledge!

☆☆ If you answered three questions correctly, great job! You've delivered the goods on this labor-intensive topic.

☆ If you answered fewer than three questions correctly, don't belabor the matter. Give the material a quick review and keep on kickin'!

Selected References

Abuogi, L., Noble, L., Smith, C., Committee on Pediatric and Adolescent HIV, & Section on Breastfeeding. (2024). Infant feeding for persons living with and at risk for HIV in the United States: Clinical report. *Pediatrics, 153*(6), e2024066843. https://doi.org/10.1542/peds.2024-066843

Alves, C., Jenkins, S., & Rapp, A. (2023). Early pregnancy loss (spontaneous abortion). In *StatPearls* [Internet]. StatPearls Publishing. https://www.ncbi.nlm.nih.gov/books/NBK560521/

Iftikhar, S., & Biswas, M. (2023). Cardiac disease in pregnancy. In *StatPearls* [Internet]. StatPearls Publishing. https://www.ncbi.nlm.nih.gov/books/NBK537261/

Luger, R., & Kight, B. (2022). Hypertension in pregnancy. In *StatPearls* [Internet]. StatPearls Publishing. https://www.ncbi.nlm.nih.gov/books/NBK430839/

Office of AIDS Research. (2023). *HIV and women (based on assigned sex at birth)*. https://hivinfo.nih.gov/understanding-hiv/fact-sheets/hiv-and-women-based-assigned-sex-birth

Office on Women's Health. (2023). Women and HIV. https://www.womenshealth.gov/hiv-and-aids/women-and-hiv

Ricci, S., Kyle, T., & Carman, S. (2021). Nursing management during the postpartum period. In *Maternity and pediatric nursing* (4th ed., pp. 536–574). Wolters Kluwer.

Silbert-Flagg, J. (2023). Nursing care of a postpartal family. In *Maternal and child health nursing* (9th ed., pp. 396–424). Wolters Kluwer.

Chapter 7

Labor and birth

Just the facts

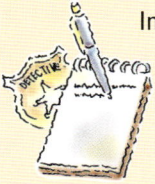

In this chapter, you'll learn:

◆ types of fetal presentations and positions

◆ ways in which labor can be stimulated

◆ signs and symptoms of labor

◆ stages and cardinal movements of labor

◆ nursing responsibilities during labor and birth, including ways to provide comfort and support.

A look at labor and birth

Labor and birth are physically and emotionally straining for patients. As the patient's body undergoes physical changes to help the fetus pass through the cervix, they may also feel discomfort, pain, panic, irritability, and loss of control. To ensure the safest outcome for the patient and child, it is important to fully understand the stages of labor and the factors affecting its length and difficulty. With an understanding of the labor and birth process, providing supportive measures that promote relaxation and help increase the patient's sense of control is easier.

Fetal presentation

Fetal presentation is the relationship of the fetus to the cervix. It can be assessed through vaginal examination, abdominal inspection and palpation, sonography, or auscultation of fetal heart tones. By knowing the fetal presentation, you can anticipate which part of the fetus will first pass through the cervix during delivery.

Factors determining fetal presentation

The primary factors determining fetal presentation during birth are fetal attitude, lie, and position.

Fetal attitude

Fetal attitude (degree of flexion) is the relationship of the fetal body parts to one another. It indicates whether the presenting parts of the fetus are in flexion or extension.

Flexion occurs as the fetal head meets resistance from the cervix, the walls of the pelvis, or the pelvic floor. In full flexion, (1) the fetal back is rounded, (2) the chin is on the chest, (3) the thighs are flexed on the abdomen, (4) the legs are flexed at the knees, and (5) the smallest diameter presents to the pelvis. Full flexion is commonly called *the fetal position* and is the most favorable for vaginal birth.

Resistance from the pelvic floor causes the fetal head to extend so that it can pass under the pubic arch. *Extension* occurs after internal rotation is complete.

Fetal lie

The relationship of the fetal spine to the maternal spine is referred to as *fetal lie*. Fetal lie can be described as longitudinal, transverse, or oblique.

Fetal position

Fetal position is the relationship of the presenting part of the fetus to a specific quadrant of the maternal pelvis.

Spelling it out

Fetal position is defined using three letters.

The first letter designates whether the presenting part faces the patient's right (R) or left (L) side. The second letter refers to the presenting part of the fetus: the occiput (O), mentum (M), sacrum (S), or scapula or acromion process (A). The third letter designates whether the presenting part is pointing to the anterior (A), posterior (P), or transverse (T) section of the patient's pelvis.

The most common fetal positions are left occiput anterior (LOA) and right occiput anterior (ROA). (See *Fetal position abbreviations*.)

Fetal position abbreviations

Here's a list of presentations that are used when documenting vertex presentations. Although it is possible to apply the same abbreviation system to breech (sacrum), face (mentum), and shoulder (acromion process) presentation, it is rarely done due to those presentations precipitating a cesarean birth.

Vertex presentations (occiput)

LOA, left occiput anterior	ROA, right occiput anterior
LOP, left occiput posterior	ROP, right occiput posterior
LOT, left occiput transverse	ROT, right occiput transverse

Duration determinant

Commonly, the duration of labor and birth is shortest when the fetus is in the LOA or ROA position. When the fetal position is posterior, such as left occiput posterior (LOP), labor tends to be longer and more painful for the patient because the fetal head puts pressure on the sacral nerves. (See *Determining fetal position.*)

Determining fetal position

Fetal position is determined by the relationship of a specific presenting part (occiput, sacrum, mentum [chin], or sinciput [forehead]) to the four quadrants (anterior, posterior, right, or left) of the maternal pelvis. For example, a fetus whose occiput (O) is the presenting part and who is located in the right (R) and anterior (A) quadrant of the maternal pelvis is identified as ROA.

These illustrations show the possible positions of a fetus in vertex presentation.

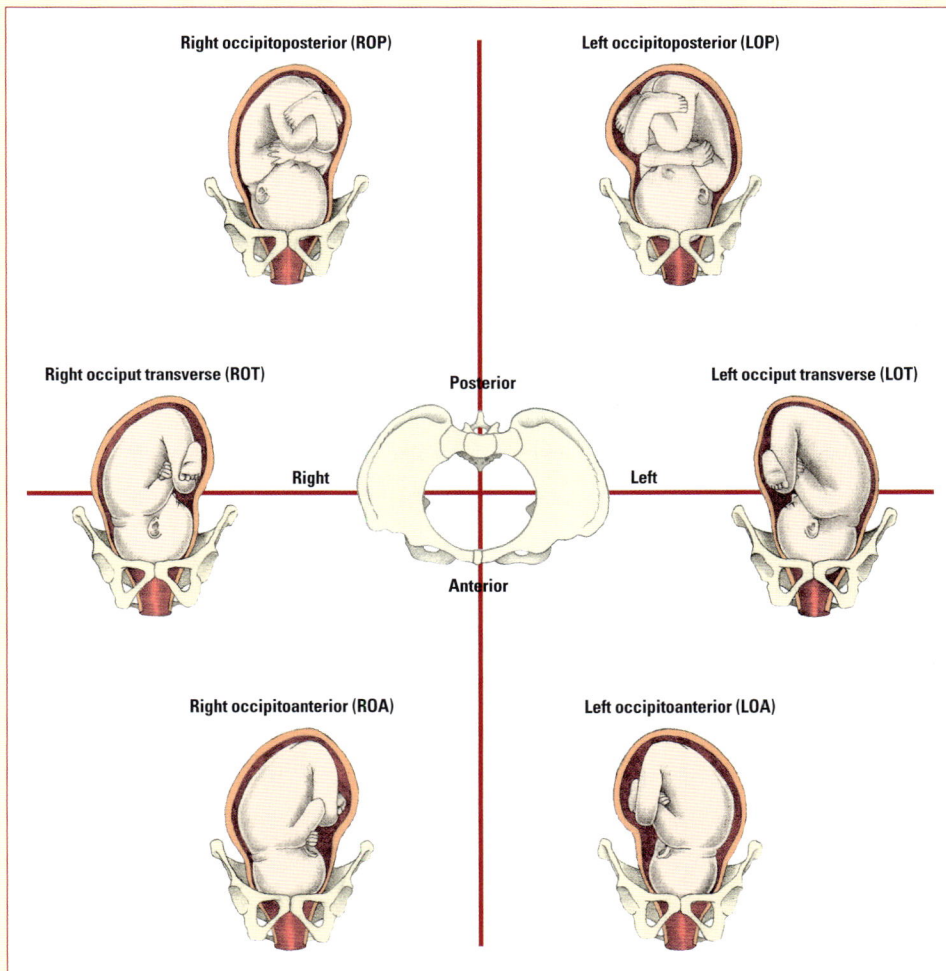

Right occipitoposterior (ROP)   Left occipitoposterior (LOP)

Right occiput transverse (ROT)   Posterior   Left occiput transverse (LOT)

Right   Left

Anterior

Right occipitoanterior (ROA)   Left occipitoanterior (LOA)

Which way do I lie?

Longitudinal	Transverse	Oblique
The fetal spine is parallel to the maternal spine.	The fetal spine is perpendicular to the maternal spine.	The fetal spine is at an angle to the bony inlet and no palpable fetal part is presenting.
Approximately 99% of all fetuses are in this position. The presenting part can be either vertex or breech.	Occurs in less than 1% of all deliveries and is considered abnormal. The presenting part can be a shoulder, an iliac crest, a hand, or an elbow.	Also considered abnormal and is rare. The presenting part can also be a shoulder, an iliac crest, a hand, or an elbow.

Types of fetal presentation

Fetal presentation refers to the part of the fetus that presents into the birth canal first. It is determined by fetal attitude, lie, and position. Fetal presentation should be determined in the early stages of labor in case an abnormal presentation endangers the birthing patient and the fetus. (See *Classifying fetal presentation*.)

Classifying fetal presentation

Fetal presentation may be broadly classified as cephalic, shoulder, or breech. Almost all births are cephalic presentations. Breech births are the second most common type.

Cephalic
In the cephalic, or head-down, presentation, the position of the fetus may be further classified by the presenting skull landmark, such as vertex, brow, sinciput (forehead), or mentum (chin).

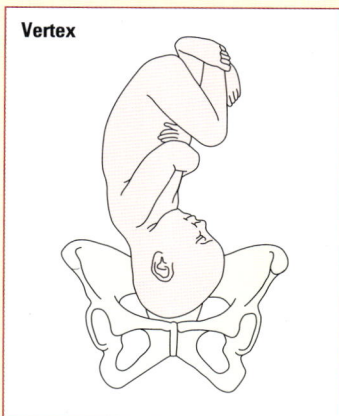

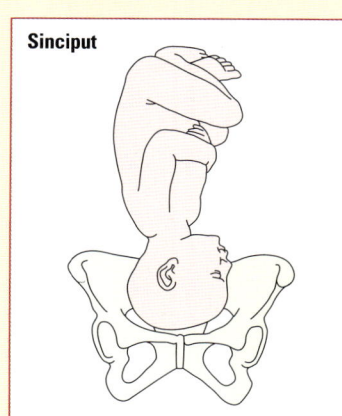

Vertex

Sinciput

Classifying fetal presentation (*continued*)

Brow

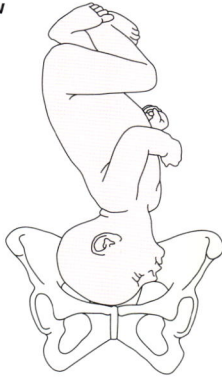

Mentum

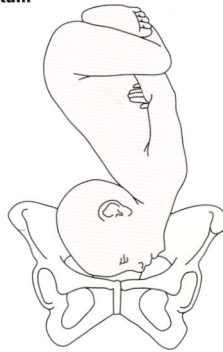

Shoulder
Although a fetus may adopt one of several shoulder presentations, examination cannot differentiate among them; thus, all transverse lies are considered shoulder presentations.

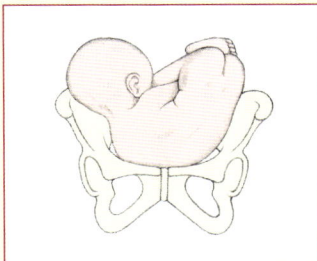

Breech
In the breech, or head-up, presentation, the position of the fetus may be further classified as *frank*, where the hips are flexed, and knees remain straight; *complete*, where the knees and hips are flexed; *kneeling*, where the knees are flexed and the hips remain extended; and *incomplete*, where one or both hips remain extended and one or both feet or knees lie below the breech; or *footling*, where one or both feet extend below the breech.

(continued)

Classifying fetal presentation (continued)

Frank

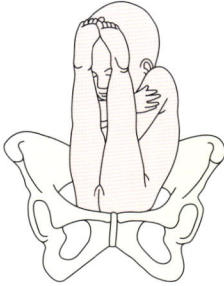

Kneeling

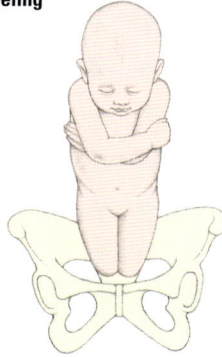

Complete

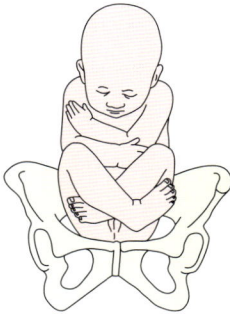

Incomplete

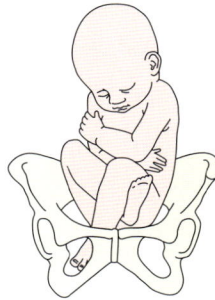

Footling

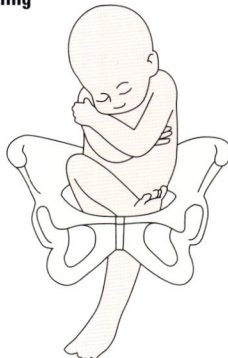

The three main types of fetal presentation are:
1. cephalic
2. breech
3. shoulder.

Cephalic presentation

When the fetus is in cephalic presentation, the head is the first part to contact the cervix and is expelled from the uterus during delivery. About 97% of all fetuses are in cephalic presentation at birth.

The four types of cephalic presentation are vertex, brow, face, and mentum (chin).

Vertex

In the vertex cephalic presentation, the most common presentation overall, the fetus is in a longitudinal lie with an attitude of full flexion. This presentation is considered optimal for fetal descent through the pelvis.

Brow

In brow presentation, the fetus's brow or forehead is the presenting part. Although this is not the optimal presentation for a fetus, few suffer serious complications from the delivery. Many brow presentations convert to vertex presentations during descent through the pelvis.

Face

The face type of cephalic presentation is unfavorable for the patient and the fetus. Because the face is the presenting part of the fetal head, severe edema and facial distortion may occur from the pressure of uterine contractions during labor.

Mentum

The mentum, or chin, type of cephalic presentation is also unfavorable for the patient and the fetus. In this presentation, the fetus is in a longitudinal lie with an attitude of complete extension. The presenting part of the fetus is the chin, which may lead to severe edema and facial distortion from the pressure of the uterine contractions during labor. Labor is usually prolonged and ineffective.

Breech presentation

Although 25% of all fetuses are in breech presentation at week 30 of gestation, most turn spontaneously at 35 to 36 weeks' gestation. However, breech presentation occurs at term in about 3% of births. Labor is usually prolonged with breech presentation because of ineffective cervical dilation caused by decreased pressure on the cervix and delayed descent of the fetus.

It gets complicated

In addition to prolonging labor, the breech presentation increases the risk of complications. In the fetus, cord prolapse; anoxia; intracranial hemorrhage caused by rapid molding of the head; neck trauma; and shoulder, arm, hip, and leg dislocations or fractures may occur. Complications that may occur in the patient include perineal tears, cervical lacerations during delivery, and infection from premature rupture of the membranes.

Once, twice, three types more

The three types of breech presentation are complete, frank, and incomplete.

Complete breech

In a complete breech presentation, the fetus's buttocks and the feet are the presenting parts. The fetus is in a longitudinal lie and is in complete flexion. Although considered an abnormal fetal presentation, complete breech is the least difficult of the breech presentations.

Frank breech

In a frank breech presentation, the fetus's buttocks are the presenting part. The fetus is in a longitudinal lie and is in moderate flexion.

Incomplete breech

In an incomplete breech presentation, also called a *footling breech*, one or both of the knees or legs are the presenting parts. If one leg is extended, then it is called a *single-footling breech* (the other leg may be flexed in the normal attitude); if both legs are extended, then it is called a *double-footling breech*. The fetus is in a longitudinal lie. A footling breech is the most difficult of the breech deliveries. Cord prolapse is common in a footling breech because of the space created by the extended leg. A cesarean birth may be necessary to reduce the risk of fetal or maternal mortality.

Shoulder presentation

Although common in multiple pregnancies, the shoulder presentation of the fetus is an abnormal presentation that occurs in 1 to 300 deliveries. The shoulder, iliac crest, hand, or elbow is the presenting part in this presentation. The fetus is in a transverse lie, and the attitude may range from complete flexion to complete extension.

Early identification and intervention are critical when the fetus is in a shoulder presentation. Abdominal and cervical examination and sonography are used to confirm whether the patient's abdomen has an abnormal or distorted shape. Attempts to turn the fetus may be unsuccessful unless the fetus is small or preterm. A cesarean birth may be necessary to reduce the risk of fetal or maternal death.

Engagement

Engagement occurs when the presenting part of the fetus passes into the pelvis to the point where, in cephalic presentation, the biparietal diameter of the fetal head is at the level of the mid-pelvis (or at the level of the ischial spines). Vaginal and cervical examinations are used to assess the degree of engagement before and during labor.

A good sign

Because the ischial spines are usually the narrowest area of the female pelvis, engagement indicates that the pelvic inlet is large enough for the fetus to pass through (because the widest part of the fetus has already passed through the narrowest part of the pelvis).

Floating away

In the primipara, nonengagement of the presenting part at the onset of labor may indicate a complication, such as cephalopelvic disproportion, abnormal presentation or position, or an abnormality of the fetal head. The nonengaged presenting part is described as *floating*. In the multipara, nonengagement is common at the onset of labor. However, the presenting part quickly becomes engaged as labor progresses.

Station

Station is the relationship of the presenting part of the fetus to the maternal ischial spines. If the fetus is at station 0, then the fetus is considered to be at the level of the ischial spines. The fetus is considered engaged when it reaches station 0.

Grand central stations

Fetal station is measured in centimeters. The measurement is called *minus* when it is above the level of the ischial spines and *plus* when it is below that level. Station measurements range from −1 to −4 cm (minus station) and from +1 to +4 cm (plus station).

A crowning achievement

When the station is measured at +4 cm, the presenting part of the fetus is at the perineum—commonly known as *crowning*. (See *Assessing fetal engagement and station*.)

Assessing fetal engagement and station

During a cervical examination, you will assess the extent of the fetal presenting part into the pelvis. This is referred to as *fetal engagement*.

After determining fetal engagement, palpate the presenting part and grade the fetal station (where the presenting part lies in relation to the ischial spines of the maternal pelvis). If the presenting part is not fully engaged into the pelvis, then you will not be able to assess station.

Station grades range from −4 (4 cm above the maternal ischial spines) to +4 (4 cm below the maternal ischial spines, causing the perineum to bulge). A zero grade indicates that the presenting part lies level with the ischial spines.

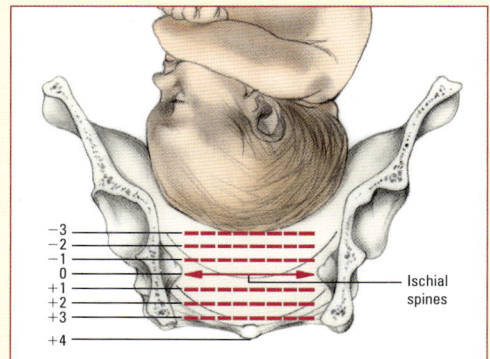

−3
−2
−1
0
+1
+2
+3
+4

Ischial spines

A look at labor stimulation

For some patients, it is necessary to stimulate labor. The stimulation of labor may involve induction (artificially starting labor) or augmentation (assisting a labor that started spontaneously).

Although induction and augmentation involve the same methods and risks, they're performed for different reasons. Many high-risk pregnancies must be induced because the safety of the patient or fetus is in jeopardy. Medical problems that justify induction of labor include preeclampsia, eclampsia, severe hypertension, diabetes, Rh sensitization, prolonged rupture of the membranes (over 24 hours), and a postmature fetus (a fetus that is 42 weeks' gestation or older). Augmentation of labor may be necessary if the contractions are too weak or infrequent to be effective.

Conditions for labor stimulation

Before stimulating labor, the fetus must be:
- in longitudinal lie (the long axis of the fetus is parallel to the long axis of the patient)
- at least 39 weeks' gestation or have fetal lung maturity established.

The ripe type

In addition to the earlier fetal criteria, the patient must have a ripe cervix before labor is induced. A ripe cervix is soft and supple to the touch rather than firm. Softening of the cervix allows for cervical effacement, dilation, and effective coordination of contractions. The Bishop score can assess whether a cervix is ripe enough for induction. (See *Bishop score*.)

Bishop score

Bishop score is a tool used to assess whether a patient is ready for labor. A score ranging from 0 to 3 is given for each of five factors: cervical dilation, length (effacement), consistency, position, and station.

If the patient's score exceeds 8, then the cervix is considered suitable for induction.

Factor	Score
Cervical dilation	
• Cervix closed	0
• Cervix dilated 1–2 cm	1
• Cervix dilated 3–4 cm	2
• Cervix dilated 5–6 cm	3
Cervical length (effacement)	
• Cervical length >4 cm (0%–30% effaced)	0
• Cervical length 3–4 cm (40%–50% effaced)	1
• Cervical length 1–2 cm (60%–70% effaced)	2
• Cervical length <1 cm (>80% effaced)	3
Cervical consistency	
• Firm cervical consistency	0
• Medium cervical consistency	1
• Soft cervical consistency	2
• Very soft cervical consistency	3
Cervical position	
• Posterior cervical position	0
• Middle cervical position	1
• Anterior cervical position	2
• Anterior cervical position	3

(*continued*)

Bishop score (*continued*)

Factor	Score
Zero station notation (presenting part level)	
• −3	0
• −2	1
• −1 or 0	2
• +1 or +2	3
Modifiers	

Add 1 point to score for:	Subtract 1 point from score for:
• Preeclampsia	• Postdates pregnancy
• Each prior vaginal delivery	• Nulliparity
	• Premature or prolonged rupture of membranes

When it isn't so great to stimulate

Stimulation of labor should be done with caution in patients aged 35 years and older and in those with grand parity or uterine scars. Labor *should not* be stimulated if, but not limited to:

- transverse fetal position
- umbilical cord prolapse
- active genital herpes infections
- patients who have had previous myomectomy (fibroid removal) from the inside of the uterus
- history of cesarean section with a classical incision
- stimulation of the uterus that increases the risk of complications such as placenta previa, abruptio placentae, uterine rupture, and decreased fetal blood supply caused by the increased intensity or duration of contractions.

Methods of labor stimulation

If labor is to be induced or augmented, then one method or a combination of methods may be used. Methods of labor stimulation include breast stimulation, amniotomy, oxytocin administration, ripening agent application, and mechanical dilation.

Breast stimulation

In breast stimulation, the nipples are massaged to induce labor. Stimulation results in the release of oxytocin, which causes contractions that sometimes result in labor.

Too much, too soon?

One drawback of breast stimulation is that the amount of oxytocin being released by the patient's body cannot be controlled. In some cases (rarely), too much oxytocin leads to excessive uterine stimulation (tachysystole or tetanic contractions), which impairs fetal or placental blood flow, causing fetal distress.

Amniotomy

Amniotomy (artificial rupturing of the membranes) is performed to augment or induce labor when the membranes haven't ruptured spontaneously. This procedure allows the fetal head to contact the cervix more directly, thus increasing the efficiency of contractions. Amniotomy is virtually painless for both the patient and the fetus because the membranes do not have nerve endings.

Let it flow, let it flow, let it flow

During amniotomy, the patient is placed in a dorsal recumbent position. An amniohook (a long, thin instrument similar to a crochet hook) is inserted into the vagina to puncture the membranes. If puncture is properly performed, then amniotic fluid gushes out. Normal amniotic fluid is clear. Bloody or meconium-stained amniotic fluid is considered abnormal and requires careful, continuous monitoring of the patient and the fetus. Bloody amniotic fluid may indicate a bleeding problem. Meconium-stained amniotic fluid may indicate fetal distress. If the fluid is meconium stained, then note whether the staining is thin, moderate, thick, or particulate. Amniotic fluid has a scent described as either a sweet smell or odorless. A foul smell indicates the presence of an infection and the patient needs further evaluation.

Prolapse potential

Amniotomy increases the risk to the fetus because there's a possibility that a portion of the umbilical cord will prolapse with the amniotic fluid. Fetal heart rate (FHR) should be monitored during and after the procedure to make sure that umbilical cord prolapse does not occur.

Oxytocin administration

Synthetic oxytocin (Pitocin) is used to induce or augment labor. It may be used in patients with gestational hypertension, prolonged gestation, diabetes, Rh sensitization, premature or prolonged rupture of membranes, and incomplete or inevitable abortion. Oxytocin is also used to evaluate for fetal distress after 31 weeks' gestation and to control bleeding and enhance uterine contractions after the placenta is delivered.

Oxytocin is always administered intravenously with an infusion pump. Throughout administration, FHR and uterine contractions should be assessed, monitored, and documented according to the National Institute of Child Health and Human Development (NICHD) criteria.

First things first

Prior to the start of an infusion, you should have at least a 15-minute strip of both FHR and uterine activity to establish a reassuring FHR. There should also be a Bishop score documented as a measure of ensuring the cervix is ripe for labor. Additionally, a set of vital signs should be taken on the patient.

Immediate action

- Because oxytocin begins acting immediately, be prepared to start monitoring uterine contractions.
- Increase the oxytocin dosage as ordered—but never increase the dose more than 1 to 2 mU/min every 15 to 60 minutes. Typically, the dosage continues at a rate that maintains a regular pattern (uterine contractions occur every 2 to 3 minutes lasting less than 2 minutes' duration).

Following through

- Continue assessing the patient's and fetal responses to the oxytocin.
- The patient's assessment should include blood pressure, pulse, and a pain assessment.
- Review the infusion rate to prevent uterine tachysystole. To manage tachysystole, discontinue the infusion and administer oxygen.

Ripening agent application

If the patient's cervix is not soft and supple, then a ripening agent may be applied to it to stimulate labor. Medications containing prostaglandin E_2—such as dinoprostone (Cervidil, Prepidil, Prostin E2)—are commonly used to ripen the cervix. These medications initiate the breakdown of the collagen that keeps the cervix tightly closed.

Mechanical dilation method

Mechanical dilation methods are effective in ripening the cervix. A common mechanical method includes inserting an indwelling (Foley) catheter (14 to 26 Fr) into the endocervical canal to ripen and dilate the cervix. The catheter is placed in the uterus, and the balloon is filled with an inflation volume of 30 to 80 mL. Direct pressure is then applied to the lower uterine segment and cervix. This direct pressure causes stress in the lower uterine segment and probably the local production of prostaglandins.

Onset of labor

True labor begins when the bloody show appears, the membranes rupture, and the patient has painful contractions of the uterus that cause effacement and dilation of the cervix. The actual mechanism that triggers this process is unknown.

Before the onset of true labor, preliminary signs appear that indicate the beginning of the birthing process. Although not considered to be a true stage of labor, these signs signify that true labor is not far away.

Preliminary signs and symptoms of labor

Preliminary signs and symptoms of labor include lightening, increased level of activity, Braxton Hicks contractions, and ripening of the cervix. Subjective signs, such as restlessness, anxiety, and sleeplessness, may also occur.

Lightening

Lightening is the descent of the fetal head into the pelvis. The uterus lowers and moves into a more anterior position, and the contour of the abdomen changes. In primiparas, these changes commonly occur about 2 weeks before birth. In multiparas, these changes can occur on the day labor begins or after labor starts.

Increased level of activity

After having endured increased fatigue for most of the third trimester, it is common for a patient to experience a sudden increase in energy before true labor starts. This phenomenon is sometimes referred to as *nesting* because, in many cases, this energy is directed toward last-minute activities, such as organizing the baby's room, cleaning, and straightening the home, and preparing other children in the household for the new arrival.

Braxton hicks contractions

Braxton Hicks contractions are mild contractions of the uterus that occur throughout pregnancy. They may become extremely strong a few days to a month before labor begins, which may cause some, especially a primipara, to misinterpret them as true labor. Several characteristics, however, distinguish Braxton Hicks contractions from labor contractions.

Patternless

Braxton Hicks contractions are irregular. There's no pattern to the length of time between them, and they vary widely in their strength. Braxton Hicks contractions can be diminished by increasing activity or by eating, drinking, or changing position. Labor contractions cannot be diminished by these activities.

Painless

Braxton Hicks contractions are commonly painless—especially early in pregnancy. Many patients feel only a tightening of the abdomen in the first or second trimester. If the patient does feel pain from these contractions, then it is felt only in the abdomen and the groin—usually not in the back. This is a major difference from the contractions of labor.

No softening or stretching

Probably the most important differentiation between Braxton Hicks contractions and true labor contractions is that Braxton Hicks contractions do not cause progressive effacement or dilation of the cervix.

Ripening of the cervix

Ripening of the cervix refers to the process in which the cervix softens to prepare for dilation and effacement. It is thought to be the result of hormone-mediated biochemical events that initiate breakdown of the collagen in the cervix, thus causing it to soften and become flexible. As the cervix ripens, it also changes position by tipping forward in the vagina.

Signs of true labor

Signs of true labor include uterine contractions, bloody show, and spontaneous rupture of membranes.

Uterine contractions

The involuntary uterine contractions of true labor help effacement and dilation of the uterus and push the fetus through the birth canal. Although uterine contractions are irregular when they begin, as labor progresses, they become regular with a predictable pattern.

Early contractions occur anywhere from 5 to 30 minutes apart and last about 30 to 45 seconds. The interval between the contractions allows blood flow to resume to the placenta, which supplies oxygen to the fetus and removes waste products. As labor progresses, the contractions increase in frequency, duration, and intensity. During the transition phase of the first stage of labor—when contractions reach their maximum intensity, frequency, and duration—they each last 60 to 90 seconds and recur every 2 to 3 minutes.

Show

Bloody show occurs as the cervix thins and begins to dilate, allowing passage of the mucus plug that seals the cervical canal during pregnancy. Mucus from the plug mixes with blood from the cervical capillaries because of the pressure of the fetus on the canal and other changes in the cervix. Consequently, the show may appear pinkish, blood-tinged, or brownish. Occasionally, in primiparas, it may be passed up to 2 weeks before labor begins.

Spontaneous rupture of membranes

Twenty-five percent of all labors begin with spontaneous rupture of the membranes. The membranes—consisting of the amniotic and chorionic membranes—cover the fetal surface of the placenta and form a sac that contains and supports the fetus and the amniotic fluid. This fluid, produced by the amniotic membrane, acts as a cushion throughout gestation, protects the fetus from temperature changes, protects the umbilical cord from pressure, and is believed to aid in fetal muscular development by allowing the fetus to move freely.

Color-coded

The amniotic fluid that is lost after the rupture of the membranes should be odorless and clear. Colored fluid usually indicates a problem. Yellow fluid indicates that the amniotic fluid is bilirubin stained from the breakdown of red blood cells, which may be caused by blood incompatibility. Green fluid indicates meconium staining, possibly from a breech presentation or fetal anoxia, and needs immediate evaluation.

Rupture or be ruptured

If a patient's membranes have not ruptured spontaneously before the transition phase of the first stage of labor, then they may rupture when the cervix becomes fully dilated at 10 cm or amniotomy may be performed. Membrane rupture shortens the duration of labor and aids in the dilation of the cervix. Intact membranes inhibit dilation of the cervix. Membranes that remain intact delay full dilation and lengthen the duration of labor because the amniotic fluid cushions the pressure of the fetal head against the cervix, preventing the contractions from exerting their full impact.

A little premature

Premature rupture of membranes (rupture that occurs more than 24 hours before labor begins) is associated with a risk of infection and umbilical cord prolapse.

Stages of labor

Labor is typically divided into four stages:
1. The first stage, when effacement and dilation occur, begins with the onset of true uterine contractions and ends when the cervix is fully dilated.
2. The second stage, which encompasses the actual birth, begins when the cervix is fully dilated and ends with the delivery of the fetus.
3. The third stage, also called the *placental stage*, begins immediately after the neonate is delivered and ends when the placenta is delivered.
4. The fourth stage begins after delivery of the placenta. During this stage, homeostasis is reestablished.

First stage

The first stage of labor begins with the onset of contractions and ends when the cervix is dilated to 10 cm (full dilation). It is divided into two phases: latent and active.

Latent phase

The latent phase of labor begins with the onset of regular contractions. Usually, the contractions during this phase are mild. They last about 30 to 45 seconds and recur every 5 to 10 minutes. Initially, the contractions may vary in intensity and duration, but they become consistent within a few hours.

Waiting for dilation

The latent phase averages about 8 hours in the primipara and 5 hours in the multipara and ends when rapid cervical dilation begins. During this phase, the cervix dilates from 0 to 6 cm and becomes fully effaced. The contractions begin irregular in frequency and gradually become more regular. Contractions usually cause mild-to-moderate discomfort. Walking can help the patient to remain relaxed and help with progressing the labor.

Technical stuff

Obtain the required blood sample and urine specimen, monitor the vital signs, monitor FHR, and explain and initiate electronic monitoring or intermittent auscultation of fetal heart tones, as ordered.

It's all about timing and intensity

During the latent phase, start timing the frequency and length (duration) of the contractions and assessing their intensity. To time the frequency of contractions, gently rest a hand on the patient's abdomen at the fundus of the uterus. Count from the beginning of one contraction to the beginning of the next. To time the length (duration), begin timing at the start of the gradual tensing and upward rising of the fundus (initially, these sensations may not be felt by the patient); end timing when the uterus has fully relaxed.

Shower me with comfort and support

Nursing care during the latent phase focuses on the psychological status of the patient as well as the physical care. Offer support and encourage the patient to use proper breathing techniques. In addition, continue to involve the labor support person in the patient's care. Placing the patient in an upright or side-lying position may provide additional comfort.

Active phase

During the active phase of labor, the release of bloody show increases and the membranes may rupture spontaneously. The contractions are stronger, the duration of each contraction lasting about 60 to 90 seconds and recurring about every 1 to 2 minutes. The increased strength of the contractions commonly causes severe pain with maximum intensity. Cervical dilation occurs more rapidly, increasing from 7 to 10 cm, and the fetus begins to descend through the pelvis at an increased rate. If the membranes are not already ruptured, then they usually rupture when the patient is 10 cm dilated and the remainder of the mucus plug is expelled from the cervix.

Whole lot of changing going on

The active phase is an emotionally charged time. The patient may be feeling excitement as well as fear. The patient also undergoes many systemic physical changes. (See *Systemic changes in the active phase of labor*.)

Systemic changes in the active phase of labor

This chart shows the systemic changes that occur during the active phase of labor.

System	Change
Cardiovascular	• Increased blood pressure • Increased cardiac output • Supine hypotension
Respiratory	• Increased oxygen consumption • Increased rate • Possible hyperventilation leading to respiratory alkalosis, hypoxia, and hypercapnia (if breathing is not controlled)
Neurologic	• Increased pain threshold and sedation caused by endogenous endorphins • Anesthetized perineal tissues caused by constant intense pressure on nerve endings
Gastrointestinal	• Dehydration • Decreased motility • Slow absorption of solid food • Nausea • Diarrhea
Musculoskeletal	• Diaphoresis • Fatigue • Backache • Joint pain • Leg cramps
Endocrine	• Decreased progesterone level • Increased estrogen level • Increased prostaglandin level • Increased oxytocin level • Increased metabolism • Decreased blood glucose
Renal	• Difficulty voiding • Proteinuria (1+ normal)

How long must this go on?

The active phase of labor averages 6 hours in a primipara and 3 hours in a multipara. If analgesic agents are given at this time, they will not slow labor. Poor fetal position and a full bladder may prolong this phase.

What they're feeling

When in the active phase, the patient may experience intense pain or discomfort as well as nausea and vomiting. They may also experience intense mood swings and feelings of anxiety, panic, irritability, and loss of control because of the intensity and duration of contractions.

What you're doing

Nursing care during the active phase includes monitoring vital signs and FHR, encouraging proper breathing techniques, and administering medications, as ordered. Arrange for a nurse to be with the patient at all times because there's a possibility that birth is imminent. Make sure to provide emotional support to the patient and their support person during this time.

Second stage

The second stage of labor starts with full dilation and effacement of the cervix and ends with the delivery of the neonate. It lasts about up to 3 hours for the primipara and 0 to 30 minutes for the multipara. During the second stage, the frequency of the contractions slows to about one every 2 to 3 minutes. However, they continue to last 60 to 90 seconds and are accompanied by the uncontrollable urge to push or bear down. The decreased frequency of the contractions gives the patient a chance to rest.

Vigilance!

During the second stage of labor (including pushing), auscultate FHR every 15 minutes for a low-risk patient and every 5 minutes for a high-risk patient.

Movin' out

Whereas the previous stage of labor primarily involved thinning and opening of the cervix, the second stage involves moving the fetus through the birth canal and out of the body.

As the uterine contractions work to accomplish this movement, the fetus pushes on the internal side of the perineum, causing the perineum to bulge and become tense. The fetal scalp becomes visible at the opening of the vagina (called *crowning*). The vaginal opening changes from a slit to an oval and then to a circle.

Getting pushy

Part of the phenomena of the second stage of labor is the urge to push or bear down. Not every patient feels this urge immediately upon becoming dilated to 10 cm.

Laboring down

Patients who lack the urge to push upon becoming fully dilated should be allowed to labor down (also known as passive fetal descent). This often occurs in those who receive regional anesthesia/analgesia. Laboring down is simply where the patient does not push with contractions but allows the contractions to do the work. Allowing a patient to labor down, especially if they have received regional anesthesia/analgesia, decreases the incidence of operative birth. Laboring down with the patient in a variety of positions also promotes passive fetal descent.

Open versus closed

Traditional closed glottis pushing (making no noise, holding one's breath for a count of 10, and quickly gasping in air and repeating) is a common occurrence in many labor rooms that has not proven to be the most effective method of pushing. Decreased venous return from the extremities, which is a result of closed glottis pushing, makes less blood available for the transport of oxygen to the fetus resulting in a greater likelihood of a non-reassuring FHR pattern.

Open glottis pushing allows a patient to make noise and bear down for 6 to 8 seconds at a time, resulting in less fetal stress and greater perineal relaxation. Pushing is also encouraged in a variety of positions in this method to help the fetus navigate the pelvis. Providing pressure in the posterior vagina (using sterile vaginal exam technique) also helps to shorten the second stage of labor.

Cardinal movements of labor

The cardinal movements of labor are fetal position changes that occur during the second stage of labor. They help the fetus pass through the birth canal. These movements are necessary because of the size of the fetal head in relation to the irregularly shaped pelvis. Specific, deliberate, and precise, the various movements allow the smallest diameter of the fetus to pass through the corresponding diameter of the patient's pelvis. (See *Cardinal movements of labor*.)

Cardinal movements of labor

These illustrations show the fetal movements that occur during the cardinal movements of labor.

Engagement, descent, flexion

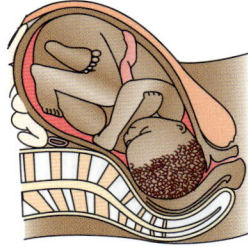

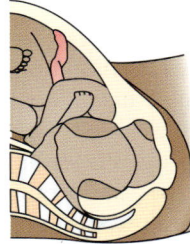

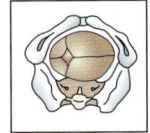

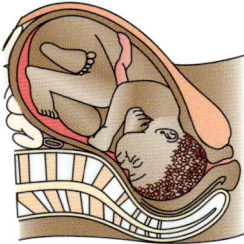

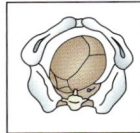

Internal rotation

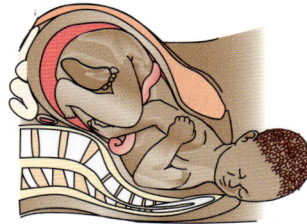

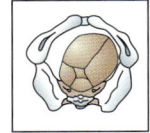

External rotation (restitution)

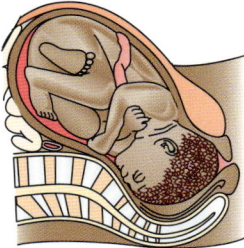

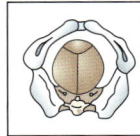

Extension beginning (rotation complete)

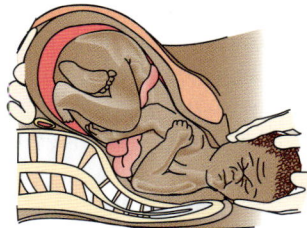

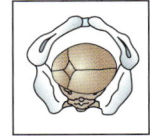

External rotation (shoulder rotation)

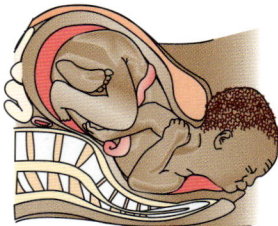

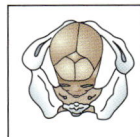

Extension complete

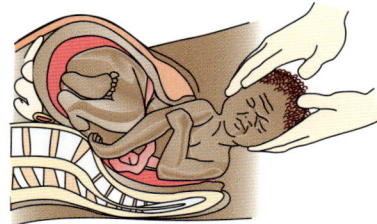

Expulsion

Descent

Descent, the first of the cardinal movements, is the downward movement of the fetus. It is determined when the biparietal diameter of the head passes the ischial spines and moves into the pelvic inlet.

Making contact

Full descent is accomplished when the fetal head passes beyond the dilated cervix and contacts the posterior vaginal floor.

Flexion

Flexion, the second of the cardinal movements, occurs during descent. It is caused by the resistance of the fetal head against the pelvic floor. The combined pressure from this resistance and uterine and abdominal muscle contractions forces the head of the fetus to bend forward so that the chin is pressed to the chest. This allows the smallest diameter of the fetal head to descend through the pelvis.

A different angle

Flexion causes the presenting diameter to change from occipitofrontal (nasal bridge to the posterior fontanel) to suboccipitobregmatic (posterior fontanel to subocciput) in an occiput anterior position. If the fetus is an occiput posterior position, then flexion is incomplete and the fetus has a larger presenting diameter, which can prolong labor.

Internal rotation

The fetal head typically enters the pelvis with its anteroposterior head diameter in a transverse (right to left) position. This position is beneficial when entering the pelvis because the diameter at the pelvic inlet is widest from right to left. However, if the head remains in the transverse position, then the shoulders are in a position where they're too wide to pass through the pelvic inlet.

Shifting toward the same plane

To allow the shoulders to pass through the pelvic inlet, the fetal head rotates about 45 degrees as it meets the resistance of the pelvic floor. With the head rotated, the anteroposterior diameter of the head is in the anteroposterior plane of the pelvis (front to back), which places the widest part of the shoulders in line with the widest part of the pelvic inlet and outlet. At this point, the face of the fetus is usually against the patient's back and the back of the fetal head is against the front of the patient's pelvis.

Extension

Extension occurs after the internal rotation is complete. As the head passes through the pelvis, the occiput emerges from the vagina and the back of the neck stops under the symphysis pubis (pubic arch). Further descent is temporarily halted because the fetus's shoulders are too wide to pass through the pelvis or under the pubic arch.

Pivotal movements

With the back of the fetal neck resting against the pubic arch, the arch acts as a pivot. The upward resistance from the pelvic floor causes the head to extend. As this occurs, the brow, nose, mouth, and chin are born.

External rotation

External rotation (also called *restitution*) is necessary because the shoulders, which previously turned to fit through the pelvic inlet, must now turn again to fit through the pelvic outlet and under the pubic arch.

Return the fetus to the transverse position . . .

After the head is born, the face, which is facing down after the completion of extension, is turned to face one of the patient's inner thighs. The head rotates about 45 degrees, returning the anteroposterior head diameter to the transverse (right to left) position assumed during descent.

. . . and prepare for shoulder delivery

The anterior shoulder (closest to the front of the patient) is delivered first with the possible assistance of downward flexion on the head. After the anterior shoulder is delivered, a slight upward flexion may be necessary to deliver the posterior shoulder.

Weighing in

During external rotation, a neonate who weighs more than 9.9 lb (4.5 kg) has a greater likelihood of experiencing shoulder dystocia than the one who weighs less. Shoulder dystocia occurs when lack of room for passage causes the shoulders to stop at the pelvic outlet. Commonly, shoulder dystocia is resolved by sharply flexing the patient's thighs against their abdomen. This movement reduces the angle between the sacrum and the spine and allows the neonate's shoulders to pass through. However, the neonate may sustain some injury to the brachial plexus.

Expulsion

After delivery of the shoulders, the remainder of the body is delivered quickly and easily. Termed *expulsion*, this step signifies the end of the second stage of labor.

Third stage

The third stage of labor, also called the *placental stage*, occurs after delivery of the neonate and ends with the delivery of the placenta. It consists of two phases: placental separation and placental expulsion. This stage of labor is important because a placenta that remains in place may cause hemorrhage, shock, infection, or even death.

From round to discoid

After the neonate has been delivered, uterine contractions commonly stop for several minutes. During this time, the uterus is a round mass located below the level of the umbilicus that feels firm to the touch. When contractions resume, the uterus takes on a discoid shape until the placenta has separated from the uterus.

Placental separation

Separation of the placenta from the uterus occurs after the uterus resumes contractions. Uterine contractions continue to occur in the wavelike pattern they assumed throughout the other stages of labor. However, in the other stages, the fetus exerted pressure on the placenta during contractions, which prevented the placenta from separating prematurely. When the fetus is no longer in the uterus, the uterine walls contract on an almost empty space. Nothing exerts reverse pressure on the placenta. As a result, the placenta folds and begins to separate from the uterine wall. This separation causes bleeding that further pushes the placenta away from the uterine wall, ultimately causing the placenta to fall to the upper vagina or lower uterine segment.

Placental expulsion

Natural bearing down by the patient or gentle pressure on the fundus of the contracting uterus (Credé maneuver) aids in the delivery of the placenta. To avoid possible eversion (turning inside out) of the uterus, which can result in gross hemorrhage, never exert pressure on the uterus when it is not contracted. Manual removal of the placenta may be indicated if it doesn't deliver spontaneously within 30 minutes of delivery.

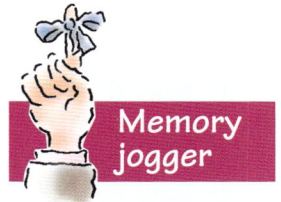

Memory jogger

To help remember which type of placenta is which, think "Shiny Schultze" and "Dirty Duncan." The Schultze placenta is shiny from the fetal membrane. The Duncan placenta exposes the maternal side and appears red and dirty, with an irregular surface.

Check it out

After delivery, examine the placenta to make sure it is intact and normal in appearance and weight. This helps determine whether any has been retained in the uterus. The placenta is usually one sixth the weight of the infant.

Additional layers

An outer area of decidua (the lining of the uterus) is expelled at the same time as the placenta. The remainder of the decidua separates into two layers:
1. The superficial layer that is shed in the lochia during the postpartum period
2. The basal layer that remains in the uterus to regenerate new endothelium

Blood volume matters

Normal bleeding occurs until the uterus contracts with enough force to seal the blood collection spaces. A blood loss of 300 to 500 mL should be expected. Blood loss exceeding 500 mL may indicate a cervical tear or a problem at the episiotomy site. It may also indicate that the uterus is not contracting properly because of retained placenta or a full bladder.

Fourth stage

The fourth stage of labor occurs immediately after the delivery of the placenta. It usually lasts for about 1 to 4 hours, and it initiates the postpartum period. During this stage, the patient should be monitored closely because their body has just undergone many changes.

Risks associated with the fourth stage of labor include hemorrhage, bladder distention, and venous thrombosis. Oxygen, type O– negative blood or blood tested for compatibility, and IV fluids must be available for 2 to 3 hours after delivery.

Monitoring

Monitor the patient's vital signs every 15 minutes for a minimum of 1 hour and then as ordered. Expect the patient's pulse, respirations, and blood pressure to be slightly increased at this time because of the birth process, excitement, and oxytocin administration. In addition, the patient may experience a normal chill and shaking sensation shortly after birth that may be caused by excess epinephrine production during labor or the sudden release of pressure on the pelvic nerves.

The incredible shrinking uterus

After delivery, the uterus gradually decreases in size and descends into its prepregnancy position in the pelvis—a process known as *involution*. To evaluate this process, palpate the uterine fundus and determine uterine size, degree of firmness, and rate of descent (which is measured in fingerbreadths above or below the umbilicus). Involution normally begins immediately after delivery, when the firmly contracted uterus lies almost at the umbilicus.

Void to avoid interference

Encourage the patient to void because a full bladder interferes with uterine contractions that work to compress the open blood vessels at the placental site. If these blood vessels are allowed to bleed freely, then hemorrhage may occur. Observe the amount, color, and consistency of the lochia and watch for its absence, which may indicate that a clot is blocking the cervical os. Sudden heavy bleeding could result if a change of position dislodges the clot.

Clot watch

Pregnant and postpartum patients have higher fibrinogen levels, which increase the possibility of clot formation. Patients have an additional risk of clot formation if they have varicose veins, a history of thrombophlebitis, or if they had a cesarean birth. Monitor closely for signs of venous thrombosis, especially if the duration of labor was abnormally long or if the patient was confined to bed for an extended period.

Nursing procedures

Nursing procedures performed during labor and delivery include monitoring of the FHR, monitoring uterine activity, and cervical examination. Monitoring of the FHR and uterine activity can be intermittent or continuous.

How often to monitor

Interpretation of FHR and uterine contractions should be conducted at regular intervals. The Association of Women's Health, Obstetric and Neonatal Nurses (AWHONN) specifies guidelines for monitoring patients who lack risk factors and monitoring of patients who have risk factors. For a patient with no risk factors, the FHR and uterine activity should be assessed every 30 minutes during the first stage of labor and every 15 minutes during the second stage of labor. The assessment of the FHR may be done via auscultation or electronically, and the assessment of uterine activity may be done via palpation or electronically. A patient with risk factors needs continuous FHR monitoring (such as an increased risk for prenatal death, cerebral palsy or neonatal encephalopathy, and the use of oxygen for labor induction or augmentation), and the assessment should be done every 15 minutes during the first stage of labor and every 5 minutes during the second stage of labor.

Intermittent monitoring of fetal status

FHR assessment

Intermittent FHR monitoring is the periodic auscultation of FHR by either a fetoscope or a handheld Doppler device. A Doppler is more commonly used because it is more sensitive to fluctuations in FHR.

Up and about

Intermittent FHR monitoring allows the patient to ambulate during the first stage of labor. Because auscultation is not done until after a contraction, this type of monitoring does not document how the fetus is responding to the stress of labor as well as continuous FHR monitoring does.

Baseline

To establish the baseline FHR, auscultate FHR for 30 to 60 seconds immediately after a contraction has ended. Assess FHR more frequently after the patient ambulates, after cervical examination, or after pain medication administration. Auscultate FHR every 30 minutes during labor for a low-risk patient and every 15 minutes for a high-risk patient.

Uterine contraction palpation

External uterine palpation can tell you the frequency, duration, and intensity of contractions and the relaxation time between them. The character of contractions varies with the stage of labor and the body's response to labor-inducing medications, if administered. As labor advances, contractions become more intense, occur more often, and last longer. In some patients, labor progresses rapidly, preventing the patient from entering a health care facility.

How fast? How long? How hard?

To assess frequency, time the interval between the beginning of one contraction and the beginning of the next. To assess duration, time the period from when the uterus begins tightening until it has relaxed completely.

To assess intensity, palpate the uterine fundus and compare the degree of tightness as described previously in the "Do you feel a nose, a chin, or a forehead?" section.

- Assess contractions in low-risk patients every 30 minutes in the latent phase and the active phases and every 15 minutes in the transition phase of the first stage of labor. More frequent assessments are required for high-risk patients. High-risk fetal status assessments should also occur every 30 minutes during the latent phase, every 15 minutes during the active phase, and every 5 minutes in the second stage. (See *Contraction without relaxation.*)

Advice from the experts

Contraction without relaxation

If any contraction lasts longer than 90 seconds and is not followed by uterine muscle relaxation, or if the relaxation period is less than 1 minute between contractions, then this may indicate tachysystole of the uterus or tetanic contractions. When the uterus doesn't relax, or the relaxation period is less than 1 minute, uteroplacental blood flow is interrupted, which can lead to fetal hypoxia and fetal distress.

If the patient's contractions last longer than 90 seconds or if the relaxation period is less than 1 minute, then follow these steps:
- Discontinue the oxytocin infusion to stop uterine stimulations (if the patient is receiving oxytocin).
- Make sure that the patient is lying on their left side; this increases uteroplacental perfusion.
- Notify the health care provider immediately.

Continuous external electronic monitoring

Continuous external electronic monitoring is an indirect, noninvasive procedure. Two devices, an ultrasound transducer and a tocotransducer, are placed on the patient's abdomen to evaluate FHR and uterine contractions during labor. These devices are held in place with an elastic stockinette or by using plastic or soft straps.

Continuous internal electronic monitoring

Internal monitoring, also called *direct monitoring*, is an invasive procedure that uses a spiral electrode attached to the presenting fetal part (usually the scalp) and an IUPC. This helps assess fetal response to uterine contractions, measures intrauterine pressure, and tracks labor progress.

Internal monitoring is indicated for high-risk pregnancies. However, it can be performed only if the amniotic sac has ruptured, the cervix is dilated at least 2 cm, and the presenting part of the fetus is at least in the −1 station. Complications of internal fetal monitoring for the patient may include uterine perforation and intrauterine infections. Fetal complications may include abscess, hematoma, and infection.

Spiral electrode

The spiral electrode, sometimes called a *fetal scalp electrode* or FSE, detects the fetal heartbeat and transmits it to the monitor, which converts the signals to a fetal electrocardiogram (ECG) waveform.

Intrauterine pressure catheter

An IUPC may be used if external uterine monitoring doesn't provide satisfactory information. It may also be necessary in high-risk pregnancies or if the patient is obese. Insertion of an IUPC is done only by specially trained health care providers. Nurses need to check the policy per institution on who is allowed to place an IUPC.

Fetal strip evaluation

Fetal strip evaluation should be done in a systematic fashion that addresses all components of the strip. The strip should be evaluated considering uterine activity/contractions, baseline FHR, variability of the FHR, periodic or episodic changes to the FHR, and changes in the FHR over time. Following the evaluation of the electronic FHR monitoring strip, the strip should be graded into one of three categories.

Reading a fetal monitor strip

Presented in two parallel recordings, the fetal monitor strip records the FHR in beats per minute in the top recording and uterine activity in millimeters of mercury in the bottom recording. Obtain information on fetal status and labor progress by reading the strips horizontally and vertically.

Reading horizontally on the FHR or the uterine activity strip, each small block represents 10 seconds. Six consecutive small blocks, separated by a dark vertical line, represent 1 minute. Reading vertically on the FHR strip, each block represents amplitude of 10 beats/min. Reading vertically on the uterine activity strip, each block represents 5 mm Hg of pressure.

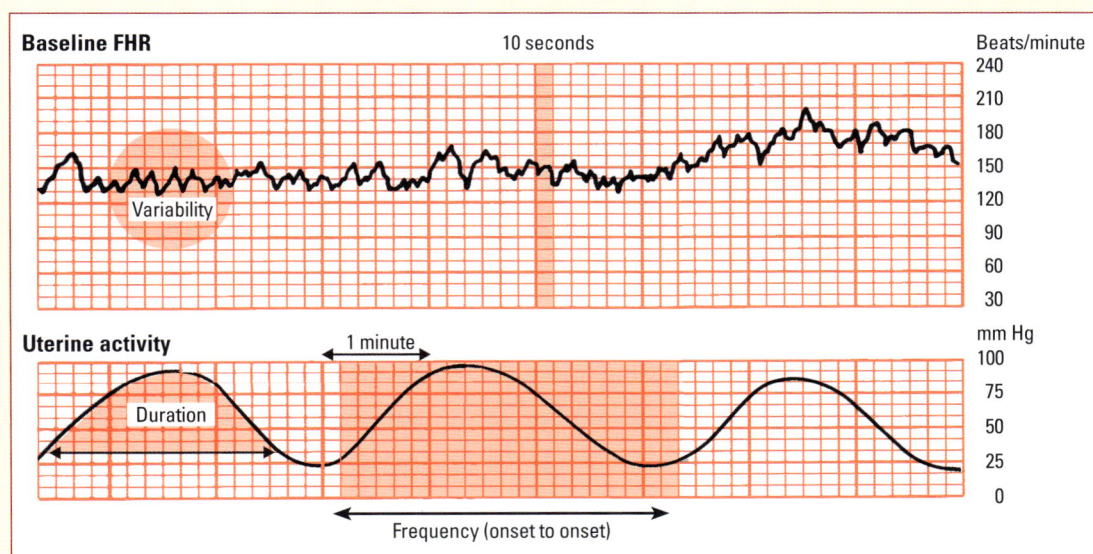

Uterine activity

Uterine contraction activity should be evaluated in segments of 10 minutes but averaged over a 30-minute window. A normal contraction pattern should mean that there are less than or equal to five contractions in 10 minutes (averaged over 30 minutes). If greater than five contractions occur in the 10-minute period, then the terminology assigned to it is tachysystole. Additional components of a uterine contraction pattern assessment include intensity of the contraction, duration of the contraction, and rest or relaxation time between contractions. Also, the assessment of the uterine activity should be considered in light of the response of the FHR.

Baseline FHR

The normal baseline FHR should range from 110 to 160 beats/min and is rounded to increments of 5 beats/min in a 10-minute window. Periodic and episodic changes are not considered when determining the baseline. An FHR in excess of 160 beats/min is defined as fetal tachycardia, and an FHR less than 110 beats/min is defined as fetal bradycardia. Sinusoidal pattern is a smooth, undulating wave pattern in which no acceleration or deceleration is noted.

FHR variability

FHR variability is a fluctuation of the baseline FHR that occurs as variations in the amplitude and frequency. This fluctuation represents the interaction between the sympathetic and parasympathetic nervous systems of the fetus. The constant interactions between these systems result in a moment-to-moment change in the FHR. It signals that both nervous systems are working. This interaction can be termed as *absent, minimal, moderate,* or *marked* and is determined by beats per minute.

Episodic or periodic

Changes to the FHR are classified as either episodic or periodic. Episodic changes are not associated with uterine contractions, and periodic changes in the baseline are temporary, recurrent changes associated with uterine contractions.

Changes to the FHR

Changes to the FHR can be reassuring or non-reassuring, depending on the change and the whole picture of FHR and uterine activity, and last less than 2 minutes. Changes that last more than 2 minutes and less than 10 minutes are considered prolonged changes, and changes that last more than 10 minutes are considered baseline changes.

In 2023, the American College of Obstetricians and Gynecologist (ACOG) reinforced that when a fetus is showing signs of distress (i.e., fetal bradycardia, fetal tachycardia, late decelerations, category II or category III), it is **not** recommended to use supplemental oxygen as an intervention.

Classifications of FHR monitoring

Classifications of FHR monitoring were developed, by the NICHD, as a means to help organize the data obtained from a systematic evaluation of the FHR. There are three categories of interpretation: category I, category II, and category III.

Category I

The tracings are normal and a solid predictor of a normal fetal acid–base balance. No actions are recommended for tracings in this category. Criteria for this category include baseline FHR within normal limits (110 to 160 beats/min), moderate variability, no late or variable decelerations, and early deceleration and acceleration may or may not be present.

Category II

The tracings are considered indeterminate, and, although not predictive of an abnormal fetal acid–base balance, they also lack the features of either category I or III. Criteria for this category include baseline FHR either tachycardic or bradycardic; absent, minimal, or marked variability; no accelerations can be induced; recurrent variable decelerations with minimal or moderate variability; variable decelerations with additional features such as a slow return to baseline or an increase in the rate before return to baseline; any prolonged deceleration (>2 and <10 minutes); and persistent late decelerations with moderate variability.

Category III

The tracings are considered abnormal and predictive of an abnormal fetal acid–base balance. Efforts to resolve the FHR pattern need to be made. Criteria for this category include absent FHR variability with recurrent late decelerations, recurrent variable deceleration or bradycardia, or sinusoidal pattern.

Cervical examination

During first-stage labor, a cervical examination may be done to assess cervical dilation and effacement; membrane status; and fetal presentation, position, and engagement. If the patient has excessive vaginal bleeding, which may signal placenta previa, then cervical examination is contraindicated.

Only practitioners and specially trained nurses can perform cervical examinations. In early labor, perform the cervical examination between contractions, focusing on the extent of cervical dilation and effacement. At the end of first-stage labor, perform the examination during a contraction to focus on assessing fetal descent.

Breathe and release

- Ask the patient to relax by taking several deep breaths and slowly releasing the air.

- Insert lubricated fingers (palmar surface up) into the vagina. Keep uninserted fingers flexed to avoid the rectum.
- Palpate the cervix, noting its consistency. The cervix gradually softens throughout pregnancy, reaching a buttery consistency before labor begins. (See *Cervical effacement and dilation*.)

Cervical effacement and dilation

As labor advances, so do cervical effacement and dilation, promoting delivery. During effacement, the cervix shortens and its walls become thin, progressing from 0% effacement (palpable and thick) to 100% effacement (fully indistinct, or effaced, and paper thin). Full effacement obliterates the constrictive uterine neck to create a smooth, unobstructed passageway for the fetus.

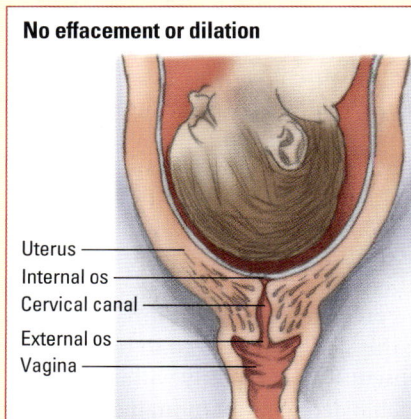

No effacement or dilation

Uterus
Internal os
Cervical canal
External os
Vagina

At the same time, dilation occurs. This progressive widening of the cervical canal—from the upper internal cervical os to the lower external cervical os—advances from 0 to 10 cm. As the cervical canal opens, resistance decreases and eases fetal descent.

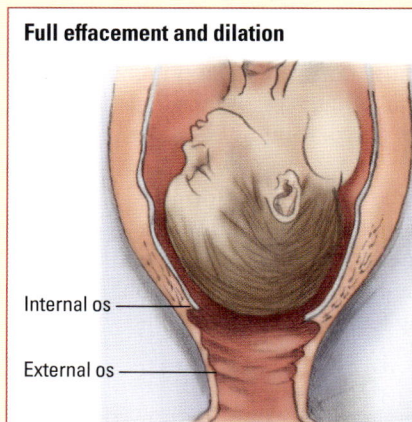

Full effacement and dilation

Internal os

External os

- After identifying the presenting fetal part and position and evaluating dilation, effacement, engagement, station, and membrane status, gently withdraw fingers.
- Help the patient clean their perineum and change the linen-saver pad, as necessary.

Flood zone

If the amniotic membrane ruptures during the examination, then record FHR and time and describe the color, odor, and approximate amount of fluid. If FHR becomes unstable, then determine fetal station and check for umbilical cord prolapse. After the membranes rupture, perform the cervical examination only when labor changes significantly to minimize the risk of introducing intrauterine infection.

Comfort and support issues

Labor and birth usually involve a significant amount of discomfort and can be emotionally draining for patients. Comfort and support measures, such as prenatal education, planning, and the presence of a birthing partner or coach, can promote relaxation and decrease or eliminate the need for analgesia or anesthesia during labor and birth.

Expect the unexpected

Although it is helpful for the patient to make decisions about the issue of pain relief during labor before the actual event, advise them to keep an open mind. The patient should be aware of the other acceptable pain relief options available in case the situation changes during labor and birth. Sometimes, it may be necessary to take the decision regarding pain relief out of the patient's hands—for example, in cases of cesarean birth. No matter what method of pain relief is used, the patient should feel comfortable with it and it should be medically safe.

To provide comfort and support during labor and birth, it is important to understand sources of pain, pain perception and how it affects the patient's response to relief measures, cultural and familial influences on responses to pain, and different approaches to relieving pain.

Sources of pain

The pain experienced during labor and birth comes from several sources.

Uterine contractions

The contraction of the uterine muscles is a prominent source of pain during labor and birth. Like the heart, stomach, and intestine, the uterus is part of an involuntary muscle group. During a contraction, the blood vessels constrict, which reduces the blood supply to the uterine and cervical cells, causing temporary hypoxia or anoxia and pain. As labor progresses and contractions increase in intensity and duration, the blood supply to the cells decreases further, thus increasing the pain.

Dilation

Dilation and stretching of the cervix and lower uterine segment also cause pain during labor. Similar to the intestinal pain caused by accumulated gas in the bowel, this pain increases as the dilation increases.

Distention

Distention of the vagina and perineum to accommodate passage of the fetal head also causes pain during labor. As the fetal head is delivered, an episiotomy or possible tearing of the perineum intensifies this pain.

Pressure on adjacent organs

Another source of pain during labor is the pressure of the presenting part on the adjacent organs, such as the bladder, urethra, or lower colon. This varies depending on the position of the fetus.

Tension

Tension also contributes to pain during labor and birth. The patient's anticipation of pain and their inability to relax commonly cause tension or constriction of the voluntary muscles, including the muscles of the abdominal wall. Tense abdominal muscles increase the pressure on the uterus by preventing the uterus from rising with the contractions.

Pain perception

Pain is a subjective symptom that is unique to each person who experiences it. What may be slight discomfort to one person may be intense, unbearable pain to another. Only the person who is experiencing the pain can describe it or know its extent. When assessing the patient in labor, watch for signs of pain, such as increased respiratory and pulse rates, clenched fists, facial tenseness, and flushed or pale areas of the skin. Many factors influence how pain is perceived.

Under the influence of endorphins

A patient's pain threshold (the amount of pain perceived at a given time) may be influenced by their level of endorphins, the opiatelike substances that are produced by the body in response to pain.

If you expect it, pain will come

A patient who expects the pain of labor to be the most horrible pain they have ever experienced commonly becomes increasingly tense with each contraction and episode of pain, which can intensify the overall perception of the pain.

Too tired and weak for distractions

Fatigue, nutritional status, and sleep deprivation can also affect pain perception. A tired or malnourished person has less energy than a rested one and cannot focus on distraction strategies.

Mind games

Psychological factors, including fear, anxiety, body image, self-concept, and feelings of having no control over the situation, also affect the perception of pain. In addition, memories of previous child-birth experiences affect how the labor pains of the current pregnancy are perceived.

More pieces to the pain puzzle

Other factors that influence pain perception during labor include the intensity of labor, pelvic size and shape, and the interventions of caregivers (which can be a positive or negative influence on pain perception).

Nonpharmacologic pain relief

Nonpharmacologic pain relief methods may be used as the only method of pain management during labor and delivery, or they may be used in conjunction with pharmacologic interventions. Be flexible when a patient chooses an alternative method of pain relief and provide support and reassurance if they find that the method they chose is not working effectively.

Nonpharmacologic pain relief methods include various relaxation techniques, breathing techniques, heat and cold application, counter-pressure, transcutaneous electrical nerve stimulation (TENS), hypnosis, acupuncture and acupressure, and yoga.

Relaxation techniques

Most childbirth education classes teach relaxation techniques. Relaxation turns the focus away from the pain, which reduces tension. The reduced tension leads to a perceived decrease in pain, further reducing tension, thus breaking the pain cycle.

Relaxation techniques include positioning, focusing and imagery, therapeutic touch and massage, music therapy, and the support of a birthing partner or coach. Many patients find these techniques helpful in the early stages of labor, even if they later decide they need supplemental analgesia or anesthesia. Usually, the amount of needed pharmacologic assistance is reduced when used in conjunction with relaxation techniques.

Doula on duty

The patient may choose to have a doula present. A *doula* is a trained professional who provides guidance and support during labor and delivery. As effective as a traditional support person, the doula can help increase the patient's self-esteem and decrease the use of pharmacologic pain relief. Using a doula as a birthing partner or coach does not prevent the patient's partner from being present, providing emotional support, or participating in the neonate's birth.

Breathing techniques

Breathing techniques are important to nonpharmacologic pain relief and are taught in most childbirth preparation classes. They distract from the pain of the contractions and help relax the abdominal muscles. When patients focus on slow-paced, rhythmic breathing, they are less likely to concentrate on the pain being experienced.

Easing pain one breath at a time

The most common breathing technique used is the Lamaze method. The method incorporates the theory that people can learn to use controlled breathing to reduce the pain felt during labor using stimulus–response conditioning.

In Lamaze, the patient is encouraged to direct their attention to a focal point, such as a spot on the wall, at the first sign of a contraction. This focus creates a visual stimulus that goes directly to the brain. The patient then takes a deep cleansing breath followed by rhythmic breathing. During the contraction, the patient's partner provides a series of commands or verbal encouragements to give an auditory stimulus to the brain.

Heat and cold application

Heat applied to the lower back is considered effective in reducing labor pain. A heating pad, moist compress, warm shower, or tub bath can significantly aid relaxation if the membranes remain intact. Applying a cool washcloth to the patient's forehead and providing ice chips to relieve dry mouth are other measures that can increase the comfort level.

Counterpressure

Counterpressure is the application of firm or forceful pressure, using the heel of the hand or fist, to the patient's lower back or sacrum during a contraction. It relieves back pain during labor by countering the pressure of the fetus against the patient's back.

Transcutaneous electrical nerve stimulation

TENS stimulates large-diameter neural fibers via electric currents to alter pain perception. Although not documented as a significant factor in reducing the pain caused by uterine contractions, TENS may be effective in reducing the extreme back pain that some patients have during contractions.

Acupuncture and acupressure

Acupuncture and acupressure are also pain relief methods that are sometimes used during labor. Acupuncture involves stimulating key trigger points with needles. The trigger points do not need to be near the affected organ because their activation releases endorphins, which reduce the perception of pain. Acupressure involves finger pressure or massage at the same trigger points. Holding and squeezing the hand of a person in labor may trigger the point most commonly used for acupuncture and acupressure during labor.

Yoga

Yoga uses a series of deep breathing exercises, body stretching postures, and meditation to promote relaxation, slow the respiratory rate, lower blood pressure, improve physical fitness, reduce stress, and ease anxiety. It may help reduce the pain of labor through the ability to relax the body and possibly through the release of endorphins that may occur.

Pharmacologic pain relief

Pharmacologic pain relief during labor includes analgesia and regional or local anesthesia. These approaches differ in the degree to which pain sensation is decreased. The main goals of using medication during labor are to relax the patient and relieve discomfort without significantly affecting the contractions, pushing efforts, or the fetus.

The right amount at the right time

Almost all medications given during labor have an effect on the fetus because they cross the placental barrier, so it is important to give as little medication as possible. It is also important that medications be given at the proper time. When given after 5 cm dilation in a primipara or after 3 cm dilation in a multipara, medications can speed the progress of labor because the patient can focus on working with the contractions rather than against them. If given too early in labor, then medications can slow or stop the contractions. If given within 1 hour of birth, then the neonate is likely to experience neuromuscular, respiratory, and cardiac depression after delivery.

Know your meds

The nurse must be familiar enough with anesthetic and analgesic agents to answer a patient's questions; assist the anesthesiologist and obstetrician; and quickly identify adverse effects on the patient, fetus, and neonate.

Parenteral analgesic agents

A variety of medications can be given during labor as a pain management strategy. Common analgesic agents used during labor are opioids (i.e., morphine), agonist–antagonists (i.e., butorphanol [Stadol], nalbuphine [Nubain]), and synthetic opioids (fentanyl [Sublimaze]). Opioid medications can cause respiratory depression, agonist–antagonists can also produce this but to a lesser degree, and synthetic opioids cause even less. The impact of the parenteral analgesic agents on the neonate is dependent on the timing of the medication and the dose related to birth time. Meperidine (Demerol) is rarely used in current practice due to its multiday impact on neonatal behavior (decreased muscle tone, poor sucking reflex, and reduced social responsiveness).

Regional anesthesia

Regional anesthesia blocks specific nerve pathways that pass from the uterus to the spinal cord. It relieves pain by making the nerve unable to conduct pain sensations. This form of anesthesia allows the patient to be completely awake, aware of what is happening, and—depending on the region anesthetized—aware of contractions, which gives the opportunity to push at the appropriate time.

Lumbar epidural anesthesia

Lumbar epidural anesthesia (also known as an *epidural block*) is the injection of an opioid medication, such as fentanyl (Sublimaze), bupivacaine (Marcaine), or a lidocaine-like drug (along with an opioid, such as fentanyl or morphine, to decrease the amount of motor blockage incurred) through a needle or catheter into the epidural space (the vacant space just outside the membrane in the lumbar region containing the cerebrospinal fluid that bathes the spinal column and brain). When the drug is administered into this space, it anesthetizes the nerves that carry pain signals from the uterus and perineum to the brain, thus dulling or eliminating the perception of pain. Those with preexisting medical conditions, such as heart disease, diabetes, and gestational hypertension, tend to choose this method because it makes labor almost pain-free, which can reduce physical and emotional stress. (See *A closer look at epidural anesthesia*.)

A closer look at epidural anesthesia

This illustration shows the placement of the epidural catheter used to inject pain-relieving medication into the epidural space.

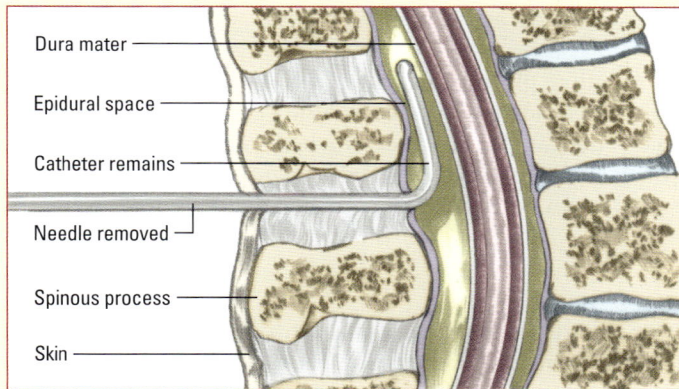

- Dura mater
- Epidural space
- Catheter remains
- Needle removed
- Spinous process
- Skin

The downside, part one

Lumbar epidural anesthesia is relatively safe, but it can lower blood pressure, which can decrease the flow of blood to the uterus and the placenta. Before receiving lumbar epidural anesthesia, the patient should receive 500 to 1,000 mL of an IV solution, such as lactated Ringer solution, to help prevent hypotension. Avoid administering a glucose solution because of the risk of causing rebound hypoglycemia in the neonate.

The downside, part two

Lumbar epidural anesthesia can also slow labor if it is given before the cervix is 5 cm dilated. It may also diminish the ability to push because the patient is unaware of the contractions, which may result in the need for forceps-assisted delivery, vacuum extraction, or cesarean birth.

How it's done

An anesthesiologist or nurse-anesthetist administers lumbar epidural anesthesia. The patient is placed on their side or in a sitting position with their back straight. This position is necessary because it reduces the possibility that the needle will pass through the epidural space into the subarachnoid space.

After the lumbar region of the patient's back is cleaned with an antiseptic and a local anesthetic is injected, a special needle is passed through the L3–L4 space into the epidural space. A catheter is then passed through the needle into the epidural space and taped in place on the skin. The needle is withdrawn, and a syringe is attached to the end of the catheter to create a closed system.

Spinal anesthesia

With spinal anesthesia, a local anesthetic is injected into the cerebro-spinal fluid in the subarachnoid space at the third or fourth lumbar interspace. Spinal anesthesia is used almost exclusively for cesarean birth.

For spinal anesthesia administration, place the patient in a side-lying or sitting position with the head bent forward and the back flexed as much as possible. If the patient is lying down, then ensure their head and upper body are higher than their abdomen and legs so that the anesthetic does not rise too high in the spinal canal.

Local anesthesia

Local anesthesia is used only for pain relief during the actual birth of the fetus because it does not provide relief from contraction pains. It is used for a vaginal delivery when there is no time for other types of anesthesia, after labor pain is relieved using opioids (which cannot be given within 1 hour of the birth), or when a patient who was using nonpharmacologic pain relief during labor needs more relief during birth.

For when labor keeps going and going and going

In most cases, the pressure of the fetal head on the perineum causes natural anesthesia, making local anesthesia administration unnecessary. However, after hours of exhaustive labor, many patients need this relief, especially if an episiotomy is to be performed.

Local infiltration

Local infiltration is the injection of a local anesthetic (usually lidocaine) into the superficial perineal nerves. It is commonly used in preparation for or before suturing an episiotomy. However, anesthesia with this method is not as effective as a pudendal block. (See *Local infiltration location*.)

Local infiltration location

Local infiltration is the injection of a local anesthetic (usually lidocaine [Xylocaine]) into the superficial perineal nerves. This illustration shows the location of the injection.

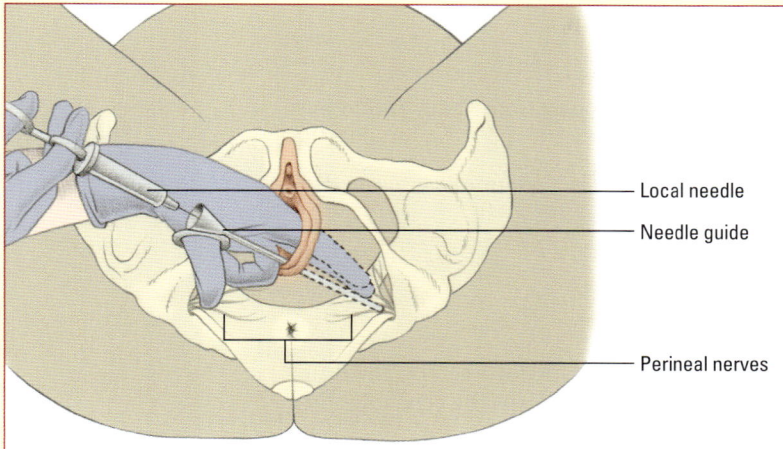

— Local needle

— Needle guide

— Perineal nerves

There are no significant risks to local infiltration, except rare allergic reactions and inadvertent intravascular injections. However, some practitioners believe that injection may weaken the perineal tissue and increase the likelihood of tearing.

Nursing interventions

Nursing interventions during labor and delivery focus on providing comfort and support. Here's what you should do:

- To promote comfort and general body cleanliness, advise the patient to take a warm shower or, if the membranes have not ruptured, a bath. If the patient cannot walk, then perform a sponge or bed bath with meticulous perineal care.
- To increase comfort and reduce the risk of infection, change the gown and sheets whenever they become soiled. Also, change the disposable underpad, especially after a cervical examination. Wipe the patient's face and neck with a cool, clean washcloth, especially during the transition phase of labor.

Quick quiz

1. In the LOA and ROA fetal positions, the presenting part is which of the following?
    A. Olecranon
    B. Chin
    C. Occiput
    D. Buttocks

Answer: C. The occiput is the presenting part in the LOA and ROA fetal positions.

2. Which of the following medications is a common cervical ripening agent?
    A. Dinoprostone (Cervidil)
    B. Oxytocin (Pitocin)
    C. Fentanyl (Sublimaze)
    D. Butorphanol tartrate (Stadol)

Answer: A. Cervidil is commonly used to ripen the cervix. The drug initiates the breakdown of the collagen that keeps the cervix tightly closed.

3. The active phase is part of which stage of labor?
    A. First stage
    B. Second stage
    C. Third stage
    D. Fourth stage

Answer: A. The first stage of labor is divided into two phases: latent and active.

4. In which order do the cardinal movements of labor occur?
    A. Flexion, extension, internal rotation, external rotation, descent, expulsion
    B. Descent, flexion, internal rotation, extension, external rotation, and expulsion
    C. Descent, internal rotation, flexion, external rotation, extension, expulsion
    D. Descent, extension, internal rotation, flexion, external rotation, expulsion

Answer: B. The cardinal movements of labor occur in this order: descent, flexion, internal rotation, extension, external rotation, and expulsion.

5. Before the administration of an epidural anesthetic, the patient should receive 500 to 1,000 mL of which IV solution?

    A.   Normal saline solution

    B.   Dextrose 5% in water (D_5W)

    C. D_5W in lactated Ringer solution

    D.   Lactated Ringer solution

Answer: D. Lactated Ringer solution should be administered before a patient receives epidural anesthesia.

Scoring

☆☆☆ If you answered all five questions correctly, terrific! You certainly delivered the goods on that challenge.

☆☆☆ If you answered four questions correctly, great! Your laboring paid off.

☆☆☆ If you answered fewer than four questions correctly, keep your head up. You'll present well in the next quiz.

Selected References

American College of Obstetricians and Gynecologists. (2022). *Oxygen supplementation in the setting of category II or III fetal heart tracings.* https://www.acog.org/clinical/clinical-guidance/practice-advisory/articles/2022/01/oxygen-supplementation-in-the-setting-of-category-ii-or-iii-fetal-heart-tracings

Association of Women's Health, Obstetric and Neonatal Nurses. (2024). Fetal heart monitoring. *Journal of Obstetric, Gynecologic, and Neonatal Nursing, 53,* e5–e9. https://doi.org/10.1016/j.jogn.2024.03.001

Hutchison, J., Mahdy H., & Hutchison, J. (2023). Stages of labor. In *StatPearls* [Internet]. StatPearls Publishing. https://www.ncbi.nlm.nih.gov/books/NBK544290/

Ricci, S., Kyle, T., & Carman, S. (2021). Labor and birth process. In *Maternity and pediatric nursing* (4th ed., pp. 437–465). Wolters Kluwer.

Ricci, S., Kyle, T., & Carman, S. (2021). Nursing management during labor and birth. In *Maternity and pediatric nursing* (4th ed., pp. 466–512). Wolters Kluwer.

Silbert-Flagg, J. (2023). Nursing care of a family during labor and birth. In *Maternal and child health nursing* (9th ed., pp. 326–372). Wolters Kluwer.

Silbert-Flagg, J. (2023). The nursing role in providing comfort during labor and birth. In *Maternal and child health nursing* (9th ed., pp. 373–395). Wolters Kluwer.

Chapter 8

Postpartum care

Just the facts

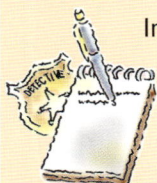

In this chapter, you'll learn:

◆ physiologic and psychological changes that occur during the postpartum period

◆ key components of a postpartum assessment

◆ nursing care measures required during the postpartum period

◆ physiologic events that occur during lactation

◆ two feeding methods, including their advantages and disadvantages.

A look at postpartum care

The postpartum period, or *puerperium*, refers to the 6- to 8-week period after delivery during which the patient's body returns to its nonpregnant state. Some people refer to this period as the *fourth trimester of pregnancy*. Many physiologic and psychological changes occur during this time. Nursing care should focus on helping the patient and their family adjust to these changes and on easing the transition to the parenting role.

Physiologic changes

Two types of physiologic changes occur during the postpartum period: retrogressive changes and progressive changes.

Getting back to normal

Retrogressive changes involve returning the body to its prepregnancy state. Retrogressive reproductive system changes include:

• shrinkage and descent of the uterus into its prepregnancy position in the pelvis

• sloughing of the uterine lining and development of lochia

• contraction of the cervix and vagina

• recovery of vaginal and pelvic floor muscle tone.

Theory of involution

After delivery, the uterus gradually decreases in size and descends into its prepregnancy position in the pelvis—a process known as *involution*. Involution normally begins immediately after delivery, when the firmly contracted uterus lies midway between the umbilicus and symphysis pubis. Soon after, the uterus rises to the umbilicus or slightly above it. After the first postpartum day, the uterus begins its descent into the pelvis at the rate of 1 cm/day (or 1 fingerbreadth/day) or slightly less for the patient who has had a cesarean birth. By the 10th postpartum day, the uterus lies deep in the pelvis—either at or below the symphysis pubis—and it cannot be palpated.

Contraction is key

If the uterus fails to contract or remain firm during involution, uterine bleeding or hemorrhage can result. At delivery, placental separation exposes large uterine blood vessels. Uterine contraction acts as a tourniquet to close these blood vessels at the placental site. Fundal massage, administration of synthetic oxytocic drugs, and release of natural oxytocic drugs during breastfeeding help maintain or stimulate contraction.

All systems undergo

Other body systems undergo retrogressive changes as well. These alterations include:

- reduction in pregnancy hormones, such as human chorionic gonadotropin, human placental lactogen, progestin, estrone, and estradiol
- extensive diuresis, which rids the body of excess fluid and reduces the added blood volume of pregnancy
- gradual rise in hematocrit, which occurs as excess fluid is excreted
- reactivation of digestion and absorption
- eventual fading of striae gravidarum (stretch marks), chloasma (pigmentation on face and neck), and linea nigra (pigmentation on abdomen)
- gradual return of tone to the abdominal muscles, wall, and ligaments
- return of vital signs to baseline/prepregnancy parameters
- weight loss due to rapid diuresis and lochial flow
- recession of varicosities (although they may never return completely to prepregnancy appearance).

In addition, estrogen and progesterone production drops abruptly after delivery, and follicle-stimulating hormone (FSH) production rises, resulting in the gradual return of ovulation and the menstrual cycle.

Making progress

Progressive changes involve building new tissues, primarily those that occur with lactation and the return of menstrual flow. In the postpartum period, fluid accumulates in the breast tissue in preparation for breastfeeding, and the size of breast tissue increases as breast milk forms. The changes associated with lactation are discussed in more detail later in this chapter.

Psychological changes

The postpartum period is a time of transition for the patient and their family. Even if the family has other children, each family member must adjust to the neonate's arrival. In addition to the changes that occur in their body, the postpartum patient undergoes many psychological changes during this time.

Don't let the phases faze you

The postpartum patient goes through three distinct phases of adjustment in the postpartum period:
1. Taking in
2. Taking hold
3. Letting go

In the past, each phase of the postpartum period encompassed a specific period, with patients progressing through the phases sequentially. However, with today's shorter hospitalizations for childbirth, patients move through the phases more quickly and sometimes even experience more than one phase at a time. (See *Phases of the postpartum period*.)

Phases of the postpartum period

This chart summarizes the three phases of the postpartum period.

Phase	Maternal behavior and tasks
Taking in (1–2 days after delivery)	• Contemplation of the recent birth experience • Assumption of passive role and dependence on others for care • Verbalization about labor and birth • Sense of wonderment when looking at the neonate
Taking hold (2–7 days after delivery)	• Increased independence in self-care • Strong interest in caring for the neonate that is often accompanied by a lack of confidence about their ability to provide care
Letting go (about 7 days after delivery)	• Adaption to parenthood and definition of new role as parent and caregiver • Abandonment of fantasized image of neonate and acceptance of real image • Recognition of neonate as a separate entity • Assumption of responsibility and care for the neonate

Building relationships

The postpartum patient and their family undergo other changes as well. Ideally, these changes lead to the development of parental love for the neonate and positive relationships among all family members.

Not all change is good

In some cases, negative psychological reactions may also occur. For example, the postpartum patient may feel let down because the neonate is now the center of attention, or they may feel disappointed because the neonate does not meet their preconceived expectations.

A postpartum patient may also feel overwhelming sadness for no discernible reason. These feelings are commonly termed *postpartum blues* or *baby blues*. A patient with postpartum blues may experience emotional lability, a let-down feeling, crying for no apparent reason, headache, insomnia, fatigue, restlessness, depression, and anger. These feelings most commonly peak around postpartum day 5 and subside by postpartum day 10. (See *Battling the baby blues*.)

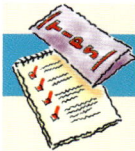

Education edge

Battling the baby blues

For many people, having a baby is a joyous experience. However, childbirth leaves some people feeling fearful, sad, depressed, angry, anxious, and afraid. Insomnia, fatigue, and difficulty concentrating are signs of baby blues. Commonly called *postpartum blues* or *baby blues*, these feelings affect about 70% to 80% of patients after childbirth. Most cases occur within 2 to 3 days postpartum and peak around days 5 to 7 after delivery. Baby blues typically resolve independently, usually around 2 weeks postpartum.

Help is on the way

To help a patient with postpartum blues, tell them to:
- get plenty of rest
- ask for help from family and friends
- take special care of themselves
- spend time with their partner
- call the practitioner if the mood does not improve after a few weeks and if there is trouble coping (this may be a sign of a more severe depression).

Be sure to explain to the postpartum patient that many new caregivers feel sadness, fear, anger, and anxiety after having a baby. These feelings do not mean that they are a failure as a caregiver. These feelings indicate the postpartum patient is adjusting to the changes that follow birth.

(continued)

Battling the baby blues (*continued*)

Blues versus depression

Unfortunately, about 6.5% to 20% of people in the postpartum period experience a more profound problem called *postpartum depression*. In these cases, feelings of depression and despair last longer than a few weeks and are so intense that they interfere with daily activities. Postpartum depression can occur after any pregnancy. It is not specifically associated with first pregnancies. It commonly requires counseling or medication to resolve.

Possible causes of postpartum depression include:

- doubt about the pregnancy
- recent stress, such as the loss of a loved one, a family illness, or a recent move
- lack of a support system
- partner violence or history of physical and emotional abuse
- unplanned cesarean birth (may leave the patient feeling like a failure)
- breastfeeding problems, especially if a patient cannot breastfeed or decides to stop
- sharp drop in estrogen and progesterone levels after childbirth, possibly triggering depression in the same way that much more minor changes in hormone levels can trigger mood swings and tension before menstrual periods
- early birth of neonate (may cause patient to feel unprepared)
- unresolved issues of not being able to be the "perfect" caregiver
- feeling of failure if the patient believes that they should instinctively know how to care for their neonate
- disappointment over sex assigned at birth of neonate or other characteristics (Neonate is not as imagined.)
- disappointment in patient's own body's appearance after delivery.

Signs and symptoms that may indicate that postpartum blues are actually postpartum depression include:

- baby blues continuing for longer than 2 weeks after delivery
- worsening insomnia
- changes in appetite; poor intake
- poor interaction with the neonate; viewing the neonate as a burden or problem
- suicidal thoughts or thoughts of harming the neonate
- feeling worthless or excessive guilt
- feelings of isolation from social contacts and support systems
- inability to care for self or neonate due to lack of energy or desire.

Those experiencing signs of postpartum depression should seek medical help as soon as possible. (See Chapter 10 for more information on postpartum depression.)

First contact

Early contact and interaction between the caregivers, the neonate, and other siblings—including rooming in and sibling visitation—encourage bonding and help integrate the neonate into the family.

Postpartum assessment

As with any assessment, a postpartum assessment consists of a patient history and a physical examination.

Patient history

A postpartum patient history should include information on the patient's pregnancy, labor, and birth events in the medical record. For example, the medical record should contain information about:
- problems experienced, such as gestational hypertension or gestational diabetes
- time of labor onset and admission to the birthing area
- types of analgesia and anesthesia used
- length of labor
- time of delivery
- time of placenta expulsion and appearance of the placenta
- laceration and repairs performed
- quantified blood loss during the delivery and recovery period
- sex, weight, and status of the neonate.

This information is needed to plan the postpartum patient's care and promote bonding.

Another reliable source

Do not rely on the medical record as a sole source of information. Always ask the patient to describe the events and fill in the details in their own words. This is also a good way to learn their emotions about pregnancy and childbirth.

Also, the patient should be asked about their family and lifestyle, including support systems, other children, other people living in the home, their occupation, their community environment, and socioeconomic level. This information can help determine whether additional support, follow-up, or education about self-care and neonatal care is needed.

Physical examination

In many cases, a complete physical examination in the postpartum period is unnecessary because the patient already had a complete assessment early in the labor process. However, there should be a complete review of systems covering the following areas:
- General appearance
- Skin
- Energy level, including level of activity and fatigue

- Pain, including location, severity, and aggravating factors, such as sitting and walking
- Gastrointestinal (GI) elimination, including bowel sounds, passage of flatus, and hemorrhoids
- Fluid intake
- Urinary elimination, including the time and amount of first voiding
- Peripheral circulation
  in addition, these four critical areas also need to be assessed:
- Breasts
- Uterus
- Lochia
- Perineum

Breasts

Inspect and then palpate the breasts, noting size, shape, and color. At first, the breasts should feel soft and secrete a thin, yellow fluid called *colostrum*. However, as they fill with milk—usually around the third postpartum day—they should begin to feel firm and warm. The entire breast may be tender, hard, and tense between feedings on palpation. A low-grade temperature (under 101°F [38.3°C]) is not uncommon between days 2 and 5, but it should not last for more than 24 hours. (See *Engorgement or something else?*)

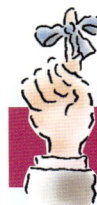

Memory jogger

To help remember what to evaluate during a postpartum assessment, think of the words **BUBBLE HE:**
Breasts
Uterus
Bowel
Bladder
Lochia
Episiotomy
Homans sign
Emotions

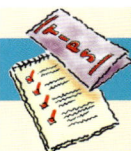

Education edge

Engorgement or something else?

Engorgement, which may result from venous and lymphatic stasis and alveolar milk accumulation, causes the entire breast to appear reddened and to feel warm, firm, and tender. The neonate will have trouble latching onto a severely engorged breast, which further complicates the situation. Encourage the patient to perform frequent and regular breastfeeding to help prevent this problem.

Something else
If the warmth, tenderness, and redness are localized to only one portion of the breast and the patient has a fever or flulike symptoms, suspect *mastitis*—inflammation of the glands or milk ducts.

Mastitis occurs in up to 20% of patients during the postpartum period. It typically results from a pathogen passing through skin breakdown or cracked nipples into the breast tissue. Teach the patient about mastitis, and teach them about signs/symptoms and to call the practitioner immediately if any signs or symptoms appear.

Land of nodule

A small, firm nodule in the breast may be caused by a temporarily blocked milk duct or milk that has not flowed into the nipple. This problem generally corrects itself when the neonate breastfeeds. Be sure to reassess the breast after the neonate feeds to determine if the problem has resolved and report your findings—including the nodule's location—to the practitioner.

Inspect the nipples for cracks, fissures, or configuration. Cracks or breaks in the skin can provide an entry for organisms and lead to infection. Also, look for other problems. Successful breastfeeding can be more challenging if the nipples are flat or inverted. A lactation consultant or a breastfeeding counselor may be helpful.

Uterus

During an examination, palpate the uterine fundus to determine uterine size, degree of firmness, and rate of descent, which are measured in fingerbreadths above or below the umbilicus. Unless the practitioner orders otherwise, perform fundal assessments every 15 minutes for the first hour after delivery, every 30 minutes for the next hour or two, every 4 hours for the rest of the first postpartum day, and then every shift until the patient is discharged. Fundal assessment will need to occur more frequently if complications are noted.

Pain at the incision site makes fundal assessment especially uncomfortable for the patient who has had a cesarean birth. In such cases, provide pain medication beforehand as ordered.

Ready, set, palpate!

Before palpating the uterus, explain the procedure to the patient and provide privacy. Wash your hands and then put on gloves. Also, ask the patient to void. A full bladder makes the uterus boggier and deviates the fundus to the right of the umbilicus or +1 or +2 cm above the umbilicus. When the bladder is empty, the uterus should be at or close to the level of the umbilicus.

Next, lower the head of the bed until the patient is lying supine or with their head slightly elevated. Expose the abdomen for palpation and the perineum for inspection. Watch for bleeding, clots, and tissue expulsion while massaging the uterus.

Performing palpation

To palpate the uterine fundus, follow these steps:

- While supporting the lower segment of the uterus with a hand placed just above the symphysis, gently palpate the fundus with the other hand to evaluate its firmness. (See *Feeling the fundus.*)

Advice from the experts

Feeling the fundus

A full-term pregnancy stretches the ligaments supporting the uterus, placing it at risk for inversion during palpation and massage. To guard against this, place one hand against the patient's abdomen at the symphysis pubis level, as shown. This steadies the fundus and prevents downward displacement. Then, place the other hand at the top of the fundus, cupping it, as shown.

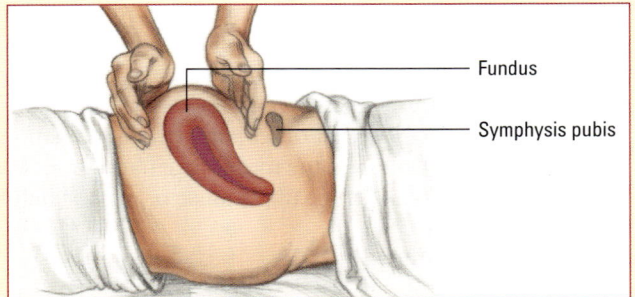

Fundus

Symphysis pubis

- Note the level of the fundus above or below the umbilicus in centimeters or fingerbreadths.
- If the uterus seems soft and boggy, gently massage the fundus with a circular motion until it becomes firm. Without digging into the abdomen, gently compress and release your fingers, always supporting the lower uterine segment with the other hand. Observe the vaginal discharge and lochia during massage.
- Massage long enough to produce firmness but not discomfort. You may also encourage the patient to massage their fundus for 10 to 15 seconds every 15 minutes. This is usually necessary only for a few hours.
- Notify the practitioner immediately if the uterus fails to contract and heavy bleeding occurs. If the fundus becomes firm after massage, keep one hand on the lower uterus and press gently toward the pubis to expel clots. (See *Complications of fundal palpation.*)

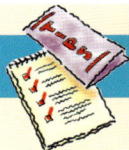

Education edge

Complications of fundal palpation

Because the uterus and its supporting ligaments are tender after birth, pain is the most common complication of fundal palpation and massage. Excessive massage can stimulate uterine contractions, causing undue muscle fatigue and leading to uterine atony or inversion. Lack of lochia may signal a clot blocking the cervical os. Heavy bleeding may result if a position change dislodges the clot. Take the patient's vital signs frequently to assess for hypovolemic shock.

Remember the bladder

When assessing the uterine fundus, also assess for bladder distention. A distended bladder can impede the downward descent of the uterus by pushing it upward and, possibly, to the right side. If the bladder is distended and the patient is unable to urinate, they may need to be catheterized.

Lochia

After birth, the outermost layer of the uterus becomes necrotic and is expelled. This vaginal discharge—called *lochia*—is similar to menstrual flow and consists of blood, fragments of the decidua, white blood cells (WBCs), mucus, and some bacteria.

Assessing lochia flow

Lochia is commonly assessed in conjunction with fundal assessment. (See *Three types of lochia.*)

Three types of lochia

Lochia color, which typically changes throughout the postpartum period, may be categorized as:
- *lochia rubra*—red vaginal discharge that occurs from approximately days 1 to 3 postpartum
- *lochia serosa*—pinkish or brownish discharge that occurs from approximately days 4 to 10 postpartum
- *lochia alba*—creamy white or colorless vaginal discharge that occurs from approximately days 10 to 14 postpartum (although it may continue for up to 6 weeks).

Help the patient into the lateral Sims position. Be sure to check under the patient's buttocks to make sure that blood is not pooling there. Then, remove the patient's perineal pad and evaluate the character and amount, color, odor, and consistency (presence of clots) of the discharge. Before removing the perineal pad, make sure that it is not sticking to any perineal stitches. Otherwise, tearing may occur, possibly increasing the risk of bleeding.

On the lookout

Here is what to look for when assessing lochia:
- *Amount*—Although it varies, the amount of lochia is typically comparable to the amount during menstrual flow. A patient who is breastfeeding may have less lochia. Also, a patient who has had a cesarean birth may have a scant amount of lochia. However, lochia

should not be absent. Lochia should be present for at least 3 weeks postpartum. Lochia flow increases with activity, for example, when the patient gets out of bed the first several times (due to pooled lochia being released) or when they lift a heavy object or walk upstairs (due to an actual increase in the amount of lochia). If a patient saturates a perineal pad in less than an hour, this is considered excessive flow, and the practitioner should be notified.

- *Color*—Lochia typically is described as lochia rubra, serosa, or alba, depending on the color of the discharge. Lochia color depends on the postpartum day. A sudden change in color—for example, from pink back to red—suggests new bleeding or retained placental fragments.
- *Odor*—Lochia should smell similar to menstrual flow. A foul or offensive odor suggests infection.
- *Consistency*—Lochia should have minimal or small clots, if any. Evidence of large or numerous clots indicates poor uterine contraction and requires further assessment.

Perineum and rectum

The pressure exerted on the perineum and rectum during birth results in edema and generalized tenderness. Some areas of the perineum may be ecchymotic, caused by the rupture of surface capillaries. Sutures from an episiotomy or laceration may also be present. Hemorrhoids are also commonly seen.

What's your position?

Assessment of the perineum and rectum mainly involves inspection and is performed at the same time as assessment of the lochia. Help the patient into the lateral Sims position. This position provides better visibility and causes less discomfort for the patient with a mediolateral episiotomy. A back-lying position can also be used for patients with midline episiotomies. Make sure there is adequate light for inspection.

Checking down under

Lift the patient's buttocks and observe for intactness of skin, positioning of the episiotomy (if one was performed), appearance of sutures (from episiotomy or laceration repair), and the surrounding rectal area. Keep in mind that the edges of an episiotomy are usually sealed 24 hours after delivery. Note ecchymosis, hematoma, erythema, edema, drainage or bleeding from sutures, a foul odor, or signs of infection. Also, observe for the presence of hemorrhoids.

Perineal care

Perineal assessment also includes perineal care. The goals of postpartum perineal care are to relieve discomfort, promote healing, and

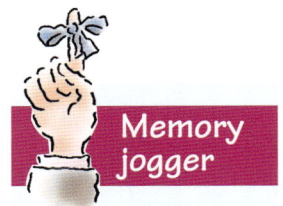

Memory jogger

To help remember what to look for when assessing an episiotomy site or a laceration, think REEDA:

Redness
Erythema and **e**cchymosis
Edema
Drainage or **d**ischarge
Approximation (of wound edges)

prevent infection by cleaning the perineal area. Assist and teach the patient how to perform perineal care in conjunction with a perineal assessment. Perineal care should be performed after the patient voids or has a bowel movement.

Two methods of providing perineal care are generally used: A water-jet irrigation system or a peri bottle is used to cleanse the perineal area.

Water-jet system

If using a water-jet irrigation system, follow these steps (after putting on gloves):
- Insert the prefilled cartridge containing the antiseptic or medicated solution into the handle, and push the disposable nozzle into the handle until it clicks into place.
- Help the patient sit on the toilet or bedpan.
- Place the nozzle parallel to the perineum and turn on the unit.
- Rinse the perineum for at least 2 minutes from front to back.
- Turn off the unit, remove the nozzle, and discard the cartridge.
- Dry the nozzle and store as appropriate for later use.

Peri bottle

If using a peri bottle for perineal care, follow these steps:
- Fill the bottle with cleaning solution (usually warm water).
- Help the patient sit on the toilet or bedpan.
- Tell them to pour the solution over the perineal area.
- After completion, help the patient off the toilet or remove the bedpan.
- Pat the perineal area dry and help the patient apply a new perineal pad.

Hot and cold comfort

During perineal care, if the patient complains of pain or tenderness, apply ice or cold packs to the area for the first 24 hours after birth. This helps reduce perineal edema and prevent hematoma formation, thereby reducing pain and promoting healing.

Cold therapy is not effective after the first 24 hours. Instead, heat is recommended because it increases circulation to the area. Forms of heat include a perineal hot pack (dry heat) or a sitz bath (moist heat).

Sitz right down

For extensive lacerations, such as third- or fourth-degree lacerations, the practitioner may order a sitz bath to aid perineal healing, provide comfort, and reduce edema. It is important to teach a patient how to use a sitz bath at home because of shortened hospitalization time. (See *Using a sitz bath*.)

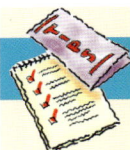

Education edge

Using a sitz bath

A sitz bath allows the postpartum patient to immerse the perineal area in warm or hot water without the bother of taking a complete bath. It relieves discomfort and promotes wound healing by cleaning the perineum and anus, increasing circulation, and reducing inflammation. It also helps relax local muscles.

How it's done
Tell the patient to follow these steps to use a sitz bath correctly:
- Assemble the equipment, and wash your hands.
- Empty your bladder.
- Fill the basin to the specified line with water at the prescribed temperature (usually 100°F to 105°F [37.8°C to 40.6°C]). Be sure to check the water temperature frequently to ensure therapeutic effects.
- Place the basin under the commode seat, clamp the irrigation tubing to block water flow, and fill the irrigation bag with water of the same temperature as that in the basin. Attach the end of the tubing in the correct groove to secure its position in the basin.
- To create flow pressure, hang the bag above your head on a hook, towel rack, or edge of a door.
- Remove and dispose your perineal pad and then sit on the basin.
- If your feet do not reach the floor and the weight of your legs presses against the edge of the equipment, place a small stool under your feet. Also, place a folded towel or small pillow against your lower back.
- Cover your shoulders and knees with blankets or a robe to prevent chilling.
- Open the clamp on the irrigation tubing to allow a stream of water to flow continuously. Refill the bag with water of the correct temperature, as needed, and continue to regulate the flow.
- After approximately 15 to 20 minutes, clamp the tubing and rest for a few minutes before arising to prevent dizziness and lightheadedness.
- Pat the perineal area dry from front to back, and apply a new perineal pad (by holding the bottom sides or ends).
- Dispose soiled materials properly. Empty and clean the sitz bath according to the manufacturer's directions.
- Report changes in drainage amount or characteristics, lightheadedness, perspiration, weakness, nausea, or irregular heart rate.

Postpartum care measures

Ongoing assessment is crucial during the postpartum period. Continue to assess the patient's vital signs, uterine fundus, lochia, breasts, and perineum as ordered. Administer medications as ordered to relieve discomfort from the episiotomy or from uterine contractions, incisional pain, or breast engorgement and assess for therapeutic effectiveness. Encourage the patient to rest after delivery and throughout the postpartum period to prevent exhaustion.

A-voiding catheterization

Assess the patient's urinary elimination. The patient should void within 6 to 8 hours after delivery. If they do not, help them urge to void by administering analgesic agents as ordered, pouring warm water over the perineum, placing the patient's hands in warm water, or running water for the patient to hear (the sound may encourage the urge to void). If all attempts fail, the patient may need to be catheterized. Closely monitor for bladder distention during this period as this may lead to increased uterine bogginess and bleeding.

Flatus foreshadows function

Finally, assess bowel function. Elimination is typically a good indicator of bowel function. The patient should have a bowel movement 1 to 2 days after delivery to avoid constipation. However, a patient who has eaten nothing by mouth for 12 to 24 hours and then has a cesarean birth may not have a bowel movement for several days. In these cases, flatus may be a better indicator of bowel function.

Encourage the patient to drink plenty of fluids and eat high-fiber foods to prevent constipation. If necessary, the practitioner may order stool softeners or laxatives. If the patient has hemorrhoids, cool witch hazel compresses may be helpful. Do not use suppositories if the patient has a third- or fourth-degree laceration.

Patient education

Because of the short length of stay for most postpartum patients, patient education is essential. Teaching should focus on self-care activities for the patient as well as neonatal care. (See *Postpartum maternal self-care*.)

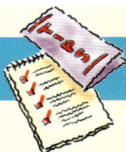

Education edge

Postpartum maternal self-care

When teaching a patient about self-care for the postpartum period, be sure to include these topic areas and instructions.

Personal hygiene
- Change perineal pads frequently, removing them from the front to the back and disposing them in a plastic bag.
- Perform perineal care each time that you urinate or move your bowels.

(continued)

Postpartum maternal self-care (*continued*)

• Monitor your vaginal discharge. It should change from red to pinkish brown to clear or white before stopping altogether. Notify your practitioner if the discharge returns to a previous color, becomes bright red or yellowish green, suddenly increases in amount, or develops an offensive odor.
• Follow your practitioner's instructions about using sitz baths or applying heat to your perineum.
• Shower daily.

Breasts
• Wear a firm, supportive bra if choosing to formula feed.
• If nipple leakage occurs, use clean gauze pads or nursing pads inside your bra to absorb the moisture.
• Inspect your nipples for cracking, fissures, or soreness, and report areas of redness, tenderness, or swelling.
• Wash breasts daily with clear water when showering and dry with a soft towel or allow to air dry. Do not use soap on your breasts or nipples because soap is drying.
• If you are breastfeeding and your breasts become engorged, use warm compresses, stand under a warm shower, or feed your baby more frequently for relief. If the baby is unable to latch on due to engorgement, using a breast pump should help. If you are not breastfeeding, apply cool compresses several times per day.

Activity and exercise
• Balance rest periods with activity, get as much sleep as possible at night, and take frequent rest periods or naps during the day.
• Check with your practitioner about when to begin exercising.
• If your vaginal discharge increases with activity, elevate your legs for about 30 minutes. If the discharge does not decrease with rest, call your practitioner.

Nutrition
• Increase your intake of protein and calories.
• Drink plenty of fluids throughout the day, including before and after breastfeeding.

Elimination
• If you have the urge to urinate or move your bowels, do not delay doing so. Urinate at least every 2 to 3 hours. This helps keep the uterus contracted and decreases the risk of excessive bleeding.
• Report difficulty urinating, burning, or pain to your practitioner.
• Drink plenty of liquids and eat high-fiber foods to prevent constipation.
• Follow your practitioner's instructions about the use of stool softeners or laxatives.

Sexual activity and contraception
• Remember that breastfeeding is not a reliable method of contraception. Discuss birth control options with your practitioner.
• Ask your practitioner when you can resume sexual activity and contraceptive measures.
• Use a water-based lubricant if necessary.
• Expect a decrease in intensity and rapidity of sexual response for about 3 months after delivery.
• Perform Kegel exercises to help strengthen your pelvic floor muscles. To do this, squeeze your pelvic muscles as if trying to stop urine flow and then release them.

Lactation

Lactation refers to the production of breast milk, the preferred source of nutrition for a neonate. All patients experience the physiologic changes that occur with lactation and breast milk production regardless of whether they plan to breastfeed.

Physiology of lactation

During pregnancy, a hormone called *prolactin* prepares the breasts to secrete milk. Other hormones (progesterone and estrogen) interact to suppress milk secretion while developing the breasts for lactation. Estrogen causes the breasts to grow by increasing their fat content. Progesterone causes lobule growth and develops the alveolar (acinar) cells' secretory capacity.

After birth, the patient's estrogen and progesterone levels drop abruptly. This drop in hormones triggers the release of prolactin from the anterior pituitary, which starts the cycle of synthesis and secretion of milk. (See *A closer look at lactation*.)

A closer look at lactation

After delivery of the placenta, the drop in progesterone and estrogen levels stimulates the production of prolactin. This hormone stimulates milk production by the acinar cells in the mammary glands.

Nerve impulses caused by the neonate sucking at the breast travel from the nipple to the hypothalamus, resulting in the production of prolactin-releasing factors. This factor leads to additional production of prolactin and, subsequently, more milk production.

Go with the flow

Milk flows from the acinar cells through small tubules to the lactiferous sinuses (small reservoirs located behind the nipple). This milk, called *foremilk*, is thin, bluish, and sugary and is constantly forming. It quenches the neonate's thirst but contains little fat and protein.

When the neonate sucks at the breast, oxytocin is released, causing the sinuses to contract. Contraction pushes the milk forward through the nipple to the neonate. In addition, the release of oxytocin causes the smooth muscles of the uterus to contract.

That let-down feeling

Movement of the milk forward through the nipple is termed the *let-down reflex* and may be triggered by things other than the infant sucking at the breast. For example, patients have reported that hearing their baby cry or thinking about them causes this reflex.

(continued)

A closer look at lactation (*continued*)

Once the let-down reflex occurs and the neonate has fed for 10 to 15 minutes, new milk—called *hindmilk*—is formed. This milk is thicker and whiter, and it contains higher concentrations of fat and protein. Hindmilk contains the calories and fat necessary for the neonate to gain weight, build brain tissue, and be more content and satisfied between feedings.

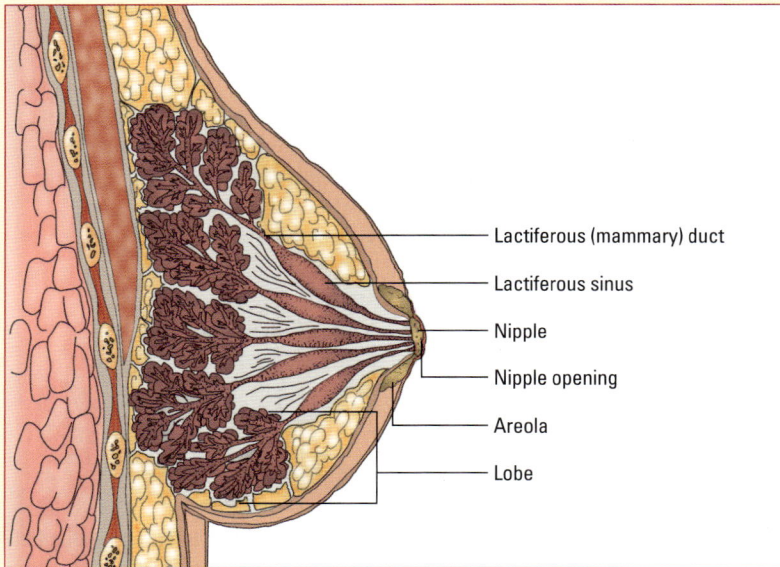

- Lactiferous (mammary) duct
- Lactiferous sinus
- Nipple
- Nipple opening
- Areola
- Lobe

Breast milk composition

From about the fourth month of pregnancy until the first 3 to 4 days after delivery, the acinar cells produce and secrete colostrum. Colostrum is a thick, sticky, golden-yellow fluid that contains protein, sugar, fat, water, minerals, vitamins, and maternal antibodies. It is easy for the neonate to digest because it is high in protein and low in sugar and fat. It also provides complete adequate nutrition for the neonate. The high protein level of colostrum aids in the binding of bilirubin and has a laxative effect, which promotes early passage of the neonate's first stool (called *meconium*).

Got milk?

On about the second to fourth postpartum day, colostrum is replaced by mature breast milk. During this time, copious amounts of breast milk are produced. The composition of this breast milk changes with each feeding, depending on the stage of breastfeeding. Transitional breast milk is replaced by true or mature breast milk by around day 10 after delivery.

Lactation and the menstrual cycle

After the placenta is delivered, estrogen and progesterone production ceases. As a result, the pituitary gland increases the production of FSH, which eventually leads to ovulation and resumption of the menstrual cycle.

Here we go again

Lactating patients begin menstruating again at various times, anywhere from 2 to 18 months. Ovulation may occur by the end of the first month postpartum, or it may not occur for one or more menstrual cycles. Patients who are not lactating usually resume menstruating in 6 to 10 weeks. Approximately one half of these patients ovulate with the first menstrual cycle.

Neonatal nutrition

Human milk consumed through breastfeeding is considered optimal for neonates. Despite this, not all patients can or choose to breastfeed. Medical conditions, cultural background, anxiety, drug misuse, and various other factors can prevent breastfeeding. Preterm or high-risk neonates may require additives or fortifiers in their breast milk to meet their unique needs while still receiving all the benefits of regular breast milk.

Breastfeeding

Breastfeeding is considered the safest, simplest, and least expensive way to provide complete infant nourishment. The American Academy of Pediatrics (AAP) recommends breastfeeding exclusively for the first 6 months of the infant's life and supports continued breastfeeding after solid foods are introduced for 2 years or beyond—as long as it is jointly desired by the breastfeeding caregiver and the infant.

Contrary to popular belief

Breastfeeding is contraindicated if the patient:
- has HIV infection that is not virally suppressed (during and after pregnancy) while on antiretroviral therapy
- has herpes lesions on their nipples

- is receiving certain medications, such as methotrexate (Folex PFS [parenteral formulation solution]) or lithium (Eskalith), that pass into the breast milk and potentially the neonate. Each unit should have resources to serve as a guide to which medication may be incompatible with breastfeeding
- is on a restricted diet that interferes with adequate nutrient intake and subsequently affects the quality of milk produced
- has breast cancer
- has a severe chronic condition, such as untreated tuberculosis, untreated brucellosis, suspected or confirmed Ebola
- uses illicit drugs (i.e., heroin, cocaine) and some prescription opioids.

Advantages

Breastfeeding is advantageous for the caregiver and the neonate. Maternal benefits include:

- protection against breast cancer and ovarian cancer
- assistance in uterine involution due to the release of oxytocin
- less preparation time and less cost than using infant formula
- reduced risk of developing rheumatoid arthritis, hypertension, and cardiovascular disease with 12 months of cumulative breastfeeding.

More good news about breastfeeding

Breast milk is also highly beneficial for the neonate. For example, it reduces the risk of infection because it contains:

- immunoglobulin A—an antibody that prevents foreign proteins from being absorbed by the neonate's GI tract
- lactoferrin—an iron-binding protein that interferes with bacterial growth
- lysozyme—an enzyme that actively destroys bacteria
- leukocytes—WBCs that protect against common respiratory infections
- macrophages—cells that produce interferon, which offers protection from viral invasion.

In addition, breastfeeding is advantageous to the neonate for these reasons:

- Breast milk promotes rapid brain growth because it contains large amounts of lactose, which is easily digested and can be rapidly converted to glucose.
- Breast milk's protein and nitrogen contents provide foundations for neurologic cell building.
- Breast milk contains adequate electrolyte and mineral composition for the neonate's needs without overloading the neonate's renal system.
- Breastfeeding improves the neonate's ability to regulate calcium and phosphorus levels.

- The sucking mechanism associated with breastfeeding reduces dental arch malformations.
- A breastfed neonate's GI tract contains large amounts of *Lactobacillus bifidus*, a beneficial bacterium that prevents the growth of harmful organisms.

On the contrary

Breastfeeding may delay ovulation but should not be considered a reliable form of contraception. In addition, evidence does not suggest that breastfeeding aids in weight loss after pregnancy.

Maternal nutrition and breastfeeding

Nutritional needs for a patient who is breastfeeding are only slightly different from those during pregnancy. Folate and iron needs decrease after giving birth, and energy requirements increase.

Fueling milk production

While breastfeeding, a healthy patient should consume 2,000 to 2,400 calories per day, based on daily lifestyle and activity level. Those with a more sedentary lifestyle may only need 1,800 to 2,000 calories per day. Continuing a prenatal vitamin supplement with docosahexaenoic acid (DHA) is recommended while breastfeeding. If caloric intake is low, which can occur when a lactating patient is trying to lose weight postpartum, the nutrient intake in the breast milk may become inadequate.

Water hydrant

Adequate hydration encourages ample milk production. Breastfeeding patients should drink a beverage before breastfeeding as well as during or after to ensure adequate fluid intake, which maintains milk production. Water is the best option for daily hydration. The breastfeeding caregiver should drink ½ oz of water for every pound of body weight and extra as needed when thirsty. Fruit juice and milk are other options for hydration.

Keep contaminants out!

Most ingested substances are secreted into the breast milk. Therefore, beverages containing alcohol and caffeine should be limited or avoided because they may be harmful to the neonate. In addition, it is important to check with a health care provider before taking medication. Some researchers believe that components of the maternal food may contribute to colic or the neonate's fussiness.

Breastfeeding assistance

Even patients who have previously breastfed can benefit from assistance and instruction. The key is helping the patient to latch the neonate properly. Breastfeeding should occur as soon as possible after birth. However, this may not be possible, especially if the patient is overly fatigued or if a complication has developed.

Don't get comfy yet

When assisting with breastfeeding, explain the procedure and provide privacy. Also, encourage them to use the bathroom and change the neonate's diaper before breastfeeding begins so that feeding is uninterrupted. Then, wash hands and instruct the patient to do the same. Help the patient find a comfortable position. (See *Breastfeeding positions*.) Inform them that uterine cramping may occur during breastfeeding until the uterus returns to its original size.

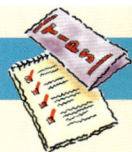

Education edge

Breastfeeding positions

The position a patient uses when breastfeeding should be comfortable and efficient. Explain that changing positions periodically alters the neonate's grasp on the nipple and helps to prevent contact friction in the same area. As appropriate, suggest these popular feeding positions.

Cradle position

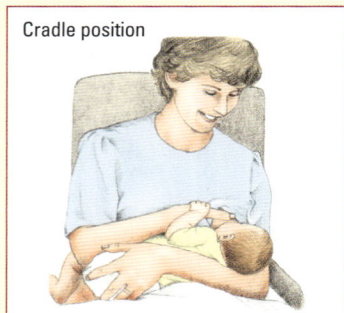

Cradle position

The patient cradles the neonate's head in the crook of their arm. Instruct them to place a pillow on their lap for the neonate to lie on. Offer to place a pillow behind their back. This provides comfort and may also assist with correct positioning.

Cross-body position

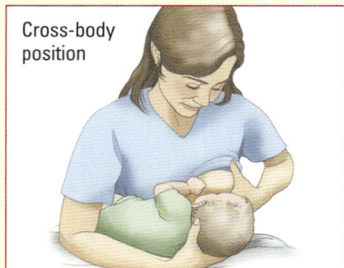

Cross-body position

Instruct the patient: "Sitting with your elbows supported by pillows, use your left hand to grasp your left breast and use your right hand to support the neonate's head. Bring the head to the left breast with the neonate's body across your body. Bring the neonate to you and do not bend over."

Breastfeeding positions (*continued*)

Side-lying position

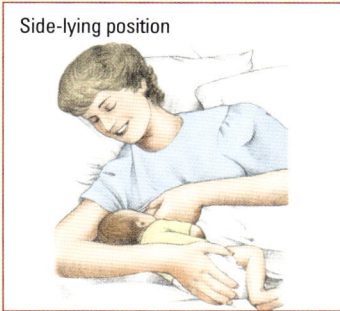

Side-lying position

Instruct the patient to lie on their side with their stomach facing the neonate. As the neonate's mouth opens, the patient should pull the baby toward the nipple. Inform the patient to place a pillow or rolled blanket behind the neonate's back to prevent them from moving or rolling away from the breast.

Biologic or laid-back position

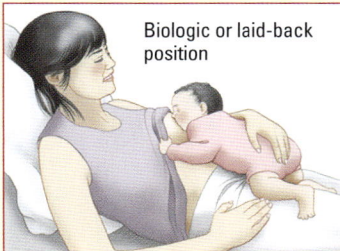

Biologic or laid-back position

Assist the patient to lie back on a bed or couch but do not lie flat. Place the neonate on the chest so that the whole front of the neonate is against the patient's skin. Allow the infant to find the breast, and the breast may or may not be held by the patient.

Football position

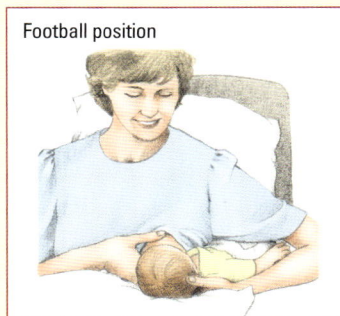

Football position

Sitting with a pillow in front, the patient places their hand under the neonate's head. As the neonate's mouth opens, the patient pulls the neonate's head near the breast. This position may be more comfortable for the patient who has had a cesarean birth.

Getting latched on

Calm babies latch on quickly. Ways to calm a baby include skin-to-skin, rocking, talking to the baby, or allowing the baby to suck on a clean finger.

There are multiple ways to help an infant latch on to the breast.

- Skin-to-skin—Place the infant, dressed in a diaper only, on patient's bare chest in between the breasts. The infant will bob their head and move closer to the breast and muzzle or lick the breast.

- Guiding the patient's hand, have them place the thumb on top of the exposed breast's areola and the first two fingers beneath it, forming a C. Have them turn the neonate so that the infant's entire body faces the breast.
- Touch the infant's mouth with the underside of the areola. When the infant's mouth is opened, promptly introduce the breast with the underside of the areola first. This allows for the nipple to be pointed toward the roof of the infant's mouth. This helps the infant to exert sufficient pressure with their lips, gums, and cheek muscles on the milk sinuses below the areola.
- Allow the infant to feed without time limits as to how long the infant should be on the breast. During the first few days of life, an infant may only nurse on one breast at a feeding. If this is the case, alternate breasts from feeding to feeding.

To make sure that both breasts receive equal stimulation, advise the patient to begin the next feeding using the breast on which the neonate finished this feeding. To help remember, the patient can put a safety pin on the bra strap on the side last used.

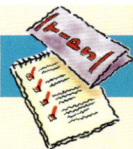

Education edge

Teach patients to observe their babies for feeding/hunger cues

Feeding/hunger cues include:
stretching
eyes opening
yawning
rooting
sticking their tongue out
crying, which is a late hunger cue.

Quelling concerns

Patients commonly have questions about breastfeeding, including how often the neonate should feed, how much the neonate is getting, and what to do if the neonate is too sleepy to breastfeed. Reassure the patient that breastfeeding schedules are not carved in stone and that developing a schedule that both the patient and the baby feel comfortable with takes time.

Feed me, feed me!

During the first few days of life, a neonate is usually fed as often as they are hungry. Feeding on demand and not on a schedule is recommended. During the first week of life, the neonate may eat as often as every 1 to 3 hours (8 to 12 times in a 24-hour period is expected). This helps to ensure that the neonate is satisfying their sucking needs and is receiving the necessary fluid and nutrients. Frequent feeding also helps initiate the patient's milk supply because frequent emptying stimulates more milk production.

A neonate's behavior and output help to determine if they are getting enough breast milk. If the infant is content between feedings, wets approximately one diaper per day of life, and has stool once per day of age, then they are getting enough milk. For example, on the first day of life, expect one wet diaper and one stool. On the second day of life, expect two wet diapers and two stools. On the third day of life, expect three wet diapers and three stools. More wet diapers or stools than expected are considered good. Once the patient's milk is evident, they can expect to see six to eight wet diapers per day and three to four stools per day. Many neonates lose weight in the days after being born (less than 10% of their body weight). The neonate should be at or above their birth weight by 2 weeks of age.

Whetting their appetite

Sometimes, neonates seem to be uninterested or fall asleep when breastfeeding. If the neonate shows little interest in breastfeeding, assist the patient in keeping the neonate awake. If the neonate is sleepy, suggest that the patient try rubbing the baby's feet, unwrapping the blanket, changing the diaper, or changing their position or the neonate's. The patient may also manually express a little milk and allow the neonate to taste it. (See *Manual breast milk expression*.) If the neonate has little success or interest in breastfeeding for several feedings, refer the patient to a lactation consultant or breastfeeding specialist.

Manual breast milk expression

Manually expressing breast milk can enhance milk production and ensure an adequate supply. It is especially helpful for patients who have problems with engorgement or those who must be away from their infants for several hours. (Someone who works outside the home or is away on a regular basis may find an electric or battery-operated pump quicker and more efficient.)

Express yourself
To help the patient manually express breast milk, follow these steps:
- Make sure that a clean collection container is available and that you and the patient have washed your hands.
- Explain the procedure to the patient, have them sit in a comfortable position, and provide privacy.
- Tell them to place their dominant hand on one breast with the thumb positioned on the top and the fingers below and at the outer limit of the areola.

(continued)

Manual breast milk expression (*continued*)

• Instruct them to press the thumb and fingers inward toward the chest while holding the collection container with the opposite hand directly under the nipple.
• Tell the patient to move the thumb and fingers forward, using gentle pressure in a milking motion. Caution the patient not to use too much pressure, as this can injure breast tissue. Milk should flow out of the nipple and into the collection container.
• Encourage the patient to move the thumb and fingers around the breast, using the same motion, to ensure complete emptying.
• Advise the patient to cover the container, and place the milk in the refrigerator if it will be used within 24 hours. If not, it should be frozen.

Keep up the good work!

Always encourage breastfeeding efforts. To boost these efforts, urge the patient to eat balanced meals, drink at least eight 8-oz glasses of fluid daily, and nap daily for at least the first 2 weeks after giving birth. Answer questions about breastfeeding, and provide instructional materials if available. Always provide a patient who is breastfeeding information and instructions related to possible complications. (See Chapter 10, Complications of the postpartum period, for more in-depth information on complications.) Contact a lactation consultant as appropriate.

Before discharge, tell the patient about local breastfeeding support groups.

Bottle-feeding with breast milk

In some cases, a patient may need to be away from the neonate but still desires to provide breast milk. The patient may also need to express breast milk when their breasts are engorged. Although breast milk can be expressed by hand, using a battery-powered or electric pump may be the most efficient method.

Breast pumping

Breast pumping involves using suction created with a manual, battery-powered, or electric pump to stimulate lactation. It is used when the postpartum patient and neonate are separated or while illness temporarily incapacitates one or the other.

A breast pump can also relieve engorgement, collect milk for a premature neonate with a weak sucking reflex, reduce pressure on sore or cracked nipples, or reestablish the milk supply. The patient can also use a pump to collect milk when they are unable to manually express it.

Preparing to pump

Before teaching the patient to use a breast pump:
- assemble the equipment according to the manufacturer's instructions
- explain the procedure to the patient
- provide privacy
- wash hands and instruct the patient to wash theirs
- help the patient into a comfortable position and urge them to relax.

Tell the patient to drink a beverage before and after pumping. If the patient's breasts are engorged, instruct them to apply warm compresses for 5 minutes, or take a warm shower before pumping.

Manual pump

To use a manual pump, instruct the patient to place the flange or shield against the breast with the nipple in the center of the device. Then, have them pump each breast by operating the device according to the manufacturer's instructions. The patients should continue until the breast is empty and then repeat the procedure on the other breast. It is also acceptable to pump for 5 minutes on one side and then switch sides and pump for 5 minutes, and then, after 5 to 10 minutes, they should switch sides again and continue pumping until milk stops flowing from each breast.

Battery-powered or electric pump

To use a battery-powered or electric pump, instruct the patient to set the suction regulator on low. Tell them to hold the collection unit upright to allow milk to flow into it. Have them place the shield against their breast with the nipple in the center. They should turn on the machine and adjust the suction regulator to a comfortable pressure.

Instruct the patient to start with the least amount of suction to prevent nipple damage and then gradually increase the suction. Advise them to check the operator's manual to see the pressure setting at which the pump functions most efficiently.

Keep on pumping

Instruct the patient to pump each breast for 15 to 20 minutes or until the milk stops spraying, which takes longer. They may wish to use a double pump, which allows for pumping both breasts at the same time.

When the patient has finished pumping, show them how to remove the shield from the breast by inserting a finger between the breast and the shield to break the vacuum seal. Then, return the suction regulator to the low setting and turn off the machine.

Freeze, store, or enjoy right now?

After using either type of pump, the patient should let their nipples air dry for about 15 minutes. They should also disassemble the pump's removable parts and clean them according to the manufacturer's directions.

If the patient plans to store or freeze the milk, have them fill a clean container (Avoid plastic bags or bags that fit into nursery bottles since they tend to leak.). Always label the collected milk with the date and the time of collection. (See *Breast milk storage.*) Write the neonate's name on the label, if necessary. If the neonate is going to drink the milk right away, show the patient how to attach a rubber nipple to the cylinder or collection unit.

Breast milk storage

Location	Temperature	Storage time frame	Additional information
Tabletop	Room temperature up to 77°F (25°C)	6–8 hours	Cover and keep as cool as possible.
Cooler bag	5°F–39°F (−15°C to 3.9°C)	24 hours	Keep ice packs in contact with milk containers.
Refrigerator	39°F (3.9°C)	5 days	Keep milk at the back of the main body.
Refrigerator freezer with common door	5°F (−15°C)	2 weeks	Keep milk at the back of the main body.
Refrigerator freezer with separate door	0°F (−17.8°C)	3–6 months	Keep milk at the back of the main body.
Deep freezer	−4°F (−20°C)	6–12 months	Keep milk at the back of the main body.

Bottle-feeding with formula

Formula-feeding is a reliable and nutritionally adequate method of feeding for neonates. Commercial formulas are designed to mimic human milk.

Types of formulas

Commercial formulas typically provide 20 calories per ounce when diluted properly and are classified as milk based, soy based, and elemental. Milk-based formulas are usually recommended. Some of these formulas are lactose-free, so they can be used for neonates with galactosemia or lactose intolerance.

Health food for babies

Soy-based formulas are used for babies who could be allergic to cow's milk protein. Elemental formulas are commonly prescribed for babies who may have protein allergies or fat malnutrition. With these formulas, the amount of fat, protein, and carbohydrates is modified.

Formula × four

Commercial formulas may be supplied in one of four forms:
- Powdered—to be combined with water
- Condensed liquid—must be diluted
- Ready to feed
- Disposable, individually prepared bottles

The powdered form is the least expensive, whereas individually prepared bottles are the most expensive but easiest to use. Most health care facilities use individually prepared bottles. Tell caregivers about the forms of formula available, so they can choose what is most convenient for them.

Formula-feeding assistance

Each day, an infant requires 2.5 to 3 oz of fluid per pound of body weight (150 to 200 mL/kg) and 50 to 55 calories per pound of body weight (100 to 120 kcal/kg). Because commercial formulas consistently provide 20 calories per ounce, only the infant's fluid needs are used to determine the amount of each feeding. Unlike breastfeeding, you can measure the amount of formula consumed.

Until about age 4 months, most infants need six feedings per day. After this, the number of feedings drops, but the amount at each feeding increases because the baby starts to eat cereal, fruits, and vegetables.

Prefeeding prep

When bottle-feeding a neonate or helping the caregiver with bottle-feeding, know the type of formula ordered and how it is supplied. If you are using a commercially prepared formula, check the expiration date, uncap the formula bottle, and make sure that the seal is not broken to ensure sterility and freshness. If the seal is broken, discard the formula. If it is not broken, remove it.

Next, screw on the nipple and cap. Keep the protective sterile cap over the nipple until the neonate is ready to feed. If preparing a formula, follow the manufacturer's directions or the health care provider's prescription. Administer the formula at room temperature or slightly warmer. Do not warm the formula in a microwave because it heats the formula unevenly resulting in "hot spots" that can scald the infant's mouth and throat.

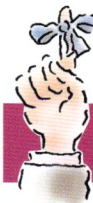

Memory jogger

To easily determine the amount of milk an infant should take in at each feeding, add 2 to 3 oz to the infant's age (in months). So, for example:

- *a 1-month-old should take 3 to 4 oz at each feeding*
- *a 4-month-old should take 6 to 7 oz*
- *a 5-month-old should take 7 to 8 oz.*

Bottle-feeding blow by blow

Teach the patient to follow these steps when bottle-feeding the neonate:

- After washing hands and preparing the formula, invert the bottle and shake some formula on the wrist to test its temperature and the patency of the nipple hole. The formula should drip freely but not stream out. If the hole is too large, the neonate may aspirate the formula. If it is too small, the extra sucking effort may tire them before they can empty the bottle.
- Sit comfortably in a semi-reclining position, and cradle the neonate in one arm to support their head and back. This position allows swallowed air to rise to the top of the stomach where it is more easily expelled. If the neonate cannot be held, sit by them, and elevate their head and shoulders slightly.
- Place the nipple in the neonate's mouth on top of their tongue but not so far back that it stimulates the gag reflex. They should begin to suck, pulling in as much nipple as is comfortable. If they do not start to suck, stroke them under the chin or on the cheek, or touch their lips with the nipple to stimulate the sucking reflex.

Tilting does the trick

- As the neonate feeds, tilt the bottle upward to keep the nipple filled with formula and to prevent them from swallowing air. Watch for a steady stream of bubbles in the bottle. This indicates proper venting and flow of formula.
- If the neonate pushes out the nipple with the tongue, reinsert the nipple. Expelling the nipple is a normal reflex and does not necessarily mean that the neonate is full.
- Always hold the bottle for a neonate. If left to feed themselves, they may aspirate formula or swallow air if the bottle tilts or empties. In older infants, experts also link bottle propping with an increased incidence of otitis media and dental caries.
- Be sure to interact with the neonate during feeding.
- Burp the neonate after each ½ oz of formula because they will usually swallow some air even when fed correctly.
- Do not worry if the neonate regurgitates some of the feedings. Neonates are prone to regurgitation because of an immature lower esophageal sphincter. Regurgitation is merely an overflow and should not be confused with vomiting—a more complete emptying of the stomach accompanied by symptoms not associated with feeding.
- Discard any remaining formula and properly dispose of all equipment.

Burping basics

Because some neonates swallow large amounts of air when feeding, encourage the patient to burp the neonate after part of the feeding and at the end of the feeding. Before burping, remind the patient to place a protective cover, such as a cloth diaper or washcloth, under the neonate's chin. The most common way to burp a neonate is to place them over one shoulder and gently pat or rub their back to help expel ingested air.

A burp is a burp is a burp

Some patients have trouble supporting the neonate's head while patting or rubbing their back. This position may be especially awkward with small neonates because they lack the ability to control their heads. In these cases, suggest the sitting position for burping. (See *Sitting up for burping.*) A third acceptable position is placing the neonate prone across the patient's lap.

Sitting up for burping

If the patient indicates that placing the neonate over their shoulder for burping is awkward, suggest this alternative:
• Hold the neonate in a sitting position on the patient's lap.
• Lean the neonate forward against one hand and support their head and neck with the index finger and thumb of that same hand, as shown in the image.

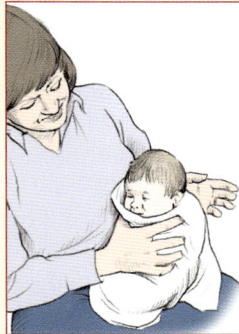

At home, go with the flow

Teach caregivers how to prepare and (if required) sterilize formula, bottles, and nipples. Although most health care facilities have a feeding schedule, advise the family to switch to a more flexible demand-feeding schedule when at home.

Breast care

A patient who plans to breastfeed after the neonate's birth will need to maintain breast tissue integrity. Although postpartum care varies for breastfeeding and non-breastfeeding patients, some guidelines are similar.

For breastfeeding patients

Provide these instructions to a patient who is breastfeeding their neonate:

- Wash breasts with water only to avoid washing away the natural oils and keratin.
- To help prevent tenderness, lubricate the nipple with a few drops of expressed breast milk before feeding.
- Place breast pads over nipples to collect milk, and replace the pads often to reduce the risk of infection. Breasts often leak during the first few weeks of breastfeeding.
- Be alert for a slight temperature elevation and an increase in breast size, warmth, and firmness 2 to 5 days after birth. This signals that breast milk is coming in.
- Apply warm compresses, massage the breasts, take a warm shower, or express some milk before feeding if breasts are engorged, and the neonate cannot latch on to the nipple.

For non-breastfeeding patients

Provide these instructions to a patient who is not breastfeeding their neonate:

- Clean breasts with water only or with soap if necessary.
- Wear a supportive bra to help minimize engorgement and decrease nipple stimulation.
- To minimize further milk production, avoid stimulating the nipples or manually expressing milk.
- Use analgesic agents (if ordered), cold compresses, and a firm supportive bra to minimize engorgement.
- Cabbage leaves can be inserted into the bra as an additional method to minimize engorgement. Wash and dry the leaves, and remove any large fibrous area prior to insertion; chill them prior to insertion into the bra, and change them every couple of hours.

Quick quiz

1. The nurse is working with a postpartum patient after delivery. Which behavior would the nurse expect to assess during the taking-in phase of the couplet?
   A. Frequent infant care questions
   B. Adapting to caregiver role
   C. Encouraging own self-care
   D. Contemplative thoughts on labor

Answer: D. During the taking-in phase, the patient is contemplative and often thinking of the labor experience and is dependent on others for care of self and infant. The other options are from the remaining phases of the postpartum period.

2. The nurse is assessing the uterine fundus in a patient 48 hours after delivery. Where would the nurse anticipate assessing for and locating the fundus?

    A.   2 cm above the umbilicus
    B.   Located at the umbilicus
    C.   2 cm below the umbilicus
    D.   Located at the symphysis pubis

Answer: C. The uterus descends at a rate of about 1 cm/day after delivery. At 48 hours (2 days) postpartum, the fundus should be located and assessed 2 cm below the umbilicus.

3. The nurse is collecting information for assessing a patient at the 6-week postpartum appointment. Which of the following does the nurse anticipate the patient reporting for current lochia?

    A.   Lochia rubra
    B.   Lochia serosa
    C.   Lochia alba
    D.   Absence of lochia

Answer: D. By 6 weeks, lochia has most often ceased. Lochia rubra typically lasts from days 1 to 3 postpartum; lochia serosa, from days 4 to 10; and lochia alba, from days 10 to 14. If the patient reports still having lochia at 6 weeks, further information is needed, and assessments should be completed.

4. The nurse is educating a patient after delivery on the process of lactation and hormones in lactation. Which of the following does the nurse teach is responsible for the stimulation of lactation?

    A.   Estrogen
    B.   Prolactin
    C.   Progesterone
    D.   FSH

Answer: B. Prolactin is the hormone responsible for stimulating lactation. The other hormones listed have different roles in the postpartum patient.

5. A postpartum patient is planning to bottle-feed their infant. Which of the following would the nurse teach the patient to use for decreasing engorgement?

    A.   Cabbage leaves
    B.   Manual expression
    C.   Warm showers
    D.   Nipple stimulation

Answer: A. For the patient who is not breastfeeding, use of cabbage leaves can be taught as one method to decrease engorgement. The other options are not appropriate for a patient who wants to dry milk supply. They are all used to decrease engorgement by engorgement of milk in breastfeeding patients.

Scoring

⭐⭐⭐ If you answered all five questions correctly, whoa! You've certainly galloped through this chapter.

⭐⭐ If you answered three to four questions correctly, giddyap! Looks like you've corralled your knowledge of postpartum care.

⭐ If you answered fewer than three questions correctly, stay steady. You're sure to be more stable the next time you go over this chapter.

Selected References

Abuogi, L., Noble, L., Committee on Pediatric and Adolescent HIV, & Section on Breast-feeding. (2024). Infant feeding for persons living with and at risk for HIV in the United States: Clinical report. *Pediatrics, 153*(6), e2024066843. https://doi.org/10.1542/peds.2024-066843

Carlson, K., Mughal, S., Azhar, Y., Siddiqui, W., & May, K. (2024). Postpartum depression (nursing). In *StatPearls*. StatPearls Publishing. https://www.ncbi.nlm.nih.gov/books/NBK568673/

Center for Disease Control and Prevention. (2022). *How much and how often to breast-feed*. https://www.cdc.gov/nutrition/infantandtoddlernutrition/breastfeeding/how-much-and-how-often.html

Healthy Children. (2022). *Amount and schedule for baby formula feeding*. Retrieved May 2022, from https://www.healthychildren.org/English/ages-stages/baby/formula-feeding/Pages/amount-and-schedule-of-formula-feedings.aspx

March of Dimes. (2021). *Baby blues after pregnancy*. https://www.marchofdimes.org/find-support/topics/postpartum/baby-blues-after-pregnancy

Ricci, S., Kyle, T., & Carman, S. (2021). Nursing management during the postpartum period. In *Maternity and pediatric nursing* (4th ed., pp. 536–574). Wolters Kluwer.

Ricci, S., Kyle, T., & Carman, S. (2021). Postpartum adaptations. In *Maternity and pediatric nursing* (4th ed., pp. 515–535). Wolters Kluwer.

Silbert-Flagg, J. (2023). Nursing care of a postpartal family. In *Maternal and child health nursing* (9th ed., pp. 396–424). Wolters Kluwer.

Chapter 9

Complications of the postpartum period

Just the facts

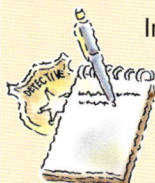

In this chapter, you'll learn:

◆ major complications that can occur during the postpartum period, including risk factors for each
◆ ways to identify complications based on key assessment findings
◆ treatments that are appropriate for each complication
◆ appropriate nursing interventions for each complication.

A look at postpartum complications

Although the postpartum period involves many physiologic and psychological changes and stressors, these changes are usually considered good—not unhealthy. During this time, the patient, the neonate, and other family members interact and grow as a family.

A cluster of complications

However, complications can develop due to a wide range of factors, such as blood loss, trauma, infection, or fatigue. Some common postpartum complications include postpartum hemorrhage, postpartum psychiatric disorders, puerperal infection, mastitis, and deep vein thrombosis (DVT). Keen nursing skills can help to prevent problems or detect them early before they cause more stress or seriously interfere with the caregiver–child relationship.

Postpartum hemorrhage

Postpartum hemorrhage—any blood loss from the uterus that exceeds 1,000 mL during a 24-hour period or when there is a loss of blood—is a major cause of mortality in the postpartum period. Many deaths from postpartum hemorrhage are preventable, and early identification and intervention are required to prevent these deaths.

After vaginal birth, blood loss of up to 500 mL is considered acceptable, although this amount may vary among health care facilities. The acceptable range for blood loss after cesarean birth is up to 1,000 mL.

Complicating the matter

A patient who has a birth complicated by any of these factors should be observed for the possibility of developing a postpartum hemorrhage:

- Abruptio placentae
- Overdistention of the uterus
- Missed abortion
- Placenta previa
- Uterine infection
- Placenta accreta
- Uterine inversion
- Severe preeclampsia
- Amniotic fluid embolism
- Intrauterine fetal death
- Precipitous labor
- Macrosomia
- Multiple gestation
- Prolonged labor
- Multiparity
- Preexisting conditions (coagulation abnormalities)
- History of a postpartum hemorrhage after a previous delivery

What a difference a day makes

Postpartum hemorrhage is classified as early or late, depending on when it occurs. *Early postpartum hemorrhage* refers to blood loss in excess of 500 mL in vaginal delivery and 1,000 mL in cesarean birth that occurs during the first 24 hours postpartum. *Late postpartum hemorrhage* refers to uterine blood loss in excess of 1,000 mL that occurs during the remaining 6-week postpartum period but after the first 24 hours.

What causes it

Uterine atony, lacerations, retained placenta or placental fragments, and disseminated intravascular coagulation (DIC) are the leading causes of postpartum hemorrhage.

Relax—don't do it!

Uterine atony is responsible for 70% to 80% of postpartum hemorrhages. Uterine atony is the failure of the myometrial muscles to contract after delivery. Any condition that interferes with the ability of the uterus to contract appropriately can lead to uterine atony and, subsequently, postpartum hemorrhage. When the uterus does not contract properly, vessels at the placental site remain open, allowing blood loss. Approximately 600 to 700 mL of blood per minute circulates to placental site. This allows for a large amount of blood loss to occur quickly after separation of the placenta. The danger of postpartum hemorrhage due to uterine atony (inadequate uterine contractions) is greatest during the first hour after birth and continues to be high for 24 hours after birth. (See *Relaxation is risky.*)

Relaxation is risky

Risk factors for uterine atony include:
- polyhydramnios
- delivery of a macrosomic neonate, usually more than 9 lb (4.1 kg)
- use of magnesium sulfate during labor
- multiple gestation
- delivery that was rapid or required operative techniques, such as forceps or vacuum suction
- injury to the cervix or birth canal, such as from trauma, lacerations, or hematoma development
- use of oxytocin to initiate or augment labor or prolonged use of tocolytic agents
- dystocia (dysfunctional labor)
- previous history of postpartum hemorrhage
- use of deep analgesia or anesthesia
- infection, such as chorioamnionitis or endometritis
- a body mass index (BMI) greater than 40.

Blame it on lacerations

Lacerations of the cervix, birth canal, or perineum can also lead to postpartum hemorrhage. Cervical lacerations may result in profuse bleeding if the uterine artery is torn. This type of hemorrhage usually occurs immediately after delivery of the placenta while the patient is still in the delivery area. Suspect lacerations when bleeding persists, but the uterus is firm.

Stuck on you

Entrapment of a partially or completely separated placenta by an hourglass-shaped uterine constriction ring (a condition that prevents the entire placenta from expelling) can cause placental fragments to be retained in the uterus. Poor separation of the placenta is common in preterm births of 20 to 24 weeks' gestation.

The reason for abnormal adherence is unknown, but it may result from implantation of the zygote in an area of defective endometrium. This abnormal implantation leaves a zone of separation between the placenta and the decidua. If the fragment is large, bleeding may be apparent in the early postpartum period. If the fragment is small, however, bleeding may go unnoticed for several days, after which time, the patient suddenly has a large amount of bloody vaginal discharge.

To clot or not to clot

DIC is a fourth cause of postpartum hemorrhage. Any patient is at risk for DIC after childbirth. However, it is more common in those with abruptio placentae, missed abortion, acute fatty liver of pregnancy, HELLP (hemolysis of red blood cells [RBCs], elevated liver enzymes, and low platelets) syndrome, placenta previa, uterine infection, placenta accreta, uterine inversion, severe preeclampsia, amniotic fluid embolism, or intrauterine fetal death.

What to look for

Bleeding is the key assessment finding for postpartum hemorrhage. It can occur suddenly in large amounts or over time as seeping or oozing of blood. Expect a patient with postpartum hemorrhage to saturate perineal pads more quickly than usual.

Soft and boggy

When uterine atony is the cause, the uterus feels soft and relaxed. The bladder may be distended, displacing the uterus to the right or left side of the midline and preventing it from contracting properly. The fundus may also be pushed upward.

A cut above

When a laceration is the cause of postpartum hemorrhage, there may be bright red blood with clots oozing continuously from the site and a uterus that remains firm.

Left behind

Bleeding caused by a retained placenta or placental fragments usually starts as a slow trickle, oozing, or frank hemorrhage. In the case of retained placental fragments, also expect to find the uterus to be soft and noncontracting.

The fourth culprit: DIC

When the patient's bleeding is continuous and uterine atony, lacerations, and retained placenta or fragments have been ruled out, coagulation problems may be the cause of the bleeding.

The shocking truth

If blood loss is severe, the patient exhibits signs and symptoms of hypovolemic shock, such as increasing restlessness, lightheadedness, and dizziness as cerebral tissue perfusion decreases. Inspection may also reveal pale skin, decreased sensorium, increased pulse rate, and rapid, shallow respirations. Urine output usually falls below 25 mL/h. Palpation may disclose rapid, thready peripheral pulses and cool skin that becomes cold and clammy.

Auscultation of blood pressure usually detects a mean arterial pressure below 60 mm Hg and narrowing pulse pressure. Capillary refill at the nail beds is delayed by 3 to 5 seconds. Remember, these are late signs of postpartum hemorrhage. The best patient outcomes result from early identification and early intervention.

What tests tell you

Diagnostic testing reveals a decrease in hemoglobin levels and hematocrit. The patient's hemoglobin level typically decreases by 1 to 1.5 g/dL, and hematocrit drops by 2% to 4% from baseline. If the patient has retained placental fragments, serum human chorionic gonadotropin levels may be elevated.

Coagulating the matter

When DIC causes postpartum hemorrhage, platelet and fibrinogen levels decrease, and clotting times (prothrombin time [PT] and partial thromboplastin time [PTT]) are prolonged. Blood tests also reveal decreased fibrinogen levels and fragmented RBCs. Fibrinolysis increases and then decreases. Coagulation factors decrease, with decreased antithrombin III, an increased D-dimer test, and a normal or prolonged euglobulin lysis time.

How it's treated

Treatment of postpartum hemorrhage focuses on correcting the underlying cause and instituting measures to control blood loss and minimizing the extent of hypovolemic shock.

Pump up the tone

For the patient with uterine atony, initiate uterine massage. The goal is to increase uterine tone and contractility to minimize blood loss. If clots are present, they should be expressed. If the patient's bladder is distended, they should try to empty their bladder because a distended bladder prevents the uterus from fully contracting. If these efforts are ineffective or fail to maintain the uterus in a contracted state, oxytocin (Pitocin) or methylergonovine (Methergine) may be given through intramuscular (IM) or intravenous (IV) routes to produce sustained uterine contractions. Prostaglandins (carboprost tromethamine) can also be given IM to promote strong, sustained uterine contractions. Cytotec can be administered rectally to help increase uterine tone. Tranexamic acid (TXA) also decreases blood loss and improves outcomes in patients with postpartum hemorrhage.

Source search

If the uterus is firm and contracted and the bladder is not distended, the source of bleeding must still be identified. Perform visual or manual inspection of the perineum, vagina, uterus, cervix, and rectum. A laceration requires sutures. If a hematoma is found, treatment may involve observation, cold therapy, ligation of the bleeding vessel, or evacuation of the hematoma. Depending on the extent of fluid loss, replacement therapy may be indicated.

Remove the stragglers

Retained placental fragments, typically, are removed manually or, if manual extraction is unsuccessful, via dilation and curettage (D&C). If the placenta is adhered to the uterine wall or has implanted into the myometrium, a hysterectomy may need to be performed to stop uterine bleeding.

Supportive to specific

Successful management of DIC requires prompt recognition and adequate treatment of the underlying disorder. Treatment may be supportive (e.g., when the underlying disorder is self-limiting) or highly specific. If the patient is not actively bleeding, supportive care alone may reverse DIC. Active bleeding may require administration of blood, fresh-frozen plasma, platelets, or packed RBCs to support hemostasis.

Heparin (Hep-loc) therapy for DIC is controversial. It may be used early in the disease to prevent microclotting but may be considered a last resort in the patient who's actively bleeding. If thrombosis occurs, heparin therapy is usually mandatory. In most cases, it is administered in combination with transfusion therapy.

Making up for lost fluids

Emergency treatment relies on prompt and adequate blood and fluid replacement to restore intravascular volume, raise blood pressure, and maintain it above 60 mm Hg. Rapid infusion of lactated Ringer solution and, possibly, albumin or other plasma expanders may be needed to expand the volume adequately until the whole blood can be matched.

What to do

Close, frequent assessment in the hour following delivery is crucial to prevent complications or allow early identification and prompt intervention should hemorrhage occur.

Here are other steps that should be taken in case of postpartum hemorrhage:

- Assess the patient's fundus and lochia every 15 minutes for 1 hour after birth to detect changes. Notify the practitioner if the fundus doesn't remain contracted or if lochia increases.
- Perform fundal massage, as indicated, to assist with uterine involution. Stay with the patient, frequently reassessing the fundus to ensure it remains firm and contracted. Keep in mind that the uterus may relax quickly when massage is completed, placing the patient at risk for continued hemorrhage.
  If postpartum hemorrhage is suspected:
- weigh perineal pads to have a more accurate quantified blood loss
- turn the patient onto their side and inspect under the buttocks for pooling of blood
- inspect the perineal area closely for oozing from possible lacerations
- monitor vital signs frequently for changes, noting trends such as a continuously rising pulse rate and a drop in blood pressure. Report changes immediately. (See *Managing low blood pressure*.)

Managing low blood pressure

If the patient's systolic blood pressure drops below 80 mm Hg, increase the oxygen flow rate, and notify the practitioner immediately. Systolic blood pressure below 80 mm Hg usually results in inadequate coronary artery blood flow, cardiac ischemia, dysrhythmia, and further complications of low cardiac output.

Another ominous sign

Notify the practitioner, and increase the infusion rate if the patient has a progressive drop in blood pressure (30 mm Hg or less from baseline) accompanied by a thready pulse. This usually signals inadequate cardiac output from reduced intravascular volume. Assess the patient's level of consciousness (LOC). As cerebral hypoxia increases, the patient becomes more restless and confused.

- Assess intake and output, and report urine output less than 30 mL/h. Encourage the patient to void frequently to prevent bladder distention from interfering with uterine involution. If they cannot void, an indwelling urinary catheter may need to be inserted.

A shocking development

Here are the steps that should be taken if the patient develops signs and symptoms of hypovolemic shock:

- Begin an IV infusion with lactated Ringer solution delivered through a large-bore (14G to 18G) catheter.
- Administer colloids (albumin) and blood products as ordered.
- Monitor the patient for fluid overload.
- Monitor for signs and symptoms of infection, such as increased temperature, foul-smelling lochia, or redness and swelling of the incision.
- Record blood pressure, pulse and respiratory rates, and peripheral pulse rates every 15 minutes until stable.
- Monitor cardiac rhythm continuously.
- During therapy, assess skin color and temperature and note changes. Cold, clammy skin may signal continuing peripheral vascular constriction and progressive shock.
- Monitor capillary refill and skin turgor.
- Watch for signs of impending coagulopathy, such as petechiae, bruising, and bleeding or oozing from gums or venipuncture sites.
- Anticipate the need for fluid replacement and blood component therapy, as ordered.
- Obtain arterial blood samples to measure arterial blood gas (ABG) levels. Administer oxygen by nasal cannula, facemask, or airway to ensure adequate tissue oxygenation. Adjust the oxygen flow rate as ABG measurements indicate.
- Obtain venous blood specimens as ordered for a complete blood count, electrolyte measurements, typing and cross-matching, and coagulation studies.
- If the patient has received IV oxytocin to treat uterine atony, continue to assess the fundus closely. Although oxytocin's action is immediate, it is short, so atony may recur. Monitor for nausea and vomiting.
- Monitor the patient for hypertension if methylergonovine is administered. This medication should not be administered if the patient's baseline blood pressure is 140/90 mm Hg or greater.
- If the practitioner orders IM administration of prostaglandin, be alert for possible adverse effects, such as nausea, diarrhea, tachycardia, headache, fever, and hypertension.
- Provide emotional support to the patient, and explain all procedures to help alleviate fear and anxiety.

- Monitor the patient's LOC for signs of hypoxia (decreased LOC).
- Prepare the patient for possible treatments, such as bimanual massage, surgical repair of lacerations, or D&C.

Postpartum psychiatric disorders

Three distinct psychiatric disorders have been recognized during the postpartum period: postpartum blues (or baby blues), postpartum depression, and postpartum psychosis. Postpartum depression and postpartum psychosis are mood disorders recognized by the American Psychiatric Association's *Diagnostic and Statistical Manual of Mental Disorders* (5th ed., text rev.).

Blue, blue, my world is blue

Baby blues are the most common of the postpartum psychiatric disorders and the least severe. Approximately 80% of all postpartum patients experience some form of baby blues. Baby blues usually occur within 2 to 3 days after birth. They are a normal, hormonally generated postpartum occurrence that is thought to foster maternal–neonatal attachment. Patients who have a history of depression, who have delivered prematurely, and those who have an infant in the newborn intensive care unit are at particularly high risk. The patient's age and obstetric complications also contribute to the risk. Baby blues typically resolve independently, usually around 2 weeks postpartum. To help a patient with postpartum blues, tell them to:

- get plenty of rest
- ask for help from family and friends
- take special care of themselves
- spend time with their partner
- call the practitioner if the mood does not improve after a few weeks and if there is trouble coping (This may be a sign of a more severe depression.).

Be sure to explain to the postpartum patient that many new parents feel sadness, fear, anger, and anxiety after having a baby. These feelings do not mean that they are a failure as a caregiver. These feelings indicate the postpartum patient adjusting to the changes that follow birth.

Postpartum depression

Postpartum depression affects 6.5% to 20% of patients postnatally. This number may be higher because many cases probably are not reported due to the stigma of a psychiatric illness. Postpartum depression has an onset before delivery in nearly 50% of patients. Not only does postpartum depression interfere with the caregiver–infant relationship, but it is thought to also interfere with child development and the relationship the child has with other children, family, and friends.

What causes it

The exact cause is unknown, but some prenatal risk factors may contribute to the development of postpartum depression.

Possible risk factors for postnatal major depression include:
- young age (e.g., below 25 years of age)
- lack of support system
- recent stress, such as loss of a loved one, a family illness, or a recent move
- unplanned cesarean birth (may leave the patient feeling like a failure)
- early birth of neonate (may cause patient to feel unprepared)
- unresolved issues of not being able to be the "perfect" parent
- feeling of failure if the patient believes that they should instinctively know how to care for their neonate
- disappointment over biologic sex of neonate or other characteristics (neonate is not as imagined)
- multiparity
- family history of postpartum depression or psychiatric illness
- intimate partner violence and lifetime history of physical or sexual abuse
- unintended/unwanted pregnancy
- negative attitudes toward pregnancy
- fear of childbirth
- poor perinatal physical health (e.g., obesity at the time of conception, pregestational or gestational diabetes, antenatal or postnatal hypertension, or infection following delivery)
- body image dissatisfaction (preconception, antenatal, and postpartum)
- personality traits, such as neuroticism (which is marked by an enduring tendency to worry and to feel anxious, angry, sad, and guilty)
- history of premenstrual syndrome or premenstrual dysphoric disorder
- sharp drop in estrogen and progesterone levels after childbirth, possibly triggering depression in the same way that much smaller changes in hormone levels can trigger mood swings and tension before menstrual periods
- perinatal anxiety symptoms and disorders
- perinatal sleep disturbance

- season of delivery (e.g., postpartum depression may increase during the time of year when daylight is diminished)
- adverse pregnancy and neonatal outcomes (e.g., including stillbirth, preterm birth, very low birth weight, and neonatal death)
- postpartum blues (subsyndromal depressive symptoms)
- breastfeeding difficulty/shorter duration/cessation
- childcare stress such as inconsolable infant crying, difficult infant temperament, or infant sleep disturbance.

Genetic and hormonal components have also been thought to play a role in the risk of developing postpartum depression.

The result

Untreated depression during pregnancy can lead to poor self-care, nonadherence with prenatal care, and a negative effect on bonding. Additionally, it can lead to a higher risk of obstetric complications, drug, tobacco, or alcohol misuse, marital struggles, abnormal infant/child development, termination of the pregnancy, and suicide.

What to look for

Some distinct signs and symptoms help distinguish postpartum depression from postpartum baby blues, including:
- feeling sad or down for longer than 2 weeks after delivery
- decreased interest in normal activities
- appetite problems and weight changes
- anxiety and agitation
- difficulty sleeping/worsening insomnia
- fatigue and reduced energy
- feeling guilty or worthless
- inability to care for self or neonate due to lack of energy or desire
- feelings of isolation from social contacts and support systems
- poor interaction with the neonate; views the neonate as a burden or problem
- feelings of suicide or thoughts of harming the infant.

The earliest postpartum depression is diagnosed in 1 to 3 weeks after birth and can occur at any point during the first year.

What tests tell you

There are no specific diagnostic tests for postpartum depression, but patients can be screened during the prenatal period for risk factors leading to the development of postpartum depression. The Edinburgh Postnatal Depression Scale tool is the most common screening tool for postpartum depression. This is a self-reporting tool, and a score of at least 12 correlates with symptoms of postpartum depression. (See *Edinburgh Postnatal Depression Scale.*)

Edinburgh Postnatal Depression Scale

As you have recently had a baby, we would like to know how you are feeling. Please UNDERLINE the answer which comes closest to how you have felt IN THE PAST 7 DAYS, not just how you feel today.

Here is an example, already completed.

I have felt happy.

Yes, all the time.
Yes, most of the time.
No, not very often.
No, not at all.

In the past 7 days:

1. I have been able to laugh and see the funny side of things.

   As much as I always could.
   Not quite so much now.
   Definitely not so much now.
   Not at all.

2. I have looked forward with enjoyment to things.

   As much as I ever did.
   Rather less than I used to.
   Definitely less than I used to.
   Hardly at all.

3. I have blamed myself unnecessarily when things went wrong.

   Yes, most of the time.
   Yes, some of the time.
   Not very often.
   No, never.

4. I have been anxious or worried for no good reason.

   No not at all.
   Hardly ever.
   Yes, sometimes.
   Yes, very often.

5. I have felt scared or panicky for no very good reason.

   Yes, quite a lot.
   Yes, sometimes.
   No, not much.
   No, not at all.

In the past 7 days:

6. Things have been getting on top of me.

   Yes, most of the time I haven't been able to cope at all.
   Yes, sometimes I haven't been coping as well as usual.
   No, most of the time I have coped quite well.
   No, I have been coping as well as ever.

7. I have been so unhappy that I have had difficulty sleeping.

   Yes, most of the time.
   Yes, sometimes.
   Not very often.
   No, not at all.

8. I have felt sad or miserable.

   Yes, most of the time.
   Yes, quite often.
   Not very often.
   No, not at all.

9. I have been so unhappy that I have been crying.

   Yes, most of the time.
   Yes, quite often.
   Only occasionally.
   No, never.

10. The thought of harming myself has occurred to me.

    Yes, quite often.
    Sometimes.
    Hardly ever.
    Never

How it's treated

Treatment can usually be accomplished on an outpatient basis. Selective serotonin reuptake inhibitors, such as paroxetine (Paxil), fluoxetine (Prozac), and sertraline (Zoloft), are one of the primary classes of medications prescribed. These agents are considered to be safe for breastfeeding patients. Psychotherapy has also been proven to be an effective treatment.

What to do

- Teach the postpartum patient about the warning signs of postpartum depression, and provide resource material.
- Include teaching about postpartum depression as part of the patient's discharge teaching plan.
- Encourage the patient to verbalize their feelings about the pregnancy.
- Help the patient understand that feeling sadness or a lack of enthusiasm about parenthood is normal.
- Instruct the patient that postpartum depression can occur at any time after delivery.
- Advise the family and the patient's support system of the warning signs of postpartum depression. Inform them that it is important not to ignore even the subtlest of signs. Urge them to report these signs to the practitioner immediately.
- Assist the patient in contacting a support group that can help to alleviate feelings of isolation.

Postpartum psychosis

Postpartum psychosis usually appears within the first 2 to 3 weeks after birth but can occur as early as the first or second day. This condition affects about 1 to 2 patients in every 1,000 births and is an emergency that requires immediate intervention.

What causes it

The exact cause is unknown but some predisposing factors may contribute to the development of postpartum psychosis. These include changing hormone levels, lack of support systems, low sense of self-esteem, financial difficulties, and major life changes.

What to look for

Signs and symptoms of postpartum psychosis may be similar to those of any psychosis. For example, the patient may experience symptoms associated with schizophrenia, bipolar disorder, or major depression. As a postpartum patient, they may also experience:

- feelings that the baby is dead or defective
- hallucinations that may include voices telling them to harm the baby or themselves

- severe agitation, irritability, or restlessness
- poor judgment and confusion
- feelings of worthlessness, guilt, isolation, or overconcern with the baby's health
- sleep disturbances
- euphoria, hyperactivity, or little concern for self or infant.

What tests tell you

There are no specific diagnostic tests for postpartum psychosis, but patients can be screened during the postpartum period using the Postpartum Depression Screening Scale (PDSS).

Postpartum Depression Screening Scale

The PDSS is a 35-item self-report Likert-type scale with a range of 1 (*strongly disagree*) to 5 (*strongly agree*) that the patient can complete in 5 to 10 minutes and is written at a third-grade level. The instrument consists of statements about how the patient feels after the baby's birth. The instrument gives the total score that determines the degree of severity of postpartum depression symptoms and indicates whether further referral is needed for diagnostic evaluation. The scale assesses the following areas:

- Eating/sleeping disturbances
- Anxiety/insecurity
- Emotional lability
- Mental confusion
- Loss of self
- Guilt/shame
- Suicidal thoughts

Scoring of the PDSS

Total score ranges 35 to 59: normal adjustment

Total score ranges 60 to 79: represents significant symptoms of postpartum depression, with a PDSS total of at least 80 indicative of major postpartum depression

How it's treated

Postpartum psychosis is a medical emergency and requires immediate hospitalization. Medications such as antipsychotic agents and antidepressant agents are used. It may also be necessary to institute suicide precautions. The patient's family and support system should also be involved in the patient's treatment plan.

What to do

- Teach the postpartum patient about the warning signs of postpartum depression and psychosis. Provide resource material.

- Include teaching about postpartum depression and psychosis as part of the patient's discharge teaching plan.
- Instruct the patient and their support system that postpartum depression and psychosis can occur at any time after delivery.
- Advise the patient's support system of the warning signs of postpartum depression and psychosis. Inform them that it is important not to ignore even the subtlest of signs. Urge them to report these signs to the practitioner immediately.

Puerperal infection

Infection during the puerperal period (immediately following childbirth) is a common cause of childbirth-related death. Puerperal infection affects the uterus and structures above it with a characteristic fever pattern. It can result in endometritis, parametritis, pelvic and femoral thrombophlebitis, and peritonitis.

In the United States, puerperal infection develops in about 6% of patients. The prognosis is good in these cases with treatment. There are also certain precautions you can take to prevent puerperal infection. (See *Preventing puerperal infection*.)

Preventing puerperal infection

Here are some steps to take to help prevent puerperal infection in a postpartum patient:
- Adhere to standard precautions at all times.
- Maintain aseptic technique when assisting with or performing a vaginal examination. Limit the number of vaginal examinations performed during labor. Wash hands thoroughly after each patient contact.
- Instruct all pregnant patients to call their practitioners immediately when their membranes rupture. Warn them to avoid intercourse after rupture of or leakage from the amniotic sac.
- Keep the episiotomy site clean and teach the patient how to maintain good perineal hygiene.
- Screen personnel and visitors to keep people with active infections away from maternity patients.

What causes it

Microorganisms that commonly cause puerperal infection include groups A, B, or G hemolytic streptococcus; *Gardnerella vaginalis*; *Chlamydia trachomatis*; and coagulase-negative staphylococci. Less common causative agents are *Clostridium perfringens, Bacteroides fragilis, Klebsiella, Proteus mirabilis, Pseudomonas, Staphylococcus aureus,* and *Escherichia coli.*

Normal unless predisposed

Most of these organisms are considered normal vaginal flora. However, they can cause puerperal infection in the presence of the following predisposing factors:

- Prolonged (more than 24 hours) or premature rupture of the membranes
- Prolonged (more than 24 hours) or difficult labor, allowing bacteria to enter while the fetus is still in utero
- Frequent or unsterile vaginal examinations or unsterile delivery
- Delivery requiring the use of instruments, which may traumatize the tissue, providing an entry portal for microorganisms
- Internal fetal monitoring, which may introduce organisms when electrodes are placed
- Retained products of conception (such as placental fragments), which cause tissue necrosis and provide an excellent medium for bacterial growth
- Hemorrhage, which weakens the patient's overall defenses
- Conditions, such as anemia, diabetes mellitus, immunosuppression, or debilitation from malnutrition, that lower the patient's ability to defend against microorganism invasion
- Cesarean birth (30% to 50% increased risk for puerperal infection)
- Existence of localized vaginal infection or other type of infection at delivery, which allows direct transmission of infection
- Bladder catheterization
- Episiotomy or lacerations
- History of urinary tract infection
- Pneumonia
- Venous thrombosis

What to look for

A characteristic sign of puerperal infection is fever (a temperature of at least 100.4°F [38°C]) that occurs during the first 10 days postpartum (except during the first 24 hours) and lasts for 2 consecutive days. The fever can spike as high as 105°F (40.6°C) and is commonly accompanied by chills, headache, malaise, restlessness, and anxiety.

Care to accompany me?

Accompanying signs and symptoms depend on the extent and site of infection and may include:

- localized perineal infection—pain; elevated temperature; edema, redness, firmness, and tenderness at the wound site; sensation of

heat; burning on urination; discharge from the wound; or separation of the wound
- endometritis—heavy, sometimes foul-smelling lochia; tender, enlarged uterus; backache; severe uterine contractions persisting after childbirth; temperature greater than 100.4°F; chills; and increased pulse rate
- parametritis (pelvic cellulitis)—vaginal tenderness and abdominal pain and tenderness (Pain may become more intense as infection spreads.).

Spreading far and wide

The inflammation may remain localized, lead to abscess formation, or spread through the blood or lymphatic system. Widespread inflammation may cause these conditions, signs, and symptoms:
- Septic pelvic thrombophlebitis—severe, repeated chills and dramatic swings in body temperature; lower abdominal or flank pain; and, possibly, a palpable tender mass over the affected area, which usually develops near the second postpartum week
- Peritonitis—rigid, boardlike abdomen with guarding (usually the first sign); elevated body temperature; tachycardia (greater than 140 beats/min); weak pulse; hiccups; nausea; vomiting; diarrhea; and constant, possibly excruciating, abdominal pain

What tests tell you

Development of the typical clinical features—especially fever for 48 hours or more after the first postpartum day—suggests a diagnosis of puerperal infection. Uterine tenderness is also highly suggestive. Typical clinical features usually suffice for a diagnosis of endometritis and peritonitis. In parametritis, pelvic examination shows induration without purulent discharge.

You're so cultured

A culture of lochia, incisional exudate (from cesarean incision or episiotomy), uterine tissue, or material collected from the vaginal cuff that reveals the causative organism may help confirm the diagnosis. However, such cultures are generally contaminated with vaginal flora and are not considered helpful. A sensitivity test is also done to determine if the proper antibiotic has been administered. Blood cultures are performed for a temperature above 101°F (38.3°C).

White cell uprising

Normal white blood cell (WBC) count during pregnancy is 5,000 to 15,000 mcL. WBCs can increase to 30,000 mcL during labor due to the stress response and then decrease after recovery. A sudden increase of 30% above the baseline WBC count over a 6-hour period or the presence of bands in the differential WBC count is a sign of infection after birth. Erythrocyte sedimentation rate may also be elevated.

How it's treated

Treatment of puerperal infection usually begins with IV infusion of a broad-spectrum antibiotic. This controls the infection and prevents its spread while you await culture results. After identifying the infecting organism, the practitioner may prescribe a more specific antibiotic. (An oral antibiotic may be prescribed after discharge.)

Ancillary measures include analgesic agents for pain, antiseptics for local lesions, and antiemetic medications for nausea and vomiting from peritonitis.

Stick to the standards

A patient with a contagious disease is usually placed in a private room and should be isolated but not from the neonate. The neonate should be isolated from other neonates and should remain in the room with the patient.

If the patient is not contagious, they do not need to be isolated. However, standard precautions should be followed. Follow Centers for Disease Control and Prevention and facility guidelines to determine whether isolation precautions are necessary.

A break from breastfeeding?

Whether the patient can continue breastfeeding, if applicable, depends on the type of antibiotic they are receiving and their physical ability to breastfeed. A patient may not be able to breastfeed if they are receiving metronidazole (Flagyl) or acyclovir (Zovirax). If they plan to breastfeed after their course of antibiotics, help them pump their breasts and discard the breast milk produced while on the medication.

Support, surgery, and drugs

Supportive care includes bed rest, adequate fluid intake, IV fluids when necessary, and measures to reduce fever. Surgery may also be necessary to remove the remaining products of conception or retained placental fragments or to drain local lesions such as an abscess in parametritis.

If the patient develops septic pelvic thrombophlebitis, treatment consists of heparin anticoagulation for about 10 days in conjunction with broad-spectrum antibiotic therapy.

What to do

If your postpartum patient develops an infection, perform these interventions:

- Monitor vital signs every 4 hours (or more frequently depending on the patient's condition).
- Assess capillary refill and skin turgor as well as mucous membranes.
- Assess intake and output closely.
- Enforce strict bed rest.
- Provide a high-calorie, high-protein diet to promote wound healing.
- Provide fluids (3,000 to 4,000 mL), unless otherwise contraindicated.
- Encourage the patient to void frequently, which empties the bladder and helps to prevent infection.
- Inspect the perineum often. Assess the fundus and palpate for tenderness (Subinvolution may indicate endometritis.). Note the amount, color, and odor of vaginal drainage, and document your observations.
- Encourage the patient to change perineal pads frequently, removing them from front to back. Help them change pads, if necessary. Be sure to wear gloves when helping the patient change a perineal pad.
- Administer antibiotics and analgesic agents, as ordered. Assess and document the type, degree, and location of pain as well as the patient's response to analgesic agents. Give the patient an antiemetic medication to relieve nausea and vomiting, as needed.
- Provide sitz baths or warm or cool compresses for local lesions, as ordered.
- Change bed linens, perineal pads, and underpads frequently.
- Provide warm blankets, and keep the patient warm.
- Thoroughly explain all procedures to the patient. Offer reassurance and emotional support.
- If the patient is separated from the neonate, reassure them often about the neonate's progress. Encourage the patient's support system to reassure the patient about the neonate's condition as well.

Mastitis

Mastitis is a parenchymatous inflammation of the mammary glands that disrupts normal lactation. It occurs postpartum in up to 20% of patients, mainly in primiparas who are breastfeeding and occasionally in nonlactating patients. The prognosis for patients with mastitis is good.

What causes it

Mastitis develops when trauma due to incorrect latching or removal from the breast allows introduction of organisms from the neonate's nose or pharynx into the patient's breast. The pathogen that most commonly causes mastitis is *S. aureus*. Less frequently, *Staphylococcus epidermidis* and beta-hemolytic streptococci are the culprits. Rarely, mastitis may result from disseminated tuberculosis or the mumps virus.

Predisposing factors include a fissure or abrasion on the nipple, blocked milk ducts, and an incomplete let-down reflex, usually due to emotional trauma. Blocked milk ducts can result from wearing a tight-fitting bra or waiting for prolonged intervals between breastfeedings.

What to look for

Mastitis may develop anytime during lactation, but it usually begins 1 to 4 weeks postpartum with fever (101°F [38.3°C] or higher in acute mastitis), chills, malaise, and flulike symptoms. Mastitis is generally unilateral and localized, but, in some cases, both breasts or the entire breast is affected.

Inspection and palpation may reveal redness, swelling, warmth, hardness, tenderness, nipple cracks or fissures, and enlarged axillary lymph nodes. Unless mastitis is treated adequately, it may progress to breast abscess.

Which kind is it?

Mastitis must be differentiated from normal breast engorgement, which generally starts with the onset of lactation (days 2 to 5 postpartum). During this time, the breasts undergo changes similar to those in mastitis, and body temperature may also be elevated.

Engorgement may be mild, causing only slight discomfort, or severe, causing considerable pain. A severely engorged breast can prevent a neonate from feeding properly because they cannot latch on to the nipple of the swollen, rigid breast.

What tests tell you

Cultures of expressed breast milk are used to confirm generalized mastitis. Cultures of breast skin are used to confirm localized mastitis. These cultures are also used to determine antibiotic therapy. Differential diagnosis should exclude breast engorgement, breast abscess, viral syndrome, and a clogged duct.

How it's treated

Antibiotic therapy, the primary treatment for mastitis, generally consists of oral cephalosporins or either cloxacillin (Cloxapen) or dicloxacillin (Dynapen) to combat staphylococcus. Azithromycin (Zithromax) or vancomycin (Vancocin) may be used for patients who are allergic to penicillin. Although symptoms usually subside after 24 to 48 hours of antibiotic therapy, antibiotic therapy should continue for 10 days.

Other appropriate measures include analgesic agents for pain and, on the rare occasions when antibiotics fail to control the infection and mastitis progresses to breast abscess, incision and drainage of the abscess. Encourage the patient to continue to breastfeed, pump, or hand express to keep the breasts empty. This will help decrease the length of time that symptoms are present.

What to do

Here's what to do to treat a patient with mastitis:
- Explain mastitis to the patient and why infection control measures are necessary.
- Establish infection control measures for the patient and neonate to prevent the spread of infection to other nursing patients.
- Obtain a complete patient history, including a drug history, especially allergy to penicillin.
- Administer antibiotic therapy, as ordered.
- Assess and record the cause and amount of discomfort. Give analgesic agents, as needed.
- Reassure the patient that breastfeeding during mastitis will not harm the neonate.
- Tell the patient to offer the neonate the affected breast first to promote complete emptying and prevent clogged ducts. However, if an open abscess develops, they must stop breastfeeding with this breast and use a breast pump until the abscess heals. They should continue to breastfeed on the unaffected side.
- Suggest applying a warm, wet towel to the affected breast or taking a warm shower to relax and improve their ability to breastfeed. Cold compresses may also be used to relieve discomfort.
- Advise the patient to wear a supportive bra.
- Provide good skin care.
- Show the patient how to position the neonate properly to prevent cracked or sore nipples.
- Tell the patient to empty the breasts as completely as possible with each feeding.
- Tell the patient to get plenty of rest and drink sufficient fluids to help combat fever.

An ounce of prevention

Before a breastfeeding patient leaves the hospital, teach them about breast care and how to prevent mastitis. (See *Preventing mastitis.*)

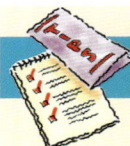

Education edge

Preventing mastitis

With today's shortened hospital stays for childbirth, postpartum teaching is more important than ever. If a patient is breastfeeding, be sure to include these instructions about breast care and preventing mastitis in the teaching plan:
- Wash hands after using the bathroom, before touching breasts, and before and after every breastfeeding.
- If necessary, apply a warm compress or take a warm shower to help facilitate milk flow.
- Properly position the neonate at the breast and ensure that they grasp the nipple and entire areola area when feeding.
- Empty breasts as completely as possible at each feeding.
- Alternate feeding positions and rotate pressure areas.
- Release the neonate's grasp on the nipple before removing them from the breast.
- Expose nipples to the air for part of each day.
- To enhance the breastfeeding experience, drink plenty of fluids, eat a balanced diet, and get sufficient rest.
- Don't wait too long between feedings, or wean the infant abruptly.

Deep vein thrombosis

DVT, also called *deep vein thrombosis*, is an inflammation of the lining of a blood vessel that occurs in conjunction with clot formation. It typically occurs at the valve cusps because venous stasis encourages accumulation and adherence of platelets and fibrin. The incidence in pregnancy and postnatal is low, at 0.1%.

Thrombophlebitis usually begins with localized inflammation (phlebitis), but this rapidly provokes thrombus formation. Rarely, venous thrombosis develops without associated inflammation of the vein (phlebothrombosis).

Any vein will do

DVT can affect small veins, such as the lesser saphenous vein, or large veins, such as the iliac, femoral, pelvic, popliteal, and vena cava. It is more serious than superficial vein thrombophlebitis because it affects the veins deep in the leg musculature that carry 90% of the venous outflow from the leg.

What causes it

DVT may be idiopathic, but it is more likely to occur along with certain diseases, treatments, injuries, or other factors. In the postpartum patient, DVT most commonly results from an extension of endometritis.

Risky business

Risk factors for developing DVT in the antepartum period include:
- multiple gestation
- varicose veins
- inflammatory bowel disease
- urinary tract infection
- diabetes
- being hospitalized for a nonpregnancy issue especially if in the hospital for 3 days or longer
- BMI of 30 or more
- maternal age of 35 years and above.

Risk factors for developing DVT in the postpartum period include:
- history of varicose veins
- high blood pressure
- stillbirth
- hemorrhage during or after delivery
- postpartum infection
- obesity
- previous DVT
- multiple gestation
- increased age (older than 30 years of age)
- family history of DVT
- smoking
- cesarean birth
- multiparity.

Compounding the risk

These risk factors are compounded by specific occurrences during labor and delivery. For example, blood clotting increases postnatally as a result of elevated fibrinogen levels. Also, pressure from the fetal head during pregnancy and delivery causes veins in the lower extremities to dilate, leading to venous stasis. Finally, lying in the lithotomy position for a long time with the lower extremities in stirrups promotes venous pooling and stasis.

Bad news × 2

During the postpartum period, two major types of DVT may occur: femoral or pelvic. Pelvic DVT runs a long course, usually 6 to 8 weeks. (See *Comparing femoral and pelvic DVT.*)

Comparing femoral and pelvic DVT

This table outlines the major differences between femoral and pelvic DVT, including the vessels affected, time of onset, assessment findings, and treatment.

Characteristic	Femoral DVT	Pelvic DVT
Vessels affected	• Femoral • Saphenous • Popliteal	• Ovarian • Uterine • Hypogastric
Onset	Approximately postpartum day 10	Approximately postpartum days 14–15
Assessment findings	• Associated arterial spasm, making leg appear milky white or drained • Edema • Fever • Malaise • Diminished peripheral pulses • Positive Homans sign • Chills • Pain • Redness and stiffness of affected leg • Shiny white skin on extremity	• Extremely high fever • Tachycardia • Chills • General malaise • Possible pelvic abscess • Abdominal and flank pain
Treatment	• Bed rest • Elevation of affected extremity • Never massaging affected area • Anticoagulant medications • Moist heat applications • Analgesic agents	• Complete bed rest • Anticoagulant medications • Antibiotics • Incision and drainage if abscess develops

What to look for

The signs and symptoms of femoral and pelvic DVT differ, but both types require careful assessment.

Femoral DVT

With femoral thrombophlebitis, the patient's temperature increases around the 10th day postpartum. Other signs and symptoms include malaise, chills, pain, stiffness, or swelling in the leg or groin.

With leg swelling, the affected extremity appears reddened or inflamed, edematous below the level of the obstruction, and possibly shiny and white. This white appearance may be related to an accompanying arterial spasm, which results in a decrease in arterial circulation to the area. When measured, the thigh and calf of the affected leg are typically larger than the unaffected extremity.

Man, Homan oh man!

Pain may occur in the calf of the affected leg when the foot is dorsiflexed. This finding—a positive Homans sign—suggests DVT but is not a reliable indicator. Even if the patient is negative for Homans sign, the possibility of an obstruction cannot be ruled out. Always elicit Homans sign passively. Active dorsiflexion could lead to embolization of a clot.

What's your sign?

A positive Rielander sign (palpable veins inside the thigh and calf) or Payr sign (calf pain when pressure is applied on the inside of the foot) also suggests femoral DVT.

Pelvic DVT

The patient with pelvic DVT appears acutely ill with a sudden onset of a high fever, severe repeated chills, and general malaise. In most cases, body temperature fluctuates widely. The patient may complain of lower abdominal or flank pain, and you may be able to palpate a tender mass over the affected area.

What tests tell you

Diagnosis of DVT is based on these characteristic test findings:
- Doppler ultrasonography identifies reduced blood flow to a specific area and obstruction to venous flow, particularly in iliofemoral DVT.
- More sensitive than ultrasonography in detecting DVT, plethysmography shows decreased circulation distal to the affected area.
- Venography usually confirms the diagnosis and shows filling defects and diverted blood flow.

How it's treated

Treatment for DVT includes bed rest, with elevation of the affected arm or leg; application of warm, moist compresses; and administration of analgesic agents, antibiotics, and anticoagulant medications. After the acute episode subsides, the patient may begin to ambulate while wearing antiembolism stockings (applied before getting out of bed).

Bring on the meds

Drug therapy typically includes anticoagulant medications to prolong clotting time, starting with heparin for 5 to 7 days and then changing to another anticoagulant, such as warfarin (Coumadin), for 3 months.

For lysis of acute, extensive DVT, treatment should include streptokinase if the risk of bleeding does not outweigh the potential benefits of thrombolytic treatment.

Kicking the treatment up a notch

Rarely, DVT may cause complete venous occlusion, which requires venous interruption through simple ligation, vein plication, or clipping. Embolectomy may be done if clots are being shed to the pulmonary and systemic vasculature, and other treatments are unsuccessful.

Caval interruption with transvenous placement of an umbrella filter can trap emboli, preventing them from traveling to the pulmonary vasculature. If the patient develops a pulmonary embolism, heparin may be initiated until the embolism resolves; then, subcutaneous heparin or an oral anticoagulant may be continued for 6 months.

Pelvic DVT in particular

In addition, treatment for pelvic DVT focuses on complete bed rest and administration of antibiotics along with anticoagulant medications. If the patient develops a pelvic abscess, a laparotomy for incision and drainage may be done. Because this procedure may cause tubal scarring and may interfere with fertility, the patient may need additional surgery later to remove the vessel before becoming pregnant again.

What to do

Prevention of DVT is key. Assess the patient for risk factors, and teach ways to reduce their risk. (See *Preventing DVT*.)

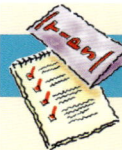

Education edge

Preventing DVT

Incorporate these instructions in the teaching plan to reduce the risk of developing DVT.
• Check with your practitioner about using a side-lying or back-lying (supine recumbent) position for birth instead of the lithotomy position (on your back with your legs in stirrups). These alternative positions reduce the risk of blood pooling in the lower extremities.
• If you must use the lithotomy position for birth, ask the practitioner to pad the stirrups well so that you put less pressure on your calves.
• Change positions frequently if on bed rest.
• Avoid deeply flexing your legs at the groin or sharply flexing your knees.

Preventing DVT (*continued*)

- Don't stand in one place for too long or sit with your knees bent or legs crossed. Elevate your legs slightly to improve venous return.
- Don't wear garters or constrictive clothing.
- Wiggle your toes and perform leg lifts while in bed to minimize venous pooling and help increase venous return.
- Use a sequential compression device or wear thigh-high stockings during and after cesarean birth until you are ambulating.
- Walk as soon as possible after birth.
- Wear antiembolism or support stockings as ordered. Put them on before getting out of bed in the morning.

In addition, because postpartum DVT commonly results from an endometrial infection:

- be alert to signs and symptoms of endometritis
- notify the practitioner if signs and symptoms of endometritis occur
- institute treatment promptly, as ordered.

Fighting back

To combat DVT, take the following measures:

- Enforce bed rest as ordered, and elevate the patient's affected arm or leg. If you use pillows for elevation of a leg, place the pillows so that they support its entire length to avoid compressing the popliteal space.
- Apply warm compresses or a covered aquathermia pad to increase circulation to the affected area and to relieve pain and inflammation.
- Give analgesic agents to relieve pain as ordered.
- Assess uterine involution and note changes in fundal consistency such as the inability to remain firm or contracted.
- Monitor vital signs closely, at least every 4 hours or more frequently if indicated. Report changes in pulse rate or blood pressure as well as temperature elevations.
- Administer IV anticoagulant medications as ordered, using an infusion monitor or pump to control the flow rate, if necessary. Have an anticoagulant antidote, such as protamine sulfate (for heparin therapy), readily available.
- Because neither heparin nor warfarin is excreted in significant amounts in breast milk, breastfeeding is allowed.
- If the patient is hospitalized, have them pump their breast milk for the neonate.
- Administer antibiotic and antipyretic therapy for the patient with pelvic DVT.
- Mark, measure, and record the circumference of the affected extremity at least once daily, and compare it to the other extremity.

To ensure accuracy and consistency of serial measurements, mark the skin over the area, and measure at the same spot daily.

- Obtain coagulation studies, such as international normalized ratio (INR), PTT, and PT, as ordered. Keep in mind that therapeutic anticoagulation values usually are considered to be one and a half to two times the control value; INR should be between 2 and 3.5.

On the lookout for lochia

- Monitor the patient for increased amounts of lochia. Encourage them to change perineal pads frequently, and weigh the pads to estimate the amount of blood loss.
- Watch for signs and symptoms of bleeding, such as tarry stools, coffee-ground vomitus, and ecchymoses. Note oozing of blood at IV sites, and assess gums for excessive bleeding. Report positive findings to the practitioner immediately.
- Assess the patient for signs and symptoms of pulmonary emboli, such as crackles, dyspnea, hemoptysis, sudden changes in mental status, restlessness, and hypotension. (See *Dealing with pulmonary embolism.*)

Dealing with pulmonary embolism

A patient with DVT is at high risk for developing a pulmonary embolism. Be alert for the classic signs and symptoms of pulmonary embolism, such as:
- chest pain
- dyspnea
- tachypnea
- tachycardia
- hemoptysis
- sudden changes in mental status
- hypotension.

Also, be vigilant in monitoring for these problems, which may occur along with the classic signs and symptoms:
- Chills
- Fever
- Abdominal pain
- Signs and symptoms of respiratory distress, including tachypnea, tachycardia, restlessness, cold and clammy skin, cyanosis, and retractions

Nip it in the bud
A pulmonary embolism is a life-threatening event that can lead to cardiovascular collapse and death. You should intervene at once if pulmonary embolism is suspected. Follow these steps:
- Elevate the head of the bed to improve the work of breathing.
- Administer oxygen via facemask at 8 to 10 L/min, as ordered.

Dealing with pulmonary embolism (*continued*)

- Begin IV fluid administration, as ordered.
- Monitor oxygen saturation rates continuously via pulse oximetry.
- Obtain ABG samples for analysis as ordered to evaluate gas exchange.
- Assess vital signs frequently, as often as every 15 minutes.
- Anticipate the need for continuous cardiac monitoring to evaluate for dysrhythmia secondary to hypoxemia and for insertion of a pulmonary artery catheter to evaluate hemodynamic status and gas exchange.
- Administer emergency drugs, such as dopamine (Intropin) for pressure support and morphine (Duramorph) for analgesia, as ordered.
- Expect the patient to be transferred to the critical care unit.
- Administer analgesic agents without aspirin for pain relief.
- Administer anticoagulant medications or thrombolytics, as ordered.

- Provide emotional support to the patient and their family, and explain all procedures and treatments.
- Prepare the patient for surgery, if indicated.
- Emphasize the importance of follow-up blood studies to monitor anticoagulant therapy.
- If the patient is discharged on heparin therapy, teach them or a family member how to give subcutaneous injections. If additional assistance is required, arrange for a home health care referral and follow-up.
- Teach the patient how to properly apply and use antiembolism stockings. Tell them to report complications, such as toes that are cold or blue.
- To prevent bleeding, encourage the patient to avoid medications that contain aspirin and to check with the practitioner before using over-the-counter medications. Teach the patient the signs and symptoms of bleeding, such as easy bruising or blood in the urine or stool.
- Tell them to use a soft toothbrush and an electric razor to prevent tissue damage and bleeding.
- Advise the patient to use contraception because oral anticoagulant medications are teratogenic.
- Tell the patient not to increase their vitamin K intake while taking oral anticoagulant medications because vitamin K counteracts the anticoagulant effects.
- Stress that the patient should report their history of DVT to the practitioner if they become pregnant again so that preventative measures can be started early.

Quick quiz

1. The nurse assesses a patient with an approximate 750 mL blood loss in the first 12 hours after a vaginal delivery of a baby with a weight of 9 lb 2 oz. What does the nurse consider as the most likely cause for blood loss in the postpartum patient?
   A. Uterine atony
   B. Perineal laceration
   C. Retained placental fragments
   D. DIC

Answer: A. Although all of the complications mentioned in the options are possible causes of postpartum hemorrhage, noted with a blood loss of more than 500 mL in a vaginal delivery, uterine atony (relaxation of the uterus) is considered the primary and most likely cause of early postpartum hemorrhage. The delivery of an infant considered large for gestational age is a primary risk factor for uterine atony.

2. Which of the following findings is most likely to be associated with the development of hypovolemic shock in a patient with postpartum hemorrhage?
   A. Respiratory rate of 18 breaths/min
   B. Pale pink, moist skin
   C. Urine output below 25 mL/h
   D. Bounding peripheral pulses

Answer: C. A urine output below 25 mL/h suggests hypovolemic shock secondary to decreased renal perfusion from overall decreased blood volume. Other findings mentioned in the options are within acceptable limits postpartum. The other signs and symptoms for possible secondary hypovolemic shock include rapid and shallow respirations; pale, cold, clammy skin; rapid, thready peripheral pulses; mean arterial pressure below 60 mm Hg; and narrowed pulse pressure.

3. The nurse educator is orienting new nurses working in the postpartum care area. The educator is discussing factors that increase the risk for puerperal infection. Which of the following does the educator include?
   A. External fetal monitoring during labor
   B. Rupture of membranes 15 hours ago
   C. Labor lasting 20 hours
   D. Cesarean birth

Answer: D. Cesarean birth increases the risk for puerperal infection by as much as 20 times. The use of internal fetal monitoring, prolonged (more than 24 hours) or premature rupture of membranes, and prolonged (more than 24 hours) or difficult labor also increase the risk for puerperal infection.

4. A patient gave birth 48 hours ago and calls the nurse to report foul-smelling lochia with worsening pain with postpartum contractions during breastfeeding. The patient's vital signs are temperature 102.2°F (39°C), heart rate 92, respiratory rate 21, blood pressure 132/82 mm Hg. On assessment, the uterus is firm and tender; abdomen is soft and no guarding with normal bowel sounds in all quadrants. What does the nurse suspect as the most likely diagnosis for this patient?

    A. Mastitis
    B. Peritonitis
    C. Endometritis
    D. Parametritis

Answer: C. Endometritis may cause heavy, foul-smelling lochia; a tender, enlarged uterus; backache; severe uterine contractions that persist after childbirth; and elevated temperature for 2 or more days after the first 24 hours postdelivery. The other options are possible infections postpartum; however, they would not present as this patient has.

5. The nurse is teaching a patient about prevention of mastitis. The nurse included education regarding handwashing to prevent transmission of which of the following organisms that is most commonly associated with mastitis?

    A. *S. aureus*
    B. *S. epidermidis*
    C. Beta-hemolytic streptococci
    D. Mumps virus

Answer: A. Although all are possible causative organisms, *S. aureus* is the most common. Mastitis caused by the mumps virus is rare.

6. A postpartum patient was on bed rest for the last 8 weeks of pregnancy before delivery of an infant after a long labor. The provider has ordered an ultrasound of the patient's left calf for possible DVT. What is the primary complication for which the nurse will monitor this patient related to the possible DVT?

    A. Endometritis
    B. Pulmonary embolism
    C. Hematoma
    D. Mastitis

Answer: B. A possible life-threatening complication and primary concern for a patient with a DVT is a pulmonary embolism. Pulmonary embolism occurs when the clot breaks off and travels to the pulmonary vascular bed, interfering with gas exchange.

Scoring

☆☆☆ If you answered all six questions correctly, great going! You've summed it up totally.

☆☆ If you answered five questions correctly, fantastic! You've added immeasurably to your knowledge of the subject.

☆ If you answered fewer than five questions correctly, no problem. Count on doing better when you read through the chapter once more.

Selected References

Beck, C., & Gable, R. (2000). Postpartum Depression Screening Scale: Development and psychometric testing. *Nursing Research, 49*, 272–282. https://doi.org/10.1097/00006199-200009000-00006

Blackmon, M. M., Nguyen, H., & Mukherji, P. (2023). Acute mastitis. In *StatPearls* [Internet]. StatPearls Publishing. https://www.ncbi.nlm.nih.gov/books/NBK557782/

Committee on Obstetric Practice. (2019). *ACOG Committee Opinion: Quantitative blood loss in obstetric hemorrhage.* https://www.acog.org/-/media/project/acog/acogorg/clinical/files/committee-opinion/articles/2019/12/quantitative-blood-loss-in-obstetric-hemorrhage.pdf

LactMed. (2018). Acyclovir. In *Drugs and Lactation Database (LactMed®)* [Internet]. National Institute of Child Health and Human Development. https://www.ncbi.nlm.nih.gov/books/NBK501195/

LactMed. (2023). Metronidazole. In *Drugs and Lactation Database (LactMed®)* [Internet]. National Institute of Child Health and Human Development. https://www.ncbi.nlm.nih.gov/books/NBK501315/

Pabinger, I., Fries, D., Schochl, H., Streif, W., & Toller, W. (2017, April). Tranexamic acid for treatment and prophylaxis of bleeding and hyperfibrinolysis. *Wiener klinische Wochenschrift, 129*(9-10), 303–316. https://www.ncbi.nlm.nih.gov/pmc/articles/PMC5429347/

Ricci, S., Kyle, T., & Carman, S. (2021). Postpartum adaptations. In *Maternity and pediatric nursing* (4th ed., pp. 515–535). Wolters Kluwer.

Ricci, S., Kyle, T., & Carman, S. (2021). Nursing management during the postpartum period. In *Maternity and pediatric nursing* (4th ed., pp. 536–574). Wolters Kluwer.

Silbert-Flagg, J. (2023). Nursing care of a family experiencing a postpartum complication. In *Maternal and child health nursing* (9th ed., pp. 647–670). Wolters Kluwer.

Wang, Y., & Zhao, S. (2010). Placental blood circulation. In *Vascular biology of the placenta.* Morgan & Claypool Life Sciences. https://www.ncbi.nlm.nih.gov/books/NBK53254/

Wilson, E., Woodd, S. L., & Benova, L. (2020, April). Incidence of and risk factors for lactational mastitis: A systemic review. *Journal of Human Lactation, 36*(4), 673–686. https://www.ncbi.nlm.nih.gov/pmc/articles/PMC7672676/

Chapter 10

Neonatal assessment and care

Just the facts

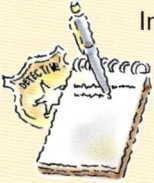

In this chapter, you'll learn:

◆ changes that occur in the neonate after birth

◆ the proper way to perform a neonatal assessment

◆ nursing interventions critical to neonatal care.

Adapting to extrauterine life

After birth, a neonate must quickly adapt to extrauterine life, even though many of the neonate's body systems are still developing. During this time of adaptation, the nurse must be aware of normal neonatal physiologic characteristics and assessment findings in order to detect possible problems and initiate appropriate interventions. (See *Physiology of the neonate.*)

Physiology of the neonate

This chart provides a summary of the physiologic characteristics of a neonate after birth, including adaptations the neonate must make to cope with extrauterine life.

Body system	Physiology after birth
Respiratory	• Onset of breathing occurs as air replaces the fluid that filled the lungs before birth.
Cardiovascular	• Functional closure of fetal shunts occurs. • Transition from fetal to postnatal circulation occurs.
Renal	• System doesn't mature fully until after the first year of life; fluid imbalances may occur.
Gastrointestinal (GI)	• System continues to develop. • Uncoordinated peristalsis of the esophagus occurs. • The neonate has a limited ability to digest fats.

(continued)

Physiology of the neonate (*continued*)

Body system	Physiology after birth
Thermogenic	• The neonate is susceptible to rapid heat loss due to acute changes in the environment and thin layer of subcutaneous fat. • Nonshivering thermogenesis occurs. • The presence of brown fat (more in the mature neonate; less in the preterm neonate) warms the neonate by increasing heat production.
Immune	• The inflammatory response of the tissues to localized infection is immature.
Hematopoietic	• Coagulation time is prolonged.
Neurologic	• Presence of primitive reflexes and time in which they appear and disappear indicate the maturity of the developing nervous system.
Hepatic	• The neonate may demonstrate jaundice.
Integumentary	• The epidermis and dermis are thin and bound loosely to each other. • Sebaceous glands are active.
Musculoskeletal	• More cartilage is present than ossified bone.
Reproductive	• Females may have a mucoid vaginal discharge and pseudomenstruation due to maternal estrogen levels. • In males, testes descend into the scrotum. • Small, white, firm cysts called *epithelial pearls* may be visible at the tip of the prepuce. • Scrotum may be edematous if the neonate presented in breech position. • Gynecomastia

Neonatal assessment

Neonatal assessment includes initial and ongoing assessments, a head-to-toe physical examination, and neurologic and behavioral assessments.

Initial assessment

The initial neonatal assessment involves assessing for any visible abnormalities and keeping accurate records. To complete an initial assessment, follow these steps:

- Wash hands and wear gloves when assessing or caring for a neonate until after the initial bath is completed to control infection.
- Ensure a proper airway by suctioning as needed and administering oxygen as needed.
- Monitor for abnormal bleeding from the cord after the provider has applied the cord clamp. Assess the number of cord vessels. Inspect the size and thickness of the cord. Assess for defects such as omphalocele or umbilical hernia.
- Observe for voiding and meconium; document the first void and stools.
- Assess for gross abnormalities and clinical manifestations of suspected abnormalities.
- Continue to assess using the appropriate criteria until the neonate is stabilized and has completed transition.
- Obtain clear footprints and fingerprints. (In some facilities, the neonate's footprints are kept on a record that also includes the birthing parent's fingerprints.)
- Follow facility protocol for neonatal identification.
- Promote bonding between the birthing parent and neonate by engaging in skin-to-skin contact (kangaroo care) or breastfeeding.

Apgar scoring

During the initial examination of a neonate, expect to calculate an Apgar score and make general observations about the neonate's appearance and behavior. Apgar scoring evaluates neonatal heart rate, respiratory effort, muscle tone, reflex irritability, and color. Evaluation of each category is performed 1 minute after birth and again at 5 minutes after birth. Each item has a maximum score of 2 and a minimum score of 0. The final Apgar score is the total of the five items; a maximum score is 10.

Evaluation at 1 minute indicates the neonate's initial adaptation to extrauterine life and whether resuscitation is necessary. The 5-minute score gives a more accurate picture of their overall status. (See *Recording the Apgar score.*)

Recording the Apgar score

Use this chart to determine the neonatal Apgar score at 1- and 5-minute intervals after birth. For each category listed, assign a score of 0 to 2, as shown. A total score of 7 to 10 indicates that the neonate is in good condition; 4 to 6, fair condition (The neonate may have moderate central nervous system depression, muscle flaccidity, cyanosis, and poor respirations.); 0 to 3, danger (The neonate needs immediate resuscitation, as ordered.). Each component should be assessed 1, 5, 10, 15, and 20 minutes after delivery, as necessary. Resuscitation efforts, such as oxygen, endotracheal intubation, chest compressions, positive pressure ventilation or nasal continuous positive airway pressure (CPAP), and epinephrine administration, should be documented.

Sign	Apgar score		
	0	**1**	**2**
Heart rate	Absent	Less than 100 beats/min	More than 100 beats/min
Respiration	Absent	Weak cry, hypoventilation	Good crying
Muscle tone	Flaccid	Some flexion	Active motion
Reflex irritability	No response	Grimace or weak cry	Cry or active withdrawal
Color	Pallor, cyanosis	Pink body, blue extremities	Completely pink

First and foremost

Assess heart rate first. If the umbilical cord still pulsates, palpate the neonate's heart rate by placing fingertips at the junction of the umbilical cord and the skin. The neonate's cord stump continues to pulsate for several hours and is a good, easy place (next to the abdomen) to check heart rate. Another method is to place two fingers or a stethoscope over the neonate's chest at the fifth intercostal space to obtain an apical pulse. For accuracy, the heart rate should be counted for 1 full minute.

Second to one

Next, check the neonate's respiratory effort, the second most important Apgar sign. Assess the neonate's cry, noting its volume and vigor. Then, auscultate the lungs using a stethoscope. Assess the respirations for depth and regularity. If the neonate exhibits abnormal respiratory responses, begin neonatal resuscitation according to the guidelines of the American Heart Association and the American Academy of Pediatrics. Afterward, use the Apgar score to judge the progress and success of resuscitation efforts. (See *Monitoring for effects of medication.*)

Advice from the experts

Monitoring for effects of medication

Closely observe a neonate whose birthing parent has received heavy sedation just before delivery or magnesium sulfate during labor. Even if the neonate has a high Apgar score at birth, they may exhibit secondary effects of sedation later. Be alert for respiratory depression or unresponsiveness. Monitor the neonate if the birthing parent received magnesium sulfate for hypotonia or analgesia during labor or if they used narcotic drugs during pregnancy.

Move along to the muscles

Determine muscle tone by evaluating the degree of flexion in the neonate's arms and legs and their resistance to straightening by extending the limbs and observing their rapid return to flexion—the neonate's normal state.

Assess reflex irritability by evaluating the neonate's cry for presence, vigor, and pitch. Initially, they may not cry, but flicking their soles should elicit a cry. The usual response is a loud, angry cry. A high-pitched or shrill cry is abnormal.

Now add a little color

Finally, observe skin color for cyanosis. A neonate usually has a pink body with blue extremities. This condition, called *acrocyanosis*, appears in about 85% of normal neonates 1 minute after birth. Acrocyanosis results from decreased peripheral oxygenation caused by the transition from fetal to independent circulation. When assessing a neonate with darker skin, observe for color changes in the mucous membranes of the mouth, lips, palms, and soles.

Gestational age and birth weight

Perinatal mortality and morbidity are related to gestational age and birth weight. Classifying a neonate by both weight and gestational age provides a more accurate method for assessing mortality risk and offers guidelines for treatment. The neonate's age and weight classifications should also be considered during future assessments.

How old are you now?

The clinical assessment of gestational age classifies a neonate as *preterm* (fewer than 37 weeks' gestation), *term* (37 to 42 weeks' gestation), or *post-term* (42 weeks' gestation or longer). The Ballard scoring system uses physical and neurologic findings to estimate a neonate's gestational age within 1 week, even in extremely preterm neonates. This evaluation can be done at any time between birth and 42 hours after birth, but the greatest reliability is between 30 and 42 hours after birth. (See *Ballard gestational age assessment tool.*)

Ballard gestational age assessment tool

To use this tool, evaluate and score the neuromuscular and physical maturity criteria, total the score, and then plot the sum in the maturity rating box to determine the neonate's corresponding gestational age.

Posture
With the neonate supine and quiet, score as follows:
- Arms and legs extended = 0
- Slight or moderate flexion of hips and knees = 1
- Moderate to strong flexion of hips and knees = 2
- Legs flexed and abducted, arms slightly flexed = 3
- Full flexion of arms and legs = 4

Square window
Flex the hand at the wrist. Measure the angle between the base of the thumb and the forearm. Score as follows:
- >90 degrees = −1
- 90 degrees = 0
- 60 degrees = 1
- 45 degrees = 2

Ballard gestational age assessment tool (*continued*)

- 30 degrees = 3
- 0 degrees = 4

Arm recoil

With the neonate supine, fully flex the forearm for 5 seconds and then fully extend by pulling the hands and releasing. Observe and score the reaction according to these criteria:
- Remains extended 180 degrees or displays random movements = 0
- Minimal flexion (140 to 180 degrees) = 1
- Small amount of flexion (110 to 140 degrees) = 2
- Moderate flexion (90 to 110 degrees) = 3
- Brisk return to full flexion (<90 degrees) = 4

Popliteal angle

With the neonate supine and the pelvis flat on the examining surface, use one hand to flex the leg and then the thigh. Then, use the other hand to extend the leg. Score the angle attained:
- 180 degrees = −1
- 160 degrees = 0
- 140 degrees = 1
- 120 degrees = 2
- 100 degrees = 3
- 90 degrees = 4
- <90 degrees = 5

Scarf sign

With the neonate supine, take their hand and draw it across the neck and as far across the opposite shoulder as possible, if needed assist the elbow by lifting it across the body. Score according to the location of the elbow:
- Elbow reaches or nears level of opposite shoulder = −1
- Elbow crosses opposite anterior axillary line = 0
- Elbow reaches opposite anterior axillary line = 1
- Elbow at midline = 2
- Elbow doesn't reach midline = 3
- Elbow doesn't cross proximate axillary line = 4

(*continued*)

Ballard gestational age assessment tool (*continued*)

Heel to ear
With the neonate supine, hold their foot with one hand and move it as near to the head as possible without forcing it. Keep the pelvis flat on the examining surface. Score as shown in the chart.

Neuromuscular Maturity

Neuromuscular maturity sign	Score		
	−1	0	1
Posture	—		
Square window (wrist)	>90 degrees	90 degrees	60 degrees
Arm recoil	—	180 degrees	140–180 degrees
Popliteal angle	180 degrees	160 degrees	140 degrees
Scarf sign			
Heel to ear			

Total neuromuscular maturity score

Neuromuscular Maturity

Score

2	3	4	5	Record score here
			—	
45 degrees	30 degrees	0 degree	—	
110–140 degrees	90–110 degrees	<90 degrees	—	
120 degrees	100 degrees	90 degrees	<90 degrees	
			—	
			—	

(*continued*)

Ballard gestational age assessment tool (*continued*)

Physical Maturity

Physical maturity sign	Score		
	−1	**0**	**1**
Skin	Sticky, friable, transparent	Gelatinous, red, translucent	Smooth, pink; visible vessels
Lanugo	None	Sparse	Abundant
Plantar surface	Heel to toe 40–50 mm: −1; <40 mm: −2	>50 mm; no crease	Faint red marks
Breast	Imperceptible	Barely perceptible	Flat areola; no bud
Eye and ear	Lids fused, loosely: −1; tightly: −2	Lids open; pinna flat, stays folded	Slightly curved pinna; soft, slow, recoil
Genitalia (male)	Scrotum flat, smooth	Scrotum empty; faint rugae	Testes in upper canal; rare rugae
Genitalia (female)	Clitoris prominent; labia flat	Prominent clitoris; small labia minora	Prominent clitoris; enlarging minora
Total physical maturity score			

Total maturity score	−10	−5	0	5	10
Gestational age (weeks)	20	22	24	26	28

		Physical Maturity					
		Score					
2	3	4		5			Record score here
Superficial peeling or rash; few visible vessels	Cracking; pale areas; rare visible vessels	Parchmentlike; deep cracking; no visible vessels		Leathery, cracked, wrinkled			
Thinning	Bald areas	Mostly bald		—			
Anterior transverse crease only	Creases over anterior two thirds	Creases over entire sole		—			
Stippled areola; 1–2-mm bud	Raised areola; 3–4-mm bud	Full areola; 5–10-mm bud		—			
Well-curved pinna; soft but ready recoil	Formed and firm; instant recoil	Thick cartilage; ear stiff		—			
Testes descending; few rugae	Testes down; good rugae	Testes pendulous; deep rugae		—			
Majora and minora equally prominent	Majora large; minora small	Majora cover clitoris and minora.		—			
15	20	25	30	35	40	45	50
30	32	34	36	38	40	42	44

Too small, too big, just right

Normal birth weight is 5 lb, 8 oz (2,500 g) or greater. Large for gestational age falls above the 90% or greater than 4.0 kg. Low birth weight is between 3 lb, 5 oz (1,500 g) and 5 lb, 8 oz (2,499 g). A neonate of very low birth weight is between 2 lb, 3 oz (1,000 g) and 3 lb, 5 oz (1,499 g). A neonate weighing less than 1,000 g has an extremely low birth weight.

Postnatal growth charts are used to assess the neonate based on head circumference, weight, length, and gestational age. Neonates who are small for gestational age have a birth weight less than the 10th percentile on postnatal growth charts; weight appropriate for gestational age signifies a birth weight within the 10th and 90th percentiles; and weight large for gestational age means a birth weight greater than the 90th percentile. (See *Caring for a preterm neonate.*)

Advice from the experts

Caring for a preterm neonate

When caring for a preterm neonate, be alert for problems—even if the neonate is of average size. A preterm neonate is more prone to respiratory distress syndrome, apnea, patent ductus arteriosus with left-to-right shunt, and infection. Neonates who are small for gestational age are more likely to experience asphyxia, hypoglycemia, and hypocalcemia.

Ongoing assessment

Ongoing neonatal physical assessment includes observing and recording vital signs and administering prescribed medications. To perform an ongoing assessment, follow these steps:

- Assess the neonate's vital signs.
- Measure and record the neonate's vital statistics.
- Administer prescribed medications such as vitamin K (phytonadione), which is a prophylactic to the transient deficiency of coagulation factors II, VII, IX, and X.
- Administer erythromycin ophthalmic ointment, the drug of choice for neonatal eye prophylaxis, to prevent damage and blindness from ophthalmia neonatorum, which is often caused if a sexually transmitted infection is transferred to the infant during birth; treatment is required by law.
- Perform laboratory tests.
- Monitor glucose levels and hematocrit (test results aid in assessing for hypoglycemia and anemia).

Caring for the large-for-gestational-age infant

Even though the infant is large for gestational age, this infant is at high risk for many physiologic conditions. Some of these problems include respiratory distress, hypoglycemia secondary to hyperinsulinemia, cardiomyopathy, and polycythemia.

Vital signs

Measuring vital signs establishes the baseline of any neonatal assessment. Vital signs include the respiratory rate, heart rate (taken apically), and the first neonatal temperature. First measure the temperature rectally to verify rectal patency, but not all nurseries routinely conduct this practice because of risks associated with perforation—especially in the premature neonate. Temperature readings are often performed using the axillary route to avoid injuring the rectal mucosa. An electronic vital signs monitor may be used. (See *Reviewing normal neonatal vital signs*.)

Reviewing normal neonatal vital signs

This list includes the normal ranges for neonatal vital signs.

Respiration
• 30 to 50 breaths/min

Heart rate (apical)
• 110 to 160 beats/min

Temperature
• Rectal: 96°F to 99.5°F (35.6°C to 37.5°C)
• Axillary: 97.5°F to 99°F (36.4°C to 37.2°C)

Blood pressure
• Systolic: 60 to 80 mm Hg
• Diastolic: 40 to 50 mm Hg

Determining respiratory rate

Observe respirations first, before the neonate becomes active or agitated. Watch and count respiratory movements for 1 minute, and record the result. A normal respiratory rate is usually between 30 and

50 breaths/min. Note any signs of respiratory distress, such as cyanosis, tachypnea, retractions, grunting, nasal flaring, or periods of apnea. Short periods of apnea (less than 15 seconds) are characteristic of the neonate. (See *Counting neonatal respirations.*)

Advice from the experts

Counting neonatal respirations

When counting a neonate's respiratory rate, observe abdominal excursions rather than chest excursions. Auscultation of the chest or placing the stethoscope in front of the mouth and nares are alternative ways to count respirations.

Assessing heart rate

Use a pediatric stethoscope to determine the neonate's apical heart rate. Place the stethoscope over the apical impulse on the fourth or fifth intercostal space at the left midclavicular line over the cardiac apex. Assess the point of maximal intensity (PMI) to assist in ruling out dextrocardia or other cardiac disorders. If PMI is not auscultated in the correct location, alert a practitioner for further evaluation. To ensure an accurate measurement, count the beats for 1 minute. A normal heart rate ranges from 110 to 160 beats/min. Variations during sleeping and waking states are normal.

Taking a rectal temperature

The technique for taking a rectal temperature in a neonate is relatively simple. With the neonate lying in a supine position, place a diaper over the penis (if applicable) and firmly grasp the ankles with the index finger between them. Then, insert a lubricated thermometer into the rectum, no more than $\frac{1}{2}$ in (1.3 cm). Placing a palm on the buttocks, hold the thermometer between the index and middle fingers. If resistance is met while inserting the thermometer, withdraw the thermometer and notify the practitioner.

Body temperature in neonates is less constant than in adults and can fluctuate without reason during the course of a day. The normal range for a rectal temperature is 96°F to 99.5°F (35.6°C to 37.5°C).

Taking an axillary temperature

To take an axillary temperature, make sure that the axillary skin is dry. Place the thermometer in the axilla, and hold it along the lateral aspect of the neonate's chest between the axillary line and the arm.

Hold the thermometer in place until the temperature registers. Normal axillary temperature is 97.5°F to 99°F (36.4°C to 37.2°C).

Reassess axillary temperature in 15 to 30 minutes if the first measurement registers outside the normal range. If the temperature remains abnormal, notify the practitioner.

The low-down on low temperatures

Decreased temperatures by either the rectal or axillary route could suggest:
- prematurity
- infection
- low environmental temperature
- inadequate clothing
- dehydration.

Why it may be high

Possible reasons for increased temperatures include:
- infection
- high environmental temperature
- excessive clothing
- proximity to heating unit or direct sunlight
- substance use disorder
- diarrhea and dehydration.

Determining blood pressure

If possible, measure a neonate's blood pressure when they are in a quiet or relaxed state. Make sure that the blood pressure cuff is small enough for the neonate (cuff width should be about one half the circumference of the neonate's arm). Then, wrap the cuff one or two fingerbreadths above the antecubital or popliteal area. With the stethoscope held directly over the chosen artery, hold the cuffed extremity firmly to provide the electronic device to inflate and deflate the cuff appropriately to keep it extended and inflate the cuff no faster than 5 mm Hg/s.

Normal systolic readings are 60 to 80 mm Hg, and normal diastolic readings are 40 to 50 mm Hg. A drop in systolic blood pressure (about 15 mm Hg) during the first hour after birth is common. Crying and movement result in blood pressure changes.

From top to bottom

Compare blood pressures in the upper and lower extremities at least once to detect abnormalities. Remember that blood pressure readings from the thigh will be approximately 10 mm Hg higher than the arm. If the blood pressure reading in the thigh is the same or lower than the arm, notify the practitioner. This could indicate coarctation of the aorta, a congenital heart defect, and should be investigated further.

Size and weight

Size and weight measurements establish the baseline for monitoring growth. They can also be used to detect disorders such as failure to thrive, hydrocephalus, microcephaly, and intrauterine growth restriction. (See *Average neonatal size and weight.*)

Average neonatal size and weight

In addition to weight, anthropometric measurements include head and chest circumferences and head-to-heel length. Together, these measurements serve as a baseline and show whether neonatal size is within normal ranges or whether there may be a significant problem or anomaly—especially if values stray far from the mean.

Average initial anthropometric ranges are:
- head circumference—13 to 14 in (33 to 35.5 cm)
- chest circumference—12 to 13 in (30.5 to 33 cm)
- head to heel—18 to 21 in (46 to 53 cm)
- weight—5 lb, 8 oz to 8 lb, 13 oz (2,500 to 4,000 g).

Head circumference   **Chest circumference**   **Head-to-heel length**

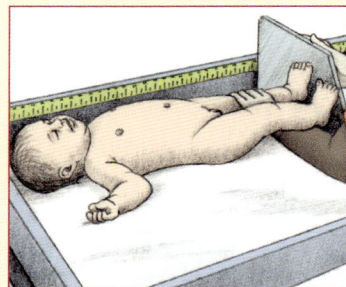

Measuring head circumference

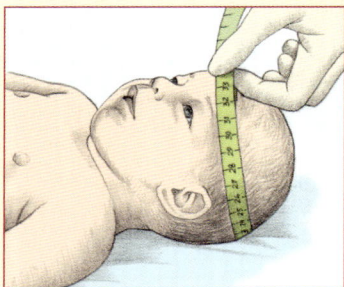

Measure head circumference by sliding the tape measure under the neonate's head at the occiput and draw the tape around snugly, just above the eyebrows. Normal neonatal head circumference is 13 to 14 in (33 to 35.5 cm). Cranial molding or caput succedaneum from a vaginal delivery may affect this measurement.

Measuring chest circumference

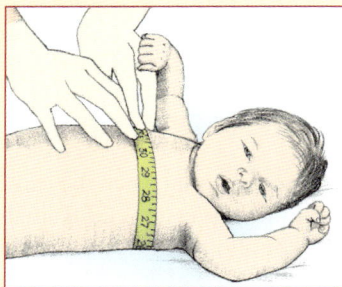

Measure chest circumference by placing the tape under the back, wrapping it snugly around the chest at the nipple line, and keeping the back and front of the tape level. Take the measurement after the neonate inspires and before they begin to exhale. Normal neonatal chest circumference is 12 to 13 in (30.5 to 33 cm).

Measuring head-to-heel length

Fully extend the neonate's legs with the toes pointing up. With the neonate's leg fully extended and toes pointed up, measure the distance from the heel to the top of the head. A length board may be used if available. Normal length is 18 to 21 in (46 to 53 cm).

Weighing the neonate

A neonate should be weighed before a feeding on a balanced scale. Remove the diaper, and place the neonate in the middle of the scale tray. Always keep one hand over the neonate to prevent them from falling off the scale; never leave the neonate unattended on the scale.

Return the neonate to the bassinet or examination table. Be sure to document if the neonate had any clothing or equipment on (such as an IV). Take the neonate's weight at the same time each day and on the same scale, if possible. Be careful to prevent heat loss.

Head-to-toe assessment

The neonate should receive a thorough physical examination of each body part. However, before each body part is examined, assess the general appearance and posture of the neonate. Neonates usually lie in a symmetrical, flexed position—the characteristic "fetal position"—as a result of their position while in utero.

Skin

In neonates, the skin may appear mottled or blotchy, especially on the extremities, for a few hours after birth. Then, it turns to its normal color.

Findings can be skin deep

Common findings in a neonatal assessment may include:

- acrocyanosis (caused by vasomotor instability, capillary stasis, and high hemoglobin level) for the first 24 hours after birth
- milia (clogged sebaceous glands) on the nose or chin
- lanugo (fine, downy hair) appearing after 20 weeks of gestation on the entire body, except the palms and soles
- vernix caseosa (a white, cheesy protective coating composed of desquamated epithelial cells and sebum)
- erythema toxicum neonatorum (a transient, maculopapular rash)
- telangiectasia (flat, reddened vascular areas) appearing on the neck, upper eyelid, or upper lip
- sudamina or miliaria (distended sweat glands), which cause minute vesicles on the skin surface, especially on the face
- pustular melanosis—vesicles, superficial pustules, and pigmented macules, which are transient and often present at birth

- hemangioma—benign self-limiting tumor of the endothelial cells lining the blood vessels; appears in the first few weeks of life and grows for the first 6 months and then decreases in size
- congenital dermal melanocytosis (formerly called Slate gray nevi)—bluish areas of pigmentation more commonly noted on the back and buttocks of neonates with darker skin tones (regardless of race).

Make general observations about the appearance of the neonate's skin in relationship to their activity, position, and temperature. Usually, the neonate is redder when crying or hot and may have transient episodes of cyanosis with crying. Cutis marmorata is transient mottling when the neonate is exposed to cooler temperatures.

Roll with it, baby

Palpate the skin to assess skin turgor. To do this, roll a fold of skin on the neonate's abdomen between the thumb and forefinger. Assess consistency, amount of subcutaneous tissue, and degree of hydration. A well-hydrated infant's skin returns to normal immediately upon release.

Head

The neonate's head is about one fourth of its body size. Six bones make up the cranium:

- The frontal bone
- The occipital bone
- Two parietal bones
- Two temporal bones

Bands of connective tissue, called *sutures*, lie between the junctures of these bones. At the junction of the sutures are wider spaces of membranous tissues, called *fontanels*.

Fontanel facts

The neonatal skull has two fontanels. The anterior fontanel is diamond shaped and located at the juncture of the frontal and parietal bones. It measures $1\frac{1}{8}$ to $1\frac{3}{8}$ in (3 to 4 cm) long and ¾ to $1\frac{1}{8}$ in (2 to 3 cm) wide and closes in about 18 months. The posterior fontanel is triangle shaped and located at the juncture of the occipital and parietal bones. It measures about ¾ in (2 cm) across and closes in 8 to 12 weeks.

In infancy, the fontanels are assessed by palpation. The fontanels should feel soft to the touch but shouldn't be depressed or bugle. The anterior fontanel may pulsate. A depressed fontanel indicates dehydration. Bulging fontanels require immediate attention because they may indicate increased intracranial pressure (ICP). The nurse may auscultate the fontanel to assess for bruits.

Locating the fontanels

The locations of the anterior and posterior fontanels are depicted in this illustration of the top of a neonatal skull.

Molding under the pressure

Molding refers to asymmetry of the cranial sutures due to difficulties during vaginal delivery; it isn't seen in neonates born by cesarean birth. There are three types of cranial abnormalities:

1. Cephalohematoma occurs when blood collects between a skull bone and the periosteum. It's caused by pressure during delivery and tends to spontaneously resolve in 3 to 6 weeks. A cephalohematoma doesn't cross cranial suture lines.
2. Caput succedaneum is a localized edematous area of the presenting part of the scalp. It's also caused by pressure during delivery but disappears spontaneously in 3 to 4 days and can cross cranial suture lines.
3. Subgaleal hemorrhage—occurs when there is bleeding between the skull periosteum and the scalp galea. This condition is an emergency and can result in death due to hemorrhage.

Heads up!

The degree of head control the neonate has should also be evaluated during this part of the examination. If neonates are placed down on a firm surface, they'll turn their heads to the side to maintain an open airway. They also attempt to keep their heads in line with their body when raised by their arms. Although head lag is normal in the neonate, marked head lag is seen in neonates with Down syndrome, brain damage, or hypoxia. No head lag can be a sign of birthing parent substance use resulting in neonatal withdrawal.

Eyes

Neonates tend to keep their eyes tightly shut. Observe the lids for edema, which is normally present for the first few days of life, and symmetry in size and shape. Note the shape of the iris. Common findings of neonatal eye examination are:

- blue or gray eyes because of scleral thinness—permanent eye color is established within 3 to 12 months
- immature lacrimal glands at birth, resulting in tearless crying for up to 2 months
- transient strabismus

- doll's eye reflex (when the head is rotated laterally, the eyes deviate in the opposite direction) that may persist for up to 10 days
- subconjunctival hemorrhages that appear from vascular tension changes during birth
- the corneal reflex—but it is generally not elicited unless a problem is suspected
- pupillary reflex and the red reflex.

Nose

Observe the neonate's nose for:
- shape
- symmetry
- placement
- patency
- bridge configuration.

Nasal passages must be kept clear to ensure adequate respiration. Neonates instinctively sneeze to remove the obstruction. Test the patency of the nasal passages by occluding each naris alternately while holding the neonate's mouth closed. (See *Monitoring for respiratory distress*.) If the infant desaturates and has cyanosis at rest but remains pink and saturated when crying, further evaluation is needed for choanal atresia.

Advice from the experts

Monitoring for respiratory distress

Nasal flaring is a serious sign of air hunger from respiratory distress. If nasal flaring or seesaw respirations; pale, gray skin; periods of apnea; bradycardia; or grunting are present, alert the practitioner. These may be signs of respiratory distress syndrome.

Mouth and pharynx

The neonate's mouth usually has scant saliva and pink lips. Inspect the mouth for its existing structures. Assess for symmetrical mouth movement, especially if there was a history of difficult delivery to ascertain if Bell palsy has occurred. The palate is usually narrow and highly arched. Inspect the hard and soft palates for clefts. Assess the philtrum and jaw size. Disorders such as Pierre Robin sequence may be present.

Pearls of wisdom on pearls

Epstein pearls (pinhead-size, white or yellow, rounded elevations) may be found on the gums or hard palate. These are caused by retained secretions and disappear within a few weeks or months. The frenulum of the upper lip may be quite thick. Precocious teeth may also be apparent. The pharynx is best assessed when the neonate is crying. Tonsillar tissue generally isn't visible. Tight frenulum can result in language disorders and, therefore, may need to be "clipped" as an infant.

Ears

Assess the neonate's ears for:
- symmetry
- placement on head
- pits or tags
- amount of cartilage
- open auditory canal
- hearing.

The neonate's ears are characterized by incurving of the pinna and cartilage deposition. The pinna is usually flattened against the side of the head from pressure in utero. The top of the ear should be above or parallel to an imaginary line from the inner to the outer canthus of the eye. Low-set ears are associated with several syndromes, including chromosomal abnormalities.

Before you go

Procedures to screen for hearing in neonates have become common practice before a neonate leaves the hospital or birthing facility. Testing can detect permanent bilateral or unilateral sensory or conductive hearing loss. (See *Universal neonatal hearing screening*.)

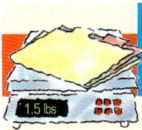

Weighing the evidence

Universal neonatal hearing screening

The Joint Committee on Infant Hearing (JCIH) Position Statement recommends early detection and intervention for infants with hearing loss.

According to JCIH recommendations:
- All infants should have hearing screening using a physiologic measure.
- Neonates who receive routine care should have access to hearing screening during their hospital birth admission.
- Neonates born in alternative care centers such as home birth settings should have access to and are referred to the hearing screening before 1 month of age.
- All neonates who require neonatal intensive care should receive hearing screening before discharge.
- All infants who do not pass the birth admission screen and any subsequent re-screening will begin appropriate audiologic and medical evaluations to confirm the presence of hearing loss before 3 months of age.

Now hear this!

Auditory assessment is performed by noninvasive, objective, physiologic measures that include otoacoustic emissions or auditory brain stem response. Both testing methods are painless and can be performed while the neonate rests. If the neonate does not pass the screening test, the test is usually repeated at age 3 months. An infant who does not pass the screening test at 3 months of age should be referred for a full audiologic evaluation. If hearing loss is present, infants should be referred to early intervention services by 6 months of age.

Neck

The neonate's neck is typically short and weak with deep folds of skin. Observe for:

- range of motion
- shape
- webbing
- abnormal masses.

Also, palpate each clavicle and sternocleidomastoid muscle. Note the position of the trachea. The thyroid gland generally is not palpable.

Chest

Inspect and palpate the chest, noting:

- shape—barrel-shaped chest
- clavicles—assess for fracture
- ribs
- nipples
- breast tissue—location of nipples and gynecomastia
- respiratory movements
- amount of cartilage in rib cage.

The neonatal chest is characterized by a cylindrical thorax (because the anteroposterior and lateral diameters are equal) and flexible ribs. Slight intercostal retractions are usually seen on inspiration. The sternum is raised and slightly rounded, and the xiphoid process is usually visible as a small protrusion at the end of the sternum.

Breast engorgement (gynecomastia) from maternal hormones may be apparent, and the secretion of "witch's milk" may occur. Supernumerary nipples may be located below and medial to the true nipples.

Lungs

Normal respirations of the neonate are abdominal with a rate between 30 and 50 breaths/min. After the first breaths to initiate respiration, subsequent breaths should be easy and fairly regular. Occasional irregularities may occur with crying, sleeping, and feeding.

Hush little baby, don't say a word

It is easiest to auscultate the lung fields when the neonate is quiet. Bilateral bronchial breath sounds should be heard. Crackles soon after birth represent the transition of the lungs to extrauterine life.

Heart

The neonate's heart rate is normally between 110 and 160 beats/min. Because neonates have a fast heart rate, it's difficult to auscultate the specific components of the cardiac cycle. Heart sounds during the neonatal period are generally of higher pitch, shorter duration, and greater intensity than in later life. The first sound is usually louder and duller than the second, which is sharp in quality. Murmurs are commonly heard, especially over the base of the heart or at the third or fourth intercostal space at the left sternal border due to incomplete functional closure of the fetal shunts.

The apical impulse (point of maximal impulse) is at the fourth intercostal space and to the left of the midclavicular line. Ascertain if there is an active precordium present. Take note of irregular heart rates. In the instance of maternal immunologic disorders, the infant is at risk for heart blocks.

Abdomen

Neonatal abdominal assessment should include:
- inspection and palpation of the umbilical cord
- evaluation of the size and contour of the abdomen
- auscultation of bowel sounds
- assessment of skin color
- observation of movement with respirations
- palpation of internal organs.

Stop, look, listen . . .

The neonatal abdomen is usually cylindrical with some protrusion. Bowel sounds are heard a few hours after birth. A scaphoid appearance indicates a diaphragmatic hernia. The umbilical cord is white and gelatinous with two arteries and one vein and begins to dry within 1 to 2 hours after delivery.

. . . and feel

The liver is normally palpable 1 in (2.5 cm) below the right costal margin. Sometimes, the tip of the spleen can be felt, but a spleen that's palpable more than $1/3$ in (1 cm) below the left costal margin warrants further investigation. Both kidneys should be palpable; this is easiest done soon after delivery, when muscle tone is lowest. The suprapubic area should be palpated for a distended bladder. The neonate should void within the first 24 hours of birth.

Femoral pulses should also be palpated at this point in the examination. Inability to palpate femoral pulses could signify coarctation of the aorta.

Genitalia

Characteristics of a male neonate's genitalia include rugae on the scrotum and testes descended into the scrotum. Scrotal edema may be present for several days after birth because of maternal hormones. Hydrocele may be noted, which is free fluid in the scrotal sac. The urinary meatus is located in one of three places:
1. At the penile tip (normal)
2. On the dorsal surface (epispadias)
3. On the ventral surface (hypospadias)

In the female neonate, the labia majora covers the labia minora and clitoris. These structures may be prominent due to maternal hormones. Vaginal discharge may also occur, and the hymenal tag is present.

Extremities

The extremities should be assessed for range of motion, symmetry, and signs of trauma. Using the Barlow and Ortolani method, the hips should be assessed for dislocation, suggestive of developmental dysplasia of the hip. Female infants who were born via cesarean birth are at higher risk for congenital hip dysplasia. Hyperflexibility of joints is characteristic of Down syndrome. Some neonates may have abnormal extremities. They may be polydactyl (more than five digits on an extremity) or syndactyl (two or more digits fused together). If edema of hands/feet is noted, it can be a clinical feature of Turner syndrome.

Note the nails

The nail beds should be pink, although they may appear slightly blue due to acrocyanosis. Persistent cyanosis indicates hypoxia or vasoconstriction.

Reading palms

The palms should have the usual creases. A bilateral transverse palmar crease, called a *simian crease*, suggests Down syndrome.

Expect resistance

Assess muscle tone. Extension of any extremity is usually met with resistance and, upon release, returns to its previously flexed position. If abnormalities in the muscle tone are noted, a neurologic evaluation should be performed.

Spine

The neonatal spine should be straight, intact, and flat, and the anus should be patent without any fissure. Dimpling at the base of the spine is commonly associated with spina bifida or tethered cord. The shoulders, scapulae, and iliac crests should line up in the same plane.

Neurologic assessment

An examination of the reflexes provides useful information about the neonate's nervous system and their state of neurologic maturation. Some reflexive behaviors in the neonate are necessary for survival, whereas other reflexive behaviors act as safety mechanisms.

Reflex revelations

Normal neonates display several types of reflexes. Abnormalities are indicated by absence, asymmetry, persistence, or weakness in these reflexes:

- Sucking—It begins when a nipple is placed in the neonate's mouth.
- Moro reflex—When the neonate is lifted above the bassinet and suddenly lowered, the arms and legs symmetrically extend and then abduct while the thumb and forefinger spread to form a "C."
- Rooting—When the neonate's cheek is stroked, the neonate turns their head in the direction of the stroke.
- Tonic neck (fencing position)—When the neonate's head is turned while they are lying in a supine position, the extremities on the same side straighten and those on the opposite side flex.
- Babinski reflex—When the sole on the side of the neonate's small toe is stroked, the toes fan upward.
- Grasping—When a finger is placed in each of the neonate's hands, the neonate's fingers grasp tightly enough to be pulled to a sitting position.
- Stepping—When the neonate is held upright with the feet touching a flat surface, they respond with dancing or stepping movements.
- Startle—A loud noise such as a hand clap elicits neonatal arm abduction and elbow flexion and the neonate's hands stay clenched.
- Trunk incurvature—When a finger is run laterally down the neonate's spine, the trunk flexes, and the pelvis swings toward the stimulated side.
- Blinking—The neonate's eyelids close in response to bright light.

Neonatal care

Physical care for the neonate includes:
- protecting from infection and injury
- maintaining a patent airway
- maintaining a stable body temperature.

Neonatal eye prophylaxis

Neonatal eye prophylaxis involves instilling 0.5% erythromycin ointment into the neonate's eyes to prevent ophthalmia neonatorum and *Neisseria gonorrhoeae* or *Chlamydia trachomatis* infections, which the neonate may have acquired from the birthing parent as they passed through the birth canal. Erythromycin provides the antimicrobial effects of a broad-spectrum antibiotic.

It's the law

Neonatal eye prophylaxis is required by law in all 50 states. Before this treatment, gonorrheal conjunctivitis was a common cause of permanent eye damage and blindness.

Break for bonding

To perform neonatal eye prophylaxis, use ophthalmic antibiotic ointment as ordered and gloves. Although the drug may be administered in the birthing room, treatment can be delayed for up to 1 hour to allow initial caregiver–child bonding. Antibiotic prophylaxis may not be effective if the infection was acquired in utero from premature rupture of the membranes.

Step by step

To perform neonatal eye prophylaxis, follow these steps:
- Wash hands, and put on gloves.
- To ensure comfort and effectiveness, shield the neonate's eyes from direct light and tilt their head slightly to the side that will receive the treatment.
- Using the nondominant hand, gently raise the neonate's upper eyelid with the index finger, and pull the lower eyelid down with the thumb.
- Using the dominant hand, instill the ointment into the lower conjunctival sac.

- Close and manipulate the eyelids to spread the medication over the eye.
- Repeat the procedure for the other eye.
- A single-dose ointment tube should be used to prevent contamination and the spread of infection.
- If the neonate's caregivers are present, explain that the procedure is required by state law.
- Complications of neonatal eye prophylaxis include chemical conjunctivitis (which may cause redness, swelling, and drainage) or discoloration of the skin around the neonate's eyes. If such complications occur, reassure the caregivers that these temporary effects will subside within a few days.

Write it down!

Be sure to document neonatal eye prophylaxis appropriately. If it is done in the delivery room, record the treatment on the delivery room form. If you perform it in the nursery, document it in your notes.

Thermoregulation

Because the neonate has a relatively large surface-to-weight ratio, reduced metabolism per unit area, and small amounts of insulating fat, they are susceptible to hypothermia. The neonate keeps warm by metabolizing brown fat, which has a greater concentration of energy-producing mitochondria in its cells, enhancing its capacity for heat production. This kind of fat is unique to neonates. Brown fat metabolism is effective but only within a very narrow temperature range.

Without careful external thermoregulation, the neonate may become chilled, which can result in:

- hypoxia
- acidosis
- hypoglycemia
- pulmonary vasoconstriction
- death.

Keep it neutral

The object of thermoregulation is to provide a neutral thermal environment that helps the neonate maintain a normal core temperature with minimal oxygen consumption and caloric expenditure. The core temperature varies with the neonate but is about 97.7°F (36.5°C). Cold stress and its complications can be prevented with proper interventions. (See *Understanding thermoregulators*.)

Understanding thermoregulators

Thermoregulators preserve neonatal body warmth in various ways. A radiant warmer maintains the neonate's temperature by radiation. An incubator maintains the neonate's temperature by conduction and convection.

Temperature settings

Radiant warmers and incubators have two operating modes: nonservo and servo. The nurse manually sets temperature on nonservo equipment; a probe on the neonate's skin controls temperature settings on servo models.

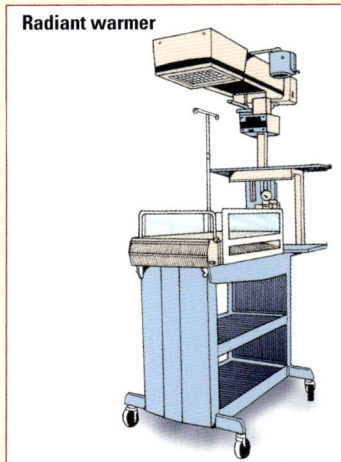

Radiant warmer

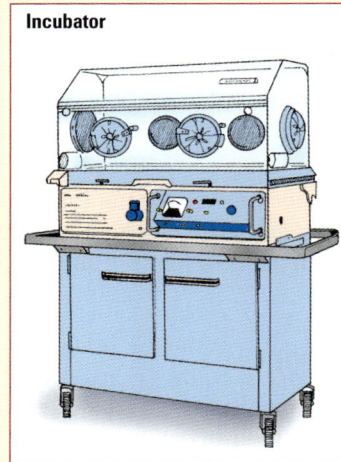

Incubator

Other features

Most thermoregulators come with alarms. Incubators have the added advantage of providing a stable, enclosed environment, which protects the neonate from evaporative heat loss.

To prevent cold stress at birth, you'll need:
- radiant warmer or incubator (if necessary)
- blankets
- washcloths or towels
- skin probe
- adhesive pad
- water-soluble lubricant
- thermometer
- clothing, including a cap.

While you wait

While preparing for the neonate's birth, turn on the radiant warmer in the delivery room, and set it to the desired temperature. Warm the blankets, washcloths, or towels under a heat source.

After the arrival

In the birthing room, follow these steps:
- Place the neonate under the radiant warmer, dry them with warm washcloths or towels, remove wet linen, and then cover their head with a cap to prevent heat loss.
- Perform required procedures quickly, and wrap them in the warmed blankets. If their condition permits, give them to their caregivers to promote bonding. Initiate breastfeeding if appropriate.

If the neonate is stable, dry them quickly, place a cap on their head, and then place the neonate skin-to-skin with a caregiver. Cover them both with a blanket. This is called *kangaroo care*. Transport the neonate to the nursery in the warmed blankets; use a transport incubator as necessary.

In the nursery, follow these steps:
- Remove the blankets and cap, and place the neonate under the radiant warmer.
- Use the adhesive pad to attach the temperature control probe to their skin in the upper right abdominal quadrant. If the neonate will lie prone, put the skin probe on their back. Don't cover the device with anything because this could interfere with the servo control.
- Take the neonate's rectal temperature on admission and then take axillary temperatures thereafter every 15 to 30 minutes until the temperature stabilizes and then every 4 hours to ensure stability. (See *Preventing heat loss*.)

Advice from the experts

Preventing heat loss

Follow these steps to prevent heat loss in the neonate.

Conduction
- Preheat the radiant warmer bed and linen.
- Warm stethoscopes and other instruments before use.
- Before weighing the neonate, pad the scale with a paper towel or a preweighed, warmed sheet.

Convection
- Place the neonate's bed out of a direct line with an open window, fan, or air-conditioning vent.

(continued)

Preventing heat loss (*continued*)

Evaporation
• Dry the neonate immediately after delivery, and remove wet linen.
• When bathing the neonate, expose only one body part at a time; wash each part thoroughly and then dry it immediately.

Radiation
• Keep the neonate and examination tables away from outside windows and air conditioners.

Sponge bathe the neonate under the warmer only after their temperature stabilizes, and their glucose level is normal. Leave them under the warmer until their temperature remains stable. If the temperature doesn't stabilize, place the neonate under a plastic heat shield or in a warmed incubator, as per facility policy. Check for signs of infection, which can cause hypothermia.

Incubator involvement

Apply a skin probe to a neonate in an incubator as you would for a neonate in a radiant warmer. Move the incubator away from cold walls or objects. Perform all required procedures quickly, and close portholes in the hood after completion. If procedures must be performed outside the incubator, do them under a radiant warmer.

To leave the facility or to move to a bassinet, a neonate must be weaned from the incubator by slowly reducing the temperature to that of the nursery. Check periodically for hypothermia. When the neonate's temperature stabilizes, dress them, put them in a bassinet, and cover them with a blanket. Also, be sure to instruct the caregivers on the importance of maintaining body temperature. (See *Maintaining the neonate's body temperature*.)

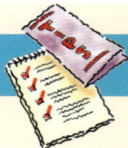

Education edge

Maintaining the neonate's body temperature

To help caregivers understand the importance of maintaining the neonate's temperature, instruct them to:
• keep the neonate wrapped in a blanket and out of drafts when they aren't in the bassinet
• avoid placing the bassinet next to a window, a fan, an air conditioner, or an air conditioner vent
• keep the stockinette cap on their head because a neonate loses considerable heat through their head
• remove any wet linens from, on, or around the neonate as soon as possible
• avoid placing the neonate on a cold surface such as a counter without first placing a towel or blanket down.

Noteworthy items

In your nursing notes, be sure to document:
- the name and temperature of the heat source used
- the neonate's temperature
- complications resulting from use of thermoregulatory equipment.

Oxygen administration

Oxygen relieves neonatal respiratory distress, which can be exhibited by cyanosis, pallor, tachypnea, nasal flaring, bradycardia, hypothermia, retractions (intercostal, subcostal marginal, suprasternal), hypotonia, hyporeflexia, or expiratory grunting. Remember, oxygen is a drug.

Too much of a good thing

No matter how it's administered, oxygen therapy can be hazardous to the neonate. When given in high concentrations and for prolonged periods, it can cause retinopathy of prematurity, which may result in blindness in preterm neonates, and can contribute to bronchopulmonary dysplasia. Because of the neonate's size and special respiratory requirements, oxygen administration commonly requires special techniques and equipment.

Hands-on in an emergency

In emergency situations, give oxygen through a manual resuscitation bag and mask of appropriate size until more permanent measures can be initiated.

A method for every occasion

When the neonate merely requires additional oxygen above the ambient concentration, it can be delivered using an oxygen hood or nasal cannula. When the neonate requires CPAP to prevent alveolar collapse at the end of an expiration, as in respiratory distress syndrome, administer oxygen through nasal prongs or an endotracheal tube (ETT) connected to a manometer. If the neonate can't breathe on their own, deliver oxygen through a ventilator via ETT. Oxygen must be warmed and humidified to prevent hypothermia and dehydration, to which the neonate is especially susceptible.

The right tools for the job

To prepare for oxygen therapy, equipment needed is:
- an oxygen source (wall, cylinder, or liquid unit)
- a compressed air source
- humidification
- flowmeters

- large- and small-bore sterile oxygen tubing
- a blood gas analyzer
- pulse oximeter
- a stethoscope
- a nasogastric (NG) tube.
  For handheld resuscitation bag and mask delivery, equipment needed is:
- a specially sized mask with handheld resuscitation bag and pressure release valve
- a manometer with connectors.
  For delivery via an oxygen hood, equipment needed is:
- an appropriate-sized oxygen hood
- an oxygen analyzer.
  For delivery through nasal prongs, other equipment includes:
- nasal prongs
- water-soluble lubricant.
  For CPAP or ETT delivery, equipment needed is:
- a manometer with connectors
- a nasopharyngeal or ETT or nasal CPAP prongs
- humidification system
- laryngoscope
- suction
- water-soluble lubricant
- hypoallergenic tape
- an exhaled CO_2 monitor.
  For delivery with a ventilator, equipment needed is:
- a ventilator unit with manometer and in-line thermometer
- specimen tubes for arterial blood gas (ABG) analysis
- an ETT
- an exhaled CO_2 monitor
- a pulse oximeter or transcutaneous oxygen monitor.

Be prepared

To prepare for oxygen administration, wash hands and gather and assemble the necessary equipment. To calibrate the oxygen analyzer, turn the analyzer on and read the results. Room air should be about 21% oxygen. Expose the analyzer probe to 100% oxygen, adjust the sensitivity, and recheck the amount of oxygen in room air.

By hand

To use a handheld resuscitation bag and mask, follow these steps:
- Place the assembled resuscitation bag and mask in the resuscitation area.
- Turn on the oxygen and compressed air flowmeters, and place the mask over the neonate's nose and mouth.

- Check pressure settings and mask size.
- Have another staff member notify the practitioner immediately.
- Provide 40 to 60 breaths/min, using enough pressure to cause a visible rise and fall of the chest. Provide enough oxygen to maintain pink nail beds and mucous membranes.
- Continuously watch the neonate's chest movements and listen to breath sounds, avoiding overventilation. If the neonate's heart rate falls below 100 beats/min, continue to use the handheld resuscitation bag until the heart rate rises to 100 beats/min or greater.
- Place pulse oximetry on infant in preductal location.
- Insert an NG tube to vent air from the neonate's stomach.
- Call for assistance from advanced trained personnel.

By hood

To use an oxygen hood, follow these steps:
- Attach the oxygen hood to the connecting tubing, and place an in-line thermometer close to the neonate.
- Activate oxygen and compressed air source, if needed, at ordered flow rates.
- Attach to a humidification source.
- Place the oxygen hood over the neonate's head.
- Measure the amount of oxygen the neonate is receiving with the oxygen analyzer. Be sure to place the analyzer probe close to the neonate's nose.
- Adjust the oxygen to the prescribed amount.

By prongs

When using nasal prongs, follow these steps:
- Match the prong size to the neonate's nose.
- Apply a small amount of water-soluble lubricant to the outside of the prongs.
- Turn on the oxygen and compressed air, if necessary.
- Connect the prongs to the oxygen source.
- Insert the prongs into the nose and secure them.
- Be sure to keep the prongs clean to ensure patency.

By CPAP

If the neonate needs CPAP to prevent alveolar collapse at the end of each breath (as in respiratory distress syndrome), they may receive this through an ETT, a nasopharyngeal tube, or nasal CPAP prongs. To use CPAP, follow these steps:
- Position the neonate on their back with a rolled towel under their neck to keep the airway open; avoid hyperextending the neck.
- Assist with intubation if necessary.
- Turn on the oxygen and compressed air source, and attach the delivery system to the ETT or nasal CPAP prongs.

- If an ETT is in place, confirm placement by using an exhaled CO_2 monitor and tape the tube in place.
- Other methods to confirm placement are equal bilateral breath sounds, condensation in the ETT, and chest x-ray (CXR) confirming placement.
- Insert an NG or orogastric tube to keep the stomach decompressed, if ordered. Leave the tube open to air unless the neonate is receiving gavage feedings.

By ventilator

To use a ventilator, follow these steps:
- Turn on the ventilator, and set the controls as ordered.
- Help with ETT insertion, and attach it to the ventilator.
- Confirm placement of the ETT with the exhaled CO_2 monitor, and tape it securely.
- Watch the manometer to maintain pressure at the prescribed level, and monitor the in-line thermometer for correct temperature.

Knowing the know-how

Know how to perform neonatal chest auscultation correctly to detect subtle respiratory changes. Also, know and identify signs of respiratory distress, and perform emergency procedures. If required, perform chest physiotherapy and percussion as ordered, and follow with suctioning to remove secretions.

Monitor ABG/capillary blood gas (CBG) levels every 15 to 20 minutes (or at prescribed intervals) after any changes in oxygen concentration or pressure. If ordered, monitor oxygen perfusion via either pulse oximetry or mixed venous oxygen saturation monitoring. Keep the practitioner aware of ABG/CBG levels, so they can order appropriate changes in oxygen concentration.

As ordered, discontinue oxygen administration when the neonate's fraction of inspired oxygen (FiO_2) is at room air level (20% to 21%) and their arterial oxygen is stable at 60 to 90 mm Hg. Repeat ABG/CBG measurements 20 to 30 minutes after discontinuing oxygen and thereafter as ordered by the practitioner or by facility policy. Monitor CO_2 levels.

On the watch

Assess the neonate for complications of oxygen administration, including:
- signs and symptoms of infection
- hypothermia
- metabolic and respiratory acidosis
- pressure injuries on the neonate's head, face, and nose
- signs of a pulmonary air leak, including pneumothorax, pneumomediastinum, pneumopericardium, and interstitial emphysema.

Safety first

When administering oxygen, always take safety precautions to avoid fire or explosion. Take measures to keep the neonate warm because hypothermia impedes respiration. (See *Hazards of oxygen therapy*.)

Hazards of oxygen therapy

No matter which system delivers the oxygen, oxygen therapy is potentially hazardous to a neonate. The gas must be warmed and humidified to prevent hypothermia and dehydration. Given in high concentrations over prolonged periods, oxygen can cause retinopathy of prematurity, leading to blindness. With low oxygen concentration, hypoxia and central nervous system damage may occur. Also, depending on how it's delivered, oxygen can contribute to bronchopulmonary dysplasia.

Other worries

Here are some other possible complications of oxygen therapy in neonates:
• Increased excessive humidification can collect in the tubing, and this can potentially impede aeration and also provide an atmosphere for infection or "drowning." Overhumidification, in turn, allows water to collect in tubing, providing a growth medium for bacteria or suffocating the neonate.
• Hypothermia can increase oxygen consumption and can result from administering cool oxygen.
• Metabolic and respiratory acidosis may follow inadequate ventilation.
• Pressure injuries may develop on the neonate's head, face, and around the nose during prolonged oxygen therapy.
• A pulmonary air leak (pneumothorax, pneumomediastinum, pneumopericardium, interstitial emphysema) may arise spontaneously with respiratory distress or result from forced ventilation.
• Decreased cardiac output may result from excessive CPAP.

For the record

When documenting oxygen administration, be sure to include:
• type of respiratory distress requiring oxygen administration
• oxygen concentration given
• oxygen delivery method used
• each change in oxygen concentration
• routine checks of oxygen concentration
• neonate's FiO_2 (as measured by the oxygen analyzer)
• ABG/CBG values, noting the time each sample was obtained
• each time suctioning is performed
• amount and consistency of mucus
• type of continuous oxygen monitoring, if any

- complications
- neonate's condition during oxygen therapy, including respiratory rate, breath sounds, and signs of additional respiratory distress.

Quick quiz

1. The nurse is preparing to attend delivery of a term neonate. When preparing for first neonatal breath, what factor does not assist in stimulation of neonatal breathing?

- A. Decreased CO_2 levels
- B. Increased CO_2 levels
- C. Decreased blood pH
- D. Decreased blood oxygen levels

Answer: A. Decreased CO_2 levels do not stimulate breathing in the neonate.

2. When assessing a neonate's umbilical cord, the nurse must look for several anatomic structures. What would the nurse document for the expected anatomy of a newborn's umbilical cord?

- A. One artery and one vein
- B. One artery and one ligament
- C. Two arteries and one vein
- D. One artery and two veins

Answer: C. The umbilical cord should consist of two arteries and one vein.

3. During transitional period after birth, neonates are assigned Apgar scores. What is included and evaluated in the scoring for Apgar?

- A. Heart rate, respiratory rate, color, blood pressure, and temperature
- B. Heart rate, respiratory effort, muscle tone, reflex irritability, and color
- C. Respiratory rate, blood pressure, reflex irritability, muscle tone, and temperature
- D. Temperature, heart rate, color, muscle tone, and blood pressure

Answer: B. Apgar scoring involves evaluating the neonate's heart rate, respiratory effort, muscle tone, reflex irritability, and color.

4. The transition from fetal to neonatal respiration is important to assess. What would be noted as a sign of respiratory distress in a neonate and require further actions by the nurse?

- A. Acrocyanosis
- B. Nasal flaring
- C. Abdominal movements
- D. Short periods of apnea (less than 15 seconds)

Answer: B. Nasal flaring is a sign of respiratory distress in the neonate. Acrocyanosis, abdominal movements, and short periods of apnea are all normal findings.

5. The nurse is educating a caregiver on the spots on the neonate's head. The nurse explains that the areas are called *fontanels*. How does the nurse describe the normal finding of the fontanels after birth to the caregiver?
   A. Soft to touch
   B. Depressed
   C. Bulging
   D. Closed

Answer: A. The fontanels should feel soft to the touch with gentle pressure/touch. The other findings indicate issues and require further assessment.

Scoring

⭐⭐⭐ If you answered all five questions correctly, give yourself a high five! Then toddle on over to the next chapter!

⭐⭐ If you answered four questions correctly, stand tall! There's no holding you back!

⭐ If you answered fewer than three questions correctly, roll with the punches! Get a leg up by revisiting this chapter!

Selected References

Gantan, E., & Wiedrich, L. (2023). Neonatal evaluation. In *StatPearls*. StatPearls Publishing. https://www.ncbi.nlm.nih.gov/books/NBK558943/

Johnson, M., Kuschel, C., & Donnan, L. (2023). Neonatal clinical examination and selective ultrasound screening are not reliable for the early diagnosis of hip dysplasia. A retrospective cohort study. *Journal of Paediatrics & Child Health*, 59, 1146–1151. https://doi.org/10.1111/jpc.16472

Meegan, S., & Martin, T. (2020). Exploring the experiences of student midwives completing the newborn infant physical examination. *British Journal of Midwifery*, 28, 115–119. https://doi.org/10.12968/bjom.2020.28.2.115

Moss, C., & Nation, H. (2024). Neonatal assessment: Put your best foot forward. *Advances in Neonatal Care*, 24, 58–64. https://doi.org/10.1097/ANC.0000000000001116

Smith, A., McGrath, R., McCallion, N., & Clarke, T. (2019). Tips for medical students and non-neonatalogists on physical examination of the newborn and important aspects of early newborn care. *Neonatology Today*, 14, 4–9.

The Joint Committee on Infant Hearing. (2019). Year 2019 position statement: Principles and guidelines for early hearing detection and intervention programs. *The Journal of Early Hearing Detection and Intervention*, 4, 1–44.

Chapter 11

High-risk neonatal conditions

Just the facts

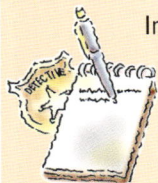

In this chapter, you'll learn:

◆ characteristics of selected neonatal disorders

◆ tests used to diagnose certain high-risk neonatal conditions

◆ medical treatments and therapies for high-risk neonatal conditions

◆ nursing interventions for high-risk neonatal conditions.

A look at the high-risk neonate

Both antenatal and postnatal factors can increase a baby's risk of complications in the immediate newborn period. Common antenatal risk factors include maternal diabetes, premature onset of labor, and chorioamnionitis. After birth, babies may become cold stressed, hypoglycemic, or have problems breathing. It is important to identify the most common issues that affect neonates with diagnostic tests, treatment strategies, and nursing interventions for each.

At risk for impaired parenting

Whenever a baby must be separated from their caregivers for observation or treatment, there is a risk of impaired parenting. Caregivers of babies who experience issues after birth may feel a sense of loss and have difficulty bonding because their neonate isn't the "perfect" child they anticipated. Families who have a baby with a serious illness or a congenital anomaly may need assistance to cope with their long-term grief in addition to referral to resources for the special care that their baby may require. Even worse, if caregivers experience a perinatal or neonatal loss, the family will need additional support in coping with their grief.

In addition to the direct care of the high-risk newborn, nurses should promote parent–infant bonding and attachment. When possible, caregivers should be allowed to be with their baby, and participate in their care, for example, feeding, holding, and diaper changes. If the baby's condition warrants intensive care, caregivers should be provided photographs after admission and be encouraged to visit and interact with the baby in the neonatal intensive care unit (NICU) as often as feasible.

Birth weight classification: AGA, SGA, LGA

Whether born preterm, at term, or post-term, neonates are classified by their birth weight as follows:
1. Babies with birth weight between the 10th and 90th percentile are considered appropriate for gestational age (AGA).
2. Those with birth weight above the 90th percentile are considered large for gestational age (LGA).
3. Small for gestational age (SGA) babies have birth weight below the 10th percentile.

Large for gestational age

Neonates born LGA have birth weights above the 90th percentile for gestational age. Babies born LGA may be large because of their family genetics. Infants of birthing parents with diabetes are at increased risk for being born LGA.

What causes it

For infants born to birthing parents with diabetes, the elevated maternal glucose levels stimulate continued insulin production by the fetus. This constant state of hyperglycemia and hyperinsulinemia in utero leads to excessive growth and fat deposition in the fetus.

What to look for

Babies born LGA generally weigh more than 8 lb, 13 oz (4,000 g) and those born to birthing parents with diabetes have head circumferences within normal limits (10th to 90th percentile). All neonates born LGA may experience hypoxia during labor and are more likely to require an assisted delivery (vacuum extraction, forceps delivery, or cesarean birth). Infants of birthing parents with diabetes are at high risk for hypoglycemia secondary to the hyperinsulinemia they experienced in utero. Babies with hypoglycemia may exhibit jitteriness, respiratory distress, lethargy, poor feeding, hypothermia, and, in rare cases, seizures. Babies born LGA are at increased risk for respiratory distress at birth from hypoglycemia, retained fetal lung fluid, surfactant deficiency, and persistent pulmonary hypertension of the newborn. They are also at increased risk for having a congenital cardiac defect.

Assessment of perfusion after birth, auscultation of heart sounds, and monitoring of vital signs are recommended elements of every newborn's care.

What tests tell you

Neonates born to birthing parents with diabetes require bedside glucose monitoring because of their risk of hypoglycemia after birth. They are also at risk for polycythemia (excess of circulating red blood cells [RBCs]) and hypocalcemia. Symptomatic infants should have a hematocrit drawn and calcium levels monitored.

How it's treated

Treatment of babies born LGA is supportive. These babies may be poor feeders and require supplemental feedings, gavage feedings, or intravenous (IV) glucose infusion. The treatment of hypoglycemia may include early initiation of feedings, supplemental feedings, dextrose buccal gel administration, or IV glucose. Supportive respiratory care of babies with respiratory distress due to hypoglycemia may be needed.

What to do

Nursing interventions for neonates born LGA include:
- assessment of cardiac and respiratory systems
- monitoring of temperature and vital signs
- close monitoring of bedside glucose levels
- monitoring of calcium levels and hematocrit for symptomatic babies
- early initiation of feeds and supplemental feeds as needed
- facilitating parent bonding
- keeping caregivers informed
- providing support to the family.

Small for gestational age

Babies with birth weights below the 10th percentile may have experienced growth restriction in utero, which can be symmetrical or asymmetrical. Those with symmetrical growth restriction have a head circumference below the 10th percentile. Babies with head-sparing, asymmetric, growth restriction have a head circumference above the 10th percentile.

What causes it

Factors that can contribute to a neonate being born SGA include:
- congenital infection
- chromosomal disorders
- gestational hypertension

- maternal diabetes that was not well controlled
- intrauterine malnutrition due to poor placental function or maternal malnutrition
- maternal smoking
- maternal drug or alcohol use
- multiple gestation.

What to look for

The classification of SGA growth is made from the baby's weight and measurements taken at birth. Babies born SGA may look wasted due to having little subcutaneous fat. Their umbilical cord is typically thin, and they can have a scaphoid abdomen. Those who experienced head-sparing growth will have a disproportionately large head with a large anterior fontanel. Physical assessment of the baby born SGA may reveal congenital anomalies, respiratory distress, or poor tone (if baby has congenital infection, hypoglycemia, or cold stress).

What tests tell you

Neonates born SGA should be monitored for:
- hypoglycemia—low blood sugar (bedside glucose monitoring)
- hypocalcemia—low calcium levels (serum calcium levels)
- hyperbilirubinemia—elevated bilirubin level (transcutaneous or serum bilirubin monitoring)
- polycythemia—elevated red blood cell count (hematocrit)
- infection (complete blood count [CBC] with differential and blood culture if warranted by maternal history or neonatal symptoms of sepsis such as lethargy, hypothermia, or respiratory distress).

How it's treated

Neonates born SGA are more likely to experience hypoxia in utero and respiratory distress after delivery. In addition, these babies may pass meconium in utero due to fetal hypoxia, which can result in meconium aspiration. They are at high risk for hypoglycemia due to decreased fat stores and may experience cold stress with their large ratio of body surface area to weight. Their treatment should be supportive and individualized with nutrition being the primary focus. SGA babies have higher caloric needs and may have difficulty feeding. They can benefit from frequent feedings and may require increased caloric density. Care of the neonate who is SGA also includes bedside glucose monitoring and careful respiratory assessments.

What to do

Nursing interventions for neonates born SGA include:
- monitoring of respiratory status
- monitoring of temperature

- providing a neutral thermal environment
- protecting the neonate from infection
- providing appropriate nutrition with frequent feeds and higher calories as needed
- assessing glucose and calcium levels
- preventing skin breakdown
- facilitating caregiver bonding
- keeping caregivers informed of the baby's condition
- providing support to the family.

Cardiac screening

Advances in prenatal diagnosis of congenital heart defects (CHDs) have improved early detection. Approximately 3 to 9 in 1,000 babies are born with a cardiac defect. Ventricular septal defects are most commonly seen and, if small, are likely to close without intervention.

What causes it

Babies born to birthing parents with diabetes, those who have immediate relatives with a CHD, and those born preterm are at increased risk for CHDs. Most cardiac defects have multifactorial causes.

What to look for

As many as half of newborns may have a physiologic murmur in the 48 hours following birth. These babies are transitioning from fetal circulation and closing their patent ductus arteriosus. Newborns with persistent murmur, cyanosis, weak pulses, or unequal upper and lower extremity pulses require further screening to rule out a critical cardiac defect.

What tests tell you

Echocardiogram is the test used to diagnose a cardiac defect. In addition, babies who are symptomatic should also have the following tests:
- Arterial blood gas—to evaluate for hypoxemia and acidosis
- Chest x-ray—to evaluate heart size and shape as well as lung fields

How it's treated

Treatment depends on the type of cardiac defect. Babies with a heart defect dependent on flow through their patent ductus arteriosus will need prostaglandin E_1 in the immediate newborn period. Babies suspected of having a cardiac defect should be seen by a pediatric cardiologist.

What to do

Universal pulse oximetry screening can lead to early recognition of newborns with cardiac defects. Screening should be done prior to the newborn's discharge but not before 24 hours of age. During the screen, the preductal (right hand) oxygen saturation is compared with the postductal (either foot) saturation. A negative screen is one where there is less than a 3% difference between the two readings, and the oxygen saturation is greater than 95% for both sites. Oxygen saturations less than 90% are considered positive, and the pediatrician should be notified immediately. For those babies whose readings fall in between, they should have a repeat screen in an hour.

Congenital neonatal infections

Newborns are at increased risk for infection due to their immature immune systems. Sepsis (blood infection) in the newborn is associated with significant morbidity and mortality. The incidence of neonatal sepsis is 1 in 5 per 1,000 births. Babies who recover are at risk for neurologic effects. Early detection and diagnosis can assist nurses in identifying at-risk newborns. Prenatal and antenatal history of newborn's birthing parent should include an assessment of risk factors such as history of infection during pregnancy, prolonged rupture of membranes (longer than 18 hours), maternal fever (101 °F or higher), foul-smelling or purulent amniotic fluid, premature onset of labor, and relevant lab results (such as group B *Streptococcus* status positive). Newborn risk factors include prematurity, need for resuscitation at birth, low 5-minute Apgar score, respiratory distress, poor perfusion, and lethargy or poor feeding.

Bacterial sepsis

What causes it

The most common bacteria causing congenital infection in the newborn are group B *Streptococcus* and *Escherichia coli*. Widespread screening of birthing parents for group B *Streptococcus* near the end of pregnancy has resulted in more birthing parents being treated with antibiotics during labor to reduce transmission of group B *Streptococcus* to their babies. In utero, the fetus may be infected by bacteria in the birthing parent's blood from the placenta, by direct contact with an infected uterus, or from bacteria ascending from the birthing parent's genital tract. After the birthing parent's membranes rupture, the baby is at risk from bacteria from the genital tract or as the baby passes through the birth canal.

What to look for

A newborn with sepsis may present with a myriad of symptoms. (See *Common clinical signs of sepsis in the newborn* for the commonly seen clinical signs of sepsis.)

Common clinical signs of sepsis in the newborn

System	Clinical signs
Thermoregulation	• Hypothermia • Temperature instability
Neurologic	• Hypotonia or hypertonia • Jitteriness • Irritability • Seizures (with associated meningitis)
Respiratory	• Respiratory distress (grunting, flaring, retractions, tachypnea) • Cyanosis • Apnea • Respiratory acidosis
Cardiovascular	• Tachycardia • Hypotension • Poor peripheral perfusion • Delayed capillary refill
Gastrointestinal	• Poor feeding • Feeding intolerance • Abdominal distention
Integumentary	• Rash • Pustules • Pallor
Metabolic	• Hypoglycemia or hyperglycemia • Metabolic acidosis

What tests tell you

Newborns with risk factors for sepsis should be screened for infection. The following tests can assist in the diagnosis of sepsis:

- CBC—Several elements of the CBC are useful in monitoring a baby with possible sepsis:
  - White blood cell (WBC)—WBC counts that are low (less than 5,000 cells/mm^3) or elevated (greater than 30,000 cells/mm^3) can be seen in babies with sepsis.
  - Differential count—An elevated immature/total neutrophil ratio (greater than 0.2) suggests infection.
  - Platelet count—Low platelet counts (less than 100,000 cells/mm^3) can be associated with sepsis in the newborn but may not present until several days after birth.
- C-reactive protein (CRP)—While CRPs may be elevated for other reasons (such as inflammation), they can be reassuring when the result is in the normal range on days 1 and 3 for babies being monitored for possible infection.
- Blood culture—The gold standard for diagnosing bacterial sepsis and identifying the causative bacteria is the blood culture.
- Cerebrospinal fluid (CSF) culture—Babies with neurologic symptoms (such as high-pitched cry, bulging fontanel, or seizures) and those with culture-positive bacterial sepsis should be screened for meningitis by sending CSF for culture and cell count.

How it's treated

Newborns suspected of having sepsis should have antibiotics started as soon as their blood culture has been obtained. Initially, broad-spectrum antibiotics are used to cover the most common organisms affecting newborns in the first week of life. Ampicillin and gentamicin are typically chosen to provide gram-positive and gram-negative coverage in the newborn suspected of having early-onset sepsis.

What to do

Newborns with suspected sepsis require close monitoring for clinical deterioration. Those who are symptomatic (having respiratory distress or temperature instability) should be admitted to the NICU for frequent monitoring of vital signs. Specific nursing care should include:

- rapid initial evaluation of vital signs and physical assessment
- thermoregulation support as needed (incubator or radiant warmer for those with low temperature)
- administration of antibiotics after blood culture is obtained
- nutritional support if baby is unable to feed orally (gavage feeds or IV glucose)

- promotion of caregiver bonding
- keeping caregivers updated on plan of care
- providing family support.

Syphilis

Syphilis is caused by the *Treponema pallidum* bacterium. Rates of congenital syphilis are rising significantly with more than 11 newborns per 1,000 affected in the United States.

What causes it

Birthing parents obtain the infection from sexual contact. Babies are infected by direct contact with lesions at birth or from transmission from the placenta in utero. Birthing parents receiving prenatal care are screened for syphilis during pregnancy and offered treatment. Birthing parents who do not receive prenatal care or decline treatment (or are reinfected during pregnancy) are at high risk for transmitting the infection to their babies.

What to look for

Symptoms at birth depend on the timing of the infection in utero. Most are not symptomatic at birth. However, the most common symptoms of congenital syphilis in the newborn are:
- nasal discharge
- fever
- skin sores/rash
- enlarged liver and spleen
- enlarged lymph nodes
- anemia—lower than normal red blood cells
- thrombocytopenia—low platelet count
- long bone abnormalities.

What tests tell you

Tests for congenital syphilis include the RPR (rapid plasma reagin; with a reactive result) or VDRL (Venereal Disease Research Laboratory) titer (with newborn's titer more than four times higher than the birthing parent's). In addition, a serum immunoglobulin M (IgM) level greater than 20 mg/dL is consistent with the diagnosis. Babies with confirmed congenital syphilis also need to have a CSF-VDRL (from spinal fluid) test and long bone x-rays.

How it's treated

Babies diagnosed with congenital syphilis need to be treated with 10 to 14 days of penicillin G (administered through intramuscular [IM] or IV routes). After discharge, babies will need to see their primary care provider to monitor RPR levels until nonreactive. For babies who had CSF involvement, referral for developmental follow-up should be made.

What to do

A thorough maternal history should be obtained to identify treatment for syphilis that the birthing parent may have obtained during their pregnancy. Babies without symptoms whose birthing parent received no or inadequate treatment during pregnancy also require treatment. Nursing interventions for newborns at risk for congenital syphilis include:

- careful physical assessment to identify skin lesions and neurologic symptoms
- contact precautions for hospitalized babies
- thermoregulation support
- administration of penicillin G
- nutritional support if baby is not able to feed orally
- promotion of caregivers bonding
- keeping caregivers updated on plan of care
- providing family support
- arranging appropriate follow-up after discharge.

Viral infections

The two most common viral organisms causing symptoms in the newborn period are cytomegalovirus (CMV) and herpes simplex virus (HSV). Approximately 1% of US-born infants acquire CMV in utero or during labor. HSV transmission occurs in 1 in 300 to 20,000 births in the United States (types 1 and 2 combined).

What causes it

Newborns whose birthing parents acquire CMV in the first trimester are most likely to be affected. HSV type 2 is typically transmitted to the newborn during delivery and can also be an ascending infection from ruptured membranes. Type 1 HSV is typically transmitted to babies after birth by direct contact with lesions or through breastfeeding (if lesions are present on the breast). Seventy-five percent of newborns with HSV infections are born to birthing parents with no known history of HSV or lesions.

What to look for

Newborns exposed to viruses in utero may exhibit symptoms like bacterial infection symptoms, such as lethargy, respiratory distress, and poor feeding. In addition, babies infected with a virus in utero may have a rash, petechiae, fever, enlarged spleen and liver, elevated liver enzymes, and early-onset jaundice. Specific findings by virus may include:

- CMV—While only 10% of babies with congenital CMV present with symptoms at birth, those who do may have "blueberry muffin" lesions, intrauterine growth restriction, and microcephaly.
- HSV types 1 and 2—Skin vesicles and those with disseminated disease may present with microcephaly, meningoencephalitis, seizures, and profound sepsis including septic shock.

What tests tell you

Babies with viral infections at birth should have screening CBCs to evaluate the parameters outlined in the "Bacterial sepsis" section. Newborns with viral infections are at increased risk for low platelet counts and should be monitored regularly. Liver function studies may be elevated and should be monitored regularly as well. Congenital CMV is diagnosed by viral culture (urine or saliva) or a CMV PCR (polymerase chain reaction) test. HSV diagnosis is made from positive cultures from fluid in vesicles or blood. All babies suspected of having congenital HSV should also be tested for meningitis using a CSF HSV PCR test.

How it's treated

Babies suspected of having HSV at birth should be started on acyclovir immediately. Duration of treatment is determined by the severity of their infection, which may be localized to skin, eyes, and mouth, localized to CSF and skin, or disseminated. Newborns with symptomatic congenital CMV may benefit from treatment with the antiviral ganciclovir (also available in the oral form, valganciclovir, for use after discharge).

What to do

Babies with congenital CMV are at high risk for developmental delays and sensorineural hearing loss. After discharge, they should be referred to an infectious disease pediatric specialist and a developmental pediatrician. Because of the risk of chorioretinitis and optic atrophy, a pediatric ophthalmologist should also follow these babies. Babies born with HSV with neurologic symptoms will need neurodevelopmental follow-up after discharge. Nursing interventions for babies born with symptomatic viral infections include:

- careful physical assessment to identify skin lesions and neurologic symptoms
- contact precautions while in the hospital
- thermoregulation support as needed
- administration of antivirals as ordered
- nutritional support if baby is unable to feed orally (gavage feeds or IV glucose)
- promotion of caregiver bonding
- keeping caregivers updated on plan of care
- providing family support
- arranging appropriate follow-up with subspecialists after discharge.

Hyperbilirubinemia

Hyperbilirubinemia is an elevated total serum bilirubin level that results in a yellow coloring of the skin and sclera known as *jaundice*. Hyperbilirubinemia may be physiologic or pathologic. Physiologic jaundice is usually seen on day 2 or 3 in the newborn and typically resolves without treatment by 7 to 10 days of life. The risk associated with a specific serum bilirubin level is dependent on the newborn's postnatal age, gestational age, and any additional risk factors. The level of risk can be determined by plotting the newborns' age in hours by their total serum bilirubin level using the nomogram developed by Bhutani. Risk levels can be easily calculated using the BiliTool (bilitool.org).

With pathologic hyperbilirubinemia, total bilirubin levels may have a rapid rate of rise (greater than 5 mg/dL/day) and be significantly increased (greater than 12 mg/dL) as early as 24 hours after birth. Excessive unconjugated bilirubin can be neurotoxic to newborns. Babies who are not treated for pathologic hyperbilirubinemia are at risk for bilirubin encephalopathy, which can lead to hearing loss and permanent neurologic impairment, including cerebral palsy.

What causes it

As erythrocytes break down at the end of their neonatal life cycle, hemoglobin separates into globin (protein) and heme (iron) fragments. Heme fragments form unconjugated bilirubin that binds with albumin and is transported to liver cells to conjugate with glucuronide and form direct bilirubin. Maternal enzymes present in breast milk can inhibit the neonate's glucuronosyltransferase conjugating activity. Conditions that increase a newborn's risk of needing treatment for hyperbilirubinemia include:

- excessive bruising at birth
- cephalohematoma
- polycythemia (excessive number of red blood cells)
- prematurity
- bacterial and viral congenital infections
- hypoxia and acidosis
- maternal–fetal blood group incompatibility (such as ABO)
- Rh incompatibility
- glucose-6-phosphate dehydrogenase deficiency (a red blood cell enzyme defect)
- East Asian or Mediterranean descent.

What to look for

The predominant sign of hyperbilirubinemia is jaundice, which doesn't become clinically apparent until serum bilirubin levels reach about 7 mg/dL. Maternal and newborn history should be reviewed for risk factors (listed earlier). Babies with untreated pathologic hyperbilirubinemia may exhibit poor feeding and lethargy.

What tests tell you

Transcutaneous bilirubin monitoring can be used in the nursery to identify babies with elevated levels. Follow-up serum total bilirubin levels can then be obtained for those at risk for needing treatment. Babies born to birthing parents who are blood type O- or Rh-negative should have their blood type tested and a direct Coombs test (direct antibody test). If the Coombs test is positive, the baby is at risk for hemolysis, and total bilirubin levels should be monitored closely. If the bilirubin levels are rising quickly or significantly elevated, further testing should include a hematocrit (to screen for anemia) and a reticulocyte count (to evaluate the degree of hemolysis).

How it's treated

Treatment options depend on the underlying cause of the jaundice.
- Newborns with physiologic hyperbilirubinemia benefit from frequent feedings (which promote the passage of meconium and decrease the enterohepatic recirculation of bilirubin).

- Phototherapy treats unconjugated hyperbilirubinemia in newborns with serum bilirubin levels in the high-risk zone or those with additional risk factors. Phototherapy works by converting bilirubin to a water-soluble form. Multiple phototherapy sources (lights or blankets) can be used as needed. (See *Performing phototherapy* for details of administering phototherapy.)

Performing phototherapy

To perform phototherapy, follow these steps:
- Set up the phototherapy unit above the neonate's bassinet according to the manufacturer's recommendations. If the neonate is in an incubator, place the phototherapy unit above the incubator according to the manufacturer's recommendations, and turn on the lights. Measure the irradiance of the light(s) with a radiometer.
- If the bilirubin level is extremely high and needs to be reduced rapidly, placing a phototherapy unit below the neonate may be necessary, in addition to the overhead phototherapy light(s).
- Explain the procedure to the caregivers.
- Record the neonate's initial bilirubin level and their axillary temperature.
- Place the eye shield over the neonate's closed eyes and fasten securely.
- Undress the neonate, and place a diaper underneath them.
- Take the neonate's axillary temperature every 2 hours, and adjust the warming unit's thermostat to keep the baby's temperature normal.
- Monitor elimination, and weigh the neonate twice daily. Watch for signs of dehydration (dry skin, poor turgor, depressed fontanels).
- Take the neonate out of the bassinet, turn off the phototherapy lights, and unmask their eyes at least every 3 to 4 hours with feedings. Assess eyes for inflammation.
- Reposition the neonate every 2 hours to expose all body surfaces to the light and to prevent head molding and skin breakdown from pressure.
- Check the bilirubin level at least once every 24 hours—more often if levels rise significantly. Turn off the phototherapy unit before drawing venous blood for testing because the lights may degrade bilirubin in the blood. Notify the practitioner if the bilirubin level nears 20 mg/dL in full-term neonates or 15 mg/dL in premature neonates.

- Babies with isoimmunization experiencing hemolysis may require treatment with multiple phototherapy sources, IV immunoglobulins, and, in the most severe cases, exchange transfusion.

Exchange transfusion

When a baby's hyperbilirubinemia has not responded to intensive phototherapy, an exchange transfusion may be needed. During the exchange, the neonate's partially hemolyzed and antibody-coated red blood cells are replaced with fresh donor blood (less than 48 hours old), thus removing some of the unconjugated bilirubin in serum. Babies must be monitored closely in the NICU for electrolyte disturbances, which can lead to dysrhythmia while receiving an exchange transfusion.

What to do

Nursing interventions for neonates with hyperbilirubinemia include:
- monitoring maternal history to ensure that Rh-negative birthing parents have received Rho(D) immune globulin during their pregnancy
- assessing every newborn for jaundice and documenting findings in the newborn record
- reporting jaundice that occurs in the first 24 hours of life and bilirubin levels in the high and high-intermediate risk zones during hospitalization to the baby's primary care provider
- encouraging frequent feeding
- reassuring caregivers that most neonates experience some degree of jaundice
- explaining hyperbilirubinemia, its causes, diagnostic tests, and treatment to parents
- advising caregivers to make a follow-up appointment with the baby's pediatrician within 48 hours after discharge.

Inborn errors of metabolism

An inborn error of metabolism interferes with a baby's ability to convert amino acids or carbohydrates into energy. Although inborn errors of metabolism are rare, they can cause rapid deterioration of newborns after birth. All states in the United States mandate newborn screening for the inborn errors of metabolism phenylketonuria (PKU) and galactosemia. These two inborn errors of metabolism can cause rapid deterioration in newborns after feedings are initiated. The initial screen should be obtained at 24 to 48 hours of age and then repeated at 7 days of age.

Phenylketonuria

PKU is the most common inborn error of amino acid metabolism, affecting 1 in 10,000 babies born. It's characterized by the body's inability to metabolize phenylalanine—an essential amino acid that's found in protein-containing foods. Excess phenylalanine can affect normal development of the brain and central nervous system (CNS) as well as levels of tyrosine—an amino acid that plays a role in the production of melanin, epinephrine, and thyroxine.

What causes it

PKU is inherited as an autosomal recessive trait. Both parents must pass the gene on for the child to be affected. In PKU, there's almost no activity of phenylalanine hydroxylase—an enzyme that helps convert phenylalanine to tyrosine. Phenylalanine accumulates in the blood and urine, resulting in low tyrosine levels. If left untreated, PKU can result in seizures and developmental delays.

What to look for

Symptoms begin after feeding a baby breast milk or formula. Clinical manifestations of PKU in a newborn may include:

- poor feeding or vomiting
- irritability
- hyperactivity
- urine odor.

What tests tell you

Newborn screening for PKU is mandatory in all states. The PKU test measures the amount of phenylalanine in the blood.

How it's treated

Treatment involves maintaining an extremely low-phenylalanine diet, such as special infant formula that does not contain phenylalanine. Birthing parents with PKU should strictly adhere to a low-phenylalanine diet before and during pregnancy because there is a strong correlation between maternal phenylalanine levels and improved fetal outcomes. Increased phenylalanine levels in utero can affect embryologic development, causing low birth weight, congenital malformations, microcephaly, and cognitive impairment.

What to do

Babies with PKU should be fed phenylalanine-free formula. After discharge, caregivers should consult with a dietitian to identify appropriate food choices as their baby grows. They should also be referred to a geneticist to guide them in future family planning.

Galactosemia

Galactosemia is an inborn error of carbohydrate metabolism, causing the baby's inability to metabolize galactose and lactose. Babies with galactosemia are at risk for speech delays, behavioral disorders and cataracts, and they may have some degree of cognitive impairment.

What causes it

Like PKU, galactosemia is an autosomal recessive condition. Galactosemia affects 1 in 60,000 live births.

What to look for

Symptoms are seen after a baby begins feeding breast milk or formula containing lactose. The most common symptoms include:

- hypoglycemia
- hyperbilirubinemia
- vomiting
- diarrhea
- jaundice
- lethargy.

What tests tell you

State-mandated newborn screens test for galactosemia. The screen looks for high levels of galactose and low galactose-1-phosphate uridyltransferase (GALT). In a baby with severe hypergalactosemia, a positive urine-reducing substance will be present. Later signs of galactosemia may include cataracts, an enlarged liver, and an enlarged spleen.

How it's treated

Newborns with galactosemia should only be fed a lactose-free formula. Caregivers should consult a nutritionist to help them maintain a lactose-free diet for babies with galactosemia as they grow. Infant diets may require vitamin D and calcium supplementation.

What to do

Caregiver education should include the importance of maintaining a lactose-free diet throughout their child's life and the need for follow-up to monitor galactose-1-phosphate levels in red blood cells. Speech therapy is often needed in children with galactosemia.

Neurologic issues

The most common neurologic symptom in newborns is seizure activity. Seizures are a symptom of an underlying problem such as hypoxia, meningitis, a structural anomaly, or a metabolic problem.

Seizures

The incidence of seizures in term babies is 2.8 per 1,000 babies born weighing more than 2,500 g. Those born prematurely are at much higher risk (57.5 per 1,000 babies with birth weight less than 1,500 g). Seizures from the most common causes occur in the first 3 days of life.

What causes it

Most newborn seizures are associated with hypoxic–ischemic encephalopathy (HIE). Hypoxia (decreased oxygen in blood) and ischemia (reduced perfusion to the brain) may occur in utero, during delivery, or right after birth. Newborns with HIE who have seizures typically present within the first 12 hours of birth. Underlying metabolic issues such as hypocalcemia and hypoglycemia can cause seizures in the newborn period. Seizures from hypocalcemia may occur at any time in the first week of life. Babies with untreated hypoglycemia who have seizures usually present early in the first 2 days of life. Newborns with sepsis who develop meningitis (bacterial or viral) are at increased risk for seizures in the first week of life. Approximately 10% of premature babies who have an intraventricular hemorrhage will have seizures in the first week of life. Less common causes of seizures in the newborn period include genetic seizure disorder, CNS malformations, inborn errors of metabolism, and neonatal abstinence syndrome (NAS). Examples of CNS defects associated with seizures include neural tube (spinal cord) defects such as meningocele and myelomeningocele.

What to look for

The most common type of seizures in the newborn period are subtle seizures, which can be seen in both term and preterm babies, and are often not identified as seizure activity. Although presentation varies, behaviors associated with subtle seizures include apnea, lip smacking, sucking, pedaling, and eye deviation. Tonic seizures are most common in extremely premature babies who have severe intraventricular hemorrhage. Findings resemble decorticate posturing in adults with tonic extension of extremities. Multifocal clonic seizures are most often seen in babies with HIE. The localized clonic (jerking) movements can move from one extremity to another without a noted pattern.

What tests tell you

Newborns who exhibit clinical signs of seizures should have an electroencephalography and a pediatric neurology consult. Babies with a history of hypoxia at birth can benefit from bedside monitoring using amplitude-integrated electroencephalography. Additional studies can identify the underlying cause of the seizure. Examples include cranial ultrasound and magnetic resonance imaging or computed tomography scans to evaluate brain structures, which can rule out intracranial hemorrhage, hydrocephalus, and other defects. Newborns with seizures should be evaluated for meningitis by obtaining a CSF culture (bacterial and viral). Serum glucose and calcium levels should be obtained to rule out hypoglycemia and hypocalcemia as potential causes of the seizures.

How it's treated

Treatment of the underlying cause of the seizures is the most important. Newborns with suspected meningitis should be treated with broad-spectrum antibiotics such as ampicillin and gentamicin until it is ruled out. Babies with hypoglycemia who have seizures should be treated with IV glucose, and those with hypocalcemia should receive calcium gluconate. Those with HIE who qualify should receive therapeutic hypothermia. Phenobarbital remains the leading drug used for the management of seizures in newborns. If seizures continue after babies receive a loading dose of phenobarbital and maintenance dosing is started, the dose may be increased or additional loading doses are given. Occasionally, babies need a second anticonvulsant agent for seizure management.

What to do

The nursing care of babies with seizures includes:
- careful physical assessment
- cardiorespiratory monitoring in the NICU
- documentation of seizure activity including the timing and duration of specific neurologic symptoms
- ensuring equipment is available to assist babies who may become apneic when they seizure
- keeping caregivers informed of their baby's condition
- encouraging caregivers to bond with their infant in the NICU
- providing emotional support to caregivers
- ensuring that the baby is referred for neurodevelopmental follow-up after discharge.

Neonatal abstinence syndrome

Although there are many medications and substances that a fetus may be exposed to in utero, opioids are most likely to cause withdrawal symptoms requiring treatment in the newborn period. Around 55% to 94% of infants exposed to opioids in utero have withdrawal symptoms. In combination, physiologic and neurobehavioral withdrawal symptoms are referred to as NAS, which affects as many as 4.8 per 1,000 babies born in urban areas and 7.5 per 1,000 babies born in rural areas.

What causes it

NAS doesn't only occur in babies whose birthing parents used illicit drugs. Increasing numbers of birthing parents are being prescribed opioid medications during their pregnancy to manage chronic pain. Examples of opioids include morphine, codeine, heroin, hydromorphone, fentanyl, and methadone. Birthing parents who seek treatment for their opioid misuse disorder during pregnancy may be treated with methadone or buprenorphine.

What to look for

The leading symptoms of NAS in the newborn are neurologic, autonomic, and gastrointestinal. The onset of symptoms varies with the type(s) of substances that the baby was exposed to in utero. Symptoms may present as early as 24 hours of age and as late as 7 days. Babies withdrawing from opioids may have any combination of these symptoms:

- High-pitched cry
- Irritability
- Tremors
- Wakefulness
- Fever
- Sweating
- Vomiting
- Loose stools
- Seizures

What tests tell you

Babies at risk for opioid withdrawal or those with a combination of symptoms that raise suspicion should be assessed using a NAS scoring tool such as Finnegan Neonatal Abstinence Scoring Tool (FNAST). Ideally, urine and meconium are tested for babies at risk for NAS soon after birth. More recently, drug testing of umbilical cord tissue has become available at some centers.

How is it treated

All babies with NAS should be treated with nonpharmacologic interventions, which may include:

- reducing environmental stimuli (being in a quiet area with lights turned low)
- swaddling
- holding
- swaying in a baby swing
- music therapy
- providing a pacifier
- feedings with increased caloric density if needed
- frequent feedings. (See *What about breastfeeding?*)

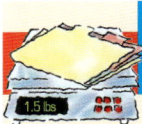

Weighing the evidence

What about breastfeeding?

Maternal substance use is not an absolute contraindication to breastfeeding. Nurses must weigh the risks and benefits to the baby if the birthing parent continues to use medications after the baby is born. Lactation consultants can provide valuable information about which medications and drugs are passed in breast milk. Caregivers who misuse drugs should avoid breastfeeding because of the baby's future neurobehavioral issues risk.

Newborns with moderate-to-severe NAS may need to be treated with oral morphine or methadone to treat their symptoms and minimize weight loss. Secondary treatment with clonidine or phenobarbital may be considered as needed.

What to do

Nursing care of the baby with NAS includes:
- monitoring for symptoms of withdrawal
- scoring of symptoms using neonatal abstinence tool
- creating a quiet, calm environment to reduce overstimulation
- providing frequent feedings of increased caloric density (See *What about breastfeeding?*)
- promoting caregiver bonding
- working with medical social worker on discharge plans
- promoting rooming in and breastfeeding when safe to do so
- keeping caregivers updated
- providing caregiver support.

Prematurity

A neonate is considered preterm if born before 37 weeks of gestation and is at risk for complications because the neonate's organ systems are immature. The degree of complications depends on gestational age. The closer the neonate is to term, the easier the transition to extrauterine life will be. Most preterm babies are born in the late preterm period after 34 weeks and before 37 weeks' gestation. One in 10 babies born in the United States is born prematurely.

What causes it

Some babies are born prematurely because of a premature rupture of membranes or premature onset of labor in the birthing parent.

In some cases of preterm labor, medications can be used to delay delivery until the baby is more mature. At other times, babies must be delivered prematurely because of negative maternal conditions affecting the birthing parent or fetus. Pregnancy-induced hypertension is a common cause of inducing labor prior to term to prevent worsening maternal complications. Birthing parents with diabetes mellitus may have babies who are macrosomic (larger than average) warranting delivery prior to term. Another contributor to preterm births is maternal infection, which can result in chorioamnionitis (bacterial infection of the fetal membranes) necessitating delivery. Multiple births may also necessitate cesarean birth prior to term.

What to look for

Physical characteristics of preterm neonates vary by gestation. Findings commonly seen in the late preterm infant are:
- low birth weight
- less subcutaneous fat than term infants
- fewer creases on palms and feet
- less muscle tone than term babies.

Because of their immature body systems, late preterm infants are at risk for:
- respiratory distress (nasal flaring, expiratory grunting, retractions)
- apnea (cessation of breathing for more than 20 seconds)
- inability to maintain body temperature in an open crib
- hyperbilirubinemia
- hypoglycemia (low blood sugar)
- inability to take all feedings by mouth (either breast or bottle).

What tests tell you

Prematurity is diagnosed by a combination of maternal history (expected date of confinement) and physical findings in the immediate newborn period. The New Ballard Score can be used to estimate gestational age. Tests for conditions that affect late preterm infants include:
- blood glucose monitoring for hypoglycemia
- arterial blood gases for those requiring oxygen
- chest x-ray to identify the cause of respiratory distress (when present)
- transcutaneous and serum bilirubin monitoring
- monitoring of electrolytes in babies requiring IV fluids to evaluate fluid balance
- infectious screening (CBC and blood culture) for babies whose maternal history places them at risk (such as premature rupture of membranes or premature onset of labor).

How it's treated

Late preterm infants may require care in the NICU after birth. When admitted to the NICU, the baby will be placed on a cardiorespiratory monitor and pulse oximeter to assess for symptoms of respiratory distress and apnea. Respiratory support is dependent on each individual baby's presentation. Late preterm babies are often cared for on a radiant warmer bed or in an isolette to help them maintain their temperature. Feedings should be started as soon as possible after birth to reduce the risk of hypoglycemia. If a baby is not able to take adequate amounts of breast milk by mouth, the baby will need to be fed using an orogastric or nasogastric tube. Babies who have significant respiratory distress may not be able to tolerate full-volume feeds. These babies, and those with hypoglycemia on feedings, require insertion of a peripheral IV for the administration of glucose. Babies receiving IV fluid are at risk for fluid imbalance and require monitoring of electrolytes.

Three goals for late preterm infants

- Maintain temperature
- Gain weight on full oral feedings
- Be free of apnea or respiratory distress for several days prior to discharge

What to do

Care of the late preterm newborn includes the following:
- Physical assessment
- Monitoring of vital signs, cardiorespiratory patterns, and oxygen saturation
- Respiratory support as needed
- Thermoregulation support with radiant warmer or isolette, if needed
- Support for oral feedings, which may include breastfeeding, bottle-feedings, or gavage feedings
- Monitoring of bedside glucose levels after birth
- Administration of IV dextrose as needed
- Monitoring of transcutaneous or serum bilirubin levels
- Providing developmentally appropriate care for gestation
- Providing breastfeeding support including information on expressing breast milk and consulting with lactation specialist
- Keeping caregivers informed
- Supporting caregivers

Teaching parents of late preterm neonates

Caregivers can experience stress, anxiety, and grief over the unexpected delivery of their baby prior to term. This can be even more difficult if the baby is close to term and requires intensive care. To help the caregivers of a late preterm neonate cope with this difficult situation, follow these guidelines:

• Orient them to the NICU environment, and introduce them to the health care team.
• Orient them to the machinery and monitors that may be attached to their neonate. Reassure them that the staff is alert to alarms as well as the cues of their child.
• Tell them what to expect for their individual baby.
• Explain to them the characteristics of a preterm neonate.
• Demonstrate to them how to handle their baby.
• Provide information on feeding, whether it's through gavage, breast, or bottle.
• Inform them of the complications that the baby is being monitored for (such as apnea).
• Include them in their baby's care whenever possible.
• Begin discharge planning early.
• Make appropriate referrals, including lactation consultant.
• Provide information on what to watch for after discharge including poor feeding, low temperature, prolonged jaundice, decreased activity, and increased work of breathing.
• Confirm that appointments with a pediatrician or nurse practitioner are made soon after discharge.

Respiratory problems

Newborns are at risk for several respiratory problems after birth, including transient tachypnea, respiratory distress syndrome (RDS), meconium aspiration syndrome (MAS), and pneumothorax. Respiratory distress is a common cause of admission to the NICU for both term and late preterm newborns.

Transient tachypnea of the newborn

Transient tachypnea of the newborn (TTN) is most seen in babies born at term or near term. TTN affects 5.7 in 1,000 babies born. It is a self-limiting process, typically resolved within a few days of life, that affects 5.7 in 1,000 babies born.

What causes it

TTN occurs when the absorption of all fetal lung fluid is delayed after birth. Newborns with TTN breathe faster to compensate for the residual lung fluid that has not yet cleared and may have other signs of respiratory distress such as grunting and retractions.

Risk factory

Newborns delivered by cesarean birth and those who are born precipitously are at increased risk for TTN. Other factors associated with TTN include:

- breech delivery
- second twin
- macrosomia (larger than average)
- maternal sedation
- male sex.

What to look for

Common signs of TTN include:

- tachypnea (breathing rate greater than 60 breaths/min)
- nasal flaring
- expiratory grunting
- retractions.

What tests tell you

Some babies with TTN symptoms resolve within a few hours of life. For those who have prolonged tachypnea and those who develop an oxygen need, the following tests can be useful:

- Arterial blood gas helps to evaluate oxygen and carbon dioxide levels in the blood.
- Chest x-ray will reveal haziness and streakiness in both lung fields and may also show mild hyperexpansion of lungs.
- Bedside glucoses should be monitored to screen for hypoglycemia, which can cause respiratory distress in the newborn.
- CBC with differential may be done to evaluate for signs of infection for a newborn whose history places them at risk.

How it's treated

Because TTN is a self-limiting process, treatment is supportive and tailored to the individual baby's symptoms. Many babies only require monitoring during the transition period, while others may need a nasal cannula or continuous positive airway pressure (CPAP) delivered via nasal prongs. The amount of supplemental oxygen should be targeted to keep the baby's oxygen saturation between 90% and 95%. It is difficult for some babies to take feedings by mouth while breathing fast, so they may require gavage feedings or an IV with glucose infusion while they are tachypneic.

What to do

Nurses caring for newborns with TTN should anticipate the following:

- Monitoring via cardiorespiratory monitor and pulse oximeter
- Administering oxygen as needed (via nasal cannula or CPAP)

- Using a radiant warmer to maintain neutral thermal environment
- Gavage feeding or placing a peripheral IV to administer glucose
- Providing parental education and emotional support

Respiratory distress syndrome

RDS is a lung immaturity disorder that causes symptoms soon after birth. Premature babies are most likely to be affected, with the most immature babies having the highest risk of RDS. Approximately half of babies with a birth weight of less than 1,000 g will have RDS.

What causes it

RDS is caused by inadequate or inactivated pulmonary surfactant that causes alveolar collapse (atelectasis), which leads to problems with oxygenation and ventilation. To overcome the atelectasis, babies exhibit increased work of breathing including nasal flaring, expiratory grunting, retractions, or tachypnea. Risk factors for RDS include:

- premature birth (especially in those babies whose birthing parents did not receive antenatal steroids)
- infant of a birthing parent with diabetes
- babies with MAS (meconium inactivates pulmonary surfactant)
- second twin
- perinatal hypoxia
- male sex
- cesarean birth without labor.

What to look for

The symptoms of RDS can appear immediately after birth or within the first few hours after birth. Common symptoms include:

- tachypnea
- nasal flaring
- retractions
- expiratory grunting
- cyanosis.

What tests tell you

Arterial blood gas monitoring reveals respiratory acidosis in a newborn with RDS. Chest x-rays show that lung fields are not well expanded. Typically, the lung fields are hazy bilaterally with a reticulogranular (ground glass) appearance that reflects the alveolar atelectasis.

Prenatal testing for lung maturity

Prenatal tests can evaluate lung maturity while the fetus is in utero by measuring the lecithin and sphingomyelin ratio of the amniotic fluid.

Lecithin and sphingomyelin are two surfactant phospholipids. Evaluation of fetal lung maturity gives insight into how the fetus will fare after birth and may precipitate treatment of the birthing parent to delay labor or to administer antenatal steroids.

How it's treated

Strategies to minimize preterm birth will reduce the number of babies born with RDS. When delay of delivery is not possible, the most immature newborns may require both respiratory support and pulmonary surfactant. Methods to administer pulmonary surfactant include administration via an endotracheal tube or through a small catheter inserted directly into the trachea and then removed. Babies with RDS require respiratory support with enough pressure to keep alveoli open and as much oxygen as needed to keep saturations in target ranges.

Respiratory remedies

Respiratory support may include:
- oxygen administration via nasal cannula
- CPAP delivered by nasal prongs
- mechanical ventilation (requiring endotracheal intubation).
  Both CPAP and mechanical ventilators generate positive end-expiratory pressure, which prevents alveolar collapse during exhalation. Ventilators also provide mechanical breaths at a higher pressure to maintain arterial blood gas levels within normal limits. There are numerous mechanical ventilators that can be used with newborns and most synchronize the mechanical breaths to each baby's own respiratory effort. Complications of oxygen therapy and mechanical ventilation may occur despite efforts to prevent them including:
- pneumothorax
- ventilator-acquired pneumonia
- bronchopulmonary dysplasia (in babies who require long-term ventilation)
- retinopathy of prematurity.

Supportive steps

Supportive treatment of premature babies with RDS includes:
- thermoregulation via an isolette or radiant warmer
- nutritional support with gradually advancing gavage feeds and IV nutrition.

What to do

Nurses have an important role in caring for babies with RDS. Frequent assessments are required to monitor breathing efforts and oxygen saturation levels. Other nursing responsibilities include:
- supporting baby's thermoregulation in an isolette or on a radiant warmer

- monitoring oxygen saturations to ensure they are within target range for baby's age
- suctioning of endotracheal tube as needed using sterile technique
- administering IV fluid and gavage feeds
- providing mouth care for babies requiring respiratory support
- educating caregivers on their baby's respiratory support
- providing developmentally appropriate care for gestation
- providing caregiver support.

Meconium aspiration syndrome

Meconium, a combination of skin cells and bile salts lining the intestines of the fetus in utero, can be expelled into the amniotic fluid when the fetus becomes stressed. This is much more likely to occur in a term or post-term newborn than a preterm one. If meconium is aspirated into the airways at birth, 3% to 12% of babies will develop MAS, although 8% to 29% of all deliveries have meconium-stained amniotic fluid.

What causes it

MAS occurs when a baby aspirates meconium creating an airway obstruction and chemical pneumonitis. The meconium may also inactivate the baby's lung surfactant. Neonates with MAS increase their respiratory efforts to create greater negative intrathoracic pressures and improve airflow to the lungs. Hyperinflation, hypoxemia, and acidemia cause increased peripheral vascular resistance. Right-to-left shunting across the patent ductus arteriosus or patent foramen ovale may occur, which worsens the hypoxia.

What to look for

Signs and symptoms of MAS include:
- meconium staining of skin, nails, and umbilical cord
- cyanosis
- respiratory distress including tachypnea, grunting, and retractions
- coarse breath sounds
- barrel-shaped chest (from hyperinflated lungs).

What tests tell you

An arterial blood gas can be used to assess a baby's oxygenation and ventilation. Babies with MAS are at risk for hypoxemia (low blood oxygen) and respiratory acidosis (elevated carbon dioxide level in blood with a low pH). Babies who have experienced fetal distress may also have metabolic acidosis. Chest x-ray will show patchy infiltrates in lung fields due to the alternating areas of hyperexpansion and atelectasis as well as hyperinflation of both lungs.

How it's treated

Newborns with MAS typically require respiratory support to maintain adequate ventilation and oxygenation. To avoid further damage to their lungs, a high-frequency jet ventilator or high-frequency oscillator can be used to deliver breaths at a faster rate and lower pressures than a conventional ventilator. Surfactant replacement therapy may be needed because meconium inactivates surfactant in the lung. Babies with MAS are at increased risk for pulmonary hypertension, which may require inhaled nitric oxide. Babies that require mechanical ventilation may need medications for pain and sedation to keep them comfortable while on the ventilator. Respiratory complications of MAS include pneumothorax, pneumonia, and persistent pulmonary hypertension.

What to do

Nursing care of the baby with MAS includes:

- monitoring of vital signs and oxygen saturation
- maintaining thermoregulation
- instituting minimal stimulation protocol (keeping environment quiet and dark when possible)
- frequent assessments of breath sounds and work of breathing
- suctioning of endotracheal tube as needed
- administration of medications for sedation and pain management as ordered
- educating and supporting caregivers.

Pneumothorax

What causes it

A pneumothorax can spontaneously occur when alveoli become overdistended and rupture. Most babies who develop a pneumothorax have a lung disorder such as RDS or MAS because lung disease and positive-pressure ventilation treatment increase the risk. However, some babies spontaneously develop a pneumothorax after birth without having received any respiratory support.

What to look for

Babies who develop a pneumothorax typically exhibit signs of respiratory distress such as tachypnea, grunting, or retractions, and they can have decreased breath sounds on the side of the affected lung. Babies receiving positive-pressure ventilation may show increased oxygen need or require increased support. A large pneumothorax may cause a drop in blood pressure because the baby's heart becomes compressed.

What tests tell you

A transilluminator can be used in a baby with pneumothorax symptoms. If a moderate or large pneumothorax is present, the affected side will "light up." A chest x-ray confirms the diagnosis, size, and location of the pneumothorax. An arterial blood gas can provide important information about oxygenation and ventilation.

How it's treated

Small pneumothoraces may resolve without treatment. Newborns receiving CPAP or mechanical ventilation may require evacuation of the pneumothorax by needle aspiration or chest tube placement. After a chest tube is placed, it should be connected to a drainage system with an underwater seal. This system can also be connected to suction to aid in resolving the pneumothorax.

What to do

Nursing care of the baby with a pneumothorax includes:
- monitoring of vital signs, oxygen saturation, and cardiorespiratory parameters
- assessment of breath sounds and breathing efforts
- ensuring that the chest tube is secured (minimizing risk of inadvertent removal)
- monitoring underwater seal chamber in the drainage system connected to chest tube
- supporting nutrition including IV fluid as needed and gavage feeds
- caregiver education and support.

Quick quiz

1. Babies born to birthing parents with diabetes are at increased risk for which of the following abnormal findings on a CBC?
    A. Polycythemia
    B. Anemia
    C. Thrombocytopenia
    D. Neutropenia

Answer: A. In utero, the fetus of a birthing parent with diabetes can experience hypoxia, leading to polycythemia (excess of red blood cells).

2. On a growth chart, a newborn has a birth weight plotted on the 8th percentile, length on the 7th percentile, and FOC (frontal occipital circumference; head circumference) on the 5th percentile. Which of the following conditions would be most likely to cause this pattern of growth?

    A. Pregnancy-induced hypertension
    B. Maternal diabetes
    C. Prematurity
    D. Intrauterine viral infection

Answer: D. Babies exposed to viral infections in utero are at increased risk for symmetric growth restriction.

3. Management of PKU includes which of the following?

    A. Blood transfusion
    B. Low-protein diet
    C. Monitoring urine for metabolites
    D. High-protein formula

Answer: B. Babies with PKU should receive special formula that does not contain phenylalanine. They will need to be on a low-protein diet for their entire life.

4. Newborns should have a cardiac screening test done at which time frame?

    A. As soon as possible after delivery
    B. 24 to 48 hours after delivery
    C. 72 hours after delivery
    D. Any time prior to discharge

Answer: B. Newborns should have a cardiac screen prior to discharge but no sooner than 24 hours after birth to increase the chance that the baby's patent ductus arteriosus has closed.

5. Maternal risk factors for congenital infection in the newborn include which of the following?

    A. Maternal temperature greater than 99°F
    B. Rupture of membranes for more than 12 hours
    C. Chorioamnionitis
    D. Clear amniotic fluid

Answer: C. Chorioamnionitis is a significant risk factor for congenital infection in the newborn. Other risk factors include maternal temperature greater than 101°F, rupture of membranes for more than 18 hours, and purulent amniotic fluid.

6. What condition causes airway obstruction in babies?
   A. MAS
   B. Pneumothorax
   C. Respiratory distress syndrome
   D. Transient TTN

Answer: A. When meconium is aspirated into the lung it creates airway obstruction and chemical pneumonitis.

7. Prolonged, untreated pathologic hyperbilirubinemia can result in which of the following?
   A. Kidney failure
   B. Liver failure
   C. Polycythemia
   D. Cerebral palsy

Answer: D. Left untreated, pathologic hyperbilirubinemia can result in encephalopathy. Manifestations of that include hearing loss, hypotonia, delayed motor skills, and cerebral palsy.

Scoring

☆☆☆ If you answered all seven questions correctly, ooh la la! You have a definite flair for neonatal care!

☆☆ If you answered five or six questions correctly, magnifique! You've outfitted yourself with a fine knowledge of high-risk neonates!

☆ If you answered fewer than five questions correctly, très bien! You can go back and look this over in your own fashion to get a better view of this chapter!

Selected References

Armentrout, D. (2021). Glucose management. In M. T. Verklan, M. Walden, & S. Forest (Eds.), *Core curriculum for neonatal intensive care nursing* (6th ed., pp. 144–151). Elsevier Saunders.

Bradshaw, W. T. (2021). Gastrointestinal disorders. In M. T. Verklan, M. Walden, & S. Forest (Eds.), *Core curriculum for neonatal intensive care nursing* (6th ed., pp. 504–542). Elsevier Saunders.

D'Apolito, K. (2021). Perinatal substance abuse. In M. T. Verklan, M. Walden, & S. Forest (Eds.), *Core curriculum for neonatal intensive care nursing* (6th ed., pp. 38–53). Elsevier Saunders.

Ditzenberger, G. (2021). Neurologic disorders. In M. T. Verklan, M. Walden, & S. Forest (Eds.), *Core curriculum for neonatal intensive care nursing* (6th ed., pp. 629–653). Elsevier Saunders.

Forest, S. (2021). Care of the extremely low birth weight infant. In M. T. Verklan, M. Walden, & S. Forest (Eds.), *Core curriculum for neonatal intensive care nursing* (6th ed., pp. 377–387). Elsevier Saunders.

Fraser, D. (2021). Respiratory distress. In M. T. Verklan, M. Walden, & S. Forest (Eds.), *Core curriculum for neonatal intensive care nursing* (6th ed., pp. 394–416). Elsevier Saunders.

Hurst, H. M. (2021). Antepartum-intrapartum complications. In M. T. Verklan, M. Walden, & S. Forest (Eds.), *Core curriculum for neonatal intensive care nursing* (6th ed., pp. 20–37). Elsevier Saunders.

Kenner, C., & Boykova, M. (2021). Families in crisis. In M. T. Verklan, M. Walden, & S. Forest (Eds.), *Core curriculum for neonatal intensive care nursing* (6th ed., pp. 288–300). Elsevier Saunders.

Lubbers, L. A. (2021). Congenital anomalies. In M. T. Verklan, M. Walden, S. Forest (Eds.), *Core curriculum for neonatal intensive care nursing* (6th ed., pp. 654–677). Elsevier Saunders.

Rudd, K. M. (2021). Infectious diseases in the neonate. In M. T. Verklan, M. Walden, & S. Forest (Eds.), *Core curriculum for neonatal intensive care nursing* (6th ed., pp. 588–616). Elsevier Saunders.

Sadowski, S. L., & Verklan, M. T. (2021). Cardiovascular disorders. In M. T. Verklan, M. Walden, & S. Forest (Eds.), *Core curriculum for neonatal intensive care nursing* (6th ed., pp. 460–503). Elsevier Saunders.

Tappero, E. (2021). Physical assessment. In M. T. Verklan, M. Walden, & S. Forest (Eds.), *Core curriculum for neonatal intensive care nursing* (6th ed., pp. 99–130). Elsevier Saunders.

Verklan, M. T. (2021). Care of the late preterm infant. In M. T. Verklan, M. Walden, & S. Forest (Eds.), *Core curriculum for neonatal intensive care nursing* (6th ed., pp. 388–393). Elsevier Saunders.

Chapter 12

Infancy and early childhood

Just the facts

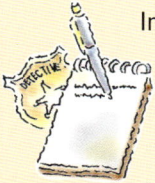

In this chapter, you'll learn:

♦ principles of growth and development for infants, toddlers, and preschoolers

♦ injury prevention for infants, toddlers, and preschoolers

♦ care of the child who has experienced maltreatment

Principles of growth and development

Growth implies an increase in size, such as height and weight, and *development* refers to the acquisition of skills and abilities that takes place throughout life.

Growth and development are essential parts of the pediatric nursing assessment. Problems that may initially seem insignificant might have severe consequences in later life if not dealt with early.

Stages of development

There are five stages of development during childhood that may overlap.

1. *Infancy* starts at birth and ends at age 1 year.
2. The *toddler stage* is from ages 1 to 3 years.
3. The *preschool stage* is from ages 3 to 6 years.
4. *School age* is from ages 6 to 12 years.
5. *Adolescence* is from ages 13 to 19 years.

Teach your children well

Beginning in infancy and throughout the early years of childhood, the nurse, caregivers, and other significant people in the child's life can teach habits of healthy eating and living, preventing serious health problems as the child grows. Other influences on growth and development include genetics and heredity as well as the child's personality or temperament.

A closer look at the infant

Infancy, the period from birth to age 1 year, is a time of many changes. During the first year of life, the infant progresses from a neonate, totally dependent on the world around them, to a baby who can interact with and process change within their surroundings. Tremendous physiologic, cognitive, and emotional development also occur.

System development

From birth to age 1 year, remarkable changes occur in the infant's neurologic, cardiovascular, respiratory, and immune systems.

Neurologic system

The central nervous system (CNS) is the fastest-growing system during infancy, as brain cells continue to develop in both size and number.

Hold your head up!

Myelinization refers to the development of a myelin sheath around nerve fibers enabling quick, efficient transmission of nerve impulses. Myelinization of the neurons occurs in a cephalocaudal (head-to-toe) direction and takes up to 2 years to complete. An infant progresses from being unable to hold their head up to holding themselves in an upright position, sitting, and keeping their head erect. As myelinization reaches the extremities, the infant can put weight on their legs and use them to stand up. As the brain and CNS develop, more sophisticated cognitive and behavioral skills follow.

Converge, stare, and search

Vision development is also tremendous. At birth, the newborn prefers facial features, but by 8 weeks, the baby is alert to moving objects and attracted to bright colors and lighted objects. Convergence and following with the eyes are jerky and inexact. By ages 4 to 6 months, the baby has bifocal vision and can stare and search. By age 1 year, distance vision and depth perception have markedly increased.

Cardiovascular and respiratory systems

The cardiovascular and respiratory systems undergo dramatic changes at birth. Because of placental oxygenation, the fetus shunts most of the blood away from the lungs while in utero.

At birth, a cascade of physiologic changes occurs. Deoxygenated blood begins to circulate to the lungs, where it receives oxygen and is then pumped out to the rest of the body through the left ventricle of the heart and aorta. Within moments, the cardiovascular and respiratory systems function essentially as those of an adult.

Immune system

The immune system develops over the first year of life. The neonate depends on maternal antibodies received via the placenta or breast milk for immunologic protection. By ages 6 to 8 weeks, an antigen–antibody response is maturing and can be triggered, for example, by immunizations, and by age 9 months, the infant is developing their own immunity.

Physical development

The physical growth and development that take place during infancy are astounding. Although patterns of growth and development will occur in a predictable order, the rate at which they occur may vary among children of the same age, and the most reliable way to interpret growth measurements is to follow trends using growth charts. Growth charts consist of a series of percentile curves that depict the distribution of selected body measurements in infants and children.

Height, weight, and head circumference

Intrauterine growth is assessed by measuring height, weight, and head circumference. These parameters form the basis of growth evaluation for the rest of the infant and toddler period.

Height

Until the child is aged 24 months, height, or length, is measured in the supine position, from the top of the head to the bottom of the heel. When measuring the infant, it is important to keep their body as straight as possible to achieve an accurate measurement. An infant's length is best measured using a stadiometer.

Trunk first, legs to follow

At the end of the first year, the infant's birth length has increased by 50%, with growth of approximately 1 in (2.5 cm) per month for the first 6 months, followed by about ½ in (1.3 cm) per month for the second 6 months. Most of this growth occurs in the trunk rather than in the legs.

Weight

Weight is the primary indicator of nutritional status and is measured on an infant scale with a bucket-type area in which the infant can lie down or sit. Changes in weight can also be used to assess hydration status. The average infant will double their birth weight by age 5 to 6 months and triple it by age 1 year.

Head circumference

A smaller head circumference, or one that lags behind the infant's height and weight, may indicate inadequate brain growth. A head circumference that increases rapidly may indicate an increase in ventricular fluid and intracranial pressure (hydrocephalus).

Teeth

Most neonates do not have teeth. Occasionally, a "natal tooth" will be present at birth and should be evaluated by a pediatric dentist because they may become loose and pose a risk of aspiration. Neonatal teeth are teeth that erupt within the first 28 days of life.

The average age at first tooth eruption is 8 months.

Gross motor development

Gross motor skills refer to the child's development of skills that require the use of large muscle groups. They include posture, head control, sitting, creeping/crawling, standing, and walking.

The infant will attain gross motor control in a cephalocaudal manner, progressing from the head to the toes. They can lift their head, then sit, stand, and, eventually, walk.

Fine motor development

Fine motor skills refer to the infant's ability to use their hands and fingers to grasp an object. As the infant grows, they begin to refine their fine motor skills to grab small objects and feed themselves.

Normal infant reflexes

Much of a neonate's behavior is controlled by reflexes. At ages 4 to 8 weeks, many of these reflexes reach their peak—especially the sucking reflex, which affords nutrition (and, therefore, survival) and psychological pleasure.

At age 3 months, the most primitive reflexes begin to disappear, except for the protective and postural reflexes (blink, parachute, cough, swallow, and gag), which remain for life. (See *Infant reflexes.*)

Psychological development

Psychological development involves language development and socialization as well as play and cognitive development.

Language development and socialization

Language development and socialization begin as soon as the neonate is born. Initially, the neonate communicates primarily through crying and socializes through some of the reflexive behaviors such as the grasp reflex.

Infant reflexes

This chart lists normal infant reflexes, how they are elicited, and the age at which they disappear.

Reflex	How to elicit	Age at disappearance
Trunk incurvature	When a finger is run laterally down the neonate's spine, the trunk flexes and the pelvis swings toward the stimulated side.	2 months
Tonic neck (fencing position)	When the neonate's head is turned while they are lying supine, the extremities on the same side extend outward, while those on the opposite side flex.	2–3 months
Grasping	When a finger is placed in each of the neonate's hands, the neonate's fingers grasp tightly enough to be pulled to a sitting position.	3–4 months
Rooting	When the cheek is stroked, the neonate turns their head in the direction of the stroke.	3–4 months
Moro (startle reflex)	When lifted above the crib and suddenly lowered (or in response to a loud noise), the arms and legs symmetrically extend and then abduct while the fingers spread to form a "C."	4–6 months
Sucking	Sucking motion begins when a nipple or gloved finger is placed in the neonate's mouth.	6 months
Babinski	When the sole on the side of the small toe is stroked, the neonate's toes fan upward.	2 years
Stepping	When held upright with the feet touching a flat surface, the neonate exhibits dancing or stepping movements.	Variable

Cry me a river

The infant cries to express needs. During the first 3 months, crying usually signals a physiologic need such as hunger. As the infant grows, they may cry for attention, from fear, or from frustration during the trials of mastering new skills. Caregivers usually become adept at translating their child's cry.

Infants who cry frequently and are difficult to console may be at increased risk for physical abuse. To help caregivers prepare for and effectively deal with crying infants, the pediatric nurse should:
- reinforce that there are times when infants cry for no reason at all
- assess how caregivers cope with fussy periods and offer support as needed

- teach caregivers comforting techniques, such as holding, swaddling, and massaging.

Smile and say "eh"

An infant's vocalization develops from cries. By age 2 months, the infant can produce single-vowel sounds, such as "ah" and "eh," and begins to develop a social smile. The social smile is the infant's first social response. It initiates social relationships, signals the beginning of thought processes, and further strengthens the bond between the caregiver and the child. By ages 3 to 4 months, the infant can coo, gurgle, and laugh in response to their environment.

Stranger danger

By age 6 months, the infant begins experimenting with sounds and attempting to imitate others. They can discern one's face from another and exhibit stranger anxiety—they are wary of strangers and cling to or clutch their caregivers. Separation anxiety may also develop at this period and peak around 9 months.

I'd like to buy a vowel

The infant can verbalize vowels and consonants by ages 7 to 9 months. They may focus intently on the mouth of someone speaking to them or imitate the expressions of others. They can recognize and respond to their own name and also understand simple commands such as the word "no."

Infant of few words

By ages 10 to 12 months, the infant begins to say words but can understand up to 100 words. They can wave goodbye and enjoy rhythm games. If the child experiences delays in vocalization, they should be evaluated for hearing loss.

Play

Play is an integral part of the socialization process. From birth to age 3 months, infants enjoy having their body parts touched and moved and looking at objects with contrasting colors. They develop the ability to grasp and move objects, so rattles are great toys now.

From ages 4 to 9 months, infants explore the world by using their senses: looking and touching. They tend to put everything within reach in their mouths. They enjoy being read to and will display more reciprocal play, such as talking back to and mimicking adult vocalizations.

Social butterfly

By ages 9 to 12 months, increased mobility allows infants to seek out new stimuli, including people, for interaction. They enjoy social games, such as peek-a-boo, tickling, and swinging.

Cognitive development

Cognitive development refers to the intellectual abilities of a child—their thinking, reasoning, and ability to problem-solve and understand. Cognitively, the infant develops the ability to perform sophisticated mental operations and process and react to stimuli in the environment around them.

Over time, they develop social skills and a sense of *object permanence* (the realization that objects continue to exist even when they cannot be seen) and *causality* (understanding that a particular action or cause leads to an effect).

Trust begins to develop during this stage. Temperament emerges as the infant displays the inborn characteristics that influence activity level, response to new people and situations, and adaptability to change.

On stage with Piaget

According to Jean Piaget's stages of early cognitive development, infants are in the sensorimotor stage, which lasts from birth to age 2. In this stage, infants discover relationships between their bodies and the environment. They rely on their senses to learn about the world around them, and they learn that the external world is not an extension of themselves.

Maintaining health

Keeping an infant healthy involves:

- providing proper nutrition
- ensuring adequate sleep and rest
- providing a safe, nurturing environment.

Nutritional guidelines

Breast milk or iron-fortified infant formula is recommended for the first 12 months of life. Human milk consumed through breastfeeding is considered nutritionally optimal for neonates. Even so, not all birthing parents can or choose to breastfeed. Medical conditions, lack of desire, cultural background, anxiety, use of certain medications, substance misuse, and other factors can prevent someone from breastfeeding. In these cases, bottle-feeding with iron-fortified infant formula is an acceptable alternative.

Breastfeeding

Breastfeeding is widely supported in the health care community. The American Academy of Pediatrics (AAP) recommends exclusive breastfeeding for approximately 6 months followed by continued breastfeeding with complementary foods for at least 2 years and beyond as mutually desired. (See *Benefits of breastfeeding*.)

Benefits of breastfeeding

Passive immunity
Human milk provides passive immunity from caregiver to infant. *Colostrum* is the first fluid secreted from the breast (within the first few days after delivery) and provides immune factor and protein to the neonate. Many components of breast milk protect against infection—it contains antibodies (especially immunoglobulin A) and white blood cells that protect the infant from some forms of infection. Breastfed babies also experience fewer allergies and food
intolerances as well as a lower risk for obesity in childhood.

Digestibility
Breast milk provides essential nutrients in an easily digestible form. It contains *lipase*, which breaks down dietary fat, making it easily available to the infant's system.

Brain development
The lipids in breast milk are high in linoleic acid and cholesterol, which are needed for brain development.

Low protein content
Cow's milk contains proportionally higher concentrations of electrolytes and protein than are needed by human
infants. It must be cleared by the immature kidneys and thus is not recommended until a baby is at least 12 months old.

Convenient and cost-free
Breastfeeding saves the money and time that would be needed to buy and prepare formula.

I demand my 10 to 15!
In general, a neonate should nurse on demand approximately eight to ten times per day for at least 10 to 15 minutes at each breast. The feeding duration may increase, and the frequency may decrease as the infant ages and after solid foods are introduced.

Caregivers should be reassured to feel confident their infant is receiving enough breast milk if they are growing appropriately. Keep in mind that intake is adequate if:
- weight loss after birth is less than 10% of birth weight
- the infant regains the weight lost after birth by age 2 weeks

- the infant has six to eight or more wet diapers per day
- there is a minimum weight gain of 0.5 oz (15 g) per day in the first 2 months of life.

Recommended vitamin supplements

Breastfed infants should receive oral supplementation of vitamin D, 400 units per day. Most newborns have sufficient iron stored in their bodies for the first 4 to 6 months of life. An infant's iron stores depend on their gestational age, maternal iron status, and the timing of umbilical cord clamping. At 6 months of age, infants require an additional source of iron such as iron-rich foods, iron-fortified cereals, or iron supplement drops because breast milk contains little iron.

Formula feeding

Formula feedings provide adequate infant nutrition. The pediatric nurse should support and never judge the person who cannot breastfeed or who chooses not to breastfeed, and reassure them about the nutritional value of infant formulas.

Infant formulas are constituted to provide the proper variety and amount of carbohydrates, protein, fats, and micronutrients needed for healthy growth and development. The U.S. Food and Drug Administration regulates infant formula composition, labeling, and inspection to ensure infant safety.

No moo cows, please

Commercially prepared formulas are recommended rather than regular cow's, goat's, or plant-based milks because these milks:
- do not meet all nutritional needs
- can be difficult to digest
- can strain the infant's kidney system.

Unlocking the secret formula

Most formulas are based on cow's milk proteins, although preparations based on soy proteins and casein hydrolysate are available for infants who cannot tolerate cow's milk–based preparations. Special formulas for infants with diseases like phenylketonuria and other metabolic disorders also exist.

Formula comes in powder, concentrated liquid, and ready-to-feed forms. Ready-to-feed formulas are convenient and prevent problems based on incorrect dilution and preparation, but they are more expensive.

Any improperly mixed or stored formula can be hazardous to the infant.

Introducing solid foods

The age at which solid foods are introduced into an infant's diet depends on factors such as the infant's nutritional need for iron, the infant's physiologic capability to digest starch, and their physical ability to swallow.

Rice is nice

By ages 4 to 6 months, an infant should be mature enough to eat solid foods. Signs an infant is ready for solid foods are sitting with support, good head and neck control, and losing the tongue thrust reflex. Rice cereal is a good food to begin with because it is easily digestible and least likely to cause allergies.

Allow the allergens

Long-term prevention of peanut allergy is possible through the early consumption of peanut products. Introducing peanut products regularly from infancy to age 5 years has been shown to reduce the rate of peanut allergy in adolescence by 71% compared to children who had early peanut avoidance.

Fingers before forks

By about age 8 or 9 months, the infant should be able to sit up and grasp objects, so introducing finger foods can help promote self-feeding. (See *Teaching points for feeding and nutrition*.)

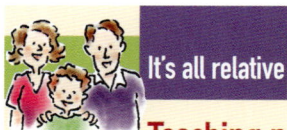

It's all relative

Teaching points for feeding and nutrition

Stress these feeding and nutritional points for infant caregivers:
• Watch for behaviors that indicate feeding preferences. If the infant rejects a food initially, offer it again later multiple times as tastes change.
• Keep the infant in an upright feeding position.
• Do not try to make the infant eat more to finish the serving or portion.
• Offer one to two teaspoons of new foods at a time.
• Introduce new foods one at a time, waiting 3 to 5 days between them so if a food allergy develops, it will be apparent which food triggered the allergic reaction.
• Use a spoon when offering new foods. Do not add foods to the infant's bottle; this can cause choking and lead to overconsumption of calories.
• Avoid grapes, grape halves, and cut-up hot dogs until the infant has adequate chewing and swallowing skills.
• Limit 100% pure fruit juice to no more than 4 oz (120 mL) per day.
• Avoid other sweetened beverages.
• Avoid honey and other unpasteurized products because they may put infants at risk for infantile botulism.

Sleep and rest guidelines

The AAP recommends that all infants be positioned on their backs for every sleep (including naps) because it significantly decreases the incidence of sudden infant death syndrome (SIDS). In addition to providing safe sleep guidelines for the prevention of SIDS, the AAP recommendations focus on safe sleeping environments to prevent sudden unexpected infant deaths (SUIDs) caused by entrapment, suffocation, and asphyxiation. Soft materials, even if covered by a sheet, should not be placed in the crib under a sleeping infant. Objects such as quilts, bumper pads, comforters, and blankets should be kept out of the infant's sleeping environment. Clothing designed to keep the infant warm without covering the head (such as a sleep sac) can be used. There is no evidence that wedges, positioners, special mattresses, and special sleep surfaces reduce the risk of SIDS or that they are safe.

Because of an increased risk of entrapment or suffocation, infants should not sleep on large beds. Room sharing without bed-sharing until the infant is 1 year of age is recommended to decrease the risk of SIDS. Bed rails should not be used due to the risk of strangulation. The sleep area should be kept free from dangling cords, window-covering cords, or electrical wires. Sitting devices such as car seats, strollers, and swings are not recommended for routine sleep. If a baby is being carried in a sling, it is essential that the head and face be visible and that the infant's nose and mouth are clear of obstructions.

To sleep, per chance to . . . wake up and eat!

Certain expectations for sleeping through the night can be made for each age group in infancy:

- From birth to age 4 months, an infant will wake to feed at night from zero to three times. Breast milk is digested faster than formula, so breastfed infants commonly will wake up to feed more frequently than bottle-fed infants.
- At 6 months of age, infants are beginning to be physiologically capable of sleeping (without feeding) for 6 to 8 hours at night. Infants may awaken during this sleep period but should be able to calm themselves and return to sleep. (See *Sleep requirements in infancy*.)

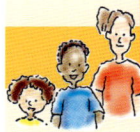

Growing pains

Sleep requirements in infancy

This chart shows the amount of sleep per 24 hours (including nighttime and naps) needed by infants from ages 1 week to 12 months.

Age	Hours of sleep per day
1 week	16½
1 month	15½
3 months	15
6 months	14½
9 months	14
12 months	13¾

Napping

From birth to age 3 months, infants may take many naps per day, but they should not be allowed to sleep longer than 4 hours at a time during the day as it will lead to more nighttime awakenings to feed.

From ages 4 to 9 months, the infant will have transitioned to two naps per day (one in the morning and one in the afternoon). Total naptime should add up to about 2 to 3 hours. By ages 9 to 12 months, most infants will have transitioned to only one nap totaling 1 to 2 hours of napping time.

Dental hygiene

Good oral health starts before the first tooth erupts. Gums should be cleaned with a soft washcloth and water twice a day. Once teeth have erupted, they should be cleaned twice daily with a small, soft-bristled toothbrush and a smear of nonfluoridated toothpaste (equal to size of grain of rice).

A dental routine should be established by 12 months of age. Fluoride supplementation may be needed if dietary or municipal drinking water is suboptimal and if the child is at risk for caries.

Preventing dental caries during infancy

In addition to being a condition associated with dietary factors, early childhood caries (ECC) can be transmitted from caregivers to baby by the bacteria *Streptococcus mutans*. To keep an infant's

smile healthy, teach the caregivers how to avoid dental caries with these tips:
- Do not put an infant to bed with a bottle at night or at naptime because pooling of carbohydrate-rich fluids (including breast milk and formula) or other sweetened liquid around the infant's teeth can cause decay.
- Do not allow the infant to carry a bottle filled with milk, formula, juice, or other sweetened liquid to use as a pacifier throughout the day. Bottles that contain liquids other than water should be offered only at mealtimes.
- Transition the infant to a cup beginning around 9 months and completed by the time of the first birthday. Cup drinking prevents pooling of liquids around the teeth.
- Do not offer the infant a pacifier dipped in sugar or honey.
- Provide regular care of the infant's teeth and gums.
- Encourage caregivers to chew gum or mints with xylitol listed as the first ingredient because xylitol has been shown to inhibit the growth of *S. mutans*.

Injury prevention

Injury prevention during infancy centers around automobile safety, preventing aspiration and falls, and childproofing the infant's environment.

Child passenger safety

The use of child restraints in automobiles reduces the risk of injury related to motor vehicle crashes. Infants and toddlers should ride in a rear-facing car safety seat as long as possible until the child achieves the highest weight or height allowed by the car seat manufacturer. Most rear-facing car safety seats have limits that allow the child to ride rear facing for at least 2 years.

Aspiration

Because infants become adept at placing objects in their mouths for exploration, they are at risk for aspiration. To prevent aspiration:
- feed infants in a slightly upright position
- cut solid foods into very small pieces when the infant starts eating solids
- avoid foods and other things that can be choking hazards such as hot dogs, nuts, popcorn, uncooked vegetables, and grapes.

Falls

As the child becomes mobile, the risk of falls increases, even a neonate is at risk for falls. To prevent falls, encourage caregivers to:
- never leave an infant unattended, especially on a changing table, bed, sofa, or counter
- place gates at the top and bottom of staircases
- install window guards or other window safety devices on windows above the first-floor level
- avoid placing infants in walkers because they can tumble over an uneven surface or fall down stairs.

Childproofing

Here are some childproofing tips for infants:
- Turn down the thermostat on the water heater to 120°F (48.9°C) or lower.
- To prevent an inadvertent scalding burn, never drink hot liquids while holding the infant.
- To prevent drowning, never leave the infant alone in the bath.
- Install both smoke and carbon monoxide detectors outside the infant's room.
- Use flame-retardant pajamas.
- If there are firearms in the home, store them in a locked safe or cabinet, use trigger locks, or lock the firearm and ammunition in separate areas.
  By age 4 months:
- Cover all electrical outlets and tape down all electrical cords (or place them behind furniture). Install childproof locks on all cabinets and place all medicines and cleaning agents in high cabinets with locks to prevent inadvertent ingestions.
- Remove all breakable items from tabletops and shelves within the infant's reach.
- Keep small toys and other small items off the floor.

Inadvertent ingestions

Inadvertent ingestions can be prevented by placing all toxic substances, such as cleaning supplies and medications, in upper or locked cabinets. The American Association of Poison Control Centers has a national poison emergency hotline that can be called toll-free 24 hours a day: 1-800-222-1222. This hotline provides guidance if a toxic substance is ingested. Every household should have this number in an easy-to-find location or saved in the phone so that it can be accessed quickly.

Toddlerhood

Toddlerhood, from ages 1 to 3 years, is the stage in which children start displaying independence and pride in their accomplishments. They intensely explore their environment, trying to figure out how things work. It is also the time when they begin to display negativism and have temper tantrums.

Physical development

During the toddler stage, physical growth slows during the second year of life. Toddlers may have limited food intake, which may concern caregivers. They need to be reassured this is within the normal range of behaviors at this age.

Height, weight, and head circumference

From ages 1 to 2 years:
- toddlers grow approximately 3½ to 5 in (9 to 12.5 cm) per year (with growth mostly in the legs, rather than in the trunk, like infants)
- toddlers can gain about 8 oz (227 g) per month
- head circumference increases about 1 in (2.5 cm) per year
- anterior fontanel usually closes (between 12 and 18 months).

Two's take off

By age 2 years:
- birth weight has usually quadrupled
- head circumference is usually equal to chest circumference
- the child is about half of their adult height.

Three's relax

From ages 2 to 3 years, toddlers:
- grow 2 to 2½ in (5 to 6.5 cm)
- gain about 3 to 5 lb (1.5 to 2.5 kg)
- show slowed increases in head circumference (less than ½ in [1.3 cm] per year).

Teeth

By approximately 33 months, all deciduous (baby) teeth have erupted and the child has about 20 teeth. The child should have their teeth brushed with a small, soft-bristled toothbrush and a scant amount of fluoride toothpaste. Fluoride supplementation may be needed if dietary and municipal drinking water fluoride levels are suboptimal and if the child is at risk for caries.

Gross motor development

Gross motor activity develops rapidly in toddlers.

Between 1 and 2 years of age, the toddler:

- learns to walk alone using a wide stance
- begins to run but may fall easily.

By age 2 years, the toddler can:

- run without falling most of the time
- throw a ball overhand without losing their balance
- walk up stairs but may have to come down backward (on their knees) or slide down on their bottoms
- use push and pull toys.

Fine motor development

Fine motor development begins slowly. However, by age 2 years, the toddler has generally mastered some complex fine motor skills.

A 1-year-old can:

- grasp a very small object.

A 2-year-old can:

- build a tower of four blocks
- scribble on paper
- drop a small pellet into a small, narrow container
- use a spoon well and drink well from a covered cup
- undress themselves.

Psychological development

A child develops a more elaborate vocabulary, a sense of autonomy, and socially acceptable play skills during the toddler stage.

Language development and socialization

As toddlers learn to understand and, ultimately, communicate with the spoken word, they develop the social skills that will allow them to interact more effectively with others.

Language

During toddlerhood, the ability to understand speech is much more developed than the ability to speak.

Now we're talking

Between the ages of 1 and 2 years, the following behaviors are observed:

- The child uses one-word sentences or *holophrases* (real words that are meant to represent entire phrases or ideas). For example,

when a toddler simply says "cookie," it is understood to mean "I want a cookie."
- The toddler has learned about four words.
- Twenty-five percent of the vocalizations are understandable.

Talk about progress!

By age 2 years, they develop the following skills:
- The number of words said has increased from about four (at age 1 year) to between 50 and 100.
- The child uses simple two-word phrases such as "more milk."
- Approximately 50% of speech is understandable by an adult who does not know the child.
- Frequent, repetitive naming of objects helps toddlers to learn appropriate words for objects.

Socialization

During toddlerhood, children develop social skills that determine the way they interact with others. As the toddler develops psychologically, they can:
- differentiate themselves from others and become less egocentric
- tolerate being separated from a caregiver
- withstand delayed gratification
- control their bodily functions (a prerequisite for toilet training)
- acquire socially acceptable behaviors
- communicate verbally.

Play

Play is the work of children. It is through play that the child learns about their own capabilities and develops the skills needed to interact with others and the environment.

Parallel play

During the toddler stage, children commonly play with others without interacting. In this type of *parallel play*, children play side by side, commonly with similar objects. Interaction is limited to the occasional comment or trading of toys. This form of play helps the toddler develop the social skills needed to move into more interactive play.

New rules, new game

During the toddler stage, the following changes are observed:
- Play changes considerably as toddlers' motor skills develop. They use their physical skills to push and pull objects, climb up, down, in, and out, and run or ride on toys.
- A short attention span requires frequent changes in toys and play media.

- Toddlers increase their cognitive abilities by manipulating objects and learning about their qualities, which makes tactile play (with water, sand, finger paints, clay) important.
- Many play activities involve imitating behaviors the child sees at home, which helps them learn new actions and skills.
- Play becomes more social but not necessarily more interactive.
- Problem-solving, creative thinking, and some understanding of cause and effect begin.

Keys to health

Guidelines for nutrition, sleep and rest, and dental hygiene should be followed to maintain a toddler's good health.

Nutrition

Nutritional guidelines for toddlers include:
- protein requirements of 1.2 g/kg/day
- caloric requirement of approximately 100 kcal/kg/day
- considerable need for vitamins and minerals, such as iron, calcium, and phosphorus.

You eat what you are

A toddler's developing eating habits are influenced by a range of factors, including:
- physiologic anorexia, a term which reflects the fact that toddlers are not growing as much as during infancy, do not need as many calories, and will therefore have less of an appetite
- need to imitate family members (toddlers may refuse to eat a particular food that caregivers or siblings choose not to eat)
- being easily overwhelmed by large portions
- inability to sit through a long meal without becoming fidgety or disruptive at times.

Sleep and rest

A consistent routine, such as a set bedtime, a light snack, reading, and a security object, helps toddlers prepare for sleep. Sleep requirements change slightly as a toddler grows and approaches the preschool stage.
- From ages 1 to 2 years, a toddler needs 10 to 15 hours of sleep every 24 hours.
- The 2- to 3-year-old needs 10 to 12 hours of sleep per night.
- During toddlerhood, naps gradually decrease to one per day. At age 3 years, many toddlers usually do not need a nap.

Dental hygiene

As soon as teeth begin to break through the gumline, a child should begin brushing their teeth with a small, soft-bristled toothbrush (with adult assistance). Fluoride toothpaste should be avoided until the child is 2 years old. If used before the child can spit out toothpaste, ingested fluoride may lead to fluorosis (a condition caused by overexposure to fluoride), which can discolor teeth.

ECC—also known as cavities—may occur when a child is routinely given a bottle of milk or juice before sleep or uses the bottle as a pacifier while awake (a bottle of water may be used if needed). Breastfeeding has also been associated with ECC when the child frequently falls asleep at the breast.

Toilet training

For toilet training to be successful, the child must display three signs of toilet training readiness:
1. First, the child must have control of the rectal and urethral sphincters.
2. Second, the child must have a cognitive understanding of what it means to hold their stool and urine until they can go to a certain place at a certain time.
3. Third, the child must have a desire to delay their immediate reward for a more socially accepted action.

Physical readiness for toilet training occurs at ages 18 to 24 months when myelinization of pyramidal tracts and conditioned reflex sphincter control are intact. Despite physical readiness, many children are not cognitively ready to begin toilet training until they are between ages 36 and 42 months.

Other signs of readiness for toilet training include:
*   periods of dryness for 2 hours or more, indicating bladder control
*   child's ability to walk well and remove clothing
*   cognitive ability to understand the task and follow simple instructions
*   facial expressions or words suggesting that the child knows when they are about to defecate and may be uncomfortable in soiled pants.

Temper tantrums

As they assert their independence, toddlers demonstrate "temper tantrums" or violent objections to rules or demands. These tantrums include behaviors such as lying on the floor and kicking their feet, screaming, and holding their breath. Tantrums can occur at any time of the day but commonly occur before bedtime. The active toddler may have trouble slowing down and, when placed in bed, resists staying there.

Dealing with tantrums

Dealing with a child's temper tantrums can be a challenge for caregivers who may be frustrated, embarrassed, and exhausted by the child's behavior. If tantrums occur in public places, caregivers may feel they are being judged by others, viewed as inept, and unable to control their child's behavior.

The nurse should reassure caregivers that temper tantrums are a normal occurrence in toddlers and that children will outgrow them as they learn to express themselves in more productive ways. This type of reassurance should be accompanied by some concrete suggestions for dealing effectively with temper tantrums:

- Provide a safe and childproof environment.
- Hold the child, if necessary, to keep them safe if their behavior is out of control.
- Give the toddler frequent opportunities to make developmentally appropriate choices.
- Know the child's limits and give the child advance warning of a request to help prevent tantrums.
- Remain calm and use simple words when dealing with a child having a tantrum.
- Ignore tantrums when the toddler is seeking attention or trying to get something they want and be sure to praise appropriate behavior.
- Help the toddler find acceptable ways to vent their anger and frustration.

When to get help
Caregivers should be advised to seek help from a health care provider when problematic tantrums:

- persist beyond age 5 years
- occur more than five times per day
- occur with a persistent negative mood
- cause property destruction
- cause harm to the child or others.

Negativism

Negativism refers to persistent negative responses to requests and is typical of toddlers as they strive for autonomy. "No" and "Me do" become the responses to almost everything, and the toddler's emotions are very strongly expressed with rapid mood swings.

No, non, nein!
Negativism commonly becomes exasperating for caregivers who may find it easier to give in to the behavior than to deal with it constructively. Unfortunately, this may reinforce the child's negative ways of interacting with others.

Apple or grape?
Negativism can usually be reduced by giving the child appropriate choices. It is hard to say "no" when the question is "Would you like apple juice or grape juice?"

Discipline

Toddlers must be directly supervised by a caregiver at all times. They must also be provided with a childproof environment because they can move quickly and skillfully and are always exploring their surroundings.

Frustration-free zone

Most discipline for toddlers involves taking measures to make the environment safe and age-appropriate, which reduces the frequency of frustration-producing situations that require a "no" from caregivers.

Tackle the triggers

Behavior management for toddlers includes reducing fatigue and hunger triggers because most inappropriate behavior occurs when the toddler is tired or hungry.

Discipline guidelines include:

- setting up routines and creating and adhering to a consistent schedule
- providing an environment that limits opportunities for negative behavior and giving positive feedback for good behavior
- using behavior modification, or positive reinforcement, for good behavior and brief time-outs (with reasonable limits) for inappropriate behavior
- recognizing individuality in the toddler's temperament
- allowing toddlers to start attempting to solve some of their own problems
- understanding and recognizing feelings of frustration, boredom, and anger
- having the patience to allow toddlers to express themselves and to provide distraction when they are bored
- avoiding physical punishment, threats, and criticism (remembering that toddlers' behaviors are generally the result of normal development, such as exploring and experimenting with their environment).

Time-outs

When using time-outs in response to a toddler's inappropriate behavior, keep these guidelines in mind:

- Make sure the child knows the rules ahead of time.
- Give the child a simple explanation of why the behavior requiring a time-out is unacceptable. For instance, "You hit your sister. Now you must sit in this chair 3 minutes."
- Place the child in a neutral or uninteresting environment.
- Limit the time-out to 1 minute per year of age (anything longer becomes frustrating and loses its intended effect).
- Reset the timer for one additional time-out if the child acts unacceptably.

- If the child is having trouble resolving their behavior problems on their own, try discussing the offense calmly and constructively and, if appropriate, helping the child determine ways to "fix" the result of the bad behavior (such as clean up a mess or apologize to a hurt friend).
- After a successful time-out, praise the child for their improved behavior.

Separation anxiety

Stranger fear and separation anxiety are expected and normal reactions from an infant with healthy attachments. As the child matures to toddler age, they may protest being left with someone other than a caregiver, close friend, or relative. Children usually progress beyond these fears with time and support.

Anxiety antidote

The following information and advice help caregivers deal with their toddler's separation anxiety:

- Toddlers should be allowed to explore at their own rate with close adult supervision. They are normally ready to venture away from their caregivers for short periods and are curious about strangers.
- A toddler should be allowed to "warm up" to a new person. To do so, the caregiver should hold or stand near the child at a "safe" distance from the stranger, allowing the child to observe the new person from the safety of their caregiver's presence. (If the caregiver welcomes the new person, the toddler will likely do the same.)

Injury prevention

Injuries are a leading cause of death in toddlers. For this reason, emphasis should be placed on injury prevention and safety awareness.

Aspiration

Aspiration can easily occur in toddlers because they may still be exploring their environments with their mouths and may ingest small objects. Preventive measures include:

- learning cardiopulmonary resuscitation (CPR) and an age-appropriate Heimlich maneuver
- avoiding large, round chunks of meat such as hot dogs (slicing them into short, lengthwise pieces is a safer option)

- avoiding fruit with pits, fish with bones, hard candy, chewing gum, nuts, popcorn, whole grapes, and marshmallows
- keeping easily aspirated objects and other choking hazards out of a toddler's environment
- being especially cautious about what toys the child plays with (choosing sturdy toys without small, removable parts).

Burns

Burns can easily occur in toddlers because they are tall enough to reach the stovetop and can walk to a fireplace or a woodstove to touch.

Hot stuff

Preventive measures include:
- setting the hot water heater thermostat at a temperature less than 120°F (49°C)
- checking bath water temperature before a child enters the tub
- keeping pot handles turned inward and using the back burners on stovetop
- keeping electrical appliances toward the backs of counters
- placing burning candles, incense, hot foods, and cigarettes out of reach
- avoiding the use of tablecloths so the toddler does not pull it to see what is on the table (possibly spilling hot foods or liquids on themselves).

Falls

Falls can easily occur as gross motor skills improve and the toddler is able to climb stairs and onto furniture.

Movin' on up

Preventive measures include:
- providing close supervision at all times during play
- keeping crib rails up and the mattress at the lowest position to prevent the child from climbing out of the crib
- placing gates across the tops and bottoms of stairways
- installing window locks on all windows to keep them from opening more than 3½ in without adult supervision
- keeping doors locked or using childproof doorknob covers at entries to stairs, high porches or decks, and laundry chutes
- avoiding the use of walkers, especially near stairs
- always restraining children in shopping carts and never leaving them unattended.

Preschool

During the preschool stage (ages 3 to 6 years), children are gaining new independence and have well-developed language skills.

Physical development

Physical development is slow and steady during the preschool stage, with most growth occurring in the long bones of the arms and legs.

Height and weight

- Preschoolers grow about 2½ to 3 in (6.5 to 7.5 cm) per year. Their average height is 37 in (94 cm).
- Weight gain is 3 to 5 lb (1.5 to 2.5 kg) per year. The average preschooler weighs 32 lb (14.5 kg).

Teeth

By the preschool years, the development of the child's primary (or *deciduous*) teeth is complete. Prepare the child and caregivers for the loss of these "baby" teeth and replacement with secondary (or *permanent*) teeth, which usually begins to occur at age 6 years.

Gross motor development

A 3-year-old can stand on one foot for a few seconds, climb stairs with alternating feet, jump in place, and kick a ball. A 4-year-old can hop, jump, and skip on one foot, throw a ball overhand, and ride a tricycle or bicycle with training wheels. A 5-year-old can skip, using alternative feet, jump rope, and balance on each foot for 4 to 5 seconds.

Fine motor development

A 3-year-old can:
- build a tower of nine to ten blocks and a three-block bridge
- copy a circle and a cross
- draw a circle with facial features (but usually not a stick figure)
- use a fork well.

A 4- or 5-year-old can:
- build a tower of ten blocks
- copy a square and trace a cross and a diamond
- draw a person or stick figure with three or more parts
- use scissors to cut out a picture following an outline.

Psychological development

During the preschool years, the child functions more socially as they are able to learn and follow rules. By this age, they may have entered a day care or nursery school setting, which enhances social development.

Many of the thought processes a preschooler goes through are essential to them for kindergarten and the school years ahead.

Language development and socialization

By the time a child reaches preschool age:
- their vocabulary increases to about 900 words by age 3 years and 2,100 words by age 5 years
- they may talk a lot and ask many "why" questions
- they usually talk in three- or four-word sentences by age 3 years. By age 5 years, they speak in longer sentences that contain all parts of speech.

Come one; come all

Socialization continues to develop as the preschooler's world expands beyond themselves and their family. Regular interaction with same-age children is necessary for the preschooler to further develop social skills.

Play

Play changes as children move into preschool years, and the parallel play of toddlerhood is essentially replaced by more interactive, cooperative play.

Ch-, ch-, ch-, ch-, changes!

Other changes in play include:
- more *associative play* in which there is interaction between the children as they play together
- better understanding of the concept of sharing
- enjoyment of large motor activities, such as swinging, riding tricycles or bicycles, and throwing balls
- more dramatic play and the child may have imaginary playmates.

Cognitive development

Preschoolers exhibit preoperational thought by using words, symbols, and objects to represent things in their environment. An example of using an object as a representation would be a child who pretends that a broom is a horse.

Piaget's cognitive theory divides the preoperational phase into two stages during the preschool years: the *preconceptual phase* and the *intuitive thought phase*.

It's all about me!

The preconceptual phase of cognitive development begins in the toddler stage and extends into the preschool stage (ages 2 to 4 years). During this phase, the child is able to:

- form beginning concepts that are not as complete or logical as adults are
- make simple classifications
- rationalize specific concepts but not the idea as a whole
- exhibit *egocentric thinking* (evaluating each situation based on their feelings or experiences, rather than the feelings of others).

Call it children's intuition

The *intuitive thought phase* begins at age 4 years and extends into school age (age 7 years). During this phase, the child:

- can classify, quantify, and relate objects (but cannot yet understand the principles behind these operations)
- uses intuitive thought processes (but is not able to fully see the viewpoints of others)
- uses many words appropriately (but without true understanding of their meaning).

Moral and spiritual development

Kohlberg's *preconventional phase* of moral development spans the preschool and school age stages, extending from ages 4 to 10 years. During this phase:

- Conscience emerges, and emphasis is on external control. The preschooler's moral standards are the same as others, and they understand that these standards must be followed to avoid punishment for inappropriate behavior or gain rewards for good or desired behavior. During this stage, children may view an illness or hospitalization as a punishment for real or perceived bad behavior.
- The preschooler behaves according to what freedom is given or what restriction is placed on their actions.

Keys to health

Guidelines for nutrition, sleep, and dental hygiene should be followed in order to maintain a preschooler's good health.

Nutrition

The caloric requirement for preschoolers is 85 to 90 kcal/kg/day or about 1,700 to 1,800 calories per day. Daily fluid intake should average 100 mL/kg, depending on the preschooler's activity level.

Make pleasant conversation

By age 5 years, the focus on the "social" aspects of eating can begin. Caregivers should encourage table conversation, good table manners, and a willingness to try a variety of foods. Preschoolers are old enough to help with meal preparation and cleanup and usually enjoy doing so.

No food fights

Caregivers should be discouraged from using food as a bribe, reward, or threat, which can set the stage for unhealthy attitudes about food and eating.

Food preferences

Many 3- to 4-year-olds have strong taste preferences. The child may want to eat only one thing, or a narrow range of foods, over and over. Emphasis should be placed on the quality of the food eaten rather than on the quantity to prevent emotional struggles over food.

To promote healthy eating habits, caregivers should encourage the child to eat fruits and vegetables.

Sleep and rest

By the time a child reaches the preschool stage, sleep patterns have likely been established during toddlerhood. Normal sleep patterns for preschoolers consist of 10 to 12 hours at night and, if not already stopped at age 3 years, one daytime nap or rest period.

Monsters under the bed

Despite these well-established patterns, sleep-related problems may reappear during preschool years:

- Dreams and nightmares become more real as magical thinking increases and a vivid imagination develops. Magical thinking is a phenomenon that leads some children to believe that a certain action they take will influence the world around them. For instance, a child may think that sleeping with a certain blanket will keep the monsters away at bedtime.
- Problems falling asleep may occur due to overstimulation, separation anxiety, fear of the dark or monsters, or use of medications such as stimulants.
- Nighttime waking may occur due to nightmares and night terrors as well as the child's inability to soothe and comfort themselves.
- Sleepwalking may occur if the child has not had enough sleep or is experiencing unusual stress.

Dental hygiene

Preschoolers have developed the fine motor skills needed to use a toothbrush properly and should be encouraged to brush twice daily. Caregivers should still supervise the child's brushing (assisting, as necessary) and perform flossing. As in toddlerhood, cariogenic foods (such as sweetened cereals and chewy candies) should be avoided.

The preschool years are an excellent time to encourage good dental hygiene habits. Caregivers should schedule a dental visit so the child can become comfortable with the routine of preventive dental care. The child should then visit the dentist at 6- to 12-month intervals.

Coping with concerns

Caregivers may be concerned about their preschoolers in the areas of discipline and fears. They may also have concerns about their child's readiness to start formal schooling.

Discipline

Caregivers commonly have questions about how best to discipline young children. Here are some pointers about appropriate methods of discipline:

- Discipline should not be confused with punishment. Discipline refers to the process of managing behaviors—good and bad—to achieve desired outcomes. Punishment is a single action taken in response to a specific behavior.
- Authority figures should administer discipline firmly, consistently, and fairly.
- The child should be given simple explanations about why a certain behavior is not appropriate. "We keep our hands to ourselves. You hit your sister, so now you have to sit in this chair for four minutes."
- Time-outs (generally 1 minute per year of age) can be used to help the child relieve intensity, regain control, and think about their inappropriate behavior.

Fears

Children experience more fears during the preschool years than at any other time. Common fears include being afraid of the dark, ghosts, and being left alone.

Who you gonna call? Ghostbusters!

No amount of logical persuasion will allay these fears, which leaves many caregivers perplexed about how to help. Caregivers can help their child overcome their fears by actively involving them in finding practical solutions to dealing with them, such as using a nightlight and keeping the closet door open or closed (to keep monsters under control). By age 6, most children will have overcome these types of fears.

Injury prevention

Injuries are a leading cause of death in the preschool-age group. For this reason, much emphasis should be placed on injury prevention and safety awareness.

Burns

Burns can easily occur in preschool-age children because they are tall enough to reach the stovetop, or can walk to a fireplace or a woodstove to touch.

Hot potato

Some pointers to help prevent burns are:
- teaching the child what "hot" means and stressing the danger of open flames
- storing matches and cigarette lighters in locked cabinets, out of reach
- burning fires in fireplaces or woodstoves with close supervision and using a fire screen when doing so
- securing safety plugs in all unused electrical outlets and keeping electrical cords tucked out of reach
- teaching preschoolers who can understand the hazards of fire to "stop, drop, and roll" if their clothes are on fire.

The great escape

Some pointers to help teach preschoolers fire safety techniques are:
- practicing escapes from home and school with preschoolers
- visiting a fire station to reinforce learning
- teaching preschoolers how to call 911 (for emergency use only).

Drowning

Toddlers and preschoolers are quite susceptible to drowning because they can walk onto docks or pool decks and stand or climb on seats in a boat. Drowning can also occur in mere inches of water, resulting from falls into buckets, bathtubs, hot tubs, toilets, and even fish tanks.

Water, water, everywhere

Preventive measures include:
- close adult supervision of any child near water, including bathtubs and toilets
- teaching children, even those who know how to swim, never to go into water without an adult and never to play near the water's edge
- using child-resistant pool covers and fences with self-closing gates around backyard pools
- emptying buckets when not in use and storing them upside down
- using U.S. Coast Guard–approved child life jackets near water and on boats.

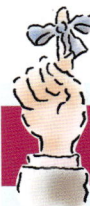

Falls

Falls can easily occur as gross motor skills improve and preschoolers are able to move chairs to climb onto counters, climb ladders, and open windows.

To prevent falls in this age group, caregivers should:
- provide close supervision during play
- install window locks on all windows to keep them from opening more than 3½ in without adult supervision
- remove unsecured scatter/throw rugs
- use a nonskid bath mat or decals in bathtub or shower
- provide safe climbing toys and choose play areas with soft ground cover and safe equipment
- teach the difference between acceptable and unacceptable places for climbing.

Motor vehicle and bicycle injuries

Motor vehicle and bicycle/tricycle injuries can easily occur in preschoolers because they may be able to unbuckle seat belts, resist riding in a car seat, or refuse to wear a bicycle helmet.

Look both ways

Preventive measures include:
- educating caregivers about the proper fit and use of bicycle helmets and requiring the child to wear a helmet every time they ride a bicycle
- teaching the preschooler never to go into a road without an adult
- not allowing a child to play on a curb or behind a parked car
- checking the area behind vehicles before backing out of the driveway (small children may not be visible in rearview mirrors because of blind spots, especially in larger vehicles)

Memory jogger

Remember tips on preventing drowning when you think of the word WATER.

Wear life jackets

Adult supervision

Teach water safety

Empty buckets

Reinforce safety with pool covers

- providing a safe, preferably enclosed, area for outdoor play (and keeping fences, gates, and doors locked)
- educating caregivers on the use of child safety seats for all motor vehicle trips and ensuring proper use by having the seats inspected. (See *Car safety seat guidelines*.)

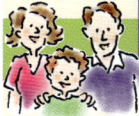

It's all relative

Car safety seat guidelines

Proper installation and use of a car safety seat are critical. In addition to the weight and age guidelines outlined in this chart, these guidelines for booster seat use will help ensure a child's safety while riding in a vehicle:
- Always make sure belt-positioning booster seats are used with both lap and shoulder belts.
- Make sure the lap belt fits low and right across the lap/upper thigh area and the shoulder belt fits snugly, crossing the chest and shoulder to avoid abdominal injuries.
- All children younger than 12 years should ride in the back seat.

Weight and age	Seat type	Seat position
Up to 2 years	Infant-only or rear-facing convertible	Rear facing
Up to 2 years	Rear-facing convertible	Rear facing
Over 2 years	Rear-facing convertible (until meeting seat manufacturer's limit for maximum weight and height) and then forward facing	Forward facing with harness, placed in back seat
4–8 years and over 40 lb (18.1 kg)	Belt-positioning booster seat	Forward facing

Poisoning

As gross motor skills improve, toddlers and preschoolers are able to climb onto chairs and reach cabinets where medicines, cosmetics, cleaning products, and other poisonous substances are stored.

Please don't eat the daisies

Preventive measures include:
- keeping medicines and other toxic materials locked away in high cupboards, boxes, or drawers
- using child-resistant containers and cupboard safety latches
- not storing a large supply of toxic agents
- teaching that medication is not a candy or treat (even though it might taste good) (This includes not referring to medicine as candy.)

- teaching the child that plants (inside or outside) are not edible
- promptly discarding empty containers that have held poisonous/hazardous materials and never reusing them to store a food or drink item or other poisonous/hazardous substance
- always keeping original labels on containers of toxic substances
- having the poison control center number (1-800-222-1222) prominently displayed on every telephone, including saved in cell phones.

Suffocation

Suffocation can easily occur in toddlers and preschoolers exposed to objects that can occlude the airway. A child may place such an object over their head or get tangled in an object such as a cord or string. Suffocation can also occur if a child becomes enclosed in a small space with a limited oxygen supply.

Preventive measures are extremely important and include:
- storing plastic bags, latex balloons, strings, and ribbons out of the child's reach
- forbidding the child to play with latex balloons, which can burst into small pieces that can be easily aspirated (supervised play with Mylar balloons is acceptable)
- keeping strings and cords (such as those on hooded clothing or window coverings) out of the child's reach
- discarding old appliances, such as refrigerators and ovens, or removing the doors from old appliances that must be stored (to prevent a child from becoming trapped)
- choosing safe toy boxes or chests without heavy, hinged lids.

Child maltreatment

Child maltreatment can include emotional neglect/abuse, physical neglect, intentional physical abuse, and sexual abuse. With emotional neglect or abuse, the child experiences a lack of affection, attention, or emotional nurturance to support normal development. A child experiences physical neglect when the caregiver fails to provide for the child's basic needs and an adequate level of care. Examples include deprivation of food, clothing, shelter, supervision, medical care, or education.

Intentional physical abuse is intentionally causing pain or harm to the child, such as with shaken baby syndrome (also known as abusive head trauma). Lastly, child sexual abuse is sexual activity with a minor as children cannot consent to any form of sexual activity. State laws vary about the age of legal consent for teenagers. Child sexual abuse does not need to include physical contact between a perpetrator and a child. Examples of childhood abuse that do not include physical contact are exhibitionism (exposing one's genitals to a minor), masturbation in the presence of a minor or forcing the minor to masturbate, and obscene conversations, phone calls, texts, or digital interactions with a minor.

What causes it

Risk factors that may predispose a child to abuse or neglect may involve the caregiver or the child. Caregiver risk factors include a history of being abused as a child, being a victim of intimate partner abuse, substance misuse, having limited social supports, or having unrealistic expectations of the child.

Risk factors for the child include being less than 3 years of age, being born prematurely, having a physical/intellectual disability, or having a mismatched temperament with the caregiver.

Other risk factors include stressful environmental factors, such as divorce, poverty, unemployment, or inadequate housing.

How it happens

Child maltreatment is a widespread problem and is part of a larger problem of violence. Many children die each day because of maltreatment. Often, people who abuse children were abused as children and may not know healthier ways to discipline a child or to show love.

It's the law

If abuse is suspected, health care providers, including doctors, nurses, and dentists, are legally required to report their suspicions to Child Protective Services.

What to look for

Physical indicators of abuse and neglect include:
- unexplained fractures (children younger than walking age rarely have fractures because their bones are still pliable)

- bruises with specific patterns, over soft-tissue areas, back, or genitals, in various stages of healing (because bruising caused by injuries most commonly occurs over bony prominences in children)
- welts from belt buckles or other distinctive instruments
- cigarette burns as well as "glove-," "sock-," or doughnut-shaped burns from dipping extremities in hot water or holding a child's bottom in hot water
- retinal hemorrhages indicating shaken baby syndrome (different from scleral hemorrhages)
- inappropriate dress, poor hygiene, or untreated medical needs
- failure to thrive.

Acting it out

Behavioral indicators include:
- withdrawn, passive, apathetic, or depressed moods
- habit-related disorders such as excessive sucking or rocking.

When things don't add up

Other findings include:
- conflicting reports from caregiver and child about how injuries occurred
- inappropriate delay in seeking treatment for injuries
- inconsistency between the history of the injury and the child's developmental level
- inappropriate response of the child to the injuries.

What tests tell you

There are no definitive tests to detect child abuse or neglect. However, some laboratory tests and x-rays may be indicated, such as:
- hemoglobin and lead levels because children who have been abused may not have had routine health care and are at higher risk for anemia and lead poisoning
- complete blood count to rule out any blood disorders
- laboratory studies to rule out sexually transmitted infections whenever sexual abuse is suspected
- x-ray studies to diagnose suspicious injury or trauma
- skeletal x-ray survey to examine the entire body for evidence of fractures occurring at various times with various levels of healing. (X-rays may indicate previous intentional trauma that is ongoing and predates the incident that brought the child to the health care provider's attention.)

Calling in the cavalry

Child Protective Services should be contacted to document the suspected injuries. When visible lesions are present, color photographs should be taken and the image should include:

- ruler for accurate measurement
- name of child
- name of person taking photo
- written description of lesion.

Complications

Complications of child abuse and neglect come in various forms depending on severity. Children can suffer a wide range of physical complications and lasting emotional effects.

How it's treated

Child maltreatment is treated by first identifying it as a problem. After the injury is treated, the child's safety must be ensured if there is any suspicion of physical abuse or violence.

What to do

The nurse should always be assessing children for signs of maltreatment. In individual instances, practice the following:

- Complete a thorough assessment of all body systems while comforting and reassuring the child to the extent possible.
- Carefully assess the child's emotional status.
- Document history and assessment objectively and with clear descriptions.
- Report suspected cases to Child Protective Services following the protocols of your facility (all health care providers are mandated reporters).
- Notify the caregiver that it is required by law to report any concerns and assessments.

The "A" team

- Collaborate with the multidisciplinary health care team about immediate- and long-term interventions to prevent further abuse.
- Work with the caregiver on changing the situation that led to the abuse and refer them to an agency or program that specializes in working with similar families.

- Teach the caregivers relevant child development principles, provide anticipatory guidance, and serve as their role model.
- Provide the child with positive attention and age-appropriate play activities.
- Reassure the child that nothing that happened was their fault and that you are there to help, not hurt them.

Quick quiz

1. When a toddler is playing, they will most likely do which of the following?
    A. Play with similar objects near, rather than with, another child
    B. Become more interactive with children around them
    C. Willingly share their toys with other children
    D. Play with one toy for a while because of their long attention span

Answer: A. During the toddler stage, children typically play with others without actually interacting. In this type of *parallel play*, children play side by side, usually with similar objects.

2. To help prevent aspiration of foods, toddlers and preschoolers should avoid which types of food?
    A. Grain products such as bread and muffins
    B. Round chunks of meat such as hot dogs
    C. Cooked vegetables, such as lima beans and corn
    D. Frozen desserts such as ice cream

Answer: B. To help prevent aspiration, avoiding large, round chunks of meat such as hot dogs is advisable. (Slicing them into short, lengthwise pieces is a safer option.)

3. Characteristics of intentional injuries in young children include which of the following?
    A. Bruises on shins and elbows
    B. Skin injuries with pattern of an object
    C. Skull fracture with history of witnessed fall
    D. Abrasions on both knees of a 2-year-old

Answer: B. Skin injuries with the pattern of an object (such as a belt or iron) are characteristics of intentional injuries in young children.

4. Which of the following finger foods is appropriate for a 9-month-old infant?
    A. Cheerios
    B. Grapes
    C. Mixed nuts
    D. Raw carrot slice

Answer: A. Cheerios are soft cereals that are easy to swallow and do not pose a choking risk. The other foods are choking hazards for small children.

5.   What is the best indicator of whether an infant is receiving enough formula or breast milk?
   A.   Burps well
   B.   Does not cry after feeding
   C.   Has six or more wet diapers per day
   D.   Sleeps all night

Answer: C. Infants receiving adequate formula or breast milk for hydration and growth will void and wet six to eight diapers daily.

6.   Which of the following interventions decreases the risk of SIDS?
   A.   Feeding the infant in an upright position
   B.   Not giving a bottle in bed at night
   C.   Putting an infant on their back to sleep
   D.   Raising the head of the crib

Answer: C. Putting the infant on their back to sleep for every sleep has decreased the overall prevalence of SIDS and will decrease the individual infant's risk of SIDS as well.

Scoring

⭐⭐⭐   If you answered all six items correctly, terrific! You've developed a strong sense of child development.

⭐⭐   If you answered four or five items correctly, good job! Treat yourself to a play break and then read on.

⭐   If you answered fewer than three items correctly, don't cry over spilled milk! Take a nap and review the chapter again.

Suggested References

American Academy of Pediatric Dentistry. (2023). *Policy on use of fluoride.* https://www.aapd.org/research/oral-health-policies--recommendations/use-of-fluoride/

American Academy of Pediatrics. (2022). *Newborn and infant breastfeeding.* https://www.aap.org/en/patient-care/newborn-and-infant-nutrition/newborn-and-infant-breastfeeding/

Centers for Disease Control and Prevention. (2021). *Vitamin D.* https://www.cdc.gov/nutrition/infantandtoddlernutrition/vitamins-minerals/vitamin-d.html

Centers for Disease Control and Prevention. (2024). *CDC's developmental milestones.* https://www.cdc.gov/ncbddd/actearly/milestones/index.html

Children's Bureau. (2024). *Child abuse and neglect.* https://www.childwelfare.gov/topics/safety-and-risk/child-abuse-and-neglect/

Du Toit, G., Huffaker, M. F., Radulovic, S., Feeney, M., Fisher, H. R., Byron, M., Dunaway, L., Calatroni, A., Johnson, M., Foong, R. X., Marques-Mejias, A., Bartha, I., Basting, M., Brough, H. A., Baloh, C., Laidlaw, T. M., Bahnson, H. T., Roberts, G., Plaut, M., … Immune Tolerance Network LEAP-Trio Trial Team. (2024). Follow-up to adolescence after early peanut introduction for allergy prevention. *NEJM Evidence, 3*(6), EVIDoa2300311. https://doi.org/10.1056/EVIDoa23003

Kaneshiro, N. (2023). *Infant reflexes.* https://medlineplus.gov/ency/article/003292.htm

Linnard-Palmer, L. (2019). Caring for neonates and infants. In L. Linnard-Palmer (Ed.), *Pediatric nursing care: A concept-based approach* (pp. 71–85). Jones & Bartlett Learning.

Nassar, H. M., Alhazzazi, T. Y., Hazzazi, L. W., & Gregory, R. L. (2021). The anticariogenic effect of xylitol on seven Streptococcus mutans strains. *Medical Science, 25,* 1681–1690.

Chapter 13

Middle childhood and adolescence

Just the facts

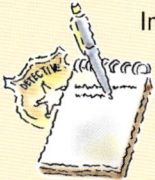

In this chapter, you'll learn:

♦ physical, psychosocial, cognitive, and moral development of school-age children and adolescents

♦ keys to health maintenance in middle childhood and adolescence

♦ common concerns of school-age children and adolescents and their caregivers

♦ injury prevention for school-age children and adolescents

♦ common health problems during middle childhood and adolescence.

School age

School age, or *middle childhood*, refers to the stage of a child's life from ages 6 to 12 years. The school-age years can be a spectacular journey filled with joys and successes as the child continues to grow and mature.

They can also be marked by challenges, as the child struggles to make sense of physical and psychological changes, their emerging identity, and the way they see themselves and are viewed by others (especially their peers).

Physical development

Physical growth at this time is relatively slow and smooth.

Height and weight

Growth slows considerably during middle childhood. During this stage, height increases by an average of 2 in (5 cm) per year, and weight increases by an average of 6 lb (2.5 kg) per year. However, during this time, the typical school-age child slims down and becomes more agile and graceful. Females tend to develop slightly faster than males, although males are, on average, taller and heavier than females until the adolescent growth spurt.

Fine motor skills

By age 7 years, the brain has completed 90% of its growth, and basic neuromuscular mechanisms are in place.

No more excuses

Development of small muscle and eye-hand coordination increases, leading to the skilled handling of tools, such as pencils and scissors for drawing and cutting. The child can then spend the remainder of this period refining physical and gross motor skills and coordination.

Pubertal changes

The pubertal growth spurt begins in females around age 10 years and in males at about age 12 years.

Jumpin' in feet first

Different areas of the body reach their peak growth at different times. Changes are easily recognized in the feet, which are the first part of the body to experience a growth spurt. Increased foot size is followed by a rapid increase in leg length and then trunk growth.

Leggy and hippy

During this time, leg growth increases more dramatically than trunk growth in males. Although females have greater hip width, males exceed females in other areas of bone growth.

No turning back

In addition to bones, gonadal hormone levels increase and cause the sexual organs to mature.

Preparation for menses

In females, the first menstruation, called *menarche*, usually starts around age 12 years but can occur as early as age 9 years and still be considered normal. The menstrual cycle may be irregular at first.

Secondary sexual characteristics also start to develop—including breasts, hips, and pubic hair—and females may experience a sudden increase in height. Nurses may find that this provides an excellent opportunity to begin educating school-age females about breast self-examination and reproductive health.

Teeth

Loss of primary teeth and eruption of the secondary teeth occur during the school-age years. Because of their size, secondary teeth may, for a while, appear disproportionately large in relation to the child's other, smaller facial features.

Psychological development

Attending school marks an acceleration in the separation of the child from their caregivers. It introduces the child to a new set of authority figures (teachers, school administrators) and strengthens peer relationships.

Psychosocial development

The school-age child enters Erikson stage of industry versus inferiority. In this stage, the child wants to work, produce and accomplish tasks. If too much is expected of them, however, or if they feel unable to measure up to set standards, the negative attributes of inadequacy and inferiority may prevail.

Language development and socialization

The school-age child has an ever-expanding vocabulary and begins to correct previous mistakes in usage. They begin to understand the double meanings of words and become proficient at giving others directions without using physical signals.

Pick a clique

In the first and second grades, peers are increasingly significant to the child. The need to find a place within a peer or social group becomes important.

Same-sex cliques are established during this period, and competition becomes more common, as does bragging over accomplishments. The child may be overly concerned with peer rules. However, caregiver's guidance continues to play an important role in the child's life.

Handle with care: sensitive to ridicule

The child's world expands as interests and activities outside the home take on an increased role in their life. They are more independent inside and outside the home. They understand the reasons for rules and become more sensitive to criticism and ridicule.

Play

The child's personality has become structured, and they are ready to be a partner in play with their friends. The child in this age group typically has two-to-three best friends, who may change frequently. Most of the child's energies are devoted to school and friends.

Cognitive development

School and learning are viewed by the school-age child as an exciting experience. The major developmental tasks at this time are achievement in school and acceptance by peers. Expectations in the classroom have intensified and require concentration, attendance, and complex auditory and visual processing.

The school-age child is in Piaget concrete-operational period, meaning the child uses thought processes to experience and understand events and actions. Children at this age are less egocentric and can see things from another's point of view.

Try to remember

Reorganization of the *frontal brain*, which is used for selective attention, occurs between ages 5 and 7 years. The ability to reason and memorize improves, and the child tends to use mnemonic strategies to remember new information. In addition, the following occurs:

- Magical thinking diminishes around this time, and the child has a much better understanding of cause and effect.
- The child begins to accept rules but may not necessarily understand them.
- Memory skills are continually improving, along with an increased attention span. The child is ready for basic reading, writing, and arithmetic.
- Abstract thinking begins to develop during the middle elementary school years.
- Caregivers remain very important during this time. Adult reassurance of the child's competence and basic self-worth is essential.

Moral and spiritual development

In general, the first level of moral thinking is put into practice at the elementary school level, and the school-age child is in Kohlberg conventional level. The child behaves according to socially acceptable norms because an authority figure tells them to do so. This obedience is compelled by the threat of punishment (external factors).

Caregiver's guidance, love, and support are essential for the development of values during this time. The child needs the opportunity to make decisions within defined boundaries. Ideally, those boundaries are set by responsible adults in the child's life.

At ages 11 to 12 years, as the child begins to approach adolescence, school and caregiver's authority are questioned. Occasionally, it is even challenged or opposed. The importance of the peer group intensifies, and rough, bold, or even brazen behavior becomes increasingly common. The peer group becomes the source of behavior standards and models.

Earthbound

Spiritual lessons should be taught in concrete terms during this stage. Children have a hard time understanding supernatural religious symbols. Repeated religious rituals, such as praying and attending church services, may comfort them.

Keys to health

During the school-age years, the child's understanding of cause and effect, coupled with the need for caregiver's and peer approval, provides an excellent opportunity to continue teaching about the need to make healthy lifestyle choices. Caregivers should continue to teach their children about the importance of:

- proper/balanced nutrition
- exercise and activity
- dental hygiene
- sleep and rest.

Nutrition

Children should be encouraged to eat a variety of healthy foods, such as proteins, fruits, vegetables, and grains, to ensure proper nutritional intake. The nurse should be sensitive to the unique dietary needs, preferences, and resources of each patient and family to create realistic and individualized recommendations. Cultural diversity, philosophical differences, and limitations due to allergies and finances among families mean that there are a variety of diets—e.g., vegetarian, vegan, religious-based, and gluten-free—of which the nurse should be aware.

Developing healthy eating habits

Establishing healthy eating habits will lay a stable foundation for adolescence, when caloric needs increase. Childhood obesity is a serious health problem in the United States. Children and their families should be educated to avoid high-fat, high-sugar, low-protein foods. (See *Encouraging proper nutrition*.)

Sleep and rest

Requirements for sleep and rest are unique and relate to the child's activity level and physical health. School-age children generally do not require an afternoon nap, and adherence at bedtime becomes easier. It is recommended that school-age children sleep 9 to 12 hours/day to best promote learning, growth, and development. Children should develop healthy sleep hygiene by avoiding screens (i.e., phone, tablet, television) or other electronic devices and by creating nighttime routines that center around calming activities such as dimming the lights, taking a warm bath, or listening to soothing music as it gets closer to bedtime.

Things that go bump in the night

Sleepwalking and sleep talking may begin during this stage, and caregivers should take measures to ensure the child's physical safety during these episodes. Nightmares are usually related to a real event in the child's life and can usually be eradicated by resolving any underlying fears the child might have.

Exercise and activity

Exercise and other forms of physical activity help the child establish healthy habits for a lifetime. Doing so may also prevent childhood obesity.

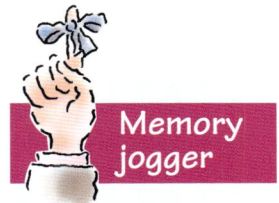

Memory jogger

When it comes to teaching children about being healthy, tell caregivers to remember PEDS:
Proper/balanced nutrition
Exercise and activity
Dental hygiene
Sleep

Children who are interested in sports can join sports teams or participate in sporting events. Those who aren't interested in team sports or whose families are unable to meet the time or financial demands can still participate in regular family play, walks, or bike rides. Children should learn the importance of daily activity, and caregivers should limit sedentary activities such as playing video games. Children should have a regular recess during school hours which allows for movement and to break up the long school day.

Clicking the remote doesn't count

Caregivers should encourage physical movement after school and on the weekends instead of more sedentary activities such as watching television or playing video games, though variations in neighborhoods, climate, and competing responsibilities may limit those opportunities.

Dental hygiene

During the school-age years the following have to be practiced:

- Teeth should be brushed at least twice a day and, if possible, after all meals.
- Drinking water should contain fluoride or fluoride supplements should be given, usually at the dentist's office.
- Flossing should be taught, and caregivers should monitor for method and adherence until the child is independent, usually around age 8 years.
- Regular dental cleanings should be scheduled every 6 months.

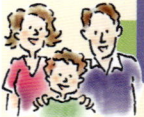

It's all relative

Encouraging proper nutrition

To ensure that children continue to develop and maintain healthy eating habits, encourage parents and caregivers to engage in the following activities:

- Stock the pantry and refrigerator with healthy choices for snacks (raw vegetables, low-sugar yogurts, fresh fruits).
- Limit meals in fast-food establishments where foods with limited nutritional value are abundant. Sit down together for family meals, preferably cooked at home. Family meals have been shown to increase healthy eating, reduce disordered eating, and contribute to normal levels of weight in children. Social benefits to the family meal have also been shown in recent years.
- Teach children how to read nutrition labels while shopping at the grocery store.
- Involve children in planning and preparing meals for the family.
- Offer candy and other sweets as an infrequent option rather than a reward for good behavior.
- Change their own eating habits to model good dietary habits for their children.

Coping with concerns

During school age, the child's life revolves around home, family, school, and peers. School-age children and their caregivers are commonly faced with concerns about school and after-school supervision. Around the age of 10 years, some children may start to stay home alone for short periods of time during daylight or early evening hours (e.g., 1 to 2 hours). Establish rules about safety, communication, emergency situations, and expectations when a child is without adult supervision.

School phobias

School phobias may also be called *school refusal* or *school avoidance*. A child's refusal to go to school may be a sign of separation anxiety. School refusal may also occur after a particular trauma, such as the death of a pet, illness within the family, or a move to a new school.

In these cases, the child may be more fearful of leaving home than they are of going to school. For example, the child might be afraid that something bad will happen to a caregiver, sibling, or pet if they are not there to protect them.

Scary school

Refusal to go to school may also be related to fear of the school itself and what the child experiences there. Caregivers should talk to their children and try to determine the underlying cause of their fear. Possible reasons for school phobias include:
- being the target of a bully
- anxiety about academic achievement
- having problems adapting to the school structure.

Stealing

Stealing is attractive to the younger school-age child who simply wants items for themselves. The child has a limited sense of what belongs to someone else and will commonly lie to cover up the offense.

Low on dough

A sense of responsibility for one's actions begins to take shape at the end of middle childhood. Stealing at the end of middle childhood is commonly a sign that something is lacking in that child's life. Possible causes include a lack of:
- financial means
- attention from a parent or caregiver
- sense of property rights.

What's yours is mine

Caregivers should recognize the child's personal property and offer some privacy in this regard, when possible. A child who knows that their own property is respected is more likely to understand the importance of respecting that of others.

Adolescence

Adolescence is defined as the developmental stage between ages 13 and 19 years.

Physical development

Adolescence is a time of great change. As physical changes occur, adolescents simultaneously struggle with the conflict between asserting independence and still relying on their caregivers.

Time for teens

Many adults anticipate the changes that occur during adolescence with great fear and trepidation. While it can be a turbulent time for the adolescent and their caregivers, it is also a time of exploration and burgeoning independence.

Height and weight

During this time, a teenager's weight almost doubles, and their height increases by 15% to 20%. Females may grow 3 to 6 in (7.5 to 15 cm)/year until age 16 years. Males may grow 3 to 6 in (7.5 to 15 cm)/year until age 18 years. Major organs double in size; the exception is the lymphoid tissue, which decreases in mass.

Males attain greater strength and muscle mass, but motor coordination lags behind growth in stature and musculature. Motor coordination catches up as strength improves.

Development of secondary sex characteristics

The pituitary gland is stimulated at puberty to produce androgen steroids responsible for secondary sex characteristics.

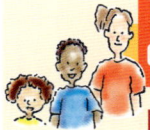

Growing pains

Beginning sexual maturity in females

Breast development and pubic hair growth are the first signs of sexual maturity in females. These illustrations show the development of the female breast and pubic hair in puberty.

Breast development
Stage 1
Only the *papilla* (nipple) elevates (not shown).

Beginning sexual maturity in females (*continued*)

Stage 2
Breast buds appear; the areola is slightly widened and appears as a small mound.

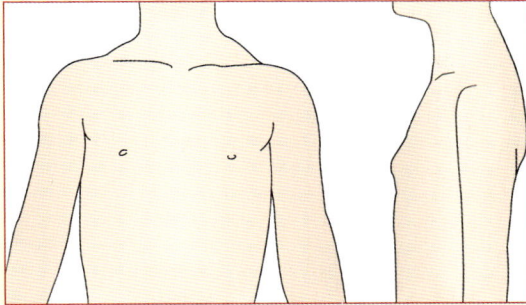

Stage 3
The entire breast enlarges; the nipple doesn't protrude.

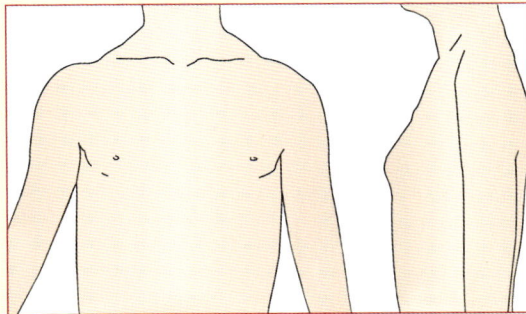

Stage 4
The breast enlarges; the nipple and the papilla protrude and appear as a secondary mound.

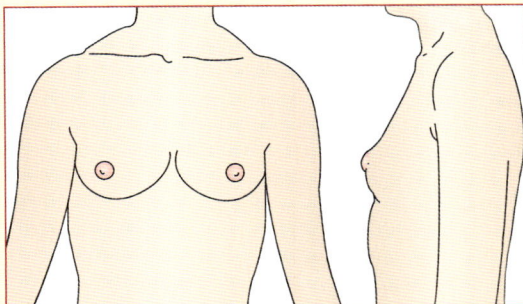

(*continued*)

Beginning sexual maturity in females (*continued*)

Stage 5
The adult breast has developed; the nipple protrudes, and the areola no longer appears separate from the breast.

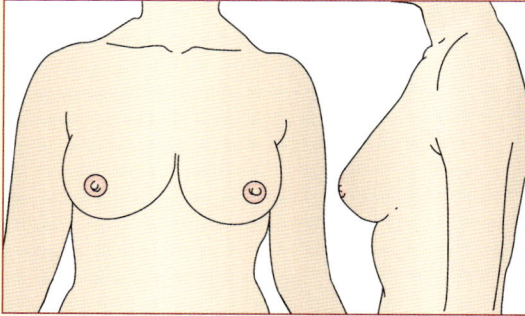

Pubic hair development
Stage 1
No pubic hair is present.

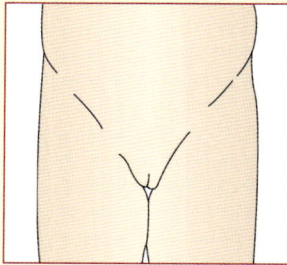

Stage 2
Straight hair begins to appear on the labia and extends between stages 2 and 3.

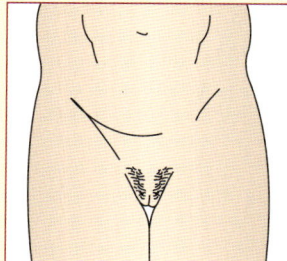

Beginning sexual maturity in females (*continued*)

Stage 3

Pubic hair increases in quantity; it appears darker, curled, and denser and begins to form the typical (but smaller in quantity) female triangle.

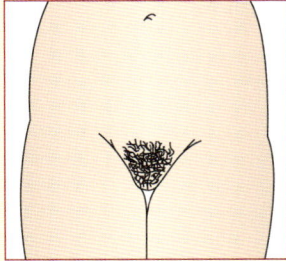

Stage 4

Pubic hair is denser and more curled; with a distribution that is more adult-like but less abundant than in adults.

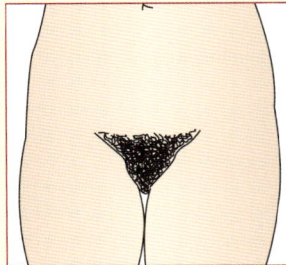

Stage 5

Pubic hair is abundant, appears in an adult female pattern, and may extend onto the medial part of the thighs.

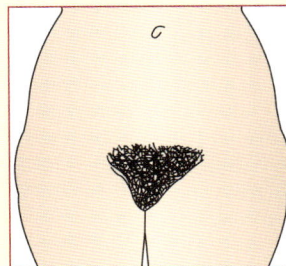

(*continued*)

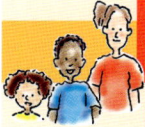

Growing pains

Beginning sexual maturity in males

Genital development and pubic hair growth are the first signs of sexual maturity in males. The following illustrations show the development of the male genitalia and pubic hair in puberty.

Stage 1
No pubic hair is present.

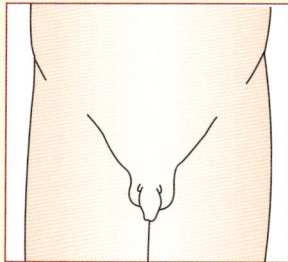

Stage 2
Downy hair develops laterally and later becomes dark; the scrotum becomes more textured, and the penis and testes may become larger.

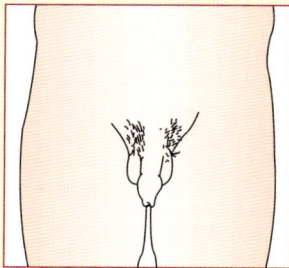

Stage 3
Pubic hair extends across the pubis; the scrotum and testes are larger; the penis enlarges in length.

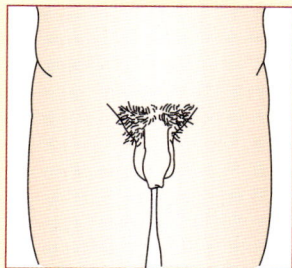

Beginning sexual maturity in males (*continued*)

Stage 4
Pubic hair becomes more abundant and curls, and the genitalia resemble those of adults; the glans penis has become larger and broader, and the scrotum becomes darker.

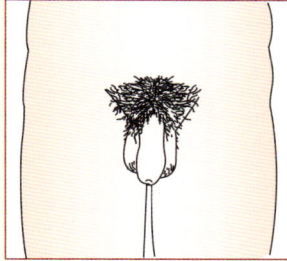

Stage 5
Pubic hair resembles adults in quality and pattern, and the hair extends to the inner borders of the thighs; the testes and scrotum reach adult size.

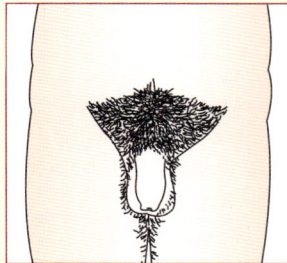

Secondary sex signs

Female secondary sexual development during puberty involves increases in the size of the ovaries, uterus, vagina, labia, and breasts. The first visible sign of sexual maturity is the appearance of breast buds (thelarche). Next, body hair appears in the pubic area and under the arms, and menarche occurs. The ovaries, present at birth, remain inactive until puberty.

Male secondary sexual development consists of genital growth and the appearance of pubic and body hair.

Androgens and estrogens

The trigger that starts puberty is unknown. What *is* clear is that, for some reason, the hypothalamus produces gonadotropin-releasing hormone, which triggers the anterior pituitary gland to produce follicle-stimulating hormone (FSH) and luteinizing hormone (LH).

FSH and LH initiate the ovulation cycle in females and promote testicular maturation and sperm production in males.

Tanner staging

The development of secondary sex characteristics occurs in an anticipated sequence for females and males and is divided into distinct stages called *Tanner stages*. Although the timing of the stages is different for each person, the sequence remains the same.

Menstruation and spermatogenesis

During early adolescence (ages 11 to 14 years), most females achieve menarche. Most males achieve active spermatogenesis at ages 12 to 15 years.

Teeth

The secondary (permanent) teeth are all present during the early adolescent years. The third molars (also known as *wisdom teeth*) may need to be extracted if impaction occurs.

Psychological development

Psychological development during adolescence revolves around socialization. As the teen ventures into the world outside their own family and is exposed to other viewpoints, peers become increasingly important, and greater independence is desired. Activities with friends start to gain importance over family-centered activities.

Psychosocial development

Adolescence is the period in which the child enters Erickson stage of identity versus role confusion. Changes in the adolescent's body are taking place rapidly, and they are preoccupied with how they look and with how others view them. While trying to meet the expectations of their peers, they are also trying to establish their own identity.

Early adolescence

During early adolescence, the teen begins to show more interest in the opposite sex, though the peer group usually consists of same-sex friends.

Rebel with a question

Conformity to peer group standards (which may conflict with family values) is of utmost importance at this time. This may lead to rebellion and questioning of caregiver's and other adult authority.

Middle adolescence

The teen becomes more self-assured during middle adolescence, and independent decision-making skills are tested.

The young and the tasteless

Activities outside the home are a priority, and teenager commonly defines themselves by whatever the peer group has determined to be important. For example, they might wear what other teens in the group wear, use the common language the peer group has decided on, and align their music tastes and other preferences with the crowd.

Late adolescence

During the late teen years, adolescent rebellion has diminished. The young adult has a fairly strong sense of who they are but may not yet have committed to a particular occupation or role in life.

Cognitive development

During adolescence, the teen moves from the concrete thinking of childhood into Piaget stage of *formal operational thought*. The teen can now reason logically about abstract concepts and derive conclusions from hypothetical premises.

I can see clearly now . . .

They can imagine events in the future instead of focusing on the present as they did in childhood. Because the future becomes a possibility, the teen may be more receptive to education that focuses on health promotion and has future benefits as a result of current behaviors.

One step forward, two steps back

Although abstract thinking becomes more refined, the teen may revert to concrete thinking during times of stress. Teens may also act impulsively or seem to disregard consequences, often behaving as though they are invincible.

Moral and spiritual development

Kohlberg conventional level of moral development continues into early adolescence. In this phase, the child does what is right because it is a socially acceptable action. The child continues to advance in moral reasoning as their cognition develops.

In with the in-crowd

The teen becomes increasingly dependent on their peer group for approval and associates good behavior with "fitting in" with the crowd. Morality may be dependent on the situation and relationship to a particular person. Peer pressure often overrides the teen's own moral reasoning.

At long last—my own person

As adolescence ends, the teen enters Kohlberg *postconventional*, or *principled, level of moral development*. They start to question and discard the status quo and choose values for themselves, not necessarily what is dictated by their peers. Although they may appreciate the peer group's opinions, they are now capable of forming a moral decision independent of the group.

What's the meaning of life?

Teens may formulate questions about the larger world as they consider religion; philosophy; and the values held by caregivers, friends, and other influential people in their lives. Adolescents may be suspicious of caregiver's religious views, and curiosity about other religious beliefs is normal. Teens sort through and adopt those religious beliefs that are consistent with their moral character.

Look, I'm legal!

A teen's worldview becomes solidified during this time. Society may consider them to be a young adult, and laws and cultural norms reinforce this perception. By the age 18 years, they are allowed to vote, and by the age 21 years, they are considered a full adult with the rights and responsibilities that go along with that status. Even so, adolescents might remain somewhat dependent on their caregivers for finances and for help in meeting adult expectations.

Keys to health

Health issues during adolescence include nutrition, sleep and rest, exercise, and dental hygiene.

Nutrition

Because physical changes are so drastic during adolescence, nutritional needs are greater than at any other time in a person's life.

Run a little, eat a lot

Activity plays a large role in a teen's caloric requirements for maintaining weight. An active teenager playing sports for several hours per day may need more than 3,000 kcal/day, whereas an inactive adolescent female may have to take in fewer than 2,000 kcal to prevent weight gain. In addition, iron and protein needs increase as females begin the menstruation cycle and males begin to develop lean muscle mass.

Got milk?

Because bone growth is so critical during adolescence, teens need to ensure the proper intake of calcium and vitamin D. From the preteen years through adolescence, daily calcium intake should be between 1,200 and 1,500 mg/day. To achieve adequate levels, teens need to consume at least three servings of calcium-fortified foods per day. Thus, it is important for providers to ask adolescents if they regularly consume dairy or other calcium-containing foods such as broccoli, spinach, tofu, or legumes.

Teens often are responsible for their own food choices and form food preferences. Caregivers should continue to offer nutritionally balanced snacks and meals that will become lifelong choices for teens. Given that breakfast and lunch are often provided by schools, caregivers and students should advocate for higher nutritional standards in the selections offered in the school setting.

Sleep and rest

Sleep needs vary from person-to-person, but teens require 8 to 10 hours of sleep each night, and those hours can't be made up or stored. Therefore, "catch-up" sleep on the weekends is not effective in replenishing a teen's sleep store.

Exercise

Physical fitness and exercise are important for several health-related reasons. With obesity in adolescents on the rise in the United States, regular aerobic exercise can help maintain a healthy weight and prevent excessive gain. It also promotes a healthy cardiovascular system by reducing and preventing high blood pressure and hyperlipidemia. Attention to strength training with weights also promotes bone health, especially in females.

Running from depression

Physical fitness may also help prevent periods of depression and help foster relationships between peers.

Dental hygiene

Good dental hygiene should consist of brushing at least twice daily, flossing once daily, and professional cleanings twice a year. Teens should avoid snacks high in sugar and sticky candies that could cause dental caries. Teens may also experience orthodontic intervention to straighten secondary teeth.

Coping with concerns

Adolescents and their caregivers are typically faced with a range of concerns that may be intensified by the teen's need for peer approval and their desire to assert their independence.

Acne

During adolescence, acne may become a problem. It is caused by blockage of follicles as a result of excessive sebum or bacteria. Acne has been associated with hormones due to the prevalence of flare-ups during a female's premenstrual period.

Acne is found primarily on the face but can also appear on the chest and back. It is usually seen by the naked eye and treated with topical agents or antibiotics for inflammatory lesions.

No laughing matter

Acne can be devastating during this time of life when appearance is of the utmost concern. Even mild to moderate acne can have lasting negative effects on self-esteem and a teen's ability and willingness to develop friendships and other relationships. In severe cases, embarrassment and isolation can lead to depression.

For these reasons, acne should be considered a serious problem that warrants intervention rather than a "phase" that a teen should simply "wait to grow out of." Treatments can include topical medications and oral antibiotics. Teens should be advised not to pick or pop acne lesions as this can contribute to scarring.

Body piercings and tattoos

Teens use body piercings and tattoos to make a "statement" about their sense of style and to express their individuality. For health reasons, such as the risk of hepatitis C, piercings and tattoos should be performed by an experienced, licensed person. Many states have age limits for these procedures. It is important not to pass judgment on the teen who chooses to get a tattoo or piercing. Rather, consider their choice as an opportunity to provide education on the subject which, in turn, helps the teen make an informed decision.

Cigarette smoking and e-cigarettes

Despite an overall decline in adolescents using nicotine products in 2019–2020, there are still 4.7 million middle and high school students using these products (approximately 1:6 children). E-cigarettes (vaping) constituted approximately 19% of all high schoolers intake of nicotine and 4% of all middle schoolers. The Centers for Disease Control and Prevention (CDC) has hypothesized that the decrease in nicotine use may be because the age to legally buy cigarettes has increased from 18 to 21 years and that the flavors of vaping liquid have become tightly regulated due to concerns for addiction and targeting of younger children. It is imperative that health promotion regarding nicotine addresses the dangers of vaping, traditional cigarettes, cigars, hookahs, chewing tobacco, and pipes.

Dangling the bait

Peer influence and family practices have a tremendous influence on teen smoking. Teens may start smoking or using e-cigarettes to "look cool" or "fit in" with their peer groups. Nearly 7 in 10 teens are exposed to advertising for cigarettes and e-cigarettes.

A slippery slope

Tobacco use can be associated with increasingly risky behaviors, such as alcohol misuse and drug misuse. The American Lung Association has instituted a voluntary program in the public school system that uses peer counseling to educate teens on the dangers and health consequences of smoking.

Injury prevention

When a child reaches school age, they are no longer under their caregivers' constant supervision. Because of this unfamiliar freedom, school-age children and adolescents can sustain a range of serious, sometimes life-threatening, injuries.

Firearms

Death by gun violence is now the leading cause of death for those under 18 years of age. Curiosity about how a gun operates coupled with easy access to firearms along with an attitude that it "won't happen to me" could have deadly consequences. Caregivers should educate teens on the safe use of a firearm but always practice safe gun storage. A loaded gun should never be stored in the home, and the ammunition and unloaded gun should be securely stored in separate areas. Caregivers should also place trigger locks on their firearms.

Motor vehicle accidents

Motor vehicle collisions are one of the leading causes of death among teens. During the late teen years, the adolescent is legally eligible for a driver's license. However, with greater privilege comes increased responsibility. Nurses can provide education that may reduce motor vehicle collisions. This includes information about distracted driving, minimizing cell phone use in a car, and the dangers of speeding as well as driving under the influence of drugs or alcohol. Teens may be reluctant to listen to their caregivers but may engage in a conversation with another trusted authority figure.

Will parallel parking be on the final exam?

State law requires teens to pass written and practical driving tests before being issued a driver's license. Some public high schools offer driver education classes as part of their curriculum. Many states have graduated driver's licenses for new teen drivers. New drivers typically must pass through three stages to receive their full driver's license: a learner's permit, a probationary license, and finally, a full driver's license. Graduated driver's licenses often limit nighttime, expressway, and unsupervised driving during the early stages. The restrictions lift with time, concluding with the teen receiving a full driver's license.

Texting while driving

Distracted driving leads to collisions. Unfortunately, about 39% of teens and young adults ages 15 to 25 years reported texting while driving. Of these teens and young adults, they also had a higher incidence of infrequent seat belt use, riding with a driver under the influence, and drinking and driving themselves than those who did not text while driving.

Buckled up for safety

A teen should be taught that wearing a seat belt, no matter what seat they are in, can drastically reduce the risk of life-threatening injuries in the event of an accident. They should also be encouraged to use a helmet when operating vehicles such as motorcycles, all-terrain vehicles (ATVs), or mopeds.

A deadly mix

Perhaps, the greatest emphasis should be placed on educating adolescents about the risks of mixing driving with alcohol or drug use. Not only is the combination illegal, but it also impairs the driver's judgment and could have deadly consequences.

Risk-taking behaviors

Teenagers are still maturing, both cognitively and emotionally. A lack of maturity may lead them to take unwise chances to be accepted by their peers.

Risky business

Teens often have an "it can't happen to me" attitude and feel they are invincible. They may take risks to seek attention and acceptance from others or to distract from failures in school, rejection by peers, neglect at home, or a combination of these factors. A teen tends to be less of a risk taker if they have established autonomy and respect their caregivers and other authority figures.

Sports injuries

Although there is the potential for injury in any sport, most injuries occur during recreational sporting events rather than during organized competitions. Serious injuries are common during recreational and individual sports.

In any case, although injuries are usually random events, the risk of injury can be decreased by improving playing conditions, demanding adherence to rules and protective equipment, and providing diligent coaching and supervision.

Injury protection

The nurse can help prevent sports injuries through education about the proper use of safety equipment and potential risks for injury. Teens need to be encouraged to use helmets when skateboarding, riding bicycles, snowmobiles, and ATVs. They should be encouraged to wear other protective equipment, such as pads and mouthguards, when playing contact sports. Pre- and postseason evaluation for concussion may be warranted in middle- and high-school-level sports. For those who have experienced a concussion, follow-up evaluation for recovery and return to normal activities should be made by a health care provider.

Slow down, you move too fast

Because a teen's body is physically maturing, they need to realize their own limitations to avoid straining or overextending themselves until their body is more able to perform a physically challenging task. After experiencing an injury, a teen must be encouraged to follow rehabilitation instructions to prevent further injury or reinjury.

Health problems

Several serious health problems can affect school-age children and adolescents. Some of these problems may be life threatening.

Alcohol and drug misuse

Alcohol misuse disorder is a chronic disorder most commonly described as the uncontrolled intake of alcoholic beverages. *Psychoactive substance misuse and dependence* is the use of illegal drugs or misuse of legal drugs, including narcotics/opioids, stimulants, depressants, antianxiety agents, and hallucinogens. Alcohol and substance misuse impair physical and mental health, social and familial relationships, and the ability to uphold responsibilities related to school and jobs.

It's old school

Today, children are not waiting to take their first drink of alcohol or "experiment" with drugs. Alcohol and drugs are readily available to school-age children, making substance misuse a problem of enormous proportions.

What causes it

Numerous biologic, psychological, and sociocultural factors may cause alcohol and substance misuse disorders. Family background may play a significant role, as the child of one caregiver with alcohol misuse disorder is three to four times more likely to develop alcohol misuse disorder than a peer without such a parent.

Psychologically speaking

Psychological factors that may lead to alcohol or drug misuse include:
- inadequate coping skills, leading to the urge to reduce anxiety and tension by using substances
- having a history of posttraumatic stress disorder (PTSD)
- having a history of attention deficit hyperactivity disorder (ADHD)
- experiencing anxiety, depression, or loneliness.

Socioculturally speaking

Sociocultural factors that may cause alcohol or drug misuse include:
- the availability of alcohol and drugs
- group or peer pressure
- societal attitudes that condone alcohol or drug use.

What to look for

Substance use disorder is defined as a maladaptive pattern of substance use leading to clinically significant impairments in health, social function, and control over substance use. These impairments may manifest as one or more of the following occurring within a 12-month period:
- Recurrent substance use resulting in a failure to fulfill major role obligations at work, school, or home

- Recurrent substance use in situations in which using the substance is physically hazardous
- Legal problems secondary to substance use
- Continued substance use despite persistent or recurrent social or interpersonal problems caused by or exacerbated by its effects

Ups and downs

People with chronic substance misuse may present with a variety of minor complaints, such as mood swings and depression, malaise, and an increased incidence of infection. They may also experience periods of sobriety that will also affect their mood and functioning.

Something smells fishy

The effects on personal appearance may include poor personal hygiene, unexplained injuries (such as cigarette burns), and nutritional deficiencies.

I've got a secret

The teen or child may be secretive about their substance use and may engage in suspicious behaviors, such as lying and stealing money, to support their habit. The school may report multiple, unexplained absences; poor classroom performance; and behavior pattern changes. When confronted about their behavior, the child may deny the problem or become angry toward others.

Acute intoxication

With acute alcohol or drug intoxication, look for one or any number of the following:
- Decreased inhibitions
- Euphoria followed by depression or hostility
- Impaired judgment
- Lack of coordination
- Respiratory depression
- Slurred speech
- Unconsciousness
- Vomiting

What tests tell you

Urine, blood, and saliva tests can confirm drug use and blood alcohol level, determine the amount and type of substance taken, and reveal some clinical complications.

Complications

Most body tissues can be adversely affected by the heavy intake of alcohol, and abrupt alcohol withdrawal can cause death. (See *Complications of alcohol misuse*.)

Complications of alcohol misuse

Alcohol can damage body tissues by its direct irritating effects, changes that take place in the body during its metabolism, aggravation of existing diseases, injuries occurring during intoxication, and interactions between alcohol and drugs. Such tissue damage can lead to a range of both short- and long-term complications, including the following.

Cardiopulmonary complications
- Cardiac dysrhythmia
- Cardiomyopathy
- Chronic obstructive pulmonary disease
- Essential hypertension
- Increased risk of tuberculosis
- Pneumonia

Hepatic complications
- Alcoholic hepatitis
- Cirrhosis
- Fatty liver

Gastrointestinal complications
- Chronic diarrhea
- Esophageal cancer
- Esophageal varices
- Esophagitis
- Gastric ulcers
- Gastritis

- Gastrointestinal (GI) bleeding
- Malabsorption
- Pancreatitis

Neurologic complications
- Alcohol-related dementia
- Alcoholic hallucinosis
- Alcohol withdrawal delirium
- Korsakoff syndrome
- Peripheral neuropathy
- Seizure disorders
- Subdural hematoma
- Wernicke encephalopathy

Psychiatric complications
- Amotivational syndrome
- Depression
- Impaired social and occupational functioning
- Misuse of multiple substances
- Suicide

Other complications
- Beriberi
- Hypoglycemia
- Leg and foot ulcers
- Prostatitis
- Fetal alcohol syndrome (from alcohol misuse while pregnant)

Chronic misuse of drugs, especially intravenous (IV) use, can lead to life-threatening complications, including:
- cardiac and respiratory arrest, subacute bacterial endocarditis, pulmonary emboli, and respiratory infections
- intracranial hemorrhage
- vasculitis, thrombophlebitis, and gangrene
- musculoskeletal dysfunction
- acquired immunodeficiency syndrome (AIDS) and hepatitis
- tetanus and septicemia
- malnutrition
- trauma
- depression, psychosis, and increased risk of suicide.

How it's treated

Treatment for alcohol and substance misuse disorders must be long term and requires the support of the child's caregivers and other significant people in their life.

Alcohol misuse disorder

Total abstinence from alcohol is commonly thought to be the most effective treatment for alcohol misuse disorder. Participation in supportive programs, including Alcoholics Anonymous, may help to produce favorable long-term results, though failure and relapse rates are high. The recovering person must also be able to fill the niche once occupied by alcohol with something constructive and meaningful.

Symptom support

Acute intoxication is treated symptomatically by:
- supporting respiration
- preventing aspiration of vomitus
- replacing fluids
- initiating emergency treatment for trauma, infection, electrolyte abnormalities, and GI bleeding.

Drug misuse

Treatment of drug dependence commonly involves a triad of care: detoxification, short- and long-term rehabilitation, and aftercare (meaning a prolonged abstinence from problematic substances). Aftercare is usually aided by participation in Narcotics Anonymous or a similar self-help group.

Slowly but surely

The teen with acute drug intoxication should receive symptomatic treatment based on the drug ingested. Detoxification with the same drug or a pharmacologically similar drug may be necessary. Depending on the dosage and the time elapsed since ingestion, additional treatment may include gastric lavage, induced emesis, activated charcoal, or forced diuresis.

What to do

- Be alert for potential problems related to alcohol and drug misuse. Ask the teen about their own use of substances and about their friends' usage. Ensure confidentiality when legally able, ask questions, and provide information in a straightforward manner to promote an open discussion.
- Be aware of signs and symptoms of intoxication with alcohol and commonly used drugs, so you will be prepared to identify them if seen in a patient.

- During an acute intoxication:
  - ○ Continuously monitor the patient's vital signs.
  - ○ Observe for complications of overdose and withdrawal, such as cardiopulmonary arrest, seizures, and aspiration.

  After an acute intoxication:
- Refer the patient for detoxification and rehabilitation as appropriate and provide a list of available community resources, such as meeting times and places for Alcoholics Anonymous and Narcotics Anonymous.
- Refer caregivers of a child in crisis to an organization such as Parents Anonymous.
- Monitor the patient for signs of depression or impending suicide.
- Encourage family members to seek professional counseling help whether or not the patient does so.

Sexually transmitted infections

An important group of infections that are transmitted through sexual contact include:
- human immunodeficiency virus (HIV) or HIV/AIDS
- chancroid
- chlamydial infections
- genital herpes
- genital warts
- gonorrhea
- lymphogranuloma venereum
- syphilis
- trichomoniasis.

They're everywhere

Sexually transmitted infections (STIs) are among the most prevalent infections around the world. The most common STIs in adolescents are gonorrhea, chlamydial infections, and genital warts, though cases of syphilis have been rising rapidly.

What causes it

The cause of an STI may be bacterial, viral, or parasitic. (See *Common STIs.*)

Common STIs

This chart lists several STIs along with their causative organisms, assessment findings, and appropriate treatments (including for patients who are pregnant).

STI	Assessment findings	Treatment
Chlamydia *Chlamydia trachomatis*	• No symptoms (commonly); suspicion should be raised if partner has been treated for nongonococcal urethritis. • Heavy, gray-white vaginal discharge • Painful urination • Positive chlamydial urine test or vaginal culture using special chlamydial test kit	• Single dose azithromycin, preferred; doxycycline for those >8 years of age is second-line treatment or for those with penicillin allergy.
Syphilis *Treponema pallidum*	• Painless ulcer on vulva or vagina (primary syphilis) • Hepatic and splenic enlargement, headache, anorexia, and maculopapular rash on the palms of the hands and soles of the feet (secondary syphilis; occurring about 2 months after initial infection) • Cardiac, vascular, and central nervous system changes (tertiary syphilis; occurring after an undetermined latent phase) • Positive Venereal Disease Research Laboratory serum test; confirmed with positive rapid plasma regain and fluorescent treponemal antibody absorption tests • Dark-field microscopy positive for spirochete	• Penicillin G benzathine (Bicillin L-A) intramuscularly (IM) (single dose) or 14-day course of doxycycline for those with penicillin allergy
Genital herpes Herpes simplex virus, type 2	• Painful, small vesicles with erythematous base on vulva, vagina, or penis, rupturing within 1–7 days to form ulcers • Low-grade fever • Dyspareunia • Positive viral culture of vesicular fluid • Positive enzyme-linked immunosorbent assay	• Acyclovir (Zovirax) orally or famciclovir or valacyclovir all for 7–10 days
Gonorrhea *Neisseria gonorrhoeae*	• May not produce symptoms • Yellow-green vaginal discharge • Male partner who experiences severe pain on urination and purulent yellow penile discharge • Positive gonorrheal urine test or culture of vaginal, rectal, or urethral secretions	• Ceftriaxone (Rocephin) as a one-time IM injection for those >45 kg For those <45 kg, ceftriaxone IV or IM 25–50 mg/kg not to exceed 250 mg IM
Condyloma acuminata Human papillomavirus (HPV)	• Discrete papillary structures that spread, enlarge, and coalesce to form large lesions; increasing in size during pregnancy • Possible secondary ulceration and infection with foul odor	• For external anogenital warts: Imiquimod 3.75% or 5% cream (patient applied) • For vaginal, cervical, or intraanal warts: cryotherapy with liquid nitrogen or surgical removal

How it happens

STIs are passed from one person to another through anal, oral, or vaginal sexual contact. The rate of transmission and, therefore, the incidence of these diseases, are rising because people may have multiple sexual partners, a lack of health promotion for condom use or abstinence, and increased reporting of new cases.

When STIs are diagnosed in children who are school age or younger, child abuse must be investigated.

What to look for

Symptoms vary depending on the infectious organism and may vary by biologic sex. Some classic symptoms of STIs include:

- pain during urination
- vaginal or penile discharge
- growths that appear on the genitalia and sores on the mouth or genitalia
- evidence of sexual abuse, such as vaginal tears, vaginal bruising, blood in the child's underwear, and difficulties voiding. (Never assume that a child of any age, including a teen, has acquired an STI by consensual sexual contact.)

What tests tell you

A sexual history provides the basis for the prevention, diagnosis, and treatment of an STI. The physical assessment, primarily a diagnostic tool, can also serve as an excellent opportunity for patient education.

Identify the STI

To help identify the infectious organism, an appropriate urine test may be ordered (for gonorrhea and chlamydia), or the suspected lesion is cultured using the appropriate method:

- A genital tract specimen from a male should contain urethral discharge or prostatic fluid.
- From a female, the specimen should contain urethral or cervical specimens.
- Two swabs should always be collected simultaneously.

Privacy is paramount

Keep in mind that examinations of this kind can be extremely difficult and embarrassing for school-age children and teens. Procedures should be explained thoroughly, and as much privacy as possible should be provided. In situations where sexual abuse is suspected, proper forensic collection and examinations should be done by specially trained nurses and health care providers.

Complications

Complications that are common to all STIs include emotional stress, infertility, ectopic pregnancies, and even death.

How it's treated

STIs may be treated with oral or IM antibiotics and antiviral medications. They are also treated symptomatically with analgesics and antipyretics. Some infections, such as herpes, genital warts, and HIV/AIDS, have no known cure but may have medications that can keep viral loads low and symptoms manageable.

What to do

Protection against and prevention of STIs should be the focus of nursing education. This information should be kept in mind when educating about STIs:

- Abstinence is the safest and most effective way to ensure that teens stay free of STIs.
- Although sex education and the availability of condoms in public schools remain controversial, the use of latex condoms for those who are sexually active can protect a teen from acquiring an STI as well as aid in pregnancy prevention.
- Teens should be strongly encouraged to seek medical treatment immediately if they suspect that they have contracted an STI as untreated infections can lead to complications if not addressed.
- If approached by a teen about treatment, remain nonjudgmental and try to address their concerns.
- Urge the teen to inform sexual contacts of their infection so they can receive medical treatment and stress the importance of remaining abstinent until the completion of treatment.
- Remind teens that neither oral contraceptive pills nor intrauterine devices (IUDs) will provide protection against STIs.
- Since 2022, there has been a 32% increase in syphilis cases and a 4% rise in the rates of chlamydia and gonorrhea. Providing support, education, testing, and treatment for teens is important for protecting health and future fertility.
- Confidentiality should be maintained. Every state and the District of Columbia recognize that no caregiver's consent is required for the testing or treatment of STIs, though some states require patients to be at least 12 years of age without needing to notify caregivers.
- Encourage routine vaccination for HPV. Males and females over the age of 9 years can prevent the most common strains of HPV which can lead to cancer later in life. This vaccination series can be initiated during annual well-child visits.

Suicide and attempted suicide

Suicide is the second leading cause of death among 15- to 24-year-olds. The rate of attempted suicides is higher in females, but males are three times more likely to die than females in their attempts. Per the CDC, suicide occurs most frequently in teens of sexual or racial minorities. Teens who identify as LGBTQIA+ or are of indigenous heritage have some of the highest suicide rates.

What to look for

Risk factors include:

- interpersonal conflict or loss
- family discord
- legal or disciplinary problems
- chronic drug or alcohol misuse
- history of physical or sexual abuse
- recent failure or disappointment
- preoccupation with death
- previous suicide attempt. (See *Suicide warning signs.*)

Advice from the experts

Suicide warning signs

During the patient interview, be alert for these signs of suicidal behavior:
- Overwhelming anxiety (the most frequent precipitant of a suicide attempt)
- Withdrawal and social isolation
- Signs and symptoms of depression, including crying, fatigue, helplessness, poor concentration, reduced interest in previously enjoyable activities, sadness, constipation, and weight loss
- Goodbyes expressed to friends and family members
- Giving away prized possessions
- Covert suicide messages and death wishes
- Obvious suicide messages such as "I'd be better off dead."

Complications

After an adolescent or school-age child attempts suicide, they are at a high risk for another attempt. Existing emotional problems may be compounded as they may be stigmatized by their peers or even by adults.

The caregivers of an adolescent or child who dies by suicide must cope with a range of emotions, including intense grief and guilt.

Caregivers are also likely to have complicated feelings even when their child survives a suicide attempt and may become excessively protective of the child.

How it's treated

Treatment for a suicide attempt is based on the underlying reason that led the child or adolescent to feel as if suicide was the only option.

Immediate hospitalization without the adolescent's consent is warranted if the threat of self-harm still exists. Treatment might also involve therapy (both group and individual), medications (such as antidepressants), remediation of social and problem-solving deficits, and family conflict resolution.

What to do

To help deter potential suicide in the child or adolescent with major depression, the nurse should keep certain guidelines in mind. (See *Suicide prevention guidelines*.)

Advice from the experts

Suicide prevention guidelines

To help deter potential suicide in patient with major depression, keep the following guidelines in mind.

Assess for clues
Watch for such clues as:
• communicating suicidal thoughts, threats, and messages and talking about death and feelings of futility
• hoarding medication
• giving away prized possessions
• describing a suicide plan
• changing behavior, especially as depression begins to lift.

Provide a safe environment
Check patient areas and correct dangerous conditions, such as:
• exposed pipes
• windows without safety glass
• access to the roof or open balconies.

Remove dangerous objects
Remove potentially dangerous objects from the patient's environment, such as:
• belts
• razors
• suspenders

(*continued*)

Suicide prevention guidelines (*continued*)

- light and window blind cords
- glass
- knives, guns, and other weapons
- nail files and clippers.

Consult with staff

Include the health care team in aspects of care and be sure to:
- recognize and document both verbal and nonverbal suicidal behaviors
- keep the health care provider informed and share data with all staff
- clarify the patient's specific restrictions
- assess the patient's risk and plan for observation
- clarify day and night staff responsibilities and frequency of consultation.

Observe the patient with suicidal behavior

Take some steps for easy observation of a patient experiencing suicidal behavior, including:
- being alert when the patient is using a sharp object (shaving), taking medication, or using the bathroom (to prevent hanging or other injury)
- assigning the patient to a room near the nurses' station
- continuously monitoring the patient through the use of a patient sitter or other staff members.

Maintain personal contact

Help the patient remain in contact with their environment by:
- reassuring the patient that they are not alone or without resources or hope
- encouraging continuity of care and consistency of primary nurses, while recognizing the professional and emotional strain that this patient population can put on the care team
- helping the patient build emotional ties to others.

Quick quiz

1. What is the first area of the body that is easily recognized as the beginning of the growth spurt in puberty?
   A. Hands, followed by lengthening of the arms
   B. Feet, followed by lengthening of the legs
   C. Shoulder width
   D. Abdominal girth

Answer: B. Different areas of the body reach their peak growth at different times. Changes are easily recognized in the feet, which are the first part of the body to experience a growth spurt. Increased foot size is followed by a rapid increase in leg length and then trunk growth.

2. Which of the following statements is true about physical growth during adolescence?
- A. Males will typically grow much faster than females.
- B. Females typically continue to grow in height until age 21 years.
- C. Most major organs will double in size.
- D. Motor coordination is even with growth in stature and musculature.

Answer: C. Major organs double in size during adolescence; the exception is the lymphoid tissue, which decreases in mass.

3. Because of the effects of menstruation, a female should increase her dietary intake of which of the following?
- A. Calcium
- B. Iron
- C. Carbohydrates
- D. Fats

Answer: B. Iron is needed in the production of the protein hemoglobin, which is vital to carrying oxygen in the blood and is lost during menses.

Scoring

⭐⭐⭐ If you answered all three items correctly, call your caregivers! They'll be proud of the abstract thinking and formal operational thought it took to master the tasks in this chapter.

⭐⭐ If you answered two items correctly, tell your peers! They'll say your understanding of middle childhood and adolescence is "way cool."

⭐ If you answered fewer than two items correctly, don't get upset! Your knowledge of middle childhood and adolescence is due for a growth spurt.

You sure are soaking up a lot of important pediatric information!

Suggested references

American Academy of Child and Adolescent Psychiatry. (2021). *Suicide in children and teens*. https://www.aacap.org/AACAP/Families_and_Youth/Facts_for_Families/FFF-Guide/Teen-Suicide-010.aspx

American Academy of Pediatric Dentistry. (2020a). *Guideline on adolescent oral health care*. http://www.aapd.org/media/Policies_Guidelines/G_Adoleshealth.pdf

American Academy of Pediatric Dentistry. (2020b). *Policy on electronic nicotine delivery systems (ENDS)*. http://www.aapd.org/media/policies_guidelines/p_electroniccig.pdf

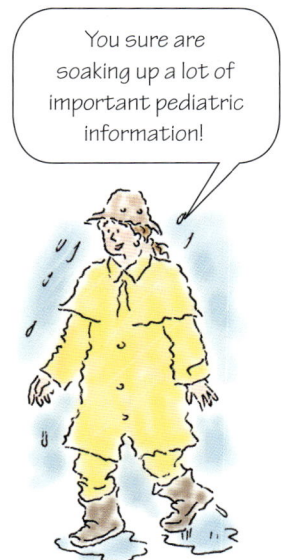

American Academy of Pediatric Dentistry. (2020c). *Policy on tobacco use.* http://www
.aapd.org/media/Policies_Guidelines/P_TobaccoUse.pdf

American Academy of Pediatric Dentistry. (2022). *Periodicity of examination, preventive
dental services, anticipatory guidance/counseling, and oral treatment for infants,
children, and adolescents.* http://www.aapd.org/media/Policies_Guidelines/
BP_Periodicity.pdf

American Academy of Pediatrics. (2023). *Recommendations for preventive pediatric health
care.* https://downloads.aap.org/AAP/PDF/periodicity_schedule.pdf

Centers for Disease Control and Prevention. (2023). *Youth Risk Behavior Survey:
2011–2021.* https://www.cdc.gov/healthyyouth/data/yrbs/pdf/YRBS_Data-
Summary-Trends_Report2023_508.pdf

Gentzke, A. S., Wang, T. W., Jamal, A., Park-Lee, E., Ren, C., Cullen, K. A., & Neff, L.
(2020). Tobacco product use among middle and high school students—
United States, 2020. *MMWR: Morbidity and Mortality Weekly Report, 69,*
1881–1888. https://doi.org/10.15585/mmwr.mm6950a1

Goldstick, J. E., Cunningham, R. M., & Carter, P. M. (2022). Current causes of death
in children and adolescents in the United States. *The New England Journal of
Medicine, 386*(20), 1955–1956. https://doi.org/10.1056/NEJMc2201761

Guttmacher Institute. (2023). *Minors' access to STI services.* https://www.guttmacher.org/
state-policy/explore/minors-access-sti-services

Hampl, S. E., Hassink, S. G., Skinner, A. C., Armstrong, S. C., Barlow, S. E., Bolling,
C. F., Avila Edwards, K. C., Eneli, I., Hamre, R., Joseph, M. M., Lunsford, D.,
Mendonca, E., Michalsky, M. P., Mirza, N., Ochoa, E. R., Sharifi, M., Staiano,
A. E., Weedn, A. E., Flinn, S. K., … Okechukwu, K. (2023). Clinical practice guideline for the evaluation and treatment of children and adolescents
with obesity. *Pediatrics, 151*(2), e2022060640. https://doi.org/10.1542/
peds.2022-060640

Workowski, K. A., Bachmann, L. H., Chan, P. A., Johnston, C. M., Muzny, C. A., Park,
I., Reno, H., Zenilman, J. M., & Bolan, G. A. (2021). Sexually transmitted
infections treatment guidelines, 2021. *MMWR: Morbidity and Mortality Weekly
Report, 70*(4), 1–187. https://doi.org/10.15585/mmwr.rr7004a1

Chapter 14

Infectious diseases

Just the facts

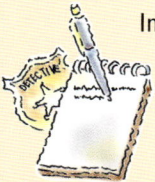

In this chapter, you'll learn:

◆ the chain of infection
◆ recommended immunization practices for infants and children
◆ common childhood infectious diseases of viral and bacterial etiology
◆ nursing interventions for the care of children with viral and bacterial illnesses.

Infection

Infection is the invasion and multiplication of microorganisms in the body. Infection can cause numerous illnesses during childhood, most of which are common, but some of which are less common or even rare.

The severity of illness caused by infection can range from subclinical to life threatening. A thorough understanding of the etiology and symptoms of infectious diseases as well as the appropriate diagnostic and therapeutic interventions will help the nurse provide optimal care.

Chain of infection

Chain of infection is a term used to describe the circle of links needed for the transmission of infectious diseases in humans. All links must be present in the following order for an infection to occur.

1. The chain begins with a pathogen that is capable of producing disease in humans, that is, bacteria, viruses, fungi, or parasites.
2. The reservoir of an infectious agent. This is where the infectious agent will live and grow. Humans are the most common reservoir. Other reservoirs include the environment, hospital settings, water supply, soil, food, and rodents or animals.
3. The third link in the chain is the portal of exit. The pathogen leaves the reservoir via mucus, blood, feces, or urine.

4. The organism is transmitted from one host to another.
5. The fifth link in the chain is the *portal of entry* (the site where disease transmission occurs), through which a pathogen can enter the body by penetrating the skin or a mucous membrane barrier by direct contact or ingestion.
6. The last link is the *host*; a susceptible host is necessary for an infectious disease to be transmitted.

Immature immunity

Infants and children are susceptible to infectious diseases because their immune systems are immature. As children mature and grow, their exposure to infectious agents increases, and they develop antibodies naturally. Subsequent infections with the same pathogen may be less severe or avoided completely.

Stages of infection

Infections follow a predictable sequence of events during transmission that results in five distinct stages of disease.

1. The *incubation stage* is the phase during which the pathogenic organism begins active reproduction in the host; the child has no clinical symptoms but may be contagious to others during this time.
2. The *prodromal stage* is the initial appearance of clinical symptoms in the host; common symptoms include fever, malaise, headache, sore throat, cough, and rhinitis.
3. During the *acute stage*, maximum symptoms are experienced by the host; toxins deposited by the pathogenic organism can produce tissue damage. (Inflammatory changes and tissue damage can also occur because of the host's immune response.)
4. The *convalescent stage* is characterized by progressive elimination of the infection (or elimination of the pathogen), healing of damaged tissue, and symptom resolution.
5. The *resolution stage* is the host's recovery from the infection without residual signs or symptoms of disease.

Cover your mouth, please

The *period of communicability* is the time when the infectious organism may move from the infected host to another person. It varies with different disease states but usually begins during the incubation phase.

Immune protection

Children receive protection from infectious diseases naturally and artificially.

Methods of obtaining immune protection

There are five different methods in which immune protection can be obtained: natural immunity, naturally acquired active immunity, naturally acquired passive immunity, artificially acquired active immunity, and artificially acquired passive immunity.

Natural (innate) immunity

Innate immunity is a combination of natural and nonspecific immunity that can protect the human body from pathogens and foreign agents. For example, the phagocytic action of white blood cells (macrophages) may be triggered by the body's innate ability to recognize and distinguish normal cells from foreign cells. The body's ability to distinguish self from nonself is natural, or innate, immunity.

Naturally acquired active immunity

Naturally acquired active immunity is obtained when the body's immune system responds to a specific pathogen. Antibodies and memory cells prevent or reduce the severity of subsequent infection with that specific pathogen. Naturally acquired active immunity persists for many years.

Naturally acquired passive immunity

Naturally acquired passive immunity involves birthing parent-to-fetus transmission of maternal antibodies.

A gift that keeps on giving . . .

The birthing parent's immunoglobulin G crosses the placenta and is transmitted to the fetus. After birth, the infant can receive passive immunity through antibodies in breast milk.

. . . for up to 2 months

Naturally acquired passive immunity differs from active immunity. Although active immunity lasts many years, or even a lifetime, passive immunity lasts only as long as the antibodies remain in the blood of the fetus or infant (usually from a few weeks to about 2 months). However, some antibodies transferred across the placenta have been isolated up to age 1 year.

Artificially acquired active immunity

Artificially acquired active immunity is achieved by the deliberate administration of a vaccine or toxoid. The vaccine or toxoid stimulates the immune system's production of antibodies against a specific antigen, but symptoms of the disease are not produced in the person receiving the vaccine.

Artificially acquired passive immunity

Artificially acquired passive immunity is conferred when antibodies developed in another person or animal donor are injected into a person. In pediatric patients, this transfer usually involves intravenous (IV) administration of a specific immunoglobulin or *antiserum*. Examples include:

- gamma-globulin (a mixture of antibodies against prevalent community diseases, pooled from human plasma donors)
- hyperimmune or convalescent serum globulin (such as tetanus antitoxin, hepatitis B immune globulin [HBIG], and varicella-zoster immune globulin).

Types of immunizations

Various immunizations are given at specific times to protect pediatric patients from certain diseases. These vaccines fall into three general categories:

- Live, attenuated vaccines
- Inactivated vaccines
- Messenger RNA (mRNA)

Live, attenuated

Live, attenuated vaccines are created from a live organism that is grown under suboptimal conditions to produce a live vaccine with reduced virulence.

Weak but stimulating

Thus, an attenuated immunization contains weakened microorganisms and stimulates immune response and production of antibodies in the host.

Measles, mumps, and rubella—itch, ouch

Examples of live, attenuated vaccines include the measles, mumps, and rubella (MMR) vaccine; the rotavirus vaccine; and the varicella vaccine.

Inactivated

- An inactivated, or *killed*, vaccine confers a weaker response than a live vaccine, necessitating frequent boosters.

Toxoids

Some bacteria, such as diphtheria, produce toxins, which cause disease. The vaccine to prevent a disease caused by a toxin is called a *toxoid*. A toxoid:

- is another form of an inactivated vaccine
- is a toxin that has been specially treated with formalin or heat to weaken its toxic effect but retain its antigenicity
- provides protection by stimulating the production of antibodies.

Inactive but popular

Examples of inactivated vaccines include:

- diphtheria and tetanus toxoids
- inactivated poliovirus vaccine (IPV)
- pertussis vaccine
- hepatitis B (HepB) vaccine.

Other vaccines

Another type of vaccine is the mRNA vaccine which produces proteins to trigger an immune response. An example of an mRNA vaccine is the COVID-19 vaccine.

Immunization schedule

Childhood immunizations include the hepatitis A and B vaccines; COVID-19 vaccine; diphtheria and tetanus toxoids and acellular pertussis (DTaP) vaccine; *Haemophilus influenzae* type B (Hib) vaccine; human papillomavirus (HPV) vaccine; influenza vaccine; IPV vaccine; meningococcal serogroup A, C, W, and Y vaccine, meningococcal B vaccine; MMR vaccine; rotavirus vaccine; varicella virus vaccine; and pneumococcal 15- or 20-valent conjugate vaccine (PCV15 or PCV20). These immunizations are usually given according to a predetermined schedule. (See *Recommended immunization schedule for children.*)

Advice from the experts

Recommended immunization schedule for children

In addition to adhering to the recommended immunization schedule for children listed in the following table, considering these simple steps will help ensure the child's safety.

Before immunization

- Obtain a history of allergic responses, especially life-threatening anaphylactic reactions to antibiotics or past vaccinations (certain vaccinations may be contraindicated in these children).
- Assess the child for moderate or severe illness. Vaccinations may be delayed in these children until they recover. However, a child with a minor illness, such as a cold, may receive immunizations.
- Keep in mind that children receiving corticosteroids for longer than 2 weeks, chemotherapy, or radiation therapy; those with human immunodeficiency virus infection, acquired immunodeficiency syndrome, or another disease that affects the immune system; and those with cancer will need special consideration for vaccination. (They may not be able to receive live virus vaccines, such as MMR, rotavirus, or varicella vaccines.)

(continued)

Recommended immunization schedule for children (*continued*)

After immunization
- Tell caregivers to watch for and report reactions other than local swelling and pain and mild temperature elevation.
- Give caregivers the child's immunization record.

General vaccine recommendations
General vaccine recommendations by the Advisory Committee on Immunization Practices, the American Academy of Pediatrics, and the American Academy of Family Physicians (http://cdc.gov/acip/vaccine-recommendations/index.html).

In the United States, immunization recommendations are governed by the Advisory Committee on Immunization Practices, the American Academy of Pediatrics, and the American Academy of Family Physicians.

COVID-19 vaccine

COVID-19 vaccine is recommended for all children starting at 6 months of age. It is effective in protecting children from serious diseases. There are currently two approved vaccines for children aged 6 months to under 12 years.

Dosing

Depending on the vaccine and the age of the child, the primary series for Moderna is a two-dose series administered 4 to 8 weeks apart or a three-dose series for Pfizer-BioNTech. Boosters are also recommended for certain patients.

Adverse reactions
- Pain at the site
- Swollen lymph nodes
- Irritability or crying
- Sleepiness
- Decrease appetite
- Headache
- Muscle or joint pain
- Chills
- Chest pain

Hepatitis A vaccine

Hepatitis A vaccine is recommended for all children starting at 12 months of age. It is also recommended for people at risk of acquiring hepatitis A. These people include:
- people who live in endemic areas
- military personnel or others traveling to high-risk areas of the world

- people at high risk (Native Americans, Alaskan natives, those with chronic liver disease or clotting factor disorders, homosexual or bisexual adolescent males, or users of injectable and illicit drugs)
- those in close contact with an international adoptee from an endemic area during the first 60 days of arrival in the United States.

Dosing

This vaccine is a series of two doses given starting at age 12 months; the two doses should be administered at least 6 months apart. Children aged 12 months to 18 years receive two doses of 0.5 mL (given at least 6 months apart). Those who are 19 years and older receive 1 mL given intramuscularly (IM) (at least 6 months apart). (See *Tips for pediatric injections*.)

Tips for pediatric injections

When giving a child an injection, the major goals should be minimizing trauma and discomfort while providing safe, efficient administration of a necessary medicine or vaccination.

Minimizing trauma

To most toddlers and preschoolers, and to many older children, the prospect of getting an injection is the most frightening part of a health care visit or even a hospitalization.

Many strategies, including those outlined in the following texts, can be used to reduce the trauma of receiving an injection while establishing trust between the child and the health care team and making future injections easier for the child (and for the nurse who is giving the injection).

Medicine to keep you healthy

- Give the child a simple, age-appropriate explanation for why the injection is being given. When a child is being vaccinated, that explanation might be "This shot will give you medicine to keep you from getting sick." (Young children may think an injection is being given as a punishment and may not even realize that medication is being given.)

- Allow the child to give a "shot" to a doll or stuffed animal; this gives them a sense of control, lets them see that the injection has a beginning and an end, and gives them a concrete understanding of what will happen.

The best policy

- Be honest; tell the child that it will hurt for a moment but that it will be over quickly. (Honesty promotes trust; if a nurse is honest about the potential for pain, the child will believe them when they tell the child something will not hurt.)

Coping and comfort

- Give the child a coping strategy, such as squeezing their caregiver's hand, counting to five, singing a song, and looking away.
- Have a caregiver hold and comfort the child while the injection is being given. A caregiver's presence reassures the child that nothing truly bad will happen. (The child may actually cry more when a caregiver is present, but this is because they feel safe enough to do so.)

Praise and cover

- When the injection has been given, tell the child that "the hurting part" is over and praise them for what a good job they did (regardless of how they reacted). Never

(*continued*)

Tips for pediatric injections (*continued*)

tell a child to "be brave," "be a good boy or be a good girl," or not to cry because these requests will set the child up for failure.

• Give the child a bandage. (A young child may not believe the "hurting part" is over until a bandage has been applied.)

• Always give injections in a designated treatment area. Avoid performing painful procedures in a playroom or, if possible, in the child's hospital room because they need to know there are places where they can feel completely safe.

Giving the injection

• Apply firm pressure at the site for 10 to 15 seconds immediately before giving the injection to decrease discomfort (a numbing patch may be used).

• When two or more injections are needed, the nurse may give them simultaneously in different extremities. Have two or more nurses to assist (and provide manual restraint, if needed) during the procedures. (The child has only one painful experience when multiple injections are given simultaneously. This is believed to be less traumatic than receiving painful injections one after the other.)

• Apply bandages to each site and immediately comfort and console the child following the injections.

• Always keep resuscitation equipment and epinephrine readily available in case of an anaphylactic response to an immunization.

Adverse reactions

Adverse reactions to the hepatitis A vaccine are rare. Administration is contraindicated for those with febrile illness or bleeding disorders.

Hepatitis B vaccine

HepB vaccine is indicated for infants, children, and adolescents to prevent hepatitis B. Acquired during childhood or adolescence, hepatitis B can cause acute illness, with anorexia, jaundice, diarrhea, vomiting, and fatigue. It can also have fatal long-term consequences from cirrhosis or liver cancer. The virus that causes hepatitis B can be spread by:

• passing of the virus from an infected birthing parent to their infant during birth
• having unprotected sexual intercourse with an infected person
• IV drug abuse or inadvertent needlestick injuries
• exposure to infected blood or body fluids.

Dosing

Various vaccine formulations are available in different strengths. Read the label carefully to determine the proper dosage for pediatric use.

Baby's first vaccine

The vaccine is given IM at birth (or before hospital discharge) and again at ages 1 to 4 months and ages 6 to 18 months, for a total of three doses. For older children and adolescents, the initial IM dose should be given as early as possible, with the second dose given 1 month later, and the third dose given 6 months after the first dose.

Positive caregiver, need an extra vaccine

Before immunizing a neonate, check the results of the birthing parent's hepatitis B surface antigen (HBsAg) test. If the birthing parent is HBsAg-positive, the vaccine must be given within 12 hours of birth, along with HBIG (also within 12 hours of birth) administered in two different sites, regardless of weight.

If the HBsAg status is unknown and the birth weight is greater than 2,000 g, administer HepB vaccine within 12 hours. If the birthing parent is HBsAg-positive, administer HBIG as soon as possible, not later than 7 days (in a separate limb). If the infant's birth weight is less than 2,000 g, administer HepB vaccine and HBIG in separate limbs within 12 hours of birth.

Adverse reactions

Common reactions are pain and redness at the site of injection and elevated liver enzymes. Mild to moderate fever may occur (more common in children and adolescents than in adults). Anaphylaxis is rare.

DTaP vaccine

The DTaP vaccine is given to protect infants and young children from acquiring diphtheria, tetanus, and pertussis. The bacterium that causes diphtheria can create a toxin that damages tissue and attacks the heart and nerves. Such an attack can be fatal. Tetanus can cause muscle spasms that can interfere with breathing, which can lead to death. Pertussis is particularly dangerous for young children, especially infants younger than age 1 year, who are most at risk for complications and death.

Dosing

The dosage for the DTaP vaccine is 0.5 mL given IM at ages 2 months, 4 months, 6 months, 15 to 18 months, and 4 to 6 years, for a total of five doses. The tetanus, diphtheria, and acellular pertussis (Tdap) vaccine is given as a booster between ages 11 and 12 years, and a tetanus and diphtheria toxoids (Td) booster is then given at 10-year intervals.

Adverse reactions

Fever, fussiness, and anorexia are common adverse reactions as well as redness, pain, and swelling at the injection site. Redness, pain, and swelling at the injection site occur more commonly after the fourth or fifth dose in the DTaP series. Anaphylaxis, fever above 102°F (38.9°C), persistent crying for 3 hours or longer, and seizures are rare but severe reactions that require emergency treatment.

Hib vaccine

The Hib vaccine is used to prevent infection with *H. influenzae* type B. This infection can lead to severe invasive illnesses, including meningitis, epiglottitis, and pneumonia. Before the vaccine, *H. influenzae* type B was the most common cause of meningitis, sepsis, epiglottitis, and pneumonia in children older than age 1 month, but vaccination with the Hib vaccine has drastically reduced the incidence.

Dosing

The Hib vaccine dosage is 0.5 mL given IM for three or four doses. Schedules for different product preparations vary. (Refer to the manufacturer's guidelines and package inserts.)

Three for PedvaxHIB . . .

For the PedvaxHIB preparation, three total doses are recommended, with the first given at age 2 months, the second at age 4 months, and the third at ages 12 to 15 months.

. . . Hiberix, Act get one dose more

For other preparations, such as ActHIB and Hiberix, four total doses are recommended, with the first given at age 2 months, the second at age 4 months, the third at age 6 months, and the fourth at ages 12 to 15 months.

Adverse reactions

Common adverse reactions are low-grade fever, localized pain, redness, and swelling at the injection site. Anaphylaxis is rare.

Human papillomavirus vaccine

The HPV vaccine is available for children aged 9 years and older to protect against HPV, which is associated with increased risk for developing certain cancers.

Dosing

HPV vaccine is 0.5 mL administered in two- or three-dose series (depending on the age started) IM. The vaccine series is usually offered around 11 to 12 years of age on a 0- and 6-month schedule. If started 15 years and older, a three-dose series schedule should be administered at 0, 1 to 2, and 6 months after the first dose.

Adverse reactions

Side effects associated with the HPV vaccine include fainting and injuries associated with falling, dizziness, pain at site, fever, and nausea. The Centers for Disease Control and Prevention (CDC) and U.S. Food and Drug Administration (FDA) recommend that patients sit or lie down for 15 minutes after the injection.

IPV

The IPV is recommended to prevent infection with the poliovirus. The live trivalent oral poliovirus vaccine (OPV) is no longer used in the United States.

Dosing

The IPV dose is 0.5 mL administered subcutaneously (SC) at ages 2 months, 4 months, 6 to 18 months, and 4 to 6 years, for a total of four doses.

Adverse reactions

Localized pain, redness, and swelling at the injection site are common adverse reactions, although IPV is safe and usually well tolerated. Anaphylaxis is rare.

MMR vaccine

The MMR vaccine stimulates immunity against measles, mumps, and rubella. Because the vaccine contains a live virus, it is contraindicated during pregnancy. Patients should not become pregnant within 1 month of immunization.

Intact immunity required

Live virus should not be administered to anyone receiving immunosuppressive therapy or to those with immunodeficiency diseases.

Dosing

The MMR vaccine dose is 0.5 mL administered SC at ages 12 to 15 months and again at ages 4 to 6 years, for a total of two doses.

Adverse reactions

Common adverse reactions to the MMR vaccine are low-grade fever for 1 week after immunization; localized pain, redness, and swelling at the injection site; rash; and joint pain. Severe reactions are rare but include viral encephalopathy and anaphylaxis.

Meningococcal vaccine

There are two available meningococcal conjugated vaccines that cover serogroup A, C, W, and Y and serogroup B and are recommended for all adolescents.

Dosing

The dose of meningococcal serogroup A, C, W, Y vaccine is given IM at ages 11 to 12 years, and a booster should be given at 16 years of age. Patients receiving their first dose between the ages of 13 and 15 need a booster between 16 and 18 years of age (minimum interval is 8 weeks). Adolescents receiving their first dose after the age of 16 years do not require a booster dose.

Serogroup B meningococcal vaccine is started at age 16 years, and patients require two doses depending on the vaccine used.

Adverse reactions

Side effects associated with the meningococcal vaccine include redness and pain at the site; fever and dizziness have been reported. It has been recommended that patients sit or lie down 15 minutes after the vaccine administration.

Pneumococcal 15- or 20-valent conjugate vaccine

PCV15 OR PCV20 is recommended for preventing and decreasing the severity of pneumococcal infections caused by *Streptococcus pneumoniae*. These invasive infections can result in otitis media, pneumonia, meningitis, and sepsis, with the most serious illness occurring in children younger than age 2 years.

Dosing

The 0.5-mL dose of PCV15 OR PCV20 is administered IM. A total of four doses are recommended, with one dose each at ages 2, 4, 6, and 12 to 15 months.

Adverse reactions

Common adverse reactions from PCV15 OR PCV20 are drowsiness, irritability, restless sleep, diarrhea, vomiting, decreased appetite, and injection site reactions (including swelling, redness, induration, inflammation, skin discoloration, and tenderness).

Rotavirus vaccine

The rotavirus is the leading cause of gastroenteritis in children younger than the age of 5 years, causing severe vomiting and watery diarrhea. Currently, there are two vaccines licensed in the United States to protect against rotavirus.

Dosing

The two vaccines RotaTeq and Rotarix are administered by mouth. RotaTeq is given in three doses at ages 2, 4, and 6 months. Rotarix is administered at 2 and 4 months of age. The maximum age for the first dose is 14 weeks and 6 days, with the maximum age for the last dose is 8 months 0 days.

Adverse reactions

Common side effects from the rotavirus vaccine include irritability, mild diarrhea, or vomiting. A small but increased risk for developing intussusception has been noted after receiving the first dose of rotavirus vaccine.

Varicella virus vaccine

Varicella virus vaccine is used to stimulate immunity to varicella (chickenpox). The vaccine contains a live virus and is contraindicated during pregnancy. It is also contraindicated in people receiving immunosuppressive therapy and in those with immunodeficiency diseases.

Dosing

Two 0.5-mL doses of varicella virus vaccine (Varivax) are given SC between ages 12 and 15 months and between 4 and 6 years of age.

Two for teens and teens for two . . .

If patients did not receive varicella vaccine as a child, adolescents aged 13 years and older receive two doses; each dose is separated by a 4- to 8-week interval.

Adverse reactions

Common adverse reactions to the varicella virus vaccine are pain, redness, localized swelling, and varicella-like rash at the injection site. Low-grade fever and irritability for 1 week after vaccine administration are also common. Anaphylaxis is rare.

Influenza vaccine

Also known as the *flu shot*, the influenza vaccine is either an inactivated or killed vaccine or a live, attenuated vaccine. Because the influenza virus changes each year, the vaccine gets updated every year in an attempt to prevent the most common strains that are circulating at that time. Therefore, the influenza vaccine needs to be given yearly.

Protection from the influenza virus should begin 2 weeks after the vaccination and may last for up to 1 year.

Who gets it?

The influenza vaccine is recommended for all children aged 6 months or older. Household contacts and caregivers of children younger than age 6 months or with a chronic health condition are encouraged to get the vaccine.

Dosing

The inactivated vaccine is administered IM once per year and is most effective when given early in the flu season, typically in October or November. For children younger than age 9 years, two doses are required for the initial influenza vaccination series and should be given 1 month apart. Children aged 6 months to 8 years who have received at least two doses before July 1, 2022, only require one dose. Children

6 to 35 months receive a dose of 0.25 to 0.5 mL (depending on the manufacturer), and those 36 months and older receive a dose of 0.5 mL.

There is an intranasal form of the influenza vaccine, which is a live, attenuated vaccine acceptable for healthy children ages 2 years and older.

Adverse reactions

The influenza vaccine typically produces only mild adverse reactions, such as soreness, redness, swelling at the injection site, fever, or body aches. Severe adverse effects such as a life-threatening allergic reaction rarely occur.

Contraindications to vaccine administration

Mild illnesses and low-grade fevers that are common in children are not contraindications to vaccine administration. However, there are several reasons to withhold or delay vaccine administration:

- Vaccination is contraindicated in patients with moderate to severe illness or a history of allergic response or anaphylaxis to the vaccine or certain antibiotics.
- Vaccination with preparations containing live or attenuated viruses should not be performed in patients who are pregnant, have an immunodeficiency disease, or are receiving immunosuppressive therapy.
- The DTaP vaccine should not be given to a child who has a progressive and active central nervous system (CNS) problem. However, a child with cerebral palsy can receive immunizations.
- The measles vaccine should be given at the same time as a tuberculin-purified protein derivative test or at least 1 month apart. The measles vaccine may weaken the skin reaction to the tuberculin test.

Bacterial infections

Bacteria are single-celled microorganisms. They have no true nucleus and reproduce by cell division. Pathogenic bacteria contain cell-damaging proteins that cause infection. These proteins come in two forms:

- Exotoxins—released during cell growth
- Endotoxins—released when the bacterial cell wall decomposes. These endotoxins cause fever and are not affected by antibiotics. (See *How bacteria damage tissue.*)

How bacteria damage tissue

The human body is constantly infected by bacteria and other infectious organisms. Some are beneficial, such as the intestinal bacteria that produce vitamins, and others are harmful, causing illnesses ranging from the common cold to life-threatening septic shock.

Invading forces

To infect a host, bacteria must first enter it. They do this by adhering to the mucosal surface and directly invading the host cell or attaching to epithelial cells and producing toxins, which invade host cells.

I will survive

To survive and multiply within a host, bacteria or their toxins adversely affect biochemical reactions in cells. The result is a disruption of normal cell function or cell death (shown in the image). For example, the diphtheria toxin damages heart muscle by inhibiting protein synthesis. In addition, as some organisms multiply, they extend into deeper tissue and eventually gain access to the bloodstream.

Clot and deprive

Some toxins cause blood to clot in small blood vessels. The tissues supplied by these vessels may be deprived of blood and may be damaged (shown in the image).

Bring down the walls

Other toxins can damage the cell walls of small blood vessels, causing leakage. This fluid loss results in decreased blood pressure, which, in turn, impairs the heart's ability to pump enough blood to vital organs (shown in the image).

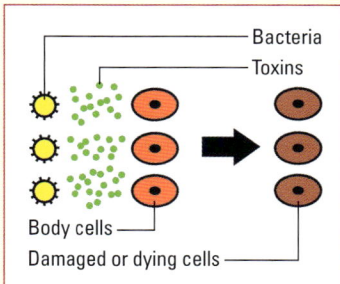

Bacteria
Toxins
Body cells
Damaged or dying cells

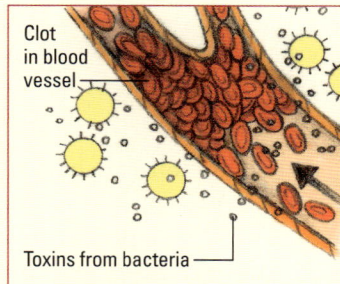

Clot in blood vessel
Toxins from bacteria

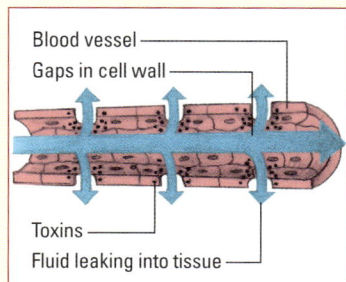

Blood vessel
Gaps in cell wall
Toxins
Fluid leaking into tissue

A class by any other class

Bacteria are classified in several other ways, such as by their shape, growth requirements, motility, and whether they're aerobic (requiring oxygen) or anaerobic (not requiring oxygen).

The young and the susceptible

Bacterial infections are common in infants and young children who haven't achieved active immunity because their immune systems have not been challenged by many pathogens. Such infections in infants include Lyme disease and pertussis. Antibiotic therapy is the treatment for bacterial infection.

Lyme disease

In the United States, Lyme disease is the most common vector-borne disorder. Although Lyme disease occurs year-round, most infections occur during warm seasons (late spring and summer). Infection with Lyme disease does not produce active immunity, so a patient may be reinfected upon reexposure.

What causes it

Lyme disease is caused by a spirochete, *Borrelia burgdorferi*, which is transmitted to humans through the bite of an infected deer tick.

How it happens

The spirochete enters the bloodstream via the tick's saliva as its bite penetrates the skin barrier.

Tick tock

The tick must feed for 36 to 72 hours or longer to transmit the infection. Most people who realize they have been bitten will remove the tick before the infection can be transmitted.

What to look for

Once infected, the skin's inflammatory response causes a localized, red, "bull's-eye" rash (*erythema migrans*) at the site of the tick bite. The rash may itch and be painful.

The rash that knows no bounds

Without treatment, the rash will expand to 6 in (15 cm) in diameter or larger. Fever, headache, malaise, and lymphadenopathy are systemic symptoms of the disease.

More reasons to treat

If the infection is left untreated, arthritic pain and swelling of the joints (Lyme arthritis), facial palsy, meningitis, and carditis may result.

What tests tell you

Diagnosis of Lyme disease is based on clinical symptoms, appearance of skin lesion (erythema migrans), and a history of exposure. The CDC recommends a two-step process confirmed by the presence of antibodies to *B. burgdorferi* in the blood. The first step is enzyme-linked immunosorbent assay (ELISA or EIA) or immunofluorescent antibody (IFA) test. If the EIA is negative, no further testing is needed. If the EIA is positive, a Western blot test is performed. If both the EIA and Western blot are positive, the patient has Lyme disease.

Complications

Symptoms of arthritis, including painful joint swelling and stiffness, are the most common complications of untreated disease. Meningitis, focal neurologic problems, and carditis are rare.

How it's treated

Amoxicillin (Amoxil) and cefuroxime (Ceftin) may be used in children younger than age 8 years. Amoxicillin and doxycycline are used for children older than 8 years of age, but doxycycline should not be used in younger children because it can cause permanent discoloration of the teeth. A full course of antibiotic therapy is administered and is continued for 14 to 21 days.

What to do

- Teach caregivers that tick-infested areas should be avoided to help prevent Lyme disease. If children must be in such areas, protective clothing should be worn, and ticks that do attach must be removed immediately. (See *Preventing tick-borne illnesses.*)
- Teach caregivers how to recognize the characteristic bull's-eye rash of Lyme disease to promote early diagnosis and treatment.

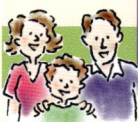

It's all relative

Preventing tick-borne illnesses

The following are measures to prevent tick-borne illnesses.

Keep 'em off

It is always preferable to stay out of tick-infested areas. Follow these tips to avoid such areas or, if unavoidable, protect yourself and others from acquiring a tick bite:

- Treat household pets that may harbor ticks (such as cats and dogs) to eliminate the ticks.
- Avoid grassy and wooded areas where ticks are abundant.

(continued)

Preventing tick-borne illnesses (*continued*)

• If children must be in such areas, dress them in appropriate protective clothing (such as long-sleeved shirts and long pants).
• Consider using insect repellents. However, repellents containing diethyltoluamide (DEET) should not be used in children younger than age 1 year. DEET is absorbed through the skin and may cause toxicity in this population.
• Check the child for ticks frequently.

Take 'em off
If a tick attaches to the skin:

• Remove it immediately using tweezers or forceps, making sure to remove the entire tick, including the mouthparts.
• Don't crush or squeeze the tick to avoid causing more organisms from the tick to enter the bite.
• Clean the site.
• Wash your hands thoroughly after cleaning the site.
• Seek prompt medical attention for initiation of antibiotic therapy if symptoms develop, such as fever, erythema, or a rash in the area of the bite.

Pertussis

Pertussis, also known as *whooping cough*, is an extremely contagious acute respiratory tract infection. It typically produces an irritating cough that becomes paroxysmal and commonly ends in a high-pitched inspiratory whoop.

Approximately 5,000 to 7,000 cases occur in the United States every year. Children who are too young to have been fully immunized and those who have not completed the immunization series are at the highest risk for serious illness.

What causes it

The pertussis infection is usually caused by the nonmotile, gram-negative coccobacillus *Bordetella pertussis.*

How it happens

The disease is transmitted through inhalation of contaminated respiratory droplets or by direct contact with contaminated articles such as soiled bed linens.

Incubation and communicability

The incubation period ranges from 3 to 12 days. The period of communicability begins about 1 week after exposure and lasts for 5 to 7 days after antibiotic therapy has begun.

What to look for

Symptoms of rhinorrhea and nasal congestion begin insidiously, followed by a nonproductive cough. These symptoms are commonly accompanied by a low-grade fever, sneezing, and watery eyes.

The cough of the giant crane

The coughing becomes increasingly more severe. Spasms of paroxysmal coughing followed by stridor on inspiration produce the characteristic "whooping" sound.

Flushing and draining

Flushing; cyanosis; and watery drainage from the nose, eyes, and mouth may accompany the coughing. Infants can have symptoms of choking and gasping for air, and vomiting may occur if the patient chokes on mucus.

What tests tell you

Isolation of *B. pertussis* in laboratory culture of respiratory secretions remains the gold standard for confirming pertussis infection. A peripheral blood smear may demonstrate leukocytosis caused by the body's response to the bacterial infection. A polymerase chain reaction (PCR) test of the nasopharyngeal specimen can also be performed.

Complications

Complications from pertussis infection are most severe, and death rates are highest in infants younger than age 6 months. Complications include:
- secondary infection, such as pneumonia and otitis media
- increased venous pressure
- anterior eye chamber hemorrhage, detached retina, and blindness
- rectal prolapse
- inguinal or umbilical hernia
- encephalopathy
- seizures.

How it's treated

Erythromycin, azithromycin, or clarithromycin given orally for 14 days is the standard treatment for pertussis infection. Trimethoprim-sulfamethoxazole (Bactrim) may be used in patients who cannot tolerate erythromycin.

What to do

To prevent pertussis, nurses should advocate active immunization beginning at age 2 months and continuing at ages 4 months, 6 months, 15 to 18 months, and 4 to 6 years, for a total of five doses. When providing care to a child with pertussis, follow these steps:
- Use droplet isolation for those with suspected or documented infection, until 5 to 7 days after antibiotic therapy has been initiated.

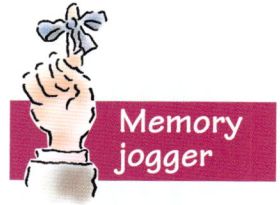

Memory jogger

To remember the complications from pertussis, just remember that the disease is highly contagious, so it IS SHARED:

Increased venous pressure

Seizures

Secondary infection

Hernia

Anterior eye chamber hemorrhage

Rectal prolapse

Encephalopathy

Death

- Closely monitor cardiorespiratory function and oxygen saturation. Maintain a patent airway; keep suctioning equipment readily available.
- Create a quiet environment to decrease coughing stimulation.
- Offer the child a small amount of fluids frequently to prevent dehydration.
- Report diagnosed disease to public health officials.
- Treat close contacts of the infected child prophylactically with oral erythromycin.

Viral infections

Viruses are the smallest known organisms and are visible only with an electron microscope. Viruses cannot replicate independently of host cells. Instead, they invade a host cell and stimulate it to participate in forming additional virus particles.

Supportive therapy is the treatment for viral infections. Antiviral medications are sometimes used to ease symptoms and potentially shorten the length of viral infections. Antibiotic therapy is not indicated for illnesses caused by viral infection but may be appropriate if a secondary bacterial infection has complicated the clinical course of the viral illness.

Rash of rashes

Common childhood rash-producing viruses include:
- fifth disease
- roseola infantum
- rubella
- rubeola
- varicella. (See *Common rash-producing infections*.)

Common rash-producing infections

Infection	Incubation (days)	Duration (days)
Fifth disease	6–14	7–21
Roseola infantum	5–15	3–6
Rubella	14–21	3
Rubeola	8–14	5
Varicella	10–21	7–14

Not so rash

Common viral infections without rash include:
- mumps
- poliomyelitis.

Fifth disease

Fifth disease is a contagious viral disease characterized by rose-colored eruptions diffused over the skin, usually starting on the cheeks.

The fifth dimension

Fifth disease got its unusual name when it was counted as the fifth of the classic, rash-producing infections of children. The other rash-producing infections referred to in this chronology were measles, scarlet fever, rubella, and another rash that is unknown to health care providers today but was referred to as "the fourth disease."

What causes it

Fifth disease is caused by human parvovirus B19.

How it happens

The virus is transmitted through infected respiratory droplet secretions and through infected blood.

Incubation and communicability

The incubation period for fifth disease is 6 to 14 days. The period of communicability lasts from several days before the appearance of a rash until the rash has appeared.

What to look for

Clinical manifestations in the prodromal phase are mild, including low-grade fever, headache, and symptoms of upper respiratory infection.

A slap in the face

The typical rash in the initial stage is described as a red facial flushing or a "slapped-cheek" appearance. The macular rash spreads rapidly to the trunk and proximal extremities. The centers of the macules fade, which gives the rash a lacy appearance.

Spare the hands, spoil the feet

The rash is not present on the palms or soles. It resolves spontaneously in 1 to 3 weeks. (See *Fifth disease*.)

What tests tell you

Diagnosis of fifth disease is usually based on reviewing the clinical presentation of the child, observing the rash, and excluding other differential diagnoses. Methods to detect the virus in laboratory studies are available, although not routinely ordered.

Complications

Complications of fifth disease are rare. Children with chronic hematologic conditions may experience transient anemias. Arthritis and joint symptoms may occur in adults but are rare in children.

Pregnant? Watch out!

Infection in a pregnant person is associated with fetal disease and may result in fetal death. However, the risk of infection is minimal for pregnant people who come into contact with the affected children.

How it's treated

No specific treatment or cure for fifth disease exists. Nursing care is supportive. No vaccine is available to prevent the illness.

What to do

Treatment is supportive and directed toward relief of symptoms:
- Antipyretic medications, such as acetaminophen or ibuprofen, are given to relieve fever.
- Soothing baths or antipruritics can be used to alleviate itching.

Don't fence me in

Fifth disease is benign and self-limiting. Because the child is not infectious to others when the rash appears, there is no reason to isolate the child.

Roseola infantum

Roseola is a common, acute, benign, presumably viral illness characterized by fever with subsequent rash. Children with roseola usually present with a high fever of an unknown origin.

What causes it

Roseola is caused by the human herpes virus 6.

How it happens

Transmission of roseola is not completely understood. The virus is detected in human saliva and is believed to be passed by oral viral shedding.

Incubation and communicability

The incubation period for roseola is 5 to 15 days. The period of communicability is unknown.

What to look for

The onset of symptoms occurs with a sudden, high fever. Children can have fevers of 103°F to 106°F (39.4°C to 41.1°C). Other than the unexplained fever, the child appears well, behaving normally. Most cases occur in infants and children younger than age 2 years, with peak incidence in children ages 6 to 12 months. The fever resolves on the third or fourth day of the illness.

Don't be rash

The febrile phase is typically followed by the development of a body rash that begins on the trunk and spreads to the neck, face, arms, and legs. The rash fades within 3 days. Some children, however, do not develop a rash.

What tests tell you

Diagnostic laboratory tests are not usually performed. It is possible to perform antibody titers to detect the virus.

Complications

Complications of roseola are rare but include extreme hyperthermia, persistent seizures, encephalitis, and hepatitis.

How it's treated

Treatment is supportive and directed at the relief of symptoms. Non-aspirin antipyretic medications, such as acetaminophen or ibuprofen, are given to relieve fever. Treating fever is important to prevent febrile seizures.

What to do

Roseola is benign and self-limiting. In addition to treatment for fever, care of a child with roseola should include:
- observation for the development of complications
- replacement of fluids and electrolytes as needed
- investigation of other common causes of high fever in young children such as otitis media.

Rubeola

Rubeola, also known as *measles*, is a highly contagious viral disease that causes a characteristic maculopapular rash.

What causes it

Rubeola infection is caused by the rubeola virus. Outbreaks of illness occur mostly in unimmunized children or in those with compromised immune systems.

How it happens

Rubeola is transmitted by airborne respiratory droplets or by direct contact with contaminated articles.

Incubation and communicability

The incubation period for rubeola is 8 to 14 days. The period of communicability begins several days before the appearance of the red rash and continues until 5 days after the rash has resolved.

What to look for

Symptoms of the prodromal phase include:

- fever
- malaise
- lethargy
- cough
- periorbital edema
- conjunctivitis
- profuse drainage from the nose
- Koplik spots, which are tiny gray-white specks surrounded by red halos that may be noted on the buccal mucosa opposite the molars about 2 days before the appearance of the body rash. (See *Spotting Koplik spots.*)

Spotting Koplik spots

Koplik spots differentiate rubeola from other rash-producing viruses. The spots appear on the buccal mucosa opposite the molars and then extend to the entire buccal surface. The raised base of the spots may join together so that the blue-white centers stand out (looking like grains of salt) on the erythematous membrane.

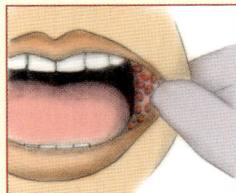

You look acute

During the acute phase of the illness, a red, blotchy, flat rash begins on the face and spreads to the trunk and extremities. The rash and other symptoms (severe cough, rhinorrhea, and lymphadenopathy) gradually subside in 5 to 7 days.

What tests tell you

Diagnosis of rubeola is usually based on clinical presentation. Laboratory tests are rarely needed.

Complications

Potential complications include:
- pneumonia
- otitis media
- encephalitis
- seizures
- secondary bacterial infections
- autoimmune reactions.

The infection can be severe or fatal in patients with impaired cell-mediated immunity. Mortality is highest in children younger than 2 years of age and in adults who can contract pneumonia secondary to the disease.

How it's treated

Maternal immunity to rubeola is active in the infant for about 1 year after birth. Immunization with MMR vaccine induces active immunity. The first vaccine is given at ages 12 to 15 months, and the second is given between ages 4 and 6 years. After the disease is diagnosed, treatment is supportive and is directed at the relief of symptoms:
- Antipyretic medications, such as acetaminophen and ibuprofen, are used to control fever.
- Antipruritic medications may be administered for itching.
- A cool mist vaporizer may be soothing to inflamed mucous membranes.
- Gentle suctioning with a bulb syringe may be needed to remove accumulated nasal secretions.

What to do

In addition to providing supportive treatment, follow these steps:
- Monitor breath sounds to detect adventitious sounds.
- Encourage fluid intake to promote hydration and decrease the viscosity of secretions.
- In the hospitalized child, maintain droplet precautions during the period of communicability.
- Report measles cases to local public health officials.

Varicella

Varicella, also called *chickenpox*, is an acute, highly contagious viral infection that can occur at any age.

What causes it

Infection with varicella-zoster virus (VZV) causes chickenpox. The virus remains latent in the dorsal root ganglia. Reactivation of the virus can cause herpes zoster infection (shingles) later in life.

How it happens

Airborne spread of respiratory secretions or, less commonly, direct contact with lesions of an infected person can cause infection in a susceptible child.

Incubation and communicability

The incubation period for chickenpox is 10 to 21 days. The period of communicability begins up to 5 days before the appearance of the body rash and continues until all lesions on the skin are crusted over.

What to look for

The onset of symptoms usually occurs 14 to 16 days after exposure. Prodromal symptoms of fever, malaise, and anorexia occur 24 to 48 hours before the development of the rash.

The clinical picture is one of a child with lesions in all stages of evolution present on the skin. The rash is pruritic. In addition, the following findings can be noted:

- The rash begins as itchy red macules on the face, scalp, or trunk that progress to papules.
- Papules develop into clear vesicles on an erythematous base (called "dewdrops on rose petals").
- Vesicles become cloudy and break easily and then scabs form.
- As initial lesions are crusting over, new lesions form on the trunk and extremities.

What tests tell you

VZV antibody tests and titers may be useful in establishing a diagnosis. Most commonly, diagnosis is based on the clinical history and presentation of a child with the characteristic vesicular rash.

Vaccination

To prevent varicella, a vaccine is given at 12 to 15 months, with a booster between 4 and 6 years of age.

Complications

Complications of varicella are rare. The disease can have significant, life-threatening complications in children who are immunocompromised.

Complications of varicella include secondary bacterial infections, such as cellulitis, lymphadenitis, abscesses, and sepsis. Other potential complications include encephalitis and meningoencephalitis, hepatitis, acute thrombocytopenia, and pneumonia.

COVID-19

COVID-19 is a viral illness caused by SARS-CoV-2, first seen in the United States in 2019–2020. It quickly spread throughout the country with most children experiencing mild symptoms, although some became severely ill.

Spread

The virus is spread by respiratory droplets and small particles, even by people without symptoms.

What to look for

Symptoms may include fever, chest pain, chills, cough, shortness of breath, respiratory distress, fatigue, muscle aches, headaches, loss of smell or taste, sore throat, congestion, rhinorrhea, nausea, vomiting, and diarrhea.

Who is at risk for serious illness

People who are older than 50 years of age, immunocompromised, physically inactive, or have preexisting conditions such as obesity, cancer, chronic kidney, liver or lung diseases, cystic fibrosis, diabetes, or hemoglobin blood disorders. Due to health disparities, the race and ethnicity of the patients may be an important factor in the risk of disease.

Testing

Antigen tests, PCRs, or nucleic acid amplification tests (NAAT) should be performed on patients with symptoms or for screening purposes.

Vaccination

Vaccination can start as young as 6 months of age requiring a two or three-dose series depending on the vaccine used.

Quick quiz

1. Which of the following statements about Lyme disease is true?
   A. Lyme disease is vaccine preventable.
   B. Lyme disease is caused by a spirochete that enters the body through a tick bite.
   C. Lyme disease is common in tropical areas where spores are found in the soil.
   D. Children with Lyme disease should be isolated from others because of the risk of disease transmission.

Answer: B. Lyme disease is caused by a spirochete, *B. burgdorferi*, which is transmitted to humans through the bite of an infected deer tick.

2. Which of the following sexually transmitted diseases is preventable through vaccination?
   A. Syphilis
   B. Gonorrhea
   C. Hepatitis A
   D. Hepatitis B

Answer: D. The HepB vaccine is given IM at birth (or before hospital discharge), at ages 1 to 4 months, and again at ages 6 to 18 months, for a total of three doses. For older children and adolescents, the initial IM dose is given, the second dose is given 1 month later, and the third dose is given 6 months after the first dose.

3. A caregiver of a child with varicella asks the nurse when the child may return to day care. The nurse correctly responds by telling the caregiver that the child can return:
   A. when the fever is resolved.
   B. 24 hours after the appearance of the rash.
   C. when all lesions are crusted over.
   D. after receiving the first dose of diphenhydramine (Benadryl).

Answer: C. The period of communicability for varicella (chickenpox) starts as early as 5 days before the appearance of the body rash. The period of communicability continues until all lesions on the skin are crusted over.

4. Which of the following is an early symptom of roseola infantum?
   A. High, unexplained fever
   B. Vomiting
   C. Development of a body rash
   D. Behavioral changes and anorexia

Answer: A. The onset of symptoms of illness occurs with sudden, high fever. Fevers of 103°F to 106°F (39.4°C to 41.1°C) can occur. Other than the unexplained fever, the child appears well, with normal behaviors.

Scoring

⭐⭐⭐ If you answered all four items correctly, bravo! Go forth and spread your understanding of viral and bacterial illnesses.

⭐⭐ If you answered three items correctly, excellent work! Your knowledge of communicable diseases is infectious.

⭐ If you answered fewer than three items correctly, don't go into isolation! Take another look at the chapter and forge ahead.

Suggested references

Akcay, N., Ogur, M., Menentoglu, M. E., Boydag Guvenc, K., Sofuoglu, A. I., & Sevketoglu, E. (2022). MIS-C and identical twins: A case series. *Pediatric Infectious Disease Journal*, *41*(1), e32–e34. https://doi.org/10.1097/INF.0000000000003392

Castellar-Lopez, J., Villamizar-Villamizar, W., Amaranto-Pallares, A., Rosales-Rada, W., De Los Angeles Velez Verbel, M., Chang, A., Jimenez, F. T., & Mendoza-Torres, E. (2021). Recent insights into COVID-19 in children and clinical recommendations. *Current Pediatric Review*, *18*(2), 121–137. https://doi.org/10.2174/1573396317666211206124347

Centers for Disease Control and Prevention. (2021). In E. Hall, A. P. Wodi, J. Hamborsky, V. Morelli, & S. Schillie (Eds.), *Epidemiology and prevention of vaccine-preventable diseases* (14th ed.). Public Health Foundation.

Centers for Disease Control and Prevention. (2022). *Clinical care of Lyme disease*. https://www.cdc.gov/lyme/hcp/clinical-care/index.html

Centers for Disease Control and Prevention. (2023). *Immunization schedules*. https://www.cdc.gov/vaccines/hcp/imz-schedules/index.html

Dufort, E. M., Koumans, E. H., Chow, E. J., Rosenthal, E. M., Muse, A., Rowlands, J., Barranco, M. A., Maxted, A. M., Rosenberg, E. S., Easton, D., Udo, T., Kumar, J., Pulver, W., Smith, L., Hutton, B., Blog, D., Zucker, H., & New York State and Centers for Disease Control and Prevention Multisystem Inflammatory Syndrome in Children Investigation Team. (2020). Multisystem inflammatory syndrome in children in New York state. *The New England Journal of Medicine*, *383*(4), 347–358. https://doi.org/10.1056/NEJMoa2021756

Lantos, P. M., Rumbaugh, J., Bockenstedt, L. K., Falck-Ytter, Y. T., Aguero-Rosenfeld, M. E., Auwaerter, P. G., Baldwin, K., Bannuru, R. R., Belani, K. K., Bowie, W. R., Branda, J. A., Clifford, D. B., DiMario, F. J., Jr., Halperin, J. J., Krause, P. J., Lavergne, V., Liang, M. H., Meissner, H. C., Nigrovic, L. E., … Zemel, L. S. (2021). Clinical practice guidelines by the Infectious Diseases Society of America, American Academy of Neurology, and American College of Rheumatology: 2020 guidelines for the prevention, diagnosis, and treatment of Lyme disease. *Neurology*, *96*(6), 262–273. https://doi.org/10.1212/WNL.0000000000011151

Maaks, D., Starr, N., Brady, M., Gaylord, N., Driessnack, M., & Duderstadt, K. (2020). *Burns' pediatric primary care* (7th ed.). Elsevier.

Naydeva-Grigorova, T., Manzoor, A., & Ahmed, M. (2015). Management of early-onset neonatal infections. *Archives of Disease in Childhood Fetal & Neonatal*, *100*(1), F93–F94. https://doi.org/10.1136/archdischild-2014-307366

Chapter 15

Neurologic problems

Just the facts

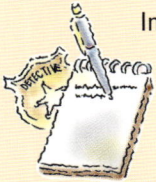

In this chapter, you'll learn:

◆ structures of the neurologic system

◆ assessment of patients with problems involving the neurologic system

◆ diagnostic tests for neurologic problems

◆ treatments and nursing interventions for children with neurologic disorders.

Anatomy and physiology

The neurologic system consists of the central nervous system (CNS), the peripheral nervous system, and the autonomic (involuntary) nervous system (ANS). Through complex and coordinated interactions, these three parts integrate all physical, intellectual, and emotional activities. Understanding how each part works is essential to conducting an accurate neurologic assessment.

Central nervous system

The CNS is composed of the brain and all its component parts, and the spinal cord. Structurally, the CNS is contained within the skull and the vertebral column.

Central command

Integration among all parts of the nervous system enables normal functioning of body parts, both voluntary and involuntary. A person's perception of oneself and their environment, reactions and interactions with the environment, and adjustment to development and environmental changes are greatly influenced by the proper integration and functioning of the nervous system.

Brain

The brain, the center of the CNS, collects, integrates, and interprets stimuli and initiates and monitors voluntary and involuntary motor activity.

The incredible expanding brain

Head circumference, which is measured in children up to ages 2 to 3 years, averages 13 to 14 in (33 to 35.5 cm) and should be ½ to 1 in (2 to 3 cm) larger than chest circumference at birth. Fifty percent of brain growth is achieved in the first year of life, 75% by age 3 years, and 90% by age 6 years. The brain comprises 12% of body weight at birth, doubles in weight in the first year, and triples by age 5 or 6 years.

Separated at birth

Because the skull protects the brain, the anterior and posterior fontanels are separated at birth to allow for brain expansion. The posterior fontanel closes between ages 4 and 8 weeks, and the anterior fontanel closes between ages 12 and 18 months.

A mass of nerves in a house of bones

Physiologically, the brain is the large, soft mass of nervous tissue housed in the cranium and protected and supported by the meninges and the skull bones. It consists of the:

- cerebrum
- cerebellum
- brain stem.

Other noteworthy figures

Other structures and elements of the brain include the:

- neurons
- meninges
- cerebrospinal fluid (CSF)
- ventricles.

Cerebrum

The cerebrum, the largest portion of the brain, is the nerve center that controls sensory and motor activities and intelligence. The outer layer of the cerebrum, the *cerebral cortex*, consists of neuron cell bodies (gray matter); the inner layers consist of axons (white matter) and basal ganglia, which control motor coordination and steadiness.

Bridging the hemispheres

A longitudinal fissure divides the cerebrum into two hemispheres connected by a wide band of nerve fibers called the *corpus callosum*. These hemispheres share information through the corpus callosum.

Because motor impulses descending from the brain cross in the medulla, the right hemisphere controls the left side of the body and the left hemisphere controls the right side of the body.

Not the piercing kind

Several fissures divide the cerebrum into lobes, each of which is associated with specific functions. (See *A look at the lobes*.)

A look at the lobes

Several fissures divide the cerebrum into hemispheres and lobes; each lobe has a specific function.

The great dividers
The *fissure of Sylvius* (lateral sulcus) separates the temporal lobe from the frontal and parietal lobes. The *fissure of Rolando* (central sulcus) separates the frontal lobes from the parietal lobe. The *parietooccipital fissure* separates the occipital lobe from the two parietal lobes.

Lovely lobes
Each lobe controls specific body functions:
• The *frontal lobe* controls voluntary muscle movements and contains motor areas (including the motor area for speech, or *Broca area*). It's the center for personality, behavioral, and intellectual functions, such as judgment, memory, and problem-solving; for autonomic functions; and for cardiac and emotional responses.
• The *temporal lobe* is the center for taste, hearing, and smell. Also, in the brain's dominant hemisphere, it interprets spoken language.
• The *parietal lobe* coordinates and interprets sensory information from the opposite side of the body.
• The *occipital lobe* interprets visual stimuli.

Passing the baton

The thalamus, a relay center below the corpus callosum, further organizes cerebral function by transmitting impulses to and from appropriate areas of the cerebrum.

The body's thermostat

The hypothalamus, which lies beneath the thalamus, is an autonomic center that regulates temperature control, appetite, blood pressure, breathing, sleep patterns, and peripheral nerve discharges that occur with behavioral and emotional expression.

Cerebellum

Beneath the cerebrum, at the base of the brain, is the cerebellum. It's responsible for smooth muscle movements, coordinating sensory impulses with muscle activity, and maintaining muscle tone and equilibrium.

Brain stem

The brain stem relays nerve impulses between the spinal cord and other parts of the brain. It houses cell bodies from most of the cranial nerves (CNs) and includes the:

- *midbrain*, which is the reflex center for the third and fourth CNs and mediates pupillary reflexes and eye movements
- *pons*, which helps regulate respirations and mediate chewing, taste, saliva secretion, hearing, and equilibrium
- *medulla oblongata*, which affects cardiac, respiratory, and vasomotor functions.

Neurons

The fundamental unit of the nervous system is the neuron, a highly specialized conductor cell that receives and transmits electrochemical nerve impulses. Neurons develop between 15 and 30 weeks' gestation.

Delicate and impulsive

Its structure contains delicate, threadlike nerve fibers that extend from the central cell body and transmit signals, or *axons*, which carry impulses away from the cell body, and *dendrites*, which carry impulses to the cell body.

Meninges

The brain is covered with three thin membranes called *meninges*:

1. The outer membrane is the *dura mater* or "hard mother"; it has various folds that separate the brain into compartments.
2. The second structure is the *arachnoid*; it has two layers of fibrous and elastic tissue and, between the layers, a spongy, cobweblike structure containing subarachnoid fluid.
3. The third structure is the *pia mater*, or "tender mother"; it is a very fine membrane that's rich in minute blood plexuses and follows the brain in all its folds. (See *Meningeal layers of the brain*.)

Meningeal layers of the brain

Three primary membranes, or meninges, help protect the CNS: the dura mater, the arachnoid membrane, and the pia mater.

Dura mater

The dura mater is a fibrous membrane that lines the skull and forms folds (reflections) that descend into the brain's fissures and provide stability. The dural folds include the:

(*continued*)

Meningeal layers of the brain (*continued*)

• falx cerebri, which lies in the longitudinal fissure and separates the hemispheres of the cerebrum
• tentorium cerebelli, which separates the cerebrum from the cerebellum
• falx cerebelli, which separates the two cerebellar lobes.
The arachnoid villi (projections of the dura mater into the superior sagittal and transverse sinuses) serve as the exit points for CSF drainage into venous circulation.

Arachnoid membrane
A fragile, fibrous layer with moderate vascularity, the arachnoid membrane lies between the dura mater and the pia mater. Injury to its blood vessels during head trauma, lumbar puncture, or cisternal puncture may cause hemorrhage.

Pia mater
An extremely thin and highly vascular membrane, the *pia mater* closely covers the brain's surface and extends into its fissures. It contains minute arteries and veins that supply the brain.

Additional layers
Three layers of space further cushion the brain and spinal cord against injury:
• The *epidural space* (a potential space) lies over the dura mater.
• The *subdural space* lies between the dura mater and the arachnoid membrane and is commonly the site of hemorrhage after head trauma.
• The *subarachnoid space*, which is filled with CSF, lies between the arachnoid membrane and the pia mater.

Cerebrospinal Fluid
The ventricles of the brain and the entire subarachnoid space around the brain and spinal cord contain CSF.

Clear liquid with a protein chaser
CSF is a clear liquid containing water and traces of organic materials (especially protein), glucose, and minerals. CSF is formed from blood in capillary networks called *choroid plexuses*, which are located primarily in the brain's lateral ventricles. The fluid is eventually reabsorbed into the venous blood through the arachnoid villi, located in dural sinuses on the brain's surface.

Better than a bubble bath
The brain floats in, and is bathed by, CSF. It acts as a shock absorber and helps reduce forces that jar or shake the brain. CSF is in contact with the entire brain and spinal cord surface as well as the surfaces of the ventricles.

Ventricles

The four ventricles are large, CSF-filled cavities within the brain. There are two lateral ventricles, one in each cerebral hemisphere. A third ventricle (located directly above the midbrain of the brain stem) communicates with both the lateral ventricles and the fourth ventricle (located in the posterior brain fossa).

Spinal cord

The spinal cord extends downward from the brain, through the vertebrae, to the level of approximately the second lumbar vertebra. It functions as a conductive pathway to and from the brain. It's also the reflex center for activities that don't require brain control such as deep tendon reflexes (the jerking reaction elicited by tapping with a reflex hammer).

Can you hear me now?

Within the spinal cord, connections are made between incoming and outgoing nerve fibers. Thirty-one pairs of spinal nerves are connected to the cord. The sensory, or ascending, tracts carry sensory impulses up the spinal cord to the brain; the motor, or descending, tracts carry motor impulses down the spinal cord and out to the peripheral nervous system.

Peripheral nervous system

The part of the nervous system outside the skull and vertebral column is considered the peripheral nervous system. It's composed of 31 spinal nerves and 12 CNs and is divided into two functional systems: the somatic nervous system and the ANS.

Spinal nerves

Messages transmitted through the spinal cord reach outlying areas through 31 pairs of segmentally arranged spinal nerves attached to the spinal cord. Spinal nerves are numbered according to their point of origin in the cord:
- Eight cervical nerves—C1 to C8
- Twelve thoracic nerves—T1 to T12
- Five lumbar nerves—L1 to L5
- One coccygeal nerve

It's rude to interrupt

After leaving the vertebral column, each spinal nerve separates into *rami* (branches), distributed peripherally, with extensive but organized overlapping. This overlapping reduces the risk of lost sensory or motor function from interruption of a single spinal nerve.

Cranial nerves

The 12 pairs of CNs transmit motor or sensory messages (or both) primarily between the brain or brain stem and the head and neck. All CNs, except the olfactory and optic nerves, exit from the midbrain, pons, or medulla oblongata of the brain stem. (See *Exit points of the CNs.*)

Exit points of the CNs

As this illustration reveals, 10 of the 12 pairs of CNs exit from the brain stem. The remaining two pairs—the olfactory and optic nerves—exit from the forebrain.

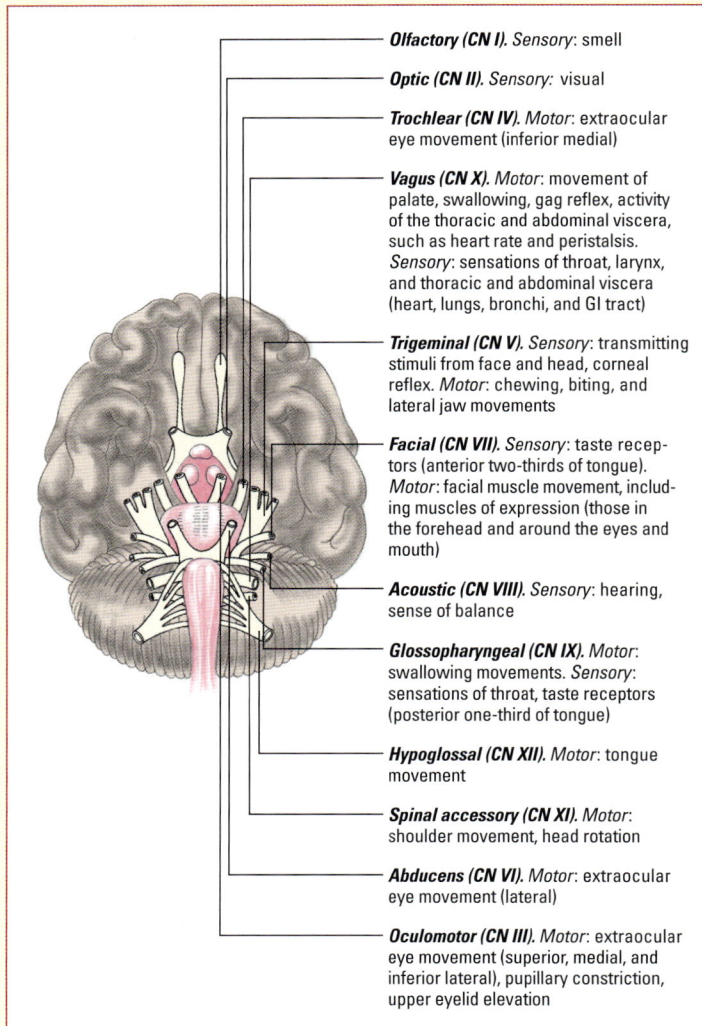

Olfactory (CN I). *Sensory*: smell

Optic (CN II). *Sensory:* visual

Trochlear (CN IV). *Motor*: extraocular eye movement (inferior medial)

Vagus (CN X). *Motor*: movement of palate, swallowing, gag reflex, activity of the thoracic and abdominal viscera, such as heart rate and peristalsis. *Sensory*: sensations of throat, larynx, and thoracic and abdominal viscera (heart, lungs, bronchi, and GI tract)

Trigeminal (CN V). *Sensory*: transmitting stimuli from face and head, corneal reflex. *Motor*: chewing, biting, and lateral jaw movements

Facial (CN VII). *Sensory*: taste receptors (anterior two-thirds of tongue). *Motor*: facial muscle movement, including muscles of expression (those in the forehead and around the eyes and mouth)

Acoustic (CN VIII). *Sensory*: hearing, sense of balance

Glossopharyngeal (CN IX). *Motor*: swallowing movements. *Sensory*: sensations of throat, taste receptors (posterior one-third of tongue)

Hypoglossal (CN XII). *Motor*: tongue movement

Spinal accessory (CN XI). *Motor*: shoulder movement, head rotation

Abducens (CN VI). *Motor*: extraocular eye movement (lateral)

Oculomotor (CN III). *Motor*: extraocular eye movement (superior, medial, and inferior lateral), pupillary constriction, upper eyelid elevation

Somatic nervous system

The somatic (voluntary) nervous system is activated by will but can function independently. It is responsible for all conscious and higher mental processes as well as subconscious and reflex actions, such as shivering.

Autonomic nervous system

The ANS regulates unconscious processes to control involuntary body functions, such as digestion, respiration, and cardiovascular function. It is usually divided into two antagonistic systems that balance each other's activities to support homeostasis under normal conditions:
- The *sympathetic nervous system* controls energy expenditure, especially in stressful situations, by releasing adrenergic catecholamines.
- The *parasympathetic nervous system* helps conserve energy by releasing the cholinergic neurohormone acetylcholine.

Neurologic assessment

A complete assessment of the neurologic system includes evaluation of:
- mental and emotional status
- CN function
- sensory function
- motor function
- reflexes.

Knowledge of the pediatric patient's physical, psychomotor, and cognitive developmental milestones is an essential assessment tool for detecting significant deviations. For toddlers and preschoolers, make a game of the assessment process when possible. Have older children assist with the assessment.

Mini assessment

Because there is not always enough time to completely assess neurologic function, a bedside assessment might focus on level of consciousness (LOC), pupillary response, motor function, reflexes, sensory functions, and vital signs.

Glasgow Coma Scale

The Glasgow Coma Scale (GCS), which assesses eye opening as well as verbal and motor responses, provides a quick, standardized account of neurologic status. A pediatric version of the scale considers the preverbal child. (See *Pediatric coma scale.*)

Pediatric coma scale

To quickly assess a patient's LOC and to uncover changes from baseline, use the pediatric coma scale. This assessment tool grades consciousness in relation to eye-opening and motor response and responses to auditory or visual stimuli. A decreased reaction score in one or more categories warns of an impending neurologic crisis. A patient scoring 8 or lower is comatose and probably has severe neurologic damage.

Test	Patient's reaction	Score
Best eye-opening response	Open spontaneously	4
	Open to sound	3
	Open to pressure	2
	No response	1
Best motor response	Obeys verbal command	6
	Localizes painful stimuli	5
	Flexion—withdrawal	4
	Flexion—abnormal (decorticate rigidity)	3
	Extension (decerebrate rigidity)	2
	No response	1
Best response to auditory and visual stimulus	For the child older than age 2 years:	
	Oriented	5
	Confused	4
	Inappropriate words	3
	Incomprehensible sounds	2
	No response	1
	OR For the child younger than age 2 years:	
	Smiles, listens, follows	5
	Cries, consolable	4
	Inappropriate persistent cry	3
	Agitated, restless	2
	No response	1
Total possible score		***3–15***

In this exam, each response receives a numerical value; the final score is the total of the values.

- A total score of 15 for all three parts is normal.
- A score of 8 or lower indicates coma.
- A score of 3, the lowest possible score, usually (but not always) indicates brain death.

Motor function

Motor function is also a good indicator of LOC and can point to CNS or peripheral nervous system damage.

Myelination mastery

The mastery of gross and fine motor skills is related to the myelination of the nervous system and follows the concept of cephalocaudal–proximodistal development. *Cephalocaudal development* is the sequence in which the greatest growth always occurs at the head and gradually works its way toward the "tail." *Proximodistal development* proceeds from the center toward the extremities.

Reflex rules

Infant activities are primarily driven by reflex, but with myelination and development, a growing child progressively performs complex tasks requiring coordinated movements.

How strong are you?

To evaluate muscle strength, follow these steps:
- Have the patient grip your hands and squeeze.
- Ask the patient to push against your palm with their foot.
- Compare muscle strength on each side to ensure the results are the same bilaterally.

Pupillary response

Brain damage is indicated by a lack of change in pupil size in response to light. Use a flashlight to assess pupillary response at the bedside. While shining the outer edge of the light into the patient's eye, observe the initial size of the pupil and the speed of the pupil's response to the light. Compare both eyes to ensure an equal bilateral response.

Diagnostic tests

Several invasive and noninvasive tests are used to diagnose neurologic disorders.

Computed tomography scan

Computed tomography (CT) scan (also called a CAT [computerized axial tomography] scan) is indicated when CNS disease is suspected. The scan uses computers and rotating x-ray machines to create cross-sectional (three-dimensional) images that can identify congenital abnormalities, fractures, brain tumors, infarction, bleeding, and hematomas as well as provide information about the ventricular system of the brain. CT scan may be done with or without contrast and provide more detailed information than normal x-ray images.

Nursing considerations

A child who knows what to expect will be less fearful and more cooperative during a CT scan. To help the child know what to expect, consider these steps:

- Explain the procedure to the child. Cooperation is necessary because the patient must lie still during the procedure.
- Show the child a picture of the CT machine to help alleviate fears. (It may be necessary to premedicate the patient.)
- Tell the child that they may hear a clicking noise as the scanner moves around their head but that the machine won't touch or hurt them.
- Explain that the child will not be able to eat or drink for 4 hours before the scan (depending on age), especially if contrast dye or anesthesia will be used.
- Assess the patient for allergy to iodinated dye or shellfish.
- Encourage the child to drink fluids after the scan, especially if dye was used because it is excreted by the kidneys.
- Remove any metal objects such as jewelry, eyeglasses, retainers, or hair accessories because they may affect the CT images. Explain that all items will be returned after the imaging.

Electroencephalogram

Electroencephalogram (EEG) is a graphic recording of the electrical activity of the brain. It is performed to identify and evaluate patients with seizures, epilepsy, head injuries, dizziness, headaches, brain tumors, and sleeping problems. EEG is also used to confirm brain death.

Nursing considerations

After explaining the procedure to the child and their caregivers, engage in the following practice:

- Reassure the child that they will not feel any pain during the test.
- Make sure the child continues to eat and drink before the test because fasting may cause hypoglycemia, which could alter the test results.

- Advise against any caffeine consumption on the morning of the test because of caffeine's stimulating effect.
- Tell the patient to remain still during the test; any movement will create interference and alter the EEG recording.

Lumbar puncture

A lumbar puncture is performed by placing a needle in the subarachnoid space of the spinal column in order to measure the pressure of that space and obtain CSF for examination and diagnosis. The needle is commonly placed between L3 and L4 (or L4 and L5). This examination may assist in the diagnosis of metastatic brain or spinal cord neoplasm, meningitis, cerebral hemorrhage, and encephalitis. The lumbar puncture may be performed under local anesthesia, intravenous (IV) sedation, or under general anesthesia.

Nursing considerations

The procedure should be explained, and written informed consent should be obtained. In addition, follow these steps:
- Apply eutectic mixture of local anesthetics (EMLA) cream to puncture site 30 to 60 minutes before the procedure to reduce pain if ordered.
- Instruct the child to empty their bladder and bowels before the procedure.
- Monitor the child's vital signs during and after the procedure.
- Explain the importance of remaining still throughout the procedure in the side-lying knee–chest position. (See *Lumbar puncture positioning.*)
- Gently hold even a cooperative child during the procedure to prevent injury from unexpected or involuntary movement.

Maintain, encourage, assess
- Keep the child flat for 1 hour after the procedure.
- Keep the child in a reclining position for up to 12 hours after the procedure to avoid the discomfort of potential postprocedural spinal headache.
- Encourage the child to drink increased amounts of fluid with a straw to replace the CSF removed during the puncture. (Drinking with a straw allows the patient to keep their head flat.)
- Assess the child for numbness, tingling, and decreased movement of the extremities; pain at the injection site; drainage of blood or CSF at the injection site; and inability to void.

Lumbar puncture positioning

When positioning a child for a lumbar puncture, follow these steps:

1. Have the child lie on their side at the edge of the bed, with their chin tucked to their chest and their knees drawn up to their abdomen.

2. Make sure the child's spine is curved and their back is at the edge of the bed. This position widens the spaces between the vertebrae, easing insertion of the needle.

3. To help the child maintain this position, place one of your hands behind their neck; place the other hand behind their knees and pull gently.

4. Hold the child firmly in this position throughout the procedure to prevent inadvertent needle displacement. (Typically, the provider inserts the needle between the third and fourth lumbar vertebrae.)

The sitting position may be used for infants. However, because the flexed position may interfere with the infant's breathing, monitor color and respiratory status closely during the procedure.

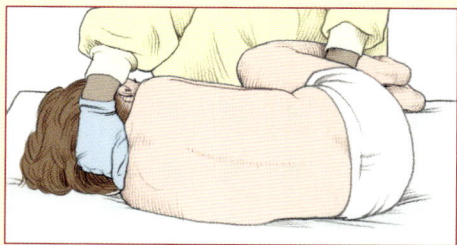

Positioning a young child

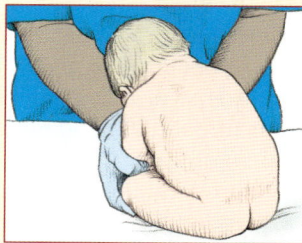

Positioning an infant

Magnetic resonance imaging

Magnetic resonance imaging (MRI) is a noninvasive diagnostic procedure using magnetic field and radio waves to create more detailed images of body organs and tissues in greater detail than a CT scan. It does not require exposure to ionizing radiation like x-ray or CT scans. MRI is indicated for the evaluation of the organs, blood vessels, and lymph nodes and is used to help diagnose a variety of conditions and to monitor certain treatments (tumors, CNS lesions, neck/back pain, heart problems, malformations of blood vessels, abnormalities of organs). MRI is sometimes used to monitor the fetus in pregnant adults and adolescents.

Nursing considerations

Begin by explaining the procedure to the patient and their family and telling them that there's no exposure to radiation during MRI. In addition, follow these steps:

- Tell the caregiver that because no radiation is used, they may read or talk to their child in the imaging room during the procedure.
- Inform the caregiver that young children may need to be sedated because of the need to remain motionless during the procedure.
- Offer ear plugs or headphones if available to distract from the tapping and thumping sounds during the MRI. Explain to the child and caregiver accompanying them that these sounds are normal.
- Tell the child that they may eat or drink as usual before and after the procedure. (No food or fluid restrictions are necessary before MRI, unless sedation is given.)
- Remove any metal objects such as jewelry, eyeglasses, retainers, or hair accessories because they may affect the MRI images or become projectile and dangerous if worn during the procedure. Explain that all items will be returned after the imaging.

Procedures and treatments

The care of a child with suspected or diagnosed neurologic problems may involve invasive procedures to monitor or treat the child's condition.

ICP monitoring

ICP pressure refers to the pressure inside the skull, representing the pressure in the brain tissue and the CSF. ICP monitoring allows assessment of the pressure exerted by the blood, brain, CSF, and any other space-occupying fluid or mass. It is used for several conditions such as traumatic brain injury, intracerebral hemorrhage, subarachnoid hemorrhage, hydrocephalus, CNS infections, and hepatic encephalopathy. Normal ICP is between 5 and 15 mm Hg; increased ICP is defined as pressure sustained at 20 mm Hg or higher.

Look closely . . .

Assessment of the child with increased ICP requires close observation because the common signs and symptoms may not appear until ICP is significantly elevated, placing the child in grave danger. ICP monitoring is done through invasive measures (intraventricular catheter or subdural screw/bolt) or noninvasive measures (epidural sensor).

- The intraventricular catheter is still considered the gold standard and most accurate of ICP monitoring, although the other monitoring techniques are sometimes preferred depending on the patient's situation. After a small burr hole is made in the skull, an external pressure transducer is connected to one of the lateral ventricles or subarachnoid space. (The catheter provides a method for measuring pressure as well as a conduit to drain off extra fluid into a drainage bag.) The drainage bag and the manometer are part of a sterile closed system. (The manometer is used to measure the ICP within the closed system.)

- If monitoring needs to be done right away, the subdural screw (bolt) is usually done where a hollow screw is placed in the subarachnoid space through a hole drilled in the skull. The top of the bolt is attached to a transducer to conduct a waveform to the monitor.
- In epidural sensor monitoring, monitoring is accomplished through a sensor inserted between the skull and dural tissue. Although less invasive than other methods, it cannot remove excess CSF.

Less invasive

In an infant, ICP monitoring can be performed without penetrating the scalp. In this external method, a photoelectric transducer with a pressure-sensitive membrane is taped to the infant's anterior fontanel. The transducer responds to pressure at the site and transmits readings to a bedside monitor and recording system.

Sorry, not for everyone

The external method is restricted to infants because pressure readings can be obtained only at the fontanels (the incompletely ossified areas of the skull). ICP monitoring from the fontanels can be inaccurate if the equipment is poorly placed or inconsistently calibrated.

Nursing considerations

Before ICP monitoring is performed, thoroughly explain the procedure to the child and their caregivers. In addition, follow these steps:
- Be familiar with the monitoring system being used and prepare the child and their family for what they can expect after placement of the selected monitoring device.
- Assess whether the child has an allergy to iodine preparations.
- Maintain sterility.
- Monitor the child closely for signs of infection.
- Monitor the amount of fluid in the drainage bag.
- Continuous assessment of the child for signs of increased ICP is required.
- Minimize activities that may elevate ICP, such as those that may cause stress, pain, or crying; bright lights, noise, and other environmental stimuli; and vigorous range of motion (ROM) exercises.

Remember that suctioning and percussion are contraindicated because they acutely elevate ICP. Suctioning may be performed if absolutely necessary by hyperoxygenating the patient with 100% oxygen before the procedure. Vibration may be used instead of percussion because it doesn't increase ICP.

Ventriculoperitoneal shunt insertion

A ventriculoperitoneal (VP) shunt is implanted in the child with hydrocephalus to prevent excess accumulation of CSF in the ventricles. The tubing diverts the CSF from the ventricles into the peritoneal cavity where it is reabsorbed. The procedure is performed under general anesthesia.

Nursing considerations

Young children may have misconceptions about procedures involving general anesthesia. When explaining this procedure (and all procedures involving general anesthesia), make sure the child understands that they will be given "a special medicine" to make sure they do not feel anything during the procedure.

A special sleep

Rather than telling a child they will be asleep (which may make them afraid to go to sleep at other times or cause them to worry that they will wake up during the procedure), tell them, "The medicine gives you a special kind of sleep that isn't like sleeping at night or naptime."

Monitor and measure

Preoperatively

Frequent neurologic assessments:
- Monitor the patient for signs of increased ICP.
- Measure head circumference daily at the occipital frontal circumference; place the tape measure just above the top of the ears, around the mid-forehead, and around the most prominent part of the occiput.
- Gently palpate fontanels and suture lines for signs of bulging, tenseness, and separation, which may indicate increased ICP or increasing ventricular size.

Postoperatively

Continue frequent neurologic assessments:
- Monitor the patient for pain and administer pain medications as ordered.
- Check orders regarding allowable activities.

- Observe the child for signs of increased ICP, which may indicate an obstructed shunt.
- Monitor the child for abdominal distention, which may indicate distal catheter displacement.
- Be alert for signs of shunt infection (fever, lethargy, irritability, redness along shunt device, abdominal discomfort, or apnea), which is the greatest postoperative risk.
- Monitor for fluid leak from the incision.
- Administer antibiotics as ordered.
- Teach caregivers to be aware of bowel patterns and recommend the use of laxatives and diet to prevent constipation, which has been associated with shunt malfunction.
- Teach caregivers signs and symptoms of shunt failure (persistent headache, emesis, lethargy, visual changes, or swelling or redness along the device).

Neurologic disorders

A diagnosis of a neurologic disorder, whether acute, chronic, or progressive, can be terrifying to a child and their caregivers. They will look to their nurses to help allay fears and concerns, answer questions, and provide ongoing support.

Bacterial meningitis

Meningitis, an inflammation of the meninges and spinal cord, is caused by either an infectious process (bacterial and viral are the most common, but can also be fungal, parasitic, and amebic) or noninfectious such as a result from complications of neurosurgery, trauma, systematic lupus, drugs, or a head injury.

What causes it

Prior to the *Haemophilus influenzae* type B vaccine (Hib vaccine), *H. influenzae* type B was the most common cause of meningitis in children older than age 1 month, but vaccination has drastically reduced its incidence. *Neisseria meningitidis* (meningococcal meningitis) and *Streptococcus pneumoniae* (pneumococcal meningitis) took the lead as the most common bacterial causes of meningitis beyond infancy. In 2001, a pneumococcal vaccine (PCV7 [now PCV20]) was added to the vaccine schedule, and since then, the incidence of meningitis caused by *S. pneumoniae* has decreased. By the end of the decade, meningococcal vaccines (MenACWY and MenB) were widely available and added to the recommended vaccines for adolescents.

Still strong

Group B streptococcus, *Escherichia coli*, and *Listeria monocytogenes* are the most common causes in infants younger than 3 months. Antibiotic resistance remains a concern among *S. pneumoniae*.

How it happens

- Bacteria reach the meninges via the bloodstream from nearby infections (e.g., sinusitis, mastoiditis, otitis media) or by communication of CSF with the exterior (e.g., myelomeningocele, penetrating injuries, or neurosurgical procedures).
- The organism becomes implanted in CSF and throughout the arachnoid space. Because CSF has relatively low levels of antibodies, complement, and white blood cells (WBCs), the infection flourishes.
- As the process continues, empyema and increased ICP develop.
- If the infection spreads to the ventricles, edema and tissue scarring around the ventricle cause obstruction of the CSF and subsequent hydrocephalus. Because CSF contains nutrients such as protein and glucose, it's an excellent medium for bacterial growth. Thus, the process of infection, edema, obstruction, and hydrocephalus can occur rapidly.

What to look for

Symptoms of bacterial meningitis are variable and depend on the child's age, pathogen, and duration of the illness before diagnosis. Findings in young infants and toddlers (between ages 3 months and 2 years) may include:

- fever
- change in feeding pattern
- vomiting or diarrhea
- bulging anterior fontanel
- irritability (becoming more so with rocking and cuddling)
- high-pitched cry
- extreme shivering
- pin-prick rash or purple bruises on body
- breathing fast or difficulty breathing
- stiff body, jerky movements, or floppy and lifeless
- seizures.

Bigger kids

In older children, look for:

- fever
- irritability
- lethargy
- confusion

- vomiting
- muscle or joint pain
- headache
- photophobia
- nuchal rigidity (resistance to neck flexion)
- opisthotonos (hyperextension of the head and neck to relieve discomfort)
- seizures
- coma
- positive Kernig or Brudzinski sign, or both. (See *Two telltale signs of meningitis.*)

Two telltale signs of meningitis

A positive response to these tests helps to establish a diagnosis of meningitis.

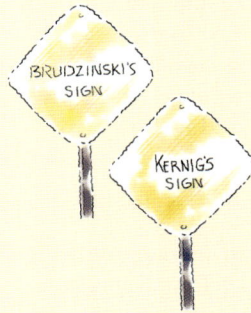

Brudzinski sign

To test for Brudzinski sign, place the patient in a dorsal recumbent position and put your hands behind their neck and bend it forward. Pain and resistance may indicate meningeal inflammation, neck injury, or arthritis. However, if the patient also flexes their hips and knees in response to the manipulation, chances are they have meningitis.

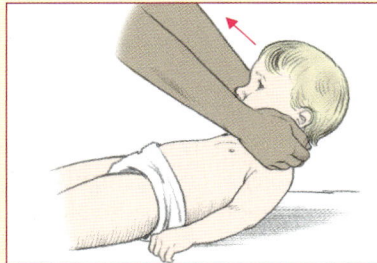

Kernig sign

To test for Kernig sign, place the patient in a supine position. Flex their leg at the hip and knee and then straighten the knee. Pain or resistance points to meningitis.

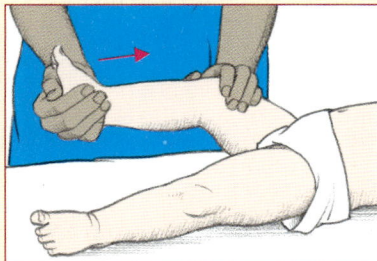

Children with a hemorrhagic rash, first appearing as petechiae and changing to purpura or large necrotic patches, may have meningococcal meningitis.

What tests tell you

Lumbar puncture is performed to evaluate the CSF for protein and glucose levels and the number of WBCs. The fluid may appear cloudy or milky white. CSF protein levels tend to be high; glucose levels may be low. Polymerase chain reaction techniques are useful when the cultures are negative because of partially treated meningitis.

A CT scan or MRI can rule out cerebral hematoma, hemorrhage, or tumor and identify an abscess. Other tests performed to aid in diagnosis include:
- blood cultures
- complete blood count (CBC)
- serum electrolytes and osmolality
- clotting factors
- nose and throat cultures.

Complications

The most common neurologic complications of meningitis are hearing loss, neurologic deficit, seizures, visual impairment, and behavioral problems. Other complications include CN dysfunction, brain abscess, and syndrome of inappropriate antidiuretic hormone (SIADH). Death occurs in 10% to 15% of patients (especially neonatal meningitis). Untreated bacterial meningitis approaches 100% mortality with neurologic sequelae among survivors.

How it's treated

Antibiotic treatment must begin immediately after lumbar puncture for blood cultures if clinical suspicion for meningitis. Gram stain and cultures can be identified in CSF up to several hours after administration of antibiotics. Evaluation includes CSF exam, CBC with differential and platelet count, two aerobic blood cultures, serum electrolytes, glucose, blood urea nitrogen, creatinine, and evaluation of clotting function (if petechial or purpuric lesions). Treatment includes the following:
- Two broad-spectrum antibiotics should be started as an initial treatment regimen.
- Antibiotics may be changed when culture and sensitivity results are known.
- Adjunctive therapy with dexamethasone (Decadron) may be provided to reduce the risk of sequelae such as hearing loss and neurologic complications.

- Isolation of the child is necessary for the first 24 hours of therapy to prevent spreading the infection.
- Assess for adequate ventilation and cardiac perfusion.
- Administer glucose if patient is hypoglycemic.
- Treat seizures if present.
- Implement fluid management as supportive therapy because fluid and electrolyte imbalances are common.
- Medications to control fever and pain/discomfort should be administered as needed.

No antibiotics needed if culture results come back negative

Treatment for viral (aseptic) meningitis is supportive; medications such as analgesics may be used to keep the child comfortable.(See *Aseptic meningitis*.) The initial symptoms of viral and bacterial meningitis are similar, so children with signs of meningitis should be treated as if it is bacterial until the culture proves otherwise.

Aseptic meningitis

Aseptic meningitis is characterized by headache, fever, vomiting, and meningeal symptoms. It results from some form of viral infection, including enteroviruses (most common), arboviruses, herpes simplex virus, mumps virus, or lymphocytic choriomeningitis virus.

Signs and symptoms

Aseptic meningitis begins suddenly with a fever up to 104°F (40°C), alterations in consciousness (drowsiness, confusion, stupor), and neck or spine stiffness, which is slight at first. (The patient experiences such stiffness when bending forward.) Other signs and symptoms include headaches, nausea, vomiting, abdominal pain, poorly defined chest pain, and sore throat.

Diagnostic tests

Patient history of recent illness and knowledge of seasonal epidemics are essential in differentiating among the many forms of aseptic meningitis. Negative bacteriologic cultures and CSF analysis showing pleocytosis and increased protein levels suggest the diagnosis. Isolation of the virus from CSF confirms it.

Treatment

Treatment is supportive and includes:
- bed rest
- maintenance of fluid and electrolyte balance
- analgesics agents for pain
- exercises to combat residual weakness
- careful handling of excretions and good handwashing technique to prevent spreading the disease.

What to do

Nursing interventions include a thorough history and careful assessment:

- Review the medical history with the patient and their family for recent illnesses, such as upper respiratory infection, head injury, otitis media, and sinusitis (or a previous lumbar puncture).
- Assess the patient for the presence or absence of headaches, hearing loss, seizure activity, change in food and fluid intake, changes in LOC, pupil reaction and size, and nuchal rigidity.
- Assess peaks and troughs of antibiotic levels to ensure adequate treatment and prevent ototoxicity.
- Ongoing assessment of LOC is the priority nursing assessment.
- Teach the caregivers about the possible complications of meningitis and about the prescribed medications.
- Question the child's caregivers about close contacts because they will need prophylactic treatment. (Close contacts should not wait for signs of meningitis to develop but should seek medical attention promptly because they could be incubating the infection.)

Brain tumors

CNS tumors are the most common solid tumors in children and cause more deaths in children than any other form of malignancy. Most brain tumors in children are *supratentorial* (above the roofline of the cerebellum); the remaining tumors are *infratentorial* (below the roofline of the cerebellum).

What causes it

The cause of brain tumors is unknown, but heredity and environmental factors have been associated with their development.

How it happens

Brain tumors are generally classified according to the tissue from which they arise: those arising inside the brain substance (such as gliomas and vascular tumors) or those arising outside the brain substance (such as meningiomas and CN tumors).

Common in kids

The most common brain tumors in children are:

- cerebellar astrocytoma
- medulloblastoma
- ependymoma
- brain stem glioma. (See *Locations of brain tumors in children.*)

Locations of brain tumors in children

Below are the most common types of brain tumor in children, along with their usual location.

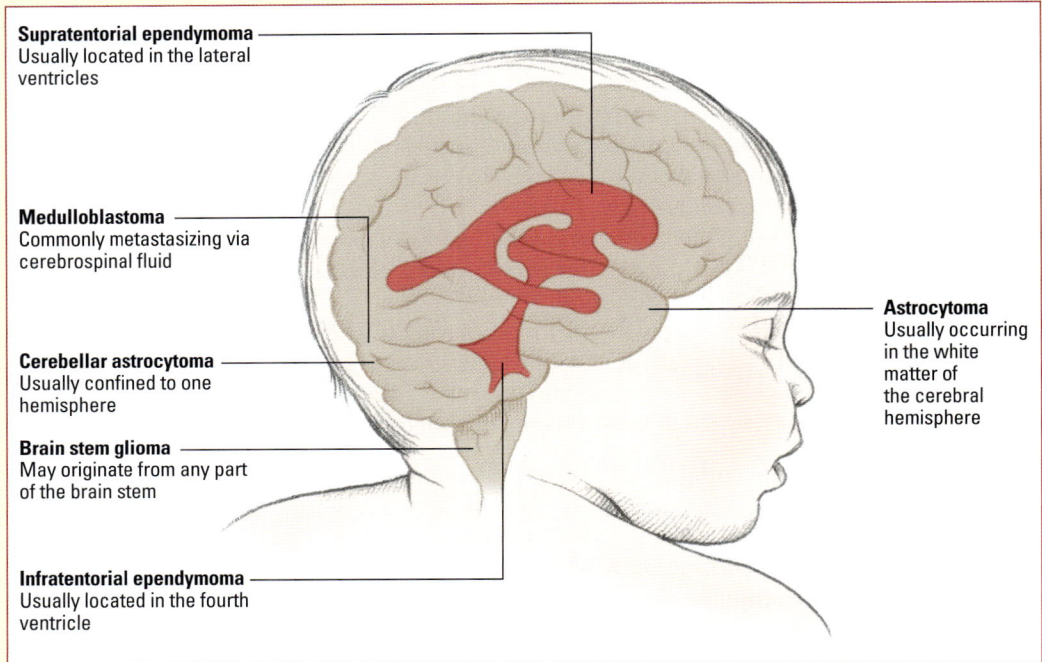

Supratentorial ependymoma
Usually located in the lateral ventricles

Medulloblastoma
Commonly metastasizing via cerebrospinal fluid

Cerebellar astrocytoma
Usually confined to one hemisphere

Brain stem glioma
May originate from any part of the brain stem

Infratentorial ependymoma
Usually located in the fourth ventricle

Astrocytoma
Usually occurring in the white matter of the cerebral hemisphere

What to look for

Signs and symptoms are directly related to the anatomic location and size of the tumor and, to some extent, the age of the child:

- The hallmark symptoms of a brain tumor are morning headache and early morning vomiting related to the child getting out of bed.
- The child may experience vision changes, such as diplopia, strabismus, and nystagmus, which may manifest as difficulties with schoolwork.
- *Papilledema* (edema of the optic disc) may be a late sign; this may be hard to evaluate in children because ophthalmic examinations require the child's cooperation.
- Enlargement of the head or bulging fontanels may be present in children before the closure of cranial sutures (at ages 12 to 18 months).
- Personality changes may be most critical and easily observable (such as crying, irritability, and not wanting to play).

- *Ataxia*, or uncoordinated gait, may be mistaken for clumsiness and is the most common sign of cerebellar involvement.

What tests tell you

History and physical and neurologic examinations provide the most important information. Diagnostic studies include:
- MRI (most common), CT scan, or PET scan showing the location and extent of the tumor
- lumbar puncture and serology of CSF to assess for the presence of tumor cells.

Complications

Some children with brain tumors experience some permanent sequelae, especially if they receive radiation therapy. They may have slowed development, incoordination, or learning disabilities. In some instances, brain tumors result in death.

How it's treated

Treatment includes:
- removing a resectable tumor
- reducing a nonresectable tumor
- relieving cerebral edema, increased ICP, and other symptoms
- preventing further neurologic damage.

The mode of therapy depends on the histologic type of the tumor, radiosensitivity, and location; it may include surgery, radiation, chemotherapy, or decompression of increased ICP with diuretics, corticosteroids, or, possibly, VP shunting of CSF.

Treatment of choice

Surgical excision is usually performed when possible. However, combination therapy (surgery and radiation with or without chemotherapy) has been proven to improve outcomes.

What to do

During your first contact with the child, perform a comprehensive assessment (including a complete neurologic evaluation) to provide baseline data and help develop your care plan. In addition, follow these steps:
- Continually assess for signs of increased ICP, including decreasing pulse and respirations, increasing systolic blood pressure, and a widening pulse pressure.
- Monitor for changes in the child's LOC. (A change in behavior is most significant in young children. A change in sleeping and waking patterns may also be significant.)
- Report changes in ocular signs, such as pupil response, shape, and size.

- Measure head circumference daily in children younger than age 2 years.
- Promote minimal sensory stimulation including quiet, dimly lit environment.
- Frequently assess pain and provide pain control as prescribed.
- Observe seizure precautions; seizures are always a possibility in a child with brain tumor.
- Always keep the bed's side rails up and assist with ambulation because CN dysfunction may lead to ataxia and weakness.
- Provide emotional support for the child and their family members; referral to a social worker, psychologist, or other health care professional may be needed to help the child and their family cope with the diagnosis.

Postoperative care

Children who undergo surgery for a brain tumor require specialized care. Positioning is important and varies with the type of surgery performed, and diligent monitoring of vital signs, neurologic status, and pain is essential. In addition, follow these steps:
- The child may be kept flat at first; positioning may be limited to a 10- to 20-degree elevation for the first 24 to 48 hours. (The doctor will prescribe the patient's position.)
- Never place the child in Trendelenburg position because it increases ICP and the risk of bleeding.
- Assess vital signs, mental status, and neurologic status frequently because the child is at risk for increased ICP related to cerebral edema, hydrocephalus, or hemorrhage.
- Prevent and assess for infection at surgical site.
- Continue monitoring and care of patient's pain.

High temp, cool blanket
- The child's temperature may be labile (usually elevated) because of edema of the brain stem; a hypothermia blanket may be used if the child becomes hyperthermic.
- Be careful not to place tension on the suture line when turning the child.
- Assess the child frequently for pain. (Analgesic agents should be provided according to the provider's orders.)

Hair today, gone tomorrow
- Body image issues (shaven head, edema, or fear of disfigurement) may be a problem for older children and adolescents; help them to work through these feelings with the help of hospital counselors.
- Provide emotional support to the caregivers; help them to work through their feelings regarding diagnosis, treatment, and

prognosis (refer them to appropriate agencies and support groups for further assistance).

Cerebral palsy

Cerebral palsy (CP) is a nonprogressive, neuromuscular disorder of varying degrees resulting from damage or developmental defects in the part of the brain that controls motor function.

Children with CP affect functional abilities but can vary greatly. Some people cannot control movements in certain parts of their bodies and may be partially paralyzed, whereas others can walk and even run. They may have completely normal intelligence and may feel as if they are trapped in a body they can't control, whereas others may have intellectual disabilities. Epilepsy, blindness, or deafness may also accompany CP diagnoses. Symptoms of CP are abnormal reflexes, floppiness, rigidity of limbs and sometimes trunk, abnormal posture and movements, problems swallowing, eye muscle imbalance, muscle stiffness, or a combination of these.

What causes it

Conditions that result in cerebral anoxia, hemorrhage, or other damage are probably responsible for CP. In most patients, the exact cause is not known.

In the womb

Prenatal conditions that may increase the risk of CP include maternal infection (such as rubella, varicella, cytomegalovirus, herpes, toxoplasmosis, syphilis, and Zika virus), radiation, anoxia, toxemia, maternal diabetes or thyroid problems, seizures or epilepsy, abnormal placental attachment, malnutrition, Rh-isoimmunization, and gene mutations that lead to abnormal brain development.

A shaky start

Perinatal and birth difficulties that increase the risk of CP include forceps delivery, breech presentation, placenta previa, abruptio placentae, metabolic or electrolyte disturbances, abnormal maternal vital signs from general or spinal anesthetic, prolapsed cord with delay in delivery of the head, premature birth, prolonged or unusually rapid labor, and multiple birth (especially infants born last in a multiple birth). Low birth weight (<5.5 lb) and babies born fewer than 37 weeks into pregnancy are at higher risk of CP.

A traumatic legacy

Infection or trauma during infancy that increases the risk of CP includes poisoning, severe kernicterus resulting from erythroblastosis fetalis, brain infection, head trauma, prolonged anoxia, brain tumor, cerebral circulatory anomalies causing blood vessel rupture, and systemic disease resulting in cerebral thrombosis or embolus. Bacterial meningitis and viral encephalitis cause inflammation in the membranes surrounding the brain and spinal cord, which can lead to CP. Severe or untreated jaundice in infancy can also cause CP.

How it happens

A perinatal anoxic episode plays the largest role in the pathologic state of brain damage. Structural or functional defects occur, impairing motor or cognitive function. Defects may not be distinguishable until several months after birth or when the child fails to meet developmental milestones.

What to look for

There are three distinct types of CP:
1. Spastic (affected part of the brain: cortex)
2. Athetoid (basal ganglia)
3. Ataxic (cerebellum)

Spastic

Spastic CP is the most common type, affecting about 70% of patients with CP. The affected area of the brain is the cortex. Typically, the child with spastic CP walks on their toes with a scissor gait, crossing one foot in front of the other. Spastic CP is characterized by:
- increased deep tendon reflexes
- hypertonia
- flexion
- tendency to have contractures
- rapid involuntary muscle contraction and relaxation
- underdevelopment of affected limbs.

Athetoid

In athetoid CP, which affects about 20% of patients with CP, involuntary, uncoordinated motion occurs with varying degrees of muscle tension. The area of injury is the basal ganglia. The child exhibits slow, writhing, uncontrolled movements involving all extremities whenever voluntary movement is attempted. Facial grimacing, poor swallowing, and drooling make speech difficult.

Ataxic

Ataxic CP accounts for about 10% of patients with CP. The affected area of the brain is the cerebellum. Its characteristics include poor balance and muscle coordination caused by disturbances in movement and balance. An unsteady, wide-based gait appears as the child begins to learn to walk; overall, the child appears clumsy.

Mixed together

Some children with CP display a combination of these clinical features:

- Delayed gross motor development makes eating, especially swallowing, difficult.
- Abnormal motor performance and coordination can manifest early in life as poor sucking and feeding difficulty.
- Spasticity of hip muscles and lower extremities makes diapering difficult.
- Posture abnormalities occur at rest or when changing position.
- Cognitive impairment occurs in varying degrees in 18% to 50% of patients (most children with CP have an IQ that is normal or higher, but they cannot demonstrate it on standardized tests).
- Seizures occur in 25% of patients with CP.
- Many children have sensory deficits related to vision (strabismus), hearing, and speech.

What tests tell you

- Developmental screening reveals delay in achieving milestones.
- EEG may identify the source of seizure activity.
- Neuroimaging studies (CT scan, MRI) determine the site of brain impairment. Cranial ultrasounds can be used as a preliminary assessment of the brain in infants.
- Cytogenetic studies (genetic evaluation of the child and other family members) and metabolic studies are performed to rule out other potential causes.

Complications

Children with CP may also have associated disorders, such as impaired intellectual development, seizures, failure to grow and thrive, and problems with vision and sense of touch.

How it's treated

CP cannot be cured, but proper treatment can help affected children reach their full potential within the limitations set by this disorder. Treatment includes the following:

- A baclofen pump may be inserted under general anesthesia to treat spasticity by delivering the skeletal muscle relaxant directly to the intrathecal space around the spinal cord (the pump usually lasts 5 years, after which a new pump must be implanted). The baclofen usually needs to be refilled every 1 to 6 months.
- Botulinum toxin A (Botox) may be used, especially for spasticity in lower extremities.
- Oral muscle relaxants may be used or neurosurgery may be required to decrease spasticity.

- Braces or splints and special appliances, such as adapted eating utensils and a low toilet seat with arms, can help the child perform activities independently.
- ROM exercises minimize contractures.
- Medications are sometimes prescribed to control drooling.
- An artificial urinary sphincter may be indicated for the incontinent child who is able to use hand controls.

Correct those contractures
- Orthopedic surgery may be indicated to correct contractures.
- Antiepileptic drugs may be used to control seizures.
- Selective dorsal rhizotomy, or severing nerves serving the spastic muscles, is done in patients with severe spasticity to help relax the muscle and reduce pain.

What to do
Care of the child with CP involves attention to diet and physical activity:
- Institute a high-calorie diet for the child with increased motor function to help them keep up with increased metabolic demands.
- Assist with locomotion, communication, and educational opportunities to enable the child to attain an optimal developmental level.
- Perform ROM exercises to minimize contractures.
- Plan activities that involve gross and fine motor skills (such as holding toys or eating utensils and positioning items to encourage reaching and rolling over).
- Provide a safe environment; have the child use protective headgear or bed pads to prevent injury.

Skilled labor of love
The nurse should also teach the family the skills needed to manage the child's care (such as medication administration, physical rehabilitation, and seizure management). Siblings should be involved in the child's care to prevent feelings of being left out.

Family members need help in setting realistic goals and managing stress. They should be referred to community agencies that will enhance the child's quality of life (early childhood stimulation programs, recreational programs for children with disabilities) and provide caregiver support.

Hydrocephalus
Hydrocephalus is an excessive accumulation of CSF within the ventricles of the brain, resulting from interference with normal circulation or absorption of the fluid.

CSF overload

As excess CSF accumulates in the ventricular system, the ventricles become dilated and the brain is compressed against the skull. If sutures are open, this results in enlargement of the skull, whereas if the sutures are fused, increased ICP signs and symptoms will present.

What causes it

Hydrocephalus that results from an obstruction in CSF flow is called *noncommunicating hydrocephalus*. Causes include faulty fetal development, infection, a tumor, a cerebral aneurysm, or a blood clot after intracranial hemorrhage.

Communicating hydrocephalus results from faulty absorption of CSF. Causes of communicating hydrocephalus include a surgical complication, adhesions, or meningeal hemorrhage. (See *Hydrocephalus and CSF circulation*.)

Hydrocephalus and CSF circulation

In noncommunicating hydrocephalus, the obstruction of CSF circulation occurs most commonly between the third and fourth ventricles, at the aqueduct of Sylvius. However, it can also occur at the outlets of the fourth ventricle (foramina of Luschka and Magendie) or, rarely, at the foramen of Monro.

Absorption distortion

In communicating hydrocephalus, faulty absorption of CSF may result from surgery, adhesions between meninges at the base of the brain, or meningeal hemorrhage. Rarely, a tumor in the choroid plexus causes overproduction of CSF, resulting in hydrocephalus.

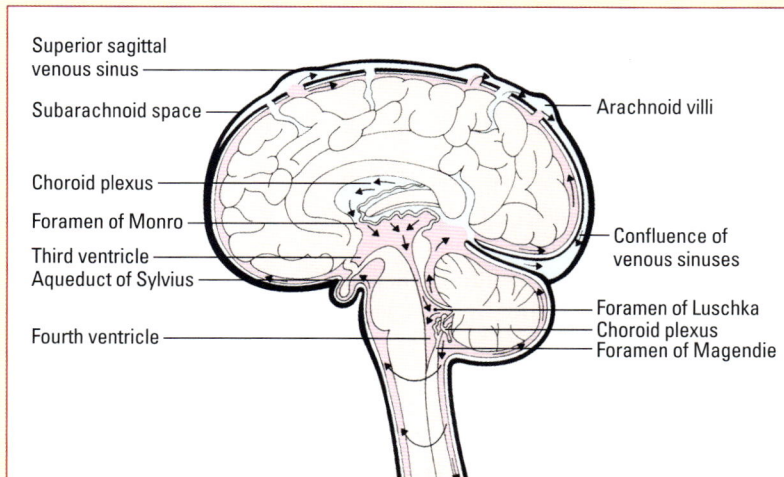

How it happens

In healthy children, CSF circulation is unimpeded:
- CSF is produced from blood in a capillary network (choroid plexus) in the brain's lateral ventricles.
- From the lateral ventricles, CSF flows through the interventricular foramen (foramen of Monro) to the third ventricle.
- From there, it flows through the aqueduct of Sylvius to the fourth ventricle, through the foramina of Luschka and Magendie, to the cisterna of the subarachnoid space.
- The fluid then passes under the base of the brain, upward over the brain's upper surfaces, and down around the spinal cord.
- Eventually, CSF reaches the arachnoid villi, where it's reabsorbed into venous blood at the venous sinuses.

What to look for

The signs and symptoms of hydrocephalus vary with the age of the child. In infants, the unmistakable sign of hydrocephalus is rapidly increasing head circumference that is clearly disproportionate to the infant's growth. Other characteristic changes include:
- widening and bulging of the fontanels
- distended scalp veins
- thin, shiny, fragile-looking scalp skin
- underdeveloped neck muscles. (See *Signs of hydrocephalus*.)

The setting sun

In severe hydrocephalus, the roof of the orbit is depressed, the eyes are displaced downward, and the sclerae are prominent. When the sclera is seen above the iris, it's called the *setting-sun sign*. Other common signs and symptoms include:
- high-pitched, shrill cry
- abnormal muscle tone of the legs
- irritability
- anorexia
- projectile vomiting.

In older children, indicators of hydrocephalus include decreased LOC, ataxia, incontinence, and impaired intellect. The most common symptoms of hydrocephalus in the older child are blurry or double vision and headaches followed by nausea and vomiting. They may also experience problems with balance, poor coordination, gait disturbance, and changes in personality or cognition.

Signs of hydrocephalus

In infants, characteristic changes in hydrocephalus include:
- marked enlargement of the head
- distended scalp veins
- thin, shiny, fragile-looking scalp skin
- weak muscles that can't support the head.

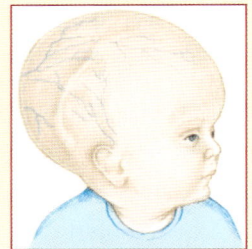

Arnold–Chiari malformation

Arnold–Chiari malformation commonly accompanies hydrocephalus, especially when a myelomeningocele is present. In this condition, an elongated or tonguelike downward projection of the cerebellum and medulla extends through the foramen magnum into the cervical portion of the spinal canal, impairing CSF drainage from the fourth ventricle.

Rigid, noisy, and irritable

Infants with this malformation also demonstrate nuchal rigidity, noisy respirations, irritability, vomiting, weak sucking reflex, and a preference for hyperextension of the neck.

What tests tell you

Diagnostic tests for hydrocephalus include:
- daily measurement of head circumference because rapid head enlargement is the first indication of the problem
- skull x-rays, which show thinning of the skull with separation of sutures and widening of the fontanels
- a CT scan and an MRI, which are used to confirm the diagnosis, assess ventricular dilatation or enlargement and demonstrate the Arnold–Chiari malformation.

Complications

Potential complications of hydrocephalus include:
- cognitive impairment or disabilities
- impaired motor function and speech
- seizures or epilepsy
- vision problems, impairment, or loss.

The most serious complication associated with shunt placement is infection. Shunt malfunction is the other major complication and is caused by such mechanical problems as kinking, plugging, migrating, and tubing separation.

How it's treated

Treatment involves removal of the obstruction (such as surgical removal of a tumor) or creation of a new CSF pathway to divert excess CSF. The goal of treatment is to bypass the obstruction and drain the fluid from the ventricles to an area where it can be reabsorbed.

It's tubular

This bypass is accomplished with insertion of a VP shunt or tube, which leads from the ventricles, out of the skull, and passes under the skin to the peritoneal cavity. (See *VP shunt.*)

VP shunt

A VP shunt drains excess CSF from the brain's lateral ventricle into the peritoneal cavity.

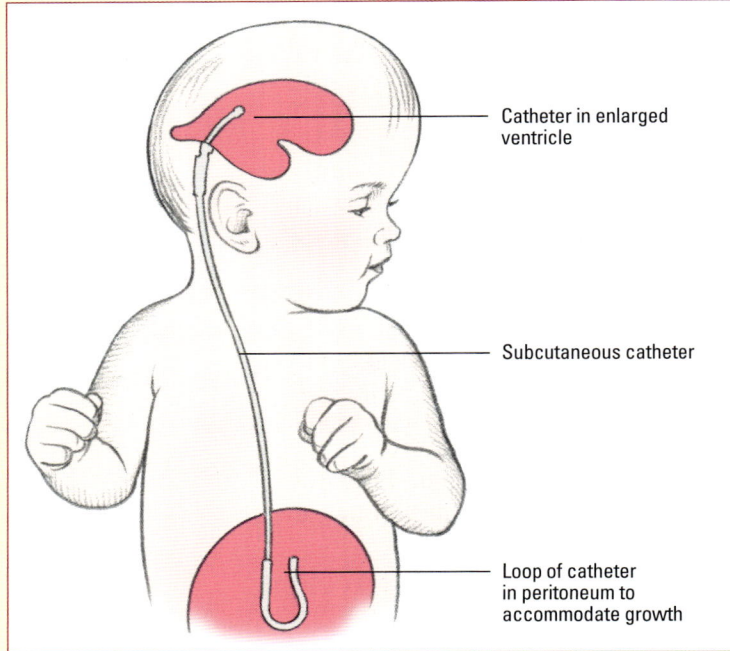

Catheter in enlarged ventricle

Subcutaneous catheter

Loop of catheter in peritoneum to accommodate growth

Straight to the heart

An alternative to the VP shunt is the less commonly used ventriculoatrial shunt, which drains the fluid from the ventricles to the right atrium of the heart.

What to do

Several preoperative and postoperative nursing interventions are indicated for the child with hydrocephalus.

Preoperative care

Preoperative care involves careful monitoring:

- Head circumference should be measured daily, watching for signs of increased ICP.
- Assess respiratory status every 4 hours or more often if necessary.
- Measure intake and output of all fluids.
- Monitor nutritional status and provide small feedings because the child is prone to vomiting. (During feedings, the child's head must be supported carefully and they must be burped frequently.)

Postoperative care

Postoperatively, the child is placed in a flat position on the nonoperative side to prevent rapid CSF drainage and pressure on the valves. If CSF is drained too rapidly, the child is at risk for subdural hematoma caused by tears in the vessels secondary to the cerebral cortex pulling away from the dura. Nursing care continues to focus on careful observation of the child's status as well as educating the caregivers about how to care for the child with the shunt in place:

- Observe for decreased LOC and vomiting.
- Observe the child for signs of shunt infection, such as fever, increased heart and respiratory rates, poor feeding or vomiting, altered mental status, seizures, and redness along the shunt tract.
- Observe for abdominal distention or discomfort because shunt placement may cause a paralytic ileus or peritonitis.
- Measure head circumference daily; any increase of more than 0.5 cm is significant and should be reported to the health care provider.

Shunt care 101

- Explain all procedures to the caregivers.
- Teach the caregivers signs and symptoms of shunt infection and malfunction and what to do if they suspect either.
- Teach the caregivers to foster normal growth and development in their child; the child should not be overprotected but should avoid contact sports.

Neural tube defects

Neural tube defects (NTDs) are serious birth defects that involve the spine or the brain. They result from failure of the neural tube to close at approximately 28 days after conception. The most common forms of NTD are:

- spina bifida (50% of patients)
- anencephaly (40%)
- encephalocele (10%).

Spina bifida

Spina bifida occulta is a visible defect with an external saclike protrusion. It is characterized by incomplete closure of one or more vertebrae without protrusion of the spinal cord or meninges.

What's in the sac?

Spina bifida cystica is a visible defect with an external saclike protrusion. It has two classifications:

- *Myelomeningocele,* in which the external sac contains meninges, CSF, and a portion of the spinal cord or nerve roots distal to the conus medullaris
- *Meningocele,* in which the sac contains only meninges and CSF and may produce no neurologic symptoms (See *Forms of spina bifida.*)

Forms of spina bifida

The most common forms of spina bifida are listed below, along with their major characteristics.

Spina bifida occulta

Spina bifida occulta is the least severe of the spinal cord defects. It's characterized by incomplete closure of one or more vertebrae without protrusion of the spinal cord or meninges.

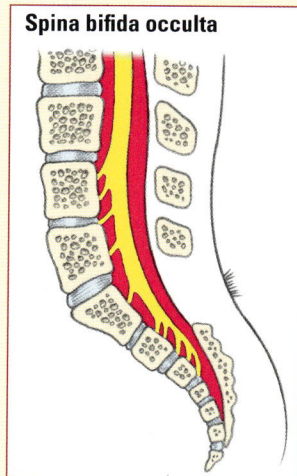

Spina bifida occulta

Spina bifida cystica

Spina bifida cystica is a visible defect with an external saclike protrusion. It has two classifications: meningocele and myelomeningocele.

Forms of spina bifida (*continued*)

Meningocele
In meningocele, the sac contains only meninges and CSF.

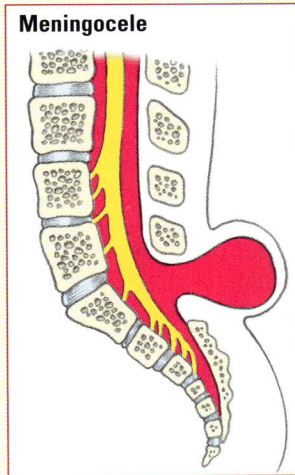

Meningocele

Myelomeningocele
In myelomeningocele, the external sac contains meninges, CSF, and a portion of the spinal cord or nerve roots distal to the conus medullaris.

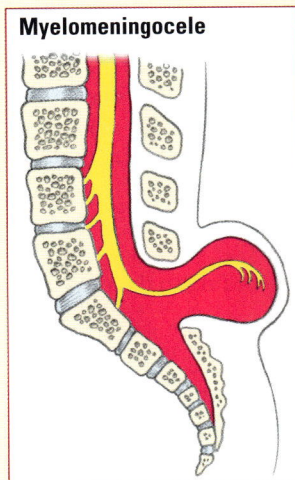

Myelomeningocele

Anencephaly

Anencephaly occurs when both cerebral hemispheres are absent. The closure defect occurs at the cranial end of the neuraxis, and, as a result, part of the entire top of the skull is missing and the brain is severely damaged. It is the most severe NTD and is incompatible with life.

Many infants with anencephaly are stillborn. If the infant does survive, there is no specific treatment. Because the infant has an intact brain stem, they can maintain vital functions, such as temperature regulation and respiratory and cardiac function. Most live for a few weeks and then die of respiratory failure.

Encephalocele

In encephalocele, a saclike portion of the meninges and brain protrudes through a defective opening in the skull.

What causes it

NTDs may be isolated birth defects, may result from exposure to a teratogen (factor that increases the risk of congenital disorder in an embryo), or may be part of a multiple malformation syndrome. It is believed that isolated NTDs (those not due to a specific teratogen or associated with other malformations) are caused by a combination of genetic and environmental factors. Although most of the specific environmental triggers are unknown, research has identified a lack of folic acid in the birthing parent's preconception diet as one of the risk factors.

How it happens

During the fourth week of gestation, ventral induction of the neural tube fails to occur. The degree of impairment depends on the size and level of the defect and whether it involves the spinal cord and nerves. Associated malformations include hydrocephalus and Arnold–Chiari malformation.

What to look for

The signs and symptoms of NTDs vary widely according to the type of the defect.

Search the sacrum

In spina bifida occulta, a depression or dimple, a small tuft of hair, a hemangioma, or a port-wine nevi in the lower lumbar or sacral area usually accompanies the defect. Because there is no herniation of the spinal cord or meninges, spina bifida occulta usually does not cause neurologic dysfunction, but it is occasionally associated with foot weakness or bowel and bladder disturbances.

Sac on the back

In myelomeningocele and meningocele, a saclike structure protrudes over the spine. Meningocele seldom causes neurologic symptoms.

Myelomeningocele is associated with permanent neurologic symptoms, such as flaccid or spastic paralysis; bowel and bladder incontinence; clubfoot; knee contractures; hydrocephalus and, possibly, cognitive impairment; Arnold–Chiari malformation; and curvature of the spine.

Poor prognosis

Clinical effects of encephalocele include paralysis, hydrocephalus, and severe cognitive impairment. Anencephaly is invariably fatal.

What tests tell you

Diagnostic tests include the following:

- Alpha-fetoprotein (AFP) screening (also known as the "quad screen" or "multiple marker" blood test) measures AFP levels in the blood at 16 to 18 weeks' gestation. AFP is a fetal-specific gamma-1 globulin in the amniotic fluid that indicates the presence of myelomeningocele. The other three parts of the quad screen involve testing the levels of human chorionic gonadotropin, estriol (typically done in the second trimester), and inhibin-A. If the AFP screen is abnormal, amniocentesis and fetal ultrasound are performed.
- Amniocentesis may reveal the presence of AFP in the amniotic fluid.
- Ultrasound may be used to detect open NTDs or ventral wall defects.
- Transillumination of a protruding spinal sac can sometimes distinguish between myelomeningocele (in which the sac transilluminates) and meningocele (in which the sac doesn't transilluminate).
- After birth, different tests such as skull x-rays, MRI, and CT scans identify the defects.

Complications

Complications of NTDs include decreased motor activity below the defect, paralysis, multiple musculoskeletal deficits, neurogenic bladder and bowel, CNS infections, hydrocephalus, and death.

Latex liability

Children with spina bifida are at high risk for developing latex allergies possibly because of frequent exposure to latex during catheterizations and multiple surgical procedures. Allergic reactions can range from mild signs and symptoms to anaphylactic shock.

How it's treated

Immediate surgical closure (within 48 hours) is the most common choice of treatment, although spina bifida occulta usually requires no surgery. The rationale for early surgical closure is to decrease the risk of infection, morbidity, and mortality and to prevent further spinal cord and spinal nerve damage. Surgery does not reverse neurologic deficits.

Scheduled for surgery

A shunt may also be needed to relieve related hydrocephalus. Treatment of encephalocele includes surgery during infancy to place protruding tissues back in the skull, excise the sac, and correct associated craniofacial abnormalities.

What to do

Nursing interventions begin prenatally and, after the child is born, continue with preoperative and postoperative care.

Prenatal care

Prenatally, care focuses on educating and supporting the caregivers:
- Refer the prospective caregivers to a genetic counselor who can provide information and support the couple's decision on how to manage the pregnancy.
- Inform people of childbearing age to take a folic acid supplement until menopause or the end of childbearing potential. Research has indicated that the risk of an open NTD may be reduced 50% to 100% in pregnant people who take folic acid.
- Provide psychological support to help the caregivers accept the diagnosis and prognosis.

Preoperative care

Before surgery, many nursing interventions focus on preventing complications associated with the sac:
- Prevent the sac from drying by covering it with warmed saline-soaked sterile dressings.
- Check for leakage from the sac, monitor for redness and infection around the sac, and assess for signs and symptoms of CNS infection.
- Assess for sensory and motor activity below the sac, including bowel and bladder function.

No pressure, please
- Prevent trauma by keeping pressure off the sac; keep the child on their abdomen with hips flexed and legs abducted.
- Institute measures to keep the sac free from infection; avoid contamination from urine and stool. (A "mud flap" can be made using a strip of plastic with adhesive backing on the top portion; this is placed directly below the defect and will prevent contamination from stool.)
- Measure head circumference to establish baseline data.
- Be aware of the increased incidence of latex allergies in these children and take appropriate precautions.

Teach and support
- Provide emotional support to the caregivers. Be aware that surgery is usually performed 24 to 48 hours after birth.

- Teach caregivers and other family members about measures to prevent contractures, pressure injuries, urinary tract infections, and other complications.

Postoperative care

After surgery, provide routine postoperative care, including monitoring vital signs, positioning, and observation of the operative site. In addition, follow these steps:

- Provide thorough skin care if paralysis is present (to prevent complications such as pressure injuries).
- Infant may be positioned on side (with order) or abdomen.
- Assess motor activity and bowel and bladder function to compare with the preoperative condition.
- Measure head circumference daily and perform ROM exercises.
- Teach clean intermittent catheterization to caregivers.
- Maintain splints, braces, and casts; use wheelchairs, walkers, and other assistive devices as needed.

Seizure disorders

A seizure is a sudden, episodic, involuntary alteration in consciousness, motor activity, behavior, sensation, or autonomic function caused by abnormal electrical discharges by the neurons in the brain. Seizures can accompany a variety of disorders, or they may occur spontaneously without apparent cause. Epilepsy is a condition in which a person has spontaneously recurring seizures.

What causes it

The most common causes of seizure during the first 6 months of life are:

- severe birth injury
- congenital defects involving the CNS
- infections
- inborn errors of metabolism.

Other causes include birth trauma (inadequate oxygen supply to the brain, blood incompatibility, or hemorrhage), infectious diseases (meningitis, encephalopathy, or brain abscess), ingestion of toxins, head trauma, metabolic disorders (hypoglycemia, hypocalcemia, hyponatremia, hypernatremia, or hyperbilirubinemia), and high fever.

How it happens

In recurring seizures (epilepsy), a group of abnormal neurons seem to undergo spontaneous firing.

Consciously electric

Electrical discharges come from central areas in the brain that affect consciousness. The discharges may be localized in one area of the brain and cause responses specific to the anatomic focus controlled by that area. They may be initiated in a localized area of the brain and then spread to other areas, resulting in a generalized response.

Cellular excitement

Hyperexcitable cells, called the *epileptogenic focus*, spontaneously release the discharges. These discharges can be triggered by either environmental or physiologic stimuli, such as emotional stress, anxiety, fatigue, infection, or metabolic disturbances.

What to look for

Seizures can take various forms, depending on their origin and whether they are localized to one area of the brain (as in partial seizures) or occur in both hemispheres (as in generalized seizures). If a partial seizure generalizes, it is still classified as a partial seizure. (See *Classifying seizures*.)

Classifying seizures

This chart lists and describes each type of seizure, along with signs and symptoms.

Type	Description	Signs and symptoms
Partial		
Simple partial	Seizure activity begins in one hemisphere or focal area. There's no change in LOC.	May have motor (change in posture), sensory (hallucinations), or autonomic (flushing, tachycardia) symptoms; no loss of consciousness
Complex partial	Seizure activity begins in one hemisphere or focal area. There's an alteration in consciousness.	Loss of consciousness, aura of visual disturbances; postictal seizures
Generalized		
Absence (petit mal)	Sudden onset; lasts 5–10 seconds; can have 100 daily; precipitated by stress, hyperventilation, hypoglycemia, fatigue; differentiated from daydreaming	Loss of responsiveness but continued ability to maintain posture control and not fall; twitching eyelids; lip smacking; no postictal symptoms
Myoclonic	Sudden, short contractures of a muscle or muscle group	No loss of consciousness; sudden, brief shock-like involuntary contraction of one muscle group
Clonic	Opposing muscles contract and relax alternately in rhythmic pattern; may occur in one limb more than others	Mucus production

Classifying seizures (*continued*)

Type	Description	Signs and symptoms
Tonic	Muscles are maintained in continuous contracted state (rigid posture).	Variable loss of consciousness; pupils dilate; eyes roll up; glottis closes; possible incontinence; may foam at mouth
Tonic–clonic (grand mal, major motor)	Violent, total-body seizure	Aura first (20–40 seconds); clonic next; postictal symptoms
Atonic	Drop-and-fall attack; needs to wear protective helmet	Loss of posture tone
Akinetic	Sudden brief loss of muscle tone or posture	Temporary loss of consciousness
Miscellaneous		
Febrile	Seizure threshold lowered by elevated temperature; only one seizure per fever; common in 4% of population under age 5; occurs when temperature is rapidly rising	Lasts <5 minutes; generalized, transient, and nonprogressive; doesn't generally result in brain damage; EEG is normal after 2 weeks.
Status epilepticus	Prolonged or frequent repetition of seizures without interruption; may result in anoxia and cardiac and respiratory arrest	Consciousness not regained between seizures; lasts >30 minutes

What tests tell you

A complete history, physical, and neurologic examination—including birth and development history, significant illnesses and injuries, family history, history of febrile seizures, and a comprehensive neurologic assessment—should be performed. Laboratory and other tests include:
- CBC and blood chemistry to detect electrolyte imbalances
- blood glucose levels to detect hypoglycemic episodes
- lumbar puncture to rule out meningitis as a cause of the seizures
- EEG to help differentiate epileptic from nonepileptic seizures (each seizure has a characteristic EEG tracing).

CT, MRI—both can help identify

If the child is taking anticonvulsant agents, blood levels should be monitored. Lead levels, toxicology screening, and radiologic tests, such as CT scanning or MRI, may be performed to identify structural lesions.

Complications

Complications from seizures include physical injury during the seizure, brain damage, and respiratory insufficiency or arrest.

How it's treated

Most children are treated with anticonvulsant agents, preferably a single medication to minimize adverse effects. Children who continue to have seizures with the single medication are treated with multiple anticonvulsant agents. Medication dosage adjustments are usually needed as the child grows since the dosage may be calculated using the child's weight. Serum drug levels are monitored to achieve therapeutic levels or when toxicity is possible. Surgery may be necessary to remove a tumor, lesion, or portion of the brain that has been identified as causing the seizure. Older children and adolescents may be candidates for a vagal nerve stimulator.

Kudos for ketogenic

A ketogenic diet may occasionally be used for children with seizures. A ketogenic diet is a high-fat, low-carbohydrate, low-protein diet that causes ketosis as the body uses fat for metabolism. Ketosis is believed to slow the electrical impulses that cause seizures. This diet is typically used in conjunction with medications. It is prescribed by a neurologist and carefully monitored by a dietitian.

Keep it cool

Children with febrile seizures may be treated with an anticonvulsant agent throughout the presenting febrile illness; long-term anticonvulsant agents are not generally used. Caregivers are taught to lower fever by administering antipyretic medications and to keep the child cool. Rectal diazepam may be given during the seizure episode.

What to do

The nurse caring for a child who has seizures should focus on maintaining airway patency, ensuring safety, administering medications, observing and treating the seizure, educating the child and their caregivers, and providing psychosocial intervention. In addition, follow these steps:

- Stay with the child during a seizure.
- Move the child to a flat surface, out of danger; if they are standing, gently assist them to the floor.
- Provide a patent airway and place the child on their side to allow saliva to drain out.
- Avoid trying to interrupt the seizure. (Instead, gently support the child's head and keep their hands from inflicting self-harm but not restrain them.)
- Pad the crib or bed rails to prevent physical injury.

Out with the noise, in with the calm

- Reduce external stimuli and environmental noise.
- Administer anticonvulsant agents as ordered.

- Record seizure activity and assess neurologic status and vital signs after the seizure subsides.
- Monitor serum levels of anticonvulsant agents to ensure therapeutic levels and prevent toxicity.

A helping hand

Having a seizure can be extremely frightening to a child; it can also be embarrassing, especially when a seizure occurs in the presence of peers. To the child's caregivers and others who witness a seizure, the experience can be terrifying. The child and their caregivers need a great deal of education and emotional support:

- Instruct the caregivers (and the child, if old enough) in all aspects of seizure control measures such as how to control fever if the child has febrile seizures.
- Stress to the caregivers the need to treat the child as normally as possible.
- Encourage the caregivers and the child to express their fears and anxieties; answer their questions honestly.

It takes a village

- Instruct the caregivers to make sure that the child's teachers, day care providers, babysitters, coaches, and other caregivers know what to do in the event of a seizure.
- If the child has had a seizure at school, suggest that the caregivers arrange to have a health care professional go to the school and talk to the child's classmates.
- Refer the family to organizations that will provide them with more information and support such as the Epilepsy Foundation.
- Remind the caregivers that their child should wear some form of medical identification such as a medical identification bracelet.

Quick quiz

1. A child who had bacterial meningitis is scheduled to have their hearing tested before discharge. The caregiver asks the nurse why the test is necessary. The most appropriate nursing response is:
   A. "It's necessary to make sure your child is developing appropriately."
   B. "The test will identify attention deficit problems related to your child's illness."
   C. "It's necessary to make sure the steroid therapy your child had in the hospital didn't affect their ability to hear."
   D. "Despite treatment, some children with bacterial meningitis suffer neurologic damage, especially to the nerve responsible for hearing."

Answer: D. The most common neurologic complications of meningitis are hearing loss, cognitive impairment, seizures, visual impairment, and behavioral problems.

2. A nurse is caring for a 2-year-old child with a VP shunt. Assessment indicates the child is afebrile but irritable and less responsive than they were previously. The most appropriate nursing action is to:
- A. lower the head of the bed and position the child on their stomach.
- B. increase the oxygen to 100%.
- C. increase the fluids the child is receiving.
- D. notify the doctor.

Answer: D. The nurse should notify the doctor of indications of increased ICP, including irritability and lethargy.

3. An 18-month-old is admitted to the emergency department with a diagnosis of seizure. Upon assessment, the child's vital signs are temperature of 104°F (40°C), respirations at 26 breaths/min, pulse at 120 beats/min, and blood pressure of 90/69 mm Hg. The nurse should:
- A. give a tepid sponge bath.
- B. administer phenytoin (Dilantin).
- C. do an Accu-Chek.
- D. aggressively hydrate the child with IV fluids.

Answer: A. An elevated temperature could lead to a febrile seizure. The nurse should intervene to lower the core body temperature by offering oral fluids, giving the child a tepid sponge bath, and administering doctor-ordered antipyretic medications.

Scoring

☆☆☆ If you answered all three items correctly, fantastic! There's no deficit in your understanding of neurologic problems.

☆☆ If you answered two items correctly, great work! Your brain is in tip-top condition.

☆ If you answered fewer than two items correctly, don't despair! Just scan the chapter again (no MRI needed).

Suggested references

Centers for Disease Control and Prevention. (2022). *Meningitis.* https://www.cdc.gov/meningitis/

Centers for Disease Control and Prevention. (2023). *Facts about Down syndrome.* https://www.cdc.gov/ncbddd/birthdefects/DownSyndrome.html

Centers for Disease Control and Prevention. (2024). *About cerebral palsy.* https://www
.cdc.gov/cerebral-palsy/about/index.html

Linnard-Palmer, L. (2019). Intracranial regulation. In L. Linnard-Palmer (Ed.),
Pediatric nursing care: A concept-based approach (pp. 295–314). Jones & Bartlett
Learning.

Miller, K. (2017). Neurologic disorders. In B. Richardson (Ed.), *Pediatric primary care:
Practice guidelines for nurses* (pp. 519–554). Jones & Bartlett Learning.

Chapter 16

Cardiovascular problems

Just the facts

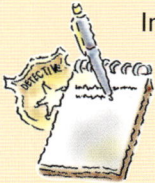

In this chapter, you'll learn:

- ♦ anatomy and physiology of the cardiovascular system
- ♦ diagnostic testing for cardiovascular problems
- ♦ treatments and procedures for cardiovascular problems
- ♦ cardiovascular system disorders that occur in children
- ♦ nursing care for the child with cardiovascular problems.

Anatomy and physiology

Understanding cardiovascular problems in children requires a sound, working knowledge of normal cardiac structure and function.

Structures of the heart

The *heart* is a muscular organ located behind the sternum in the chest and covered by a sac called the *pericardium*. Its main purpose is to pump blood throughout the body by continuous rhythmic contractions. The heart is composed of four chambers (two atria and two ventricles) and four valves.

Heart chambers

The four chambers of the heart are the right and left atria and the right and left ventricles.

Atria

The atria serve as reservoirs during ventricular contraction (systole) and as pumps during ventricular relaxation (diastole). The right atrium and the left atrium are separated by an *atrial septum*.

Ventricles

The left ventricle propels blood through the aorta to the rest of the body. The right ventricle sends blood through the pulmonary artery to the lungs. The ventricles are separated by an *interventricular septum*.

A look inside the heart

Within the heart lies four chambers (two atria and two ventricles) and four valves (two atrioventricular and two semilunar valves). A system of blood vessels carries blood to and from the heart.

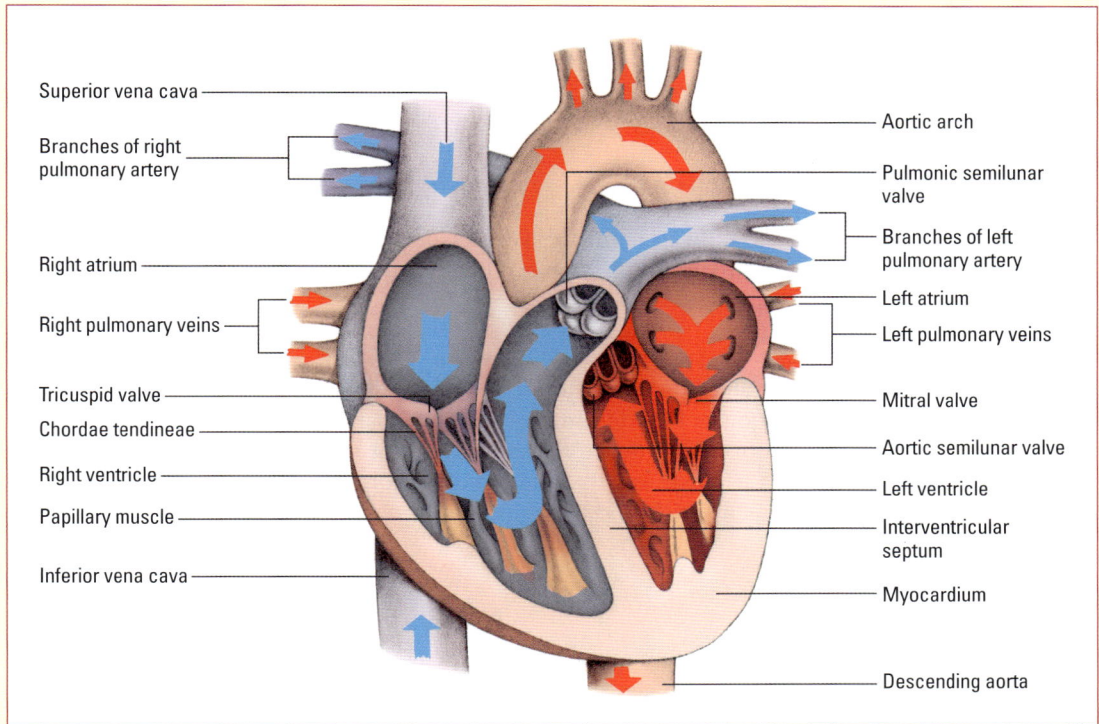

- Superior vena cava
- Branches of right pulmonary artery
- Right atrium
- Right pulmonary veins
- Tricuspid valve
- Chordae tendineae
- Right ventricle
- Papillary muscle
- Inferior vena cava

- Aortic arch
- Pulmonic semilunar valve
- Branches of left pulmonary artery
- Left atrium
- Left pulmonary veins
- Mitral valve
- Aortic semilunar valve
- Left ventricle
- Interventricular septum
- Myocardium
- Descending aorta

Equal at birth

At birth, the ventricles are relatively equal in size because of low resistance placental circulation. When the left ventricle begins functioning against systemic resistance that increases after birth, however, it becomes thicker than the right ventricle. (See *A look inside the heart.*)

Heart valves

The heart has four valves:

1. Tricuspid valve
2. Mitral valve
3. Aortic valve
4. Pulmonic valve

Tricuspid and mitral valves

The tricuspid and mitral valves are known as the *atrioventricular (AV) valves*. They prevent blood backflow from the ventricles to the atria during ventricular contraction.

Location, leaflets, and muscles

The tricuspid valve is located between the right atrium and the ventricle. It has three leaflets, or cusps, and three papillary muscles. The mitral valve is situated between the left atrium and the ventricle. It has two leaflets and two papillary muscles.

Lovely leaflets

The leaflets of both the tricuspid and mitral valves are attached to the papillary muscles of the ventricles by thin, fibrous bands called *chordae tendineae*.

Aortic and pulmonic valves

The aortic and pulmonic valves are known as the *semilunar valves*. These valves prevent backflow of blood from the aorta and pulmonary artery into the ventricles during ventricular relaxation. The aortic valve is located between the left ventricle and the aorta. The pulmonic valve is located between the right ventricle and the pulmonary artery.

Circulation

Blood is returned to the heart via the veins. *Veins* are small, thin-walled blood vessels that carry deoxygenated blood from the capillaries to the heart.

A long day's journey

Blood enters the right atrium from the inferior (IVC) and superior (SVC) venae cavae and then goes into the right ventricle. From there, it's pumped into the pulmonary artery to the lungs, where it gains oxygen and loses carbon dioxide.

Return to sender

The pulmonary veins bring the oxygenated blood from the lungs to the left atrium. The oxygenated blood then passes into the left ventricle, is pumped into the aorta, and is delivered to the rest of the body via the arteries. *Arteries* are large, thick-walled blood vessels that distribute oxygenated blood to the capillaries.

Pulmonary role reversal

The pulmonary artery is the only artery in the body that carries deoxygenated blood. The pulmonary veins are the only veins in the body that carry oxygenated blood.

Conduction system

The heart's conduction system is an electrical system that initiates myocardial contractions to move blood through the heart and maintain its rhythmic pumping action. This system is composed of several specialized cells:

- The *sinoatrial node* (also called *the pacemaker of the heart*) is located within the right atrial wall near the opening of the SVC. It initiates electrical impulses and sends them throughout the atria.
- The *AV node* is located within the right atrium near the lower end of the septum. It transmits impulses from the atria to the ventricle.

Bundles and branches

- The *AV bundle* (bundle of His) extends from the AV node to each side of the interventricular septum and divides into right and left bundle branches. It facilitates rapid conduction of the impulses through the ventricles.
- The *Purkinje fibers* extend from the AV bundle into the walls of the ventricles and rapidly conduct impulses through the heart muscle.

Cardiac physiology

The heart's primary purpose is to pump the blood that delivers oxygen and nutrients to tissues throughout the body and to remove waste products, such as carbon dioxide. To do this, the heart must maintain an adequate cardiac output.

Cardiac output is the amount of blood ejected by the heart in 1 minute. Cardiac output can be determined by multiplying the heart rate in 1 minute by the stroke volume. *Stroke volume* is the amount of blood ejected by the heart at each heartbeat (or contraction).

Stroke volume is affected by three factors:

1. *Preload,* or the stretch of the myocardial fibers, is simply the circulating blood volume.
2. *Afterload* is the resistance against which the ventricle must pump during its contraction, which can be affected by blood pressure. (Hypertension will increase afterload, as the heart must pump harder to force blood into circulation.)
3. *Contractility* is the force of left ventricular ejection.

Chillin' with homeostasis

To maintain homeostasis, the body will make many adjustments to the factors that contribute to cardiac output.

Cardiac adaptations at birth

During fetal circulation, blood is oxygenated and waste products are removed from the placenta. Blood is shunted away from those organs that aren't yet fully functional, such as the lungs and the liver.

Perfusion only—no exchange

In the fetus, the lungs are filled with fluid and aren't yet the site of gas exchange. The amount of blood that passes through the lungs is just enough to perfuse lung tissue.

Farewell placenta, hello lungs!

At birth, however, the neonate must transition from a reliance on the placenta to a reliance on their lungs for oxygenation. This transition is normally accomplished within the first few breaths after birth.

Many keys, one lock

Key structures that maintain fetal circulation include:
- *umbilical vein*, which carries oxygenated blood from the placenta to the fetus
- *umbilical arteries*, which carry deoxygenated blood from the fetus to the placenta
- *foramen ovale*, which serves as the septal opening between the atria of the fetal heart
- *ductus arteriosus*, which connects the pulmonary artery to the aorta, allowing blood to bypass the fetal lungs
- *ductus venosus*, which carries oxygenated blood from the umbilical vein to the IVC, bypassing the liver.

Out with fluid, in with air

Cardiac adaptations at birth occur gradually, resulting from structural and pressure changes in the lungs, heart, and major vessels. With the first few breaths after birth, the fluid in the neonate's lungs is absorbed and replaced with air. Inspired oxygen dilates the pulmonary vessels, resulting in decreased pulmonary vascular resistance and increased pulmonary blood flow as the lungs expand and fill with air. More blood will now travel to and from the lungs.

The drama unfolds

The pressure in the right atrium, right ventricle, and pulmonary artery decreases. Simultaneously, a gradual increase in systemic vascular resistance occurs when the umbilical cord is clamped and the low resistance placental circulation is removed. At that point, left atrial pressure increases more than right atrial pressure. The foramen ovale, which was a one-way door, closes as a result of this unequal pressure. The ductus arteriosus begins to close because of increased pulmonary blood flow and the dramatic reduction in pulmonary vascular resistance. Later, the ductus arteriosus (and ductus venosus) will become ligaments and will be closed structurally.

Out of a job

The function of the foramen ovale ceases immediately or soon after birth. Ductus arteriosus functioning ceases after the infant is about 4 days old. Anatomic closure, however, takes considerably longer. If the foramen ovale or ductus arteriosus fails to close, persistent shunting of fetal blood away from the lungs will result. (See *From fetal to neonatal circulation*.)

From fetal to neonatal circulation

These illustrations show the changes in circulation that occur at birth, allowing all neonatal blood to pass through the lungs.

Fetal circulation

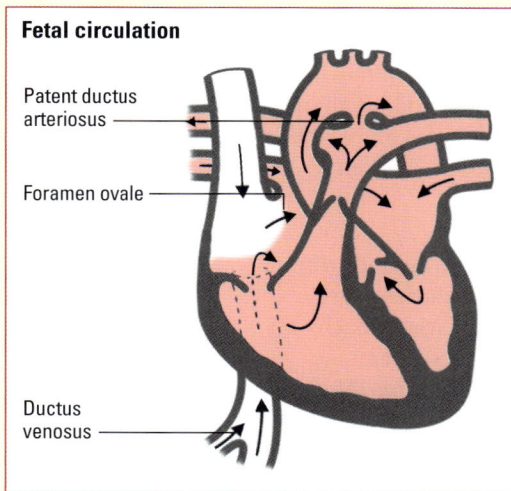

Fetal circulation

Patent ductus arteriosus

Foramen ovale

Ductus venosus

Neonatal circulation

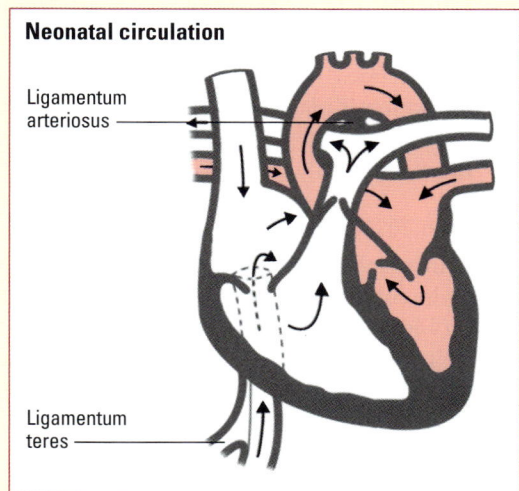

Neonatal circulation

Ligamentum arteriosus

Ligamentum teres

Murmurs

Murmurs are produced by vibrations within the chambers of the heart or major arteries from the back-and-forth flow of blood through these structures. In children, murmurs may be called:

- *innocent*, when there is no anatomic or physiologic cause
- *functional*, when there is a physiologic cause, such as anemia, but no anatomic abnormality

- *organic*, when there is some anatomic defect in the heart, with or without the existence of a physiologic abnormality.

Sit, stand, recline

When auscultating for murmurs, position the child in the sitting and reclining positions. Also, auscultate the heart with the child standing, sitting while leaning forward, and in a left-side–lying position. (See *Grading murmurs*.)

Diagnostic tests

Diagnostic tests of the cardiovascular system in children include:
- echocardiography
- electrocardiography (ECG)
- magnetic resonance imaging (MRI).

Echocardiography

Echocardiography is used to evaluate cardiac structures and functions using echoes from pulsed, high-frequency sound waves. An ultrasound transducer is placed on the chest, and the sound waves produce an image of the heart. The test is noninvasive and painless and is one of the most commonly used tests to detect cardiac problems in children.

Ultrasound–endoscopy combo

Transesophageal echocardiography (TEE) combines ultrasound with endoscopy. It's an alternative method for detecting cardiovascular problems in children and is used when the transthoracic approach isn't possible or would be difficult. During the procedure, the transducer is passed into the esophagus to an area behind the atria. The procedure is more complicated than the transthoracic approach and may require sedation and intubation to preserve the airway in young children.

Nursing considerations

Explain the procedure to the child and their caregivers; tell the child what they will see, hear, and feel, and be honest about any pain or discomfort they might experience. In addition, follow these steps:
- Stress the importance of holding still during the test and assist as necessary. (Tell the child that holding still is a "very important job.")
- Administer mild sedation if needed. Use distractions such as a video to help calm the child.

Grading murmurs

Use the system outlined here to describe the intensity of a murmur. When recording your findings, use Roman numerals as part of a fraction, always with "VI" as the denominator. For example, a grade III murmur would be recorded as "grade III/VI."

1. Grade I is a barely audible murmur.
2. Grade II is audible but quiet and soft.
3. Grade III is moderately loud, without heaves or thrills.
4. Grade IV is loud, with a thrill.
5. Grade V is very loud, with a heave or a thrill.
6. Grade VI is loud enough to be heard before the stethoscope is placed on the chest.

- For TEE, administer sedation as ordered and assist with endotracheal intubation as necessary. Explain that the child must have nothing to eat or drink before the procedure.

Electrocardiography

ECG provides a graphic representation of the heart's electrical activity. It is used to detect the presence of ischemia, injury, necrosis, bundle branch block, fascicular blocks, conduction delay, chamber enlargement, and dysrhythmia.

Nursing considerations

Explain the test to the child and their caregivers, stressing that there is no pain involved. In addition, follow these steps:
- Describe the equipment that will be used for the test; show the child a picture, or if possible, the actual equipment.
- Explain that the child may have to lie on their left side, inhale and exhale slowly, or hold their breath at intervals during the test.
- Encourage the child to be still during the test; the child may sit on their caregiver's lap if necessary.

Magnetic resonance imaging

MRI uses magnetic fields and radio frequencies to show a cross-sectional view of the heart and its structures. It is useful in identifying some congenital heart defects. MRI is generally a noninvasive test. However, contrast media may be used.

Nursing considerations

When explaining the test to the child, show them a picture of the scanner or, whenever possible, let the child see the actual scanner. Tell the child that no pain is involved; prepare them if contrast media must be used. In addition, follow these steps:
- Tell the child that their caregivers may stay in the room with them during the scan.
- Prepare the child for the movements and the loud, clicking noises made by the scanner; reassure the child that the machine will not touch them.
- Because no metal can go in the scanner, assist the child in removing hair clips, jewelry, and other metal items as necessary.
- If necessary, provide sedation to ensure that the child remains still during the test.
- Assess for a history of iodine or seafood allergies before the procedure if a contrast medium is to be used.

Exercise testing

Exercise testing may be done for some children, depending on their age and general condition. With it, the child's doctor can evaluate the extent of disease from any heart or lung disease that may be present. In addition, it can help to determine what kinds of activity ease or aggravate the child's condition as well as their conditioning, both aerobic and musculoskeletal. Either a treadmill or a stationary bike may be used while the child's heart and respiratory rate are monitored. The blood pressure and pulse oximetry are also monitored during the exercise test.

Nursing considerations

Most children know what a bicycle looks like, but they may not be familiar with the concept of a stationary bike. They may not recognize a treadmill at all. So, good instructions and explanations may be necessary. Pictures or other visual aids may be helpful. Let the child know that there will be monitoring equipment, which may contain several wires that may be attached to them. Assure the child that there is no pain involved. In addition, follow these steps:

- The child's caregivers may remain in the room with the child, unless the child prefers to test alone (a possibility for an older school-age child or an adolescent).
- Be sure the child knows to notify the health care provider right away if there is any discomfort or if there is any difficulty keeping up with the exercise.

Treatments and procedures

Treatments and procedures used for cardiac problems in childhood include:

- valve replacement
- cardiac catheterization
- cardiac surgery
- cardiac transplantation.

Teach expectations

Many of the treatments and procedures done for children with cardiac problems involve surgery. When a child knows what to expect before a surgical procedure, they may be less frightened, more cooperative, and more trusting of the nurses who provide their care. (See *Preparing children for surgery*.)

Preparing children for surgery

Many of the interventions performed for cardiac problems involve major surgery. What a child imagines about surgery is likely much more frightening than the reality. A child who knows what to expect ahead of time will be less fearful and more cooperative and will learn to trust their caregivers. A child who is well prepared for medical procedures is much less likely to experience emotional trauma, which can have long-lasting effects.

Developmental concerns

Many of the concerns that children may have about hospitalization and surgery relate to their stage of development.

Infants, toddlers, and preschoolers

• Infants and toddlers are most concerned about separation from their caregivers. Stranger anxiety may make a necessary separation (during surgery) especially difficult.

• Showing is a necessary adjunct to telling when preparing a toddler for surgery.

• Preschoolers may view medical procedures, including surgeries, as punishments for some type of perceived bad behavior.

• Preschoolers are also likely to have many misconceptions about what will happen during surgery.

School-age children

• School-age children have concerns about fitting in with peers and may view surgery as something that sets them apart from their friends.

• A desire to appear "grown up" may make the school-age child reluctant to express their fears.

• Because children are especially curious and interested in learning at this age, school-age children are very receptive to preoperative teaching and will likely ask many important questions (although they may need to be given the "permission" to do so).

Adolescents

• Adolescents struggle with the conflict between wanting to assert their independence and needing their

caregivers (and other adults) to take care of them during illness and treatment.

• Adolescents may want to discuss their illness and treatment without a caregiver present.

• In addition, adolescents may have a hard time admitting that they are afraid or experiencing pain or discomfort.

Before surgery

Whenever the situation permits, arrange for the child to visit the hospital before they are admitted for surgery. Ideally, the formal preparation for surgery is done during the preadmission visit.

Explanations should be honest and age appropriate and should involve the caregivers (unless the adolescent would rather be prepared alone). The explanation should focus on what the child will see, hear, and feel; where their caregivers will be waiting for them; and when they will be reunited.

If a child will initially be cared for in an intensive care setting, allow them to visit the area ahead of time and to meet some of the nurses who will be caring for them. Prepare them for the equipment and the other patients they will see.

Principles of preparation

Here are some principles to keep in mind when preparing a child for surgery:

• Begin by asking the child to tell you what they think is going to happen during the surgery.

• Ask the child about worries or fears. They may be worried about something that is not going to happen.

• Provide a developmentally appropriate explanation of why the surgery is being performed; encourage the child to ask questions. Pictures or illustrations can be very helpful in assisting the child to understand the explanations.

• Reassure the child that they will not wake up during the surgery but that the doctor knows how and when to wake them up afterward.

• Show the child an induction mask (if it will be used) and allow them to "practice" by placing it on their face (or yours).

(*continued*)

Preparing children for surgery (*continued*)

• Prepare the child for equipment (e.g., monitors, drains, and intravenous [IV] injections) they will wake up with.
• Tell the child about the sights and sounds of the operating room.
• Tell the child that their doctor and nurse will be in the operating room with them. Reassure them that the doctor or nurse will talk to them and tell them what is happening.

• If possible, show the child where they will be waking up in the recovery room and where their caregivers will be waiting for them.
• Tell the child it is perfectly fine to be afraid and to cry.
• After the surgery, encourage the child to talk about the experience; they may also express their feelings through art or play.

Cardiac catheterization

Cardiac catheterization is performed with a radiopaque catheter that is passed through the femoral artery directly into the heart and lungs. It may also be performed in conjunction with an angiogram, in which a radiopaque contrast medium is injected through the catheter into the circulation, allowing visualization of blood circulation through the heart chambers.

Measure for measure

Cardiac catheterization is used to evaluate ventricular function and measure heart chamber pressures and oxygen saturation in the blood. It also serves as a method for obtaining cardiac muscle biopsy specimens and for performing electrophysiologic studies.

Complications

Complications of cardiac catheterization include acute hemorrhage, transient dysrhythmia, temporarily diminished circulation to the catheterized extremity because of clot or hematoma formation, allergic reaction to the contrast medium, nausea and vomiting, and the possibility of infection.

Nursing considerations

Nursing interventions for cardiac catheterization begin when the procedure is scheduled and continue throughout the recovery period.

Before the procedure

Before catheterization, nursing interventions focus on preparing the child for the procedure, both physically and emotionally.

• Describe to the child and caregivers the procedure room as well as the equipment that will be used during the procedure. Show the child where on their body the catheter will be inserted, using doll play to prepare them, as necessary.

- Tell the child that the lights in the room will be dimmed after the catheter is placed. Reassure them that you will be right there with them and will talk to them throughout the procedure.
- Tell the child that they may feel warm after the contrast medium is injected.
- Weigh the child and take their vital signs.
- Assess the child's color, temperature of their extremities, and pedal pulses. Mark the dorsalis pedis and posterior tibial pulses with indelible ink before the procedure, allowing for easy assessment after the procedure.

After the procedure

After catheterization, nursing care focuses on preventing complications, monitoring the catheterized extremity, and ensuring adequate fluid intake.

- Keep the affected extremity immobile to prevent hemorrhage, usually for 4 to 6 hours after the procedure.
- Keep the catheter site clean and dry; monitor for bleeding and hematoma formation.
- Compare postcatheterization assessment data to precatheterization baseline data, paying special attention to pulses and neurovascular status in the catheterized extremity.
- Ensure adequate fluid intake (IV and oral) to compensate for blood loss during the procedure and the diuretic action of some contrast media used. Doing so will also aid in flushing the contrast medium from the circulation.
- Because cardiac catheterization is commonly done on an outpatient basis, provide thorough postprocedural teaching for the caregivers. (See *Instructions after cardiac catheterization.*)

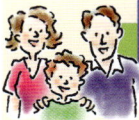

It's all relative

Instructions after cardiac catheterization

Cardiac catheterizations are commonly performed on an outpatient basis. Provide caregivers with these clear instructions about caring for their child at home:
- Remove the pressure dressing the day after the procedure.
- Keep the site covered with an adhesive bandage for several days after the procedure.
- Keep the insertion site clean and dry; give only sponge baths until the site is healed.
- Observe the site for redness, swelling, drainage, and bleeding.
- Monitor the child's temperature and report fever promptly.
- Have the child avoid strenuous exercise.
- Provide a regular diet for the child.
- Administer acetaminophen or ibuprofen as needed for discomfort or pain.
- Keep follow-up appointments.

Cardiac surgery

Treatment of almost all congenital heart defects is achieved through cardiac surgery. The specific procedure performed will depend on the defect. Even so, certain methods are used, no matter which procedure is performed.

Heart—lung vacation

Cardiopulmonary bypass machines are typically used to oxygen-ate body tissues because surgery may necessitate stopping the heart. During the procedure, the patient is placed in a hypothermic state to minimize blood loss (which enhances patient recovery) and to reduce the body's need for oxygen. An incision into the chest (thoracotomy) is commonly performed, and chest tubes are placed.

Complications

Complications of cardiac surgery may include dysrhythmia, acid–base and electrolyte imbalances, hypoxia, and trauma to the conduction pathways of the heart.

Nursing considerations

Prepare the child and their caregivers for what they will see, hear, and feel after surgery. When a child and their caregivers know ahead of time that certain events are "normal," those events will be less stress-ful and frightening when they occur.

- Monitor the patient's heart rate closely. (It will normally increase after surgery.) Changes in regularity and rhythm should be re-ported to the doctor immediately.
- Auscultate the lungs every hour, assessing for diminished or absent breath sounds, which may require further medical evaluation and intervention.

Keep the heat

- Keep the child warm to prevent heat loss. (Infants may be placed under radiant heat warmers.)
- Monitor body temperature closely. It may rise to about 100°F (37.8°C) in the first 48 hours after surgery due to the inflamma-tory process initiated by tissue trauma. Further temperature eleva-tion may indicate an infection, requiring immediate action to determine the cause.
- Maintain mechanical ventilation of the child in the immediate postoperative period. Extubation may occur in the operating room or in the early postoperative period.

- After extubation, an oxygen mask, hood, or tent or nasal cannula is used to deliver humidified oxygen. If the patient is in an oxygen tent, change their linens and clothes frequently to keep them dry, preventing excessive chilling that would increase metabolic needs and, consequently, increase cardiac and oxygen demand.

Turn and breathe

- Implement turning and deep breathing hourly, using adjunct analgesic agents and splinting of the incision to minimize discomfort and pain. Firm stuffed animals can be used effectively for incisional support during deep-breathing and spirometry exercises.
- Prepare the child for chest tube removal (typically between the first and third postoperative day), which can be a painful and frightening procedure for a child. Topical anesthetics or analgesic agents are commonly administered before removal. (See *Chest tube removal.*)

Advice from the experts

Chest tube removal

Follow these guidelines to prepare the child for chest tube removal and to reduce complications:
- Tell the child they will experience momentary sharp pain as the chest tube is removed.
- Administer anesthetics or analgesic agents as ordered.
- Instruct the child to take a deep breath. (The tube should be removed at the end of inspiration.)
- Cover the wound with sterile petroleum gauze, topped with a clear, occlusive film dressing, such as Tegaderm, making sure all sides are securely attached to the skin for an airtight seal.
- Monitor the site for drainage, bleeding, and infection. Change the dressing according to your facility's policy.

Rx: TLC

- Provide emotional support and comfort because surgery can be frightening as well as painful to the child. Encourage the caregiver's involvement in the child's care to foster feelings of comfort and security.
- Provide detailed discharge teaching. (See *Teaching about cardiac surgery.*)

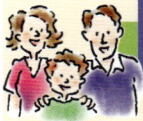

It's all relative

Teaching about cardiac surgery

Be sure to include these points in your teaching plan for the caregivers of a child who has undergone cardiac surgery:

- Dietary restrictions, if any
- Fluid requirements and restrictions
- Activity and exercise restrictions
- Operative site care and inspection
- Medication regimen
- Follow-up tests and doctor visits
- Home care needs
- Importance of encouraging the child to talk and express their feelings about the surgery and hospitalization

---

Cardiac transplantation

For infants and children with worsening heart failure and limited life expectancy, heart transplantation has become an option. Indications for transplantation in children include cardiomyopathy and end-stage congenital heart disease.

One of two

There are two surgical options for cardiac transplantation:

- *Orthotopic procedure*, in which the diseased heart is removed in its entirety and a new, healthy heart from a deceased donor is implanted.
- *Heterotopic procedure* (rarely performed in children), in which the patient's own heart is kept in place and a "piggyback" heart is implanted to serve as an additional pumping organ to assist the diseased heart.

Who knows United Network for Organ Sharing?

The process begins by placing the child on the United Network for Organ Sharing (UNOS) list to match a donor with the recipient. Due to limited donor supply, some infants and children on the UNOS list die before a new heart can be found for them. In 2024, nearly 3,400 people were on the waiting list for a cardiac transplant.

Crucial 6 months

Complications are most common during the first 6 months to 1 year after transplantation. During this period, the family must adjust to a totally new lifestyle that will require lifelong management. The leading cause of demise after heart transplantation is organ rejection. Because lifelong immunosuppressive therapy is required, infection is always a risk.

Nursing considerations

The child and their caregivers must be prepared thoroughly for this major procedure. Preparation should include a brief visit to the coronary intensive care unit (CICU), and, if possible, the child should be introduced to the nurses who will be providing their care. Caregivers should be made aware of the visiting policies in the CICU and should be assisted in making arrangements (in the hospital and at home) to spend as much time with their child as possible. Siblings can be included in the preparation so that they are aware of the changes that may take place.

The hard part is over

Postoperative care involves:
- monitoring the patient closely for signs of rejection, infection, and adverse reactions from immunosuppressive therapy
- restricting fluids as ordered to prevent hypervolemia and heart strain
- providing adequate rest periods with gradual activity increases to further decrease the workload of the heart
- encouraging adherence with the complex drug regimen required, especially in adolescents
- providing emotional support to the child and family and offering resources for additional support
- helping the caregivers (and the child, if age appropriate) come to terms with the reality that someone had to die for a heart to become available. (This concept is too confusing and upsetting for most young children; caregivers should be encouraged to provide age-appropriate explanations when the child begins to ask where their new heart came from.)

Congenital heart defects that increase pulmonary blood flow

Congenital heart defects that increase pulmonary blood flow include atrial septal defect (ASD), patent ductus arteriosus (PDA), and ventricular septal defect (VSD).

Atrial septal defect

In a child with ASD, an opening between the left and right atria allows blood to flow from the left side of the heart to the right side, resulting in ineffective pumping of the heart, thus increasing the risk of heart failure. (See *Looking at ASD*.)

Looking at ASD

An ASD is an opening between the left and right atria that allows blood to flow from the left side of the heart to the right side, as shown here.

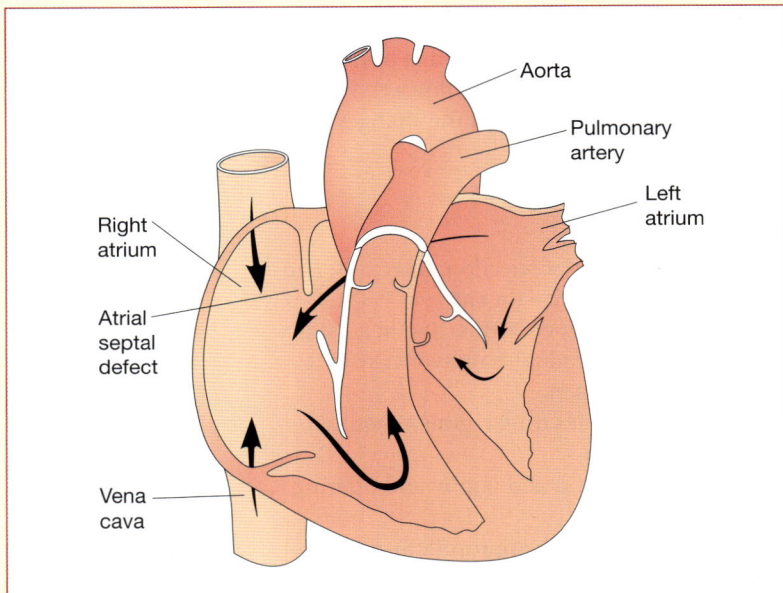

ASDs come in threes

The three types of ASDs are:
1. *ostium secundum defect*, the most common type, which occurs in the region of the fossa ovalis at the center of the atrial septum and, occasionally, extends inferiorly, close to the venae cavae
2. *sinus venosus defect*, which occurs in the superior–posterior portion of the atrial septum, sometimes extends into the venae cavae and is almost always associated with abnormal drainage of pulmonary veins into the right atrium

3. *ostium primum defect*, which occurs in the inferior portion of the septum primum and is usually associated with AV valve abnormalities (cleft mitral valve) and conduction defects.

Benign when small

ASD accounts for about 10% of congenital heart defects and is almost twice as common in females as in males, with a strong familial tendency. Although an ASD may be without symptoms during infancy and childhood, delayed development of symptoms and complications makes it one of the most common congenital heart defects diagnosed in adults. Adults with untreated ASD may present with exertional dyspnea, fatigue, palpitations, and sustained dysrhythmia.

The prognosis is excellent for patients without symptoms and for those with uncomplicated surgical repair. The prognosis is poor, however, in patients with cyanosis caused by large, untreated defects.

What causes it

The cause of ASD is unknown. Ostium primum defects commonly occur in patients with Down syndrome.

How it happens

In ASD, blood shunts from the left atrium to the right atrium because the left atrial pressure is normally slightly higher than the right atrial pressure. The difference in pressure forces large amounts of blood through the defect. This shunt results in right heart volume overload, affecting the right atrium, right ventricle, and pulmonary arteries.

Enlarge and dilate

Eventually, the right atrium enlarges, and the right ventricle dilates to accommodate the increased blood volume. If pulmonary artery hypertension develops, increased pulmonary vascular resistance and right ventricular hypertrophy follow.

What to look for

Signs and symptoms of ASD include:
- fatigue after exertion
- early to midsystolic murmur at the second or third left intercostal space
- low-pitched diastolic murmur at the lower left sternal border (more pronounced on inspiration)
- fixed, widely split S_2 due to delayed closure of the pulmonic valve
- systolic click or late systolic murmur at the apex
- clubbing and cyanosis if a right-to-left shunt develops. (See *Cyanosis and crying*.)

Cyanosis and crying

An infant may be cyanotic because they have a cardiac or pulmonary disorder. Cyanosis that worsens with crying is most likely associated with cardiac causes because crying increases pulmonary resistance to blood flow, resulting in an increased right-to-left shunt. Cyanosis that improves with crying is most likely due to pulmonary causes because deep breathing improves tidal volume.

What tests tell you

A history of increasing fatigue and characteristic physical features suggests ASD. No specific laboratory tests are recommended in the workup of ASD. These tests confirm the diagnosis:

- Chest x-ray shows an enlarged right atrium and right ventricle, a prominent pulmonary artery, and increased pulmonary vascular markings.
- ECG results may be normal but commonly show right-axis deviation, prolonged PR interval, varying degrees of right bundle branch block, right ventricular hypertrophy, atrial fibrillation, and, in ostium primum defect, left-axis deviation.
- Echocardiography measures right ventricular enlargement, may locate the defect, and shows volume overload in the right side of the heart. (It may also reveal right ventricular and pulmonary artery dilation.) TEE may be needed to diagnose a sinus venosus defect.
- Two-dimensional echocardiography with color Doppler flow and contrast echocardiography have supplanted invasive techniques such as cardiac catheterization as the confirming tests for ASD. Cardiac catheterization may be used if inconsistencies exist in the clinical data or if significant pulmonary hypertension is suspected.
- MRI may be used to identify the size and position of an ASD. MRI is most useful for small defects.

Complications

Complications of ASD may include physical underdevelopment, respiratory infections, heart failure, atrial dysrhythmia, and mitral valve prolapse.

How it's treated

Operative repair is advised for uncomplicated ASD with evidence of significant left-to-right shunting. Ideally, this is performed when the patient is between ages 2 and 4 years. An operative repair shouldn't be performed on a patient with a small defect and trivial left-to-right shunt.

Procrastination preferred

Because ASD seldom produces complications in an infant or toddler, surgery can be delayed until preschool or early school age. A large defect may need immediate surgical closure with sutures or a patch graft. Alternatively, placement of an atrial occluder during cardiac catheterization is becoming a more common intervention than open-heart surgery.

What to do

Before cardiac catheterization, explain pretest and posttest procedures to the child and their caregivers. Whenever possible, use drawings or other visual aids to enhance the explanation.

- If needed, teach the caregivers (and child) about antibiotic prophylaxis to prevent infective endocarditis.
- If surgery is scheduled, prepare the child and their caregivers for what they will experience in the intensive care unit and introduce them to the staff. Show the caregivers where they can wait during the operation and explain postoperative procedures, tubes, dressings, and monitoring equipment.
- After surgery, closely monitor the patient's vital signs, central venous and intra-arterial pressures, and intake and output. (Watch for atrial dysrhythmia, which may remain uncorrected.)
- Patients may be treated with daily aspirin for 6 months after a surgical repair in order to prevent thrombus formation.

Patent ductus arteriosus

The ductus arteriosus is a fetal blood vessel that connects the pulmonary artery to the descending aorta, just distal to the left subclavian artery. Normally, the ductus closes within days after birth. In PDA, the lumen of the ductus remains open after birth. This defect creates a left-to-right shunt of blood from the aorta to the pulmonary artery and results in recirculation of blood through the lungs.

Postdated PDA

Initially, PDA may not produce clinical effects. Over time, however, it can precipitate pulmonary vascular disease, causing symptoms to appear by age 40 years. PDA affects twice as many females as males. (See *Looking at PDA.*)

Looking at PDA

In PDA, the lumen of the ductus arteriosus stays open after birth, causing a left-to-right shunt of blood from the aorta to the pulmonary artery, resulting in recirculation of arterial blood through the lungs. This shunt reversal (from fetal circulation) occurs because of the lower pressure in the lungs and pulmonary artery after birth.

(continued)

Looking at PDA (*continued*)

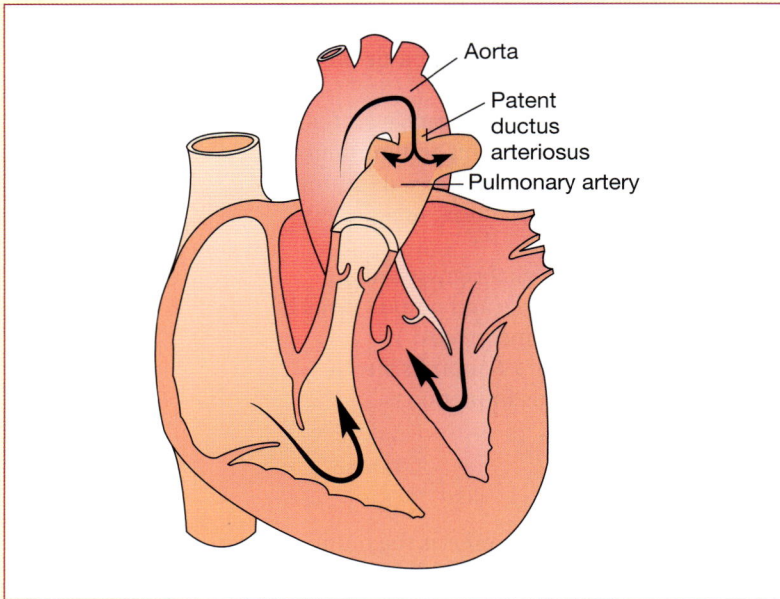

Aorta

Patent ductus arteriosus

Pulmonary artery

Smaller is better

In PDA, prognosis is good if the shunt is small or surgical repair is effective. Otherwise, PDA may advance to intractable heart failure, which may be fatal.

What causes it

PDA is associated with:
- premature birth, probably because of abnormalities in oxygenation or the relaxant action of prostaglandin E, which prevents ductal spasm and contracture necessary for closure
- rubella syndrome
- coarctation of the aorta
- VSD
- pulmonic and aortic stenosis
- living at high altitudes.

How it happens

The ductus arteriosus normally closes as prostaglandin levels from the placenta fall and oxygen levels rise. This process should begin as soon as the neonate takes their first breath but may take as long as 3 months in some children.

Back to the aorta

In PDA, relative resistance in pulmonary and systemic vasculature and the size of the ductus determine the quantity of blood that's shunted from left to right. Because of increased aortic pressure, oxygenated blood is shunted from the aorta through the ductus arteriosus to the pulmonary artery and the lungs. The blood returns to the left side of the heart and is pumped out to the aorta once more.

The left atrium and left ventricle must accommodate the increased pulmonary venous return by increasing filling pressure and workload on the left side of the heart. This compensation causes left-sided hypertrophy and, possibly, heart failure.

Reverse to cyanosis

In the final stages of untreated PDA, the left-to-right shunt leads to chronic pulmonary artery hypertension that becomes fixed and unreactive. This condition causes the shunt to reverse so that unoxygenated blood enters systemic circulation, causing cyanosis.

What to look for

Signs and symptoms of PDA may include:
- respiratory distress with signs of heart failure in infants, especially those who are premature
- classic machinery murmur (Gibson murmur), a continuous murmur heard throughout systole and diastole
- thrill palpated at the left sternal border
- prominent left ventricular impulse
- bounding peripheral pulses
- widened pulse pressure
- slow motor development
- failure to thrive
- fatigue and dyspnea on exertion, which may develop in adults with undetected PDA.

What tests tell you

These tests help diagnose PDA:
- Echocardiography (two-dimensional) is the preferred imaging method for confirming the diagnosis of PDA. It detects and estimates the size of a PDA. It also reveals an enlarged left atrium and left ventricle or right ventricular hypertrophy from pulmonary vascular disease.
- Chest x-rays in people with PDA may be normal. In some patients, it may show increased pulmonary vascular markings, prominent pulmonary arteries, and enlargement of the left ventricle and aorta.

- ECG may be normal or may indicate left atrial or ventricular hypertrophy and, in pulmonary vascular disease, biventricular hypertrophy.
- Computed tomography scans can detect a PDA. However, they are not recommended because they expose the child to ionizing radiation and are invasive, requiring IV contrast.
- MRI is of limited value in diagnosing PDA in pediatrics and is not recommended.

Complications

Possible complications of PDA may include infective endocarditis, congestive heart failure, and recurrent pneumonia.

How it's treated

Correction of PDA may involve:
- indomethacin (Indocin), a prostaglandin inhibitor, to induce ductus spasm and closure in premature infants
  - As an alternative to indomethacin (Indocin), some facilities are using IV ibuprofen for the treatment of PDA in neonates and preterm infants, with findings of equally good closure of the PDA but fewer renal side effects and complications.
- left thoracotomy to ligate the ductus if medical management cannot control heart failure (Infants with PDA who have no symptoms do not require immediate treatment; if symptoms are mild, surgical ligation of the PDA is usually delayed until the child is 1 year old.)
- video-assisted thoracoscopic surgery (VATS) to ligate the ductus as an alternative to surgery with a thoracotomy (VATS may be done at the bedside or in a procedure room and involves three small incisions in the left chest through which a clip is placed on the ductus.)
  - Alternatively, procedures can be done through a cardiac catheterization to block the flow of blood through the ductus by inserting umbrella or coil-type devices into the ends of the ductus, thus blocking the shunt.
- prophylactic antibiotics to protect against infective endocarditis
- treatment of heart failure with fluid restriction, diuretics, and digoxin.

What to do

PDA necessitates careful monitoring, patient and family teaching, and emotional support.
- Watch carefully for signs of PDA in all premature neonates.
- Be alert for respiratory distress symptoms resulting from heart failure, which may develop rapidly in a premature neonate.

Frequently assess vital signs, ECG, electrolyte levels, and intake and output and document the child's response to diuretics and other therapy.
- If the infant receives indomethacin for ductus closure, watch for possible adverse effects, such as diarrhea, jaundice, bleeding, and kidney dysfunction. Obtain blood tests before each dose of indomethacin as ordered.

Explain, prepare, meet, and greet
- Before surgery, carefully explain all treatments and tests to the caregivers and child, if age appropriate.
- Arrange for the family to meet the intensive care unit staff. Discuss the expected IV lines, monitoring equipment, and postoperative procedures.
- Immediately after surgery, the child may have a central venous pressure catheter and an arterial line in place. Carefully assess vital signs, intake and output, and arterial and venous pressures. Provide pain relief as needed.

Tell one, tell all
- Stress the need for regular medical follow-up examinations and advise the caregivers to inform any health care provider who treats their child about their history of surgery for PDA—even if the child is being treated for an unrelated medical problem.
- Before discharge, review instructions with the caregivers about activity restrictions based on the child's tolerance and energy levels. (Advise the caregivers to avoid becoming overprotective as their child's tolerance for physical activity increases.)

Ventricular septal defect

In the child with VSD, an opening in the septum between the ventricles allows blood to shunt between the left and right ventricles. This opening results in ineffective pumping of the heart and increases the risk of heart failure. (See *Looking at VSD*.)

VSDs account for up to 20% of all congenital heart defects. The prognosis is good for defects that close spontaneously or are correctable surgically.

What causes it

VSD may be associated with:
- Down syndrome and other autosomal trisomies
- kidney anomalies
- PDA and coarctation of the aorta
- prematurity.

Looking at VSD

In a VSD, an opening in the interventricular septum allows blood to shunt between the left and right ventricles.

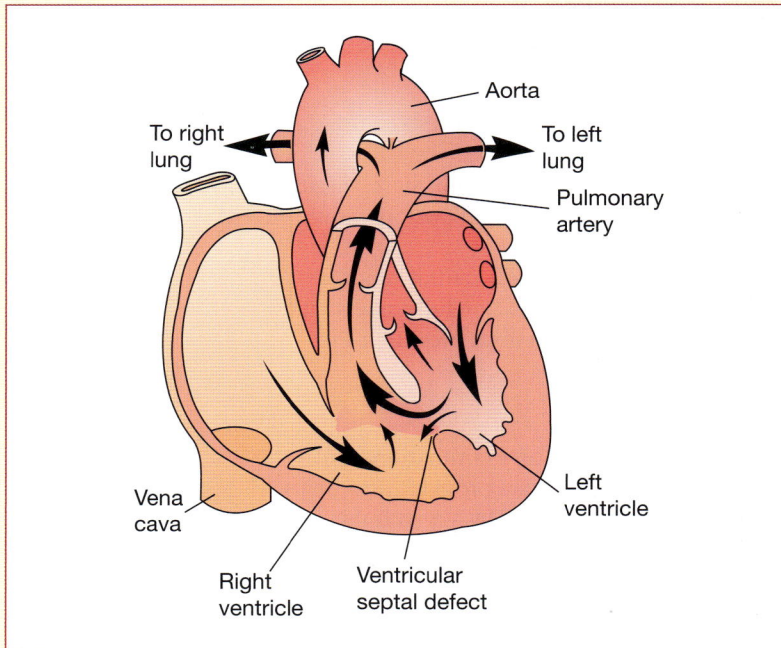

How it happens

In infants with VSD, the ventricular septum fails to close completely by gestation week 8. VSDs are located in the membranous or muscular portion of the ventricular septum and vary in size. Some defects close spontaneously; in other defects, the septum is entirely absent, creating a single ventricle. Small VSDs are likely to close spontaneously. Large VSDs should be surgically repaired before pulmonary vascular disease occurs or while it's still reversible.

Undercover VSD

VSD is not readily apparent at birth because right and left pressures are approximately equal and pulmonary artery resistance is elevated. Alveoli are not yet completely opened, so blood doesn't shunt through the defect. As the pulmonary vasculature gradually relaxes between 4 and 8 weeks after birth, right ventricular pressure decreases, allowing blood to shunt from the left to the right ventricle.

Leading with the left

Initially, large VSD shunts cause left atrial and left ventricular hypertrophy. Later, an uncorrected VSD causes right ventricular hypertrophy due to increasing pulmonary resistance. Eventually, right- and left-sided heart failure and cyanosis (from reversal of the shunt direction) occur. Fixed pulmonary hypertension may occur much later in life with right-to-left shunting, causing cyanosis and clubbing of the nail beds.

What to look for

Signs and symptoms of VSD may include:
- thin, small infant who gains weight slowly (when a large VSD is present)
- loud, harsh, widely transmitted systolic murmur heard best along the left sternal border at the third or fourth intercostal space
- palpable thrill
- loud, widely split pulmonic component of S_2
- point of maximal impulse displacement to the left
- prominent anterior chest
- liver, heart, and spleen enlargement
- feeding difficulties
- diaphoresis; tachycardia; and rapid, grunting respirations
- cyanosis and clubbing if right-to-left shunting occurs later in life.

What tests tell you

These tests help diagnose VSD:
- Echocardiography (two-dimensional) is the procedure of choice to detect and diagnose a VSD. This imaging test can be used to determine the size and location of almost all VSDs. Additional physiologic information such as right ventricular pressure and intraventricular pressure differences may be provided by Doppler echocardiography.
- Chest x-rays may reveal various sizes of VSDs, normal heart size, and an enlarged left atrium (on a lateral radiograph). Small VSDs may not be noted on a chest x-ray.
- ECG may be normal with small VSDs, whereas in large VSDs, it may show left and right ventricular hypertrophy, suggesting pulmonary hypertension.
- MRI is used as an adjunct tool in diagnosing VSDs. It can be used when echocardiography is not feasible or when it is not diagnostic.
- Cardiac catheterization is used to determine the size and exact location of the VSD and the extent of pulmonary hypertension. It is also useful for assessing pulmonary-to-systemic flow ratios—which can assist in the determination of whether surgery is indicated.

Complications

Complications of VSD may include pulmonary hypertension, infective endocarditis, pneumonia, and heart failure.

How it's treated

Many VSDs (20% to 60%) may close spontaneously during the first year of life, especially small VSDs. Correction of VSD may involve:
- early surgical correction for a large VSD, usually performed using a patch graft, before heart failure and irreversible pulmonary vascular disease develop
- placement of a permanent pacemaker, which may be necessary after VSD repair if complete heart block develops from interference with the bundle of His during surgery
- surgical closure of small defects using sutures (such defects may not be surgically repaired if the patient has normal pulmonary artery pressure and a small shunt)
- pulmonary artery banding to normalize pressures and flow distal to the band and to prevent pulmonary vascular disease if the child has other defects and will benefit from delaying surgery
- digoxin, sodium restriction, and diuretics before surgery to prevent heart failure
- prophylactic antibiotics before and after surgery to prevent infective endocarditis.

What to do

Although the caregivers of an infant with VSD commonly suspect something is wrong with their child before diagnosis, they may need psychological support to help them accept the reality of a serious cardiac disorder. Also, because surgery may take place months after diagnosis, caregiver teaching is vital to prevent complications until the child is scheduled for surgery or the defect closes. Thorough explanations of all tests are also essential. In addition, follow these steps:
- Instruct the caregivers to watch for signs of heart failure, such as poor feeding, sweating, and heavy breathing.
- If the child is receiving digoxin or other medications, tell the caregivers how to administer it and how to recognize adverse effects. (Caution them to keep medications out of the reach of all children.)
- Teach the caregivers how to recognize and report early signs of infection and to avoid exposing the child to people with obvious infections.
- Encourage the caregivers to let the child engage in normal activities.
- Stress the importance of prophylactic antibiotics before and after surgical procedures.

Congenital obstructive defects

Defects that obstruct the flow of blood out of the heart include coarctation of the aorta, aortic stenosis, and pulmonic stenosis.

Coarctation of the aorta

Coarctation is a narrowing of the aorta, usually just below the left subclavian artery, near the site where the ligamentum arteriosum (the remnant of the ductus arteriosus) joins the pulmonary artery to the aorta.

Coarctation may occur with aortic valve stenosis (usually of a bicuspid aortic valve), PDA, and VSD and with severe cases of hypoplasia of the aortic arch. The obstruction to blood flow results in ineffective pumping of the heart and increases the risk of heart failure. (See *Looking at coarctation of the aorta*.)

Looking at coarctation of the aorta

In coarctation of the aorta, a narrowing of the aorta occurs, usually near the site of insertion of the ductus arteriosus.

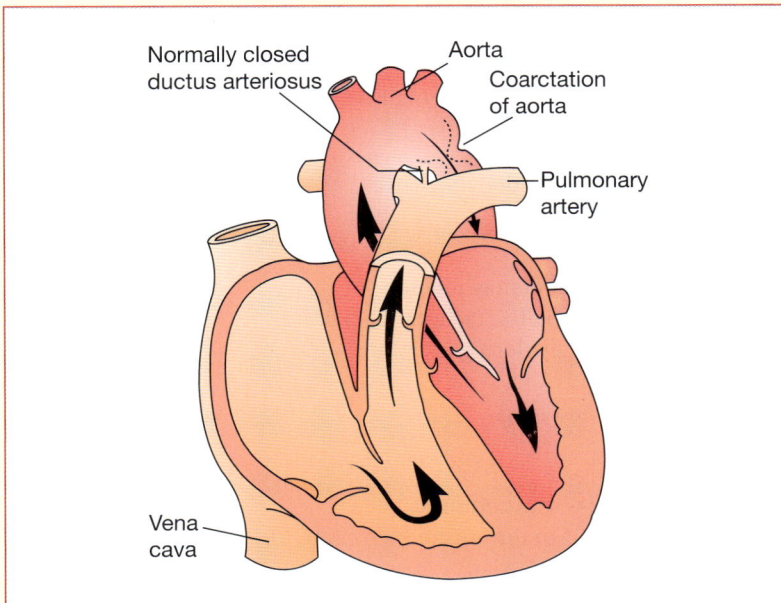

What causes it

Although the cause of this defect is unknown, it may be associated with Turner syndrome. Turner syndrome is a chromosome abnormality affecting only females, caused by the complete or partial deletion of the X chromosome.

How it happens

Coarctation of the aorta may develop because of spasm and constriction of the smooth muscle in the ductus arteriosus as it closes. This contractile tissue may extend into the aortic wall, causing narrowing. The obstructive process causes hypertension in the aortic branches above the constriction (arteries that supply the arms, neck, and head) and diminished pressure in the vessel below the constriction (that supplies the trunk and lower extremities).

Under pressure

Restricted blood flow through the narrowed aorta increases the pressure load on the left ventricle and causes dilation of the proximal aorta and ventricular hypertrophy.

A leggy problem

As oxygenated blood leaves the left ventricle, a portion travels through the arteries that branch off the aorta proximal to the coarctation. If PDA is present, the rest of the blood travels through the coarctation, mixes with deoxygenated blood from the PDA, and travels to the legs. If the PDA is closed, the legs and lower portion of the body must rely solely on the blood that gets through the coarctation.

Untreated, this condition may lead to left-sided heart failure. If coarctation remains in infancy without symptoms, it usually remains so throughout adolescence as collateral circulation develops to bypass the narrowed segment.

What to look for

Signs and symptoms of coarctation of the aorta may include:
- tachypnea, dyspnea, pulmonary edema, pallor, tachycardia, failure to thrive, cardiomegaly, and hepatomegaly during an infant's first year of life
- claudication (cramping pain in arms and legs)
- hypertension in the upper body
- headache, vertigo, and epistaxis
- pink upper extremities and cyanotic lower extremities
- bounding pulses in the arms and absent or diminished femoral pulses
- in most cases, normal heart sounds unless a coexisting cardiac defect is present

- more developed chest and arms than legs
- upper extremity blood pressure greater than lower extremity blood pressure.

What tests tell you

Physical examination reveals the cardinal signs of coarctation of the aorta, including resting systolic hypertension in the upper body, absent or diminished femoral pulses, and a wide pulse pressure. In addition, these tests may indicate the condition:

- Chest x-rays may reveal cardiomegaly, pulmonary edema, congestive heart failure, a wide ascending and descending aorta, and notching of the undersurfaces of the ribs due to erosion by collateral circulation.
- ECG may reveal left ventricular hypertrophy.
- Echocardiography may show increased left ventricular muscle thickness, coexisting aortic valve abnormalities, and the coarctation site.
- Cardiac catheterization may be used as an adjunct to help determine the severity of the coarctation.

Complications

Possible complications may include heart failure, severe hypertension, cerebral aneurysms and hemorrhage, rupture of the aorta, aortic aneurysm, and infective endocarditis.

How it's treated

Correction of coarctation of the aorta may involve:

- digoxin, diuretics, oxygen, and sedatives in infants with heart failure
- prostaglandin infusion to keep the ductus open
- antibiotic prophylaxis against infective endocarditis before and after surgery
- antihypertensive therapy for children with previous undetected coarctation until surgery is performed.

Resect, patch, ligate

Surgery may be performed early for infants with heart failure or hypertension, or it may be delayed until the preschool years. Options include:

- end-to-end anastomosis, in which the area of coarctation is resected and the distal and proximal aorta are anastomosed end to end
- patch aortoplasty, in which the area of coarctation is incised and an elliptical Dacron patch is sutured in place to widen the diameter

- subclavian flap aortoplasty, in which the distal subclavian artery is divided and the flap of the proximal portion of this vessel is used to expand the coarcted area.

What to do

When providing care to an infant, follow these steps:
- If coarctation requires rapid digitalization, monitor vital signs closely and watch for digoxin toxicity (poor feeding and vomiting).
- Monitor intake and output carefully, especially if the infant is receiving diuretics with fluid restriction.
- Weigh the child daily.

Bigger and bigger

For an older child:
- assess blood pressure in their extremities regularly, explain exercise restrictions, stress the need to take medications properly and to watch for adverse effects, and teach them about tests and other procedures.

Postop checklist

After corrective surgery, follow these steps:
- Monitor blood pressure closely using an intra-arterial line. Take blood pressure in all extremities.
- Monitor intake and output.
- If the patient develops hypertension and requires antihypertensives, administer the medication as ordered. Watch for severe hypotension and regulate the dosage carefully.
- Provide pain relief as needed and encourage a gradual increase in activity.
- Stress the importance of continued endocarditis prophylaxis if prescribed.

Stenosis, aortic

In aortic stenosis, narrowing or fusion of the aortic valve interferes with left ventricular outflow to the aorta. This defect, which is most common in males, causes left ventricular hypertrophy, causing pulmonary venous and arterial hypertension. (See *Looking at aortic stenosis.*)

What causes it

Aortic stenosis may result from congenital aortic bicuspid valves, congenital stenosis of valve cusps, or rheumatic fever.

Looking at aortic stenosis

In aortic stenosis, narrowing or fusion of the aortic valve causes left ventricular hypertrophy and interferes with ventricular outflow to the aorta.

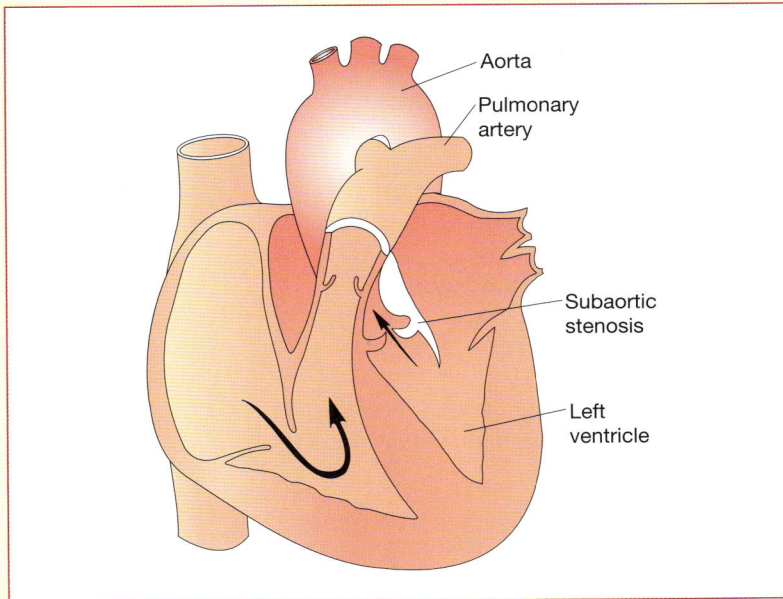

How it happens

Increased left ventricular pressure attempts to overcome the resistance of the narrowed valvular opening. The added workload increases the demand for oxygen, and diminished cardiac output causes poor coronary artery perfusion, ischemia of the left ventricle, and left-sided heart failure. If left-sided heart failure develops, increased pressure in the left atrium with resulting increased pressure in the pulmonary veins can cause pulmonary edema.

What to look for

Signs and symptoms of aortic stenosis may include:

- rough, systolic murmur heard loudest at the second intercostal space
- diminished carotid pulses
- systolic thrill

- syncope
- hypotension
- poor feeding
- anginalike chest pain on activity and exercise intolerance.

What tests tell you

Tests used to diagnose aortic stenosis and determine its severity include:

- chest x-ray, which shows left ventricular hypertrophy and prominent pulmonary vasculature
- ECG, which shows left ventricular hypertrophy in patients with severe aortic stenosis
- echocardiography, which shows a thickened aortic valve and left ventricular wall
- cardiac catheterization, which demonstrates the degree of stenosis.

Complications

Complications of aortic stenosis may include infective endocarditis, pulmonary edema, heart failure, and sudden death due to myocardial ischemia.

How it's treated

Digoxin and diuretics are given for signs of heart failure. Anticoagulant therapy is used to prevent thrombus formation around the stenotic or replaced valve. Prophylactic antibiotics are given to prevent infective endocarditis.

Surgery may involve aortic valvulotomy or prosthetic valve replacement. Balloon angioplasty, done through a cardiac catheterization, may be used to dilate the stenotic valve.

What to do

When caring for a child with aortic stenosis, ensure the following:

- Watch closely for signs of heart failure, pulmonary edema, and adverse effects of drug therapy.
- Teach the patient (and their caregivers) about the importance of the medications and consistent follow-up care.

Postsurgical steps

If the patient has had surgery, follow these steps:

- Watch for hypotension, dysrhythmia, and thrombus formation.
- Monitor vital signs, ABG values, intake and output, daily weights, blood chemistries, chest x-rays, and pulmonary artery catheter readings.

Pulmonic Stenosis

In pulmonic stenosis, a narrowing or fusing of pulmonic valve leaflets at the entrance of the pulmonary artery interferes with right ventricular outflow to the lungs, decreasing blood flow to the lungs. (See *Looking at pulmonic stenosis*.)

Looking at pulmonic stenosis

In pulmonic stenosis, a narrowing or fusing of the pulmonic valve interferes with right ventricular outflow to the lungs.

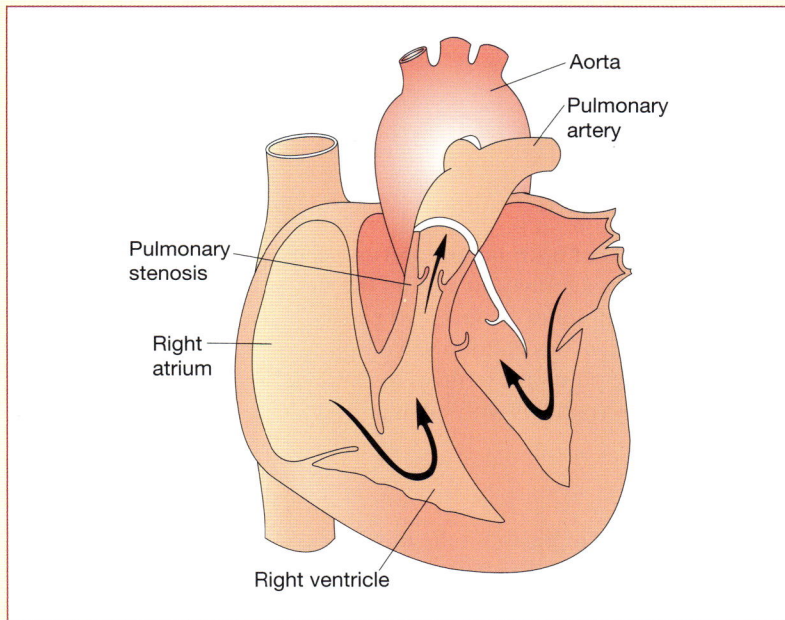

What causes it

Pulmonic stenosis results from congenital stenosis of the valve cusp and is associated with more complicated congenital heart diseases. It is one of the four defects present that comprise tetralogy of Fallot.

How it happens

Obstructed right ventricular outflow causes right ventricular hypertrophy, eventually resulting in right-sided heart failure.

What to look for

Patients with pulmonic stenosis may be without symptoms, or they may show:

- cyanosis
- signs of heart failure
- systolic murmur heard loudest at the upper left sternal border and a split S_2.

What tests tell you

Evidence of right ventricular hypertrophy may be seen on chest x-ray, ECG, and echocardiography. Echocardiography provides a definitive diagnosis of pulmonic stenosis. Cardiac catheterization is an invasive procedure and generally not needed if the diagnosis is confirmed using echocardiography.

Complications

Complications of pulmonic stenosis may include infective endocarditis and heart failure.

How it's treated

Digoxin and diuretics are given for signs of heart failure, and anticoagulant therapy is used to prevent thrombus formation around the stenotic or replaced valve. Prophylactic antibiotics are given, as needed, to prevent infective endocarditis. Percutaneous balloon valvuloplasty is the initial intervention used to relieve pulmonic stenosis in children, but in some cases, surgical valvulotomy (patients with valvular dysplasia) may be necessary.

What to do

The child and their caregivers should be taught about the importance of medications and consistent follow-up care. The patient must be watched closely for signs of heart failure or pulmonary edema and for adverse effects of drug therapy.

If the patient has had surgery, follow these steps:

- Watch for hypotension, dysrhythmia, and thrombus formation.
- Monitor vital signs, ABG values, intake and output, daily weight, blood chemistries, chest x-rays, and pulmonary artery catheter readings.

Mixed congenital heart defects

In defects that cause mixed blood flow, oxygenated and deoxygenated blood mix in the heart or great vessels. Such defects include hypoplastic left heart syndrome and transposition of the great arteries.

Hypoplastic left heart syndrome

Hypoplastic left heart syndrome refers to underdevelopment of the left side of the heart. The defects of this syndrome include:

- aortic valve atresia or stenosis
- mitral valve atresia or stenosis
- diminutive or absent left ventricle
- severe hypoplasia of the ascending aorta and aortic arch. (See *Looking at hypoplastic left heart syndrome*)

Looking at hypoplastic left heart syndrome

Hypoplastic left heart syndrome consists of these defects:
- Aortic valve atresia or stenosis
- Mitral valve atresia or stenosis
- Diminutive or absent left ventricle
- Severe hypoplasia of the ascending aorta and aortic arch

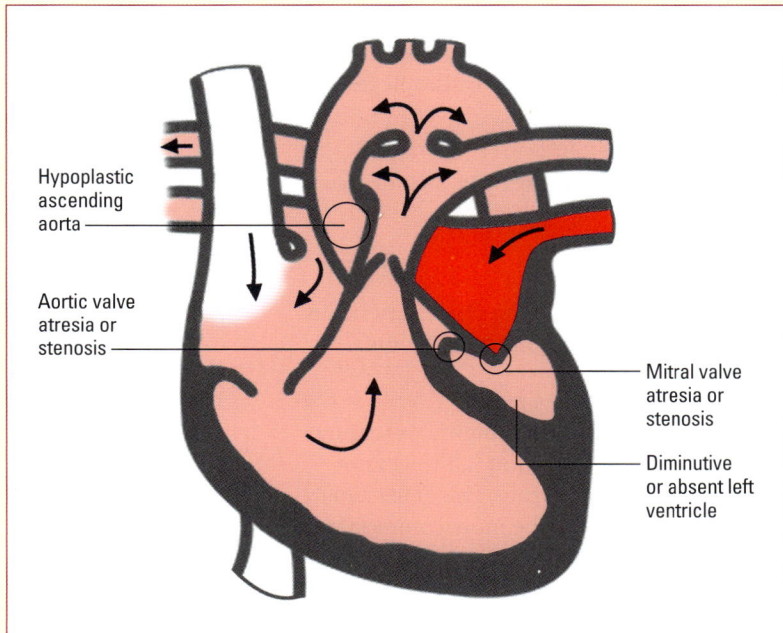

What causes it

The cause of hypoplastic left heart syndrome is unknown.

How it happens

Blood from the left atrium travels through a patent foramen ovale to the right ventricle and pulmonary artery, entering the systemic circulation via the ductus arteriosus. Patency of the ductus arteriosus, which allows blood flow to the systemic circulation, is necessary to sustain life.

What to look for

Signs and symptoms may include:
- cyanosis
- weak or absent pulses
- signs of heart failure, such as tachycardia, sweating, cardiomegaly, tachypnea, cyanosis, and peripheral edema.

Close call

If the ductus arteriosus closes, the infant will progressively deteriorate with worsening cyanosis, decreased cardiac output, and eventual cardiovascular collapse.

What tests tell you

Echocardiography is the imaging test of choice and provides a visualization of the defect. A chest x-ray may reveal cardiomegaly.

Complications

Complications of hypoplastic left heart syndrome can include heart failure and death.

How it's treated

Prostaglandin E is used to maintain patency of the ductus arteriosus. Digoxin and diuretics are administered to control heart failure.

Certain surgery

Without surgery, death will occur in early infancy. Surgical procedures include heart transplantation in the neonatal period (although not common because of the shortage of neonate organs, risk of rejection, and need for chronic immunosuppression) or the more commonly performed *staged reconstruction*, which is a series of surgeries to restructure the heart to be as efficient as possible without an adequately functioning left ventricle. Typically, three procedures are performed in stages:
- Norwood procedure (performed soon after birth)—Blood flow from the right ventricle is rerouted to provide systemic circulation (a task normally performed by the left ventricle). Because the right ventricle is now providing circulation to the rest of the body instead of to the lungs, an alternative source of pulmonary circulation must be provided. An aortopulmonary shunt is created to

connect the aorta to the main pulmonary artery to provide pulmonary blood flow.

- Bidirectional Glenn procedure (also called a hemi-Fontan) (performed at ages 4 to 6 months)—The pulmonary arteries are disconnected from their existing blood supply (e.g., a shunt created during a Norwood procedure). The SVC, which carries blood returning from the upper body, is disconnected from the heart and instead redirected into the pulmonary arteries. The IVC, which carries blood returning from the lower body, continues to connect to the heart.
- Modified Fontan procedure (the final stage performed at ages 2 to 3 years)—The blood from the IVC is redirected to the lungs. At this point, the oxygen-poor blood from upper and lower body flows through the lungs without being pumped (driven only by the pressure that builds up in the veins). This corrects the hypoxia associated with hypoplastic left heart and leaves the single ventricle responsible only for supplying blood to the body.

The ultimate goal of these surgeries is to make it possible for the right ventricle (fully functioning) to work as two normal ventricles would and to allow the separation of oxygenated and deoxygenated blood as the blood passes through the pulmonary and systemic circulations.

What to do

Explain the heart defect to the caregivers, prepare the child for surgery, and answer any questions. In addition, follow these steps:

- Monitor vital signs, pulse oximetry, and intake and output to assess kidney function and detect changes.
- Assess cardiovascular and respiratory status to detect early signs of decompensation.
- Take the patient's apical pulse for 1 minute before giving digoxin and withhold the drug to prevent toxicity if the heart rate is below 90 to 110 beats/min in infants and young children (<70 beats/min in older children).
- Monitor fluid status, enforcing fluid restrictions as appropriate to prevent fluid overload. Weigh the child daily.
- Organize nursing care activities around long periods of uninterrupted rest to decrease the child's oxygen demands.

Transposition of the great arteries

In transposition of the great arteries, the aorta rises from the right ventricle and the pulmonary artery rises from the left ventricle. This defect produces two noncommunicating circulatory systems. (See *Looking at transposition of the great arteries*.)

Looking at transposition of the great arteries

In transposition of the great arteries, the aorta rises from the right ventricle and the pulmonary artery from the left ventricle, producing two noncommunicating circulatory systems.

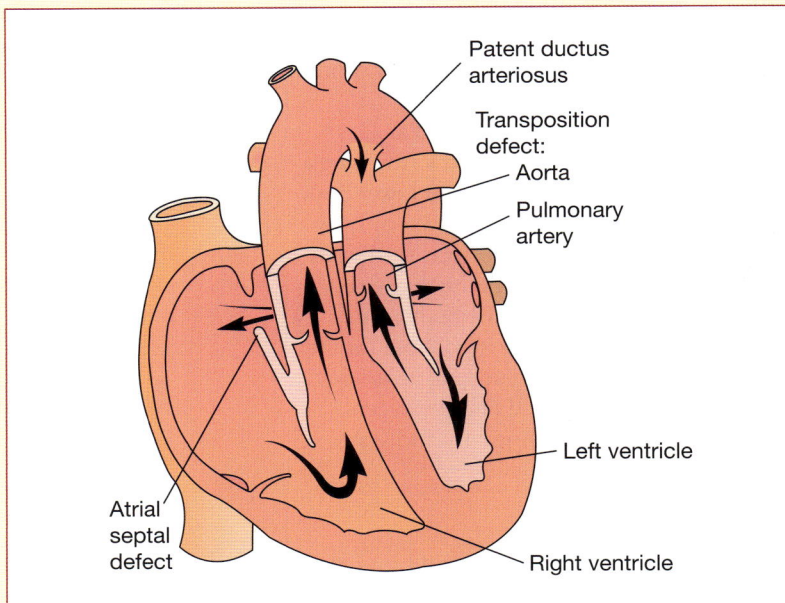

- Patent ductus arteriosus
- Transposition defect:
  - Aorta
  - Pulmonary artery
- Left ventricle
- Right ventricle
- Atrial septal defect

What causes it

The cause of transposition of the great arteries is unknown.

How it happens

The transposed pulmonary artery carries oxygenated blood back to the lungs rather than to the left side of the heart. The transposed aorta returns unoxygenated blood to the systemic circulation rather than to the lungs.

Communication between the pulmonary and systemic circulation is necessary for survival; the presence of other congenital defects, such as PDA, ASD, and VSD, allows for such communication. These defects cause holes in the heart that allow blood to flow from one side of the heart to the other so that oxygenated and deoxygenated blood can mix and flow to the lungs and the rest of the body, which is necessary to sustain life.

What to look for

Signs and symptoms of transposition of the great arteries include:
- cyanosis from birth and tachypnea (worsening with crying)
- gallop rhythm
- tachycardia
- dyspnea
- cardiomegaly
- hepatomegaly
- murmurs of ASD, VSD, or PDA and loud S_2 diminished exercise tolerance
- fatigue
- clubbing of the fingers and toes.

What tests tell you

Chest x-rays may show increased pulmonary vascular markings; right atrial and ventricular enlargements give the heart a characteristic oblong appearance. In addition, other tests may be used to evaluate the following findings:
- ECG may help determine the presence of dysrhythmia.
- Echocardiography is diagnostic of the transposition of great arteries and demonstrates the reversed position of the aorta and pulmonary artery and may detect other cardiac defects such ASD, VSD, and PDA.
- MRI is useful in determining risk of adverse clinical outcomes after the atrial switch procedure.

Complications

Complications of transposition of the great arteries may include infective endocarditis and death.

How it's treated

Prostaglandin E is given to maintain patency of the ductus arteriosus. Prophylactic antibiotics may be needed to prevent infective endocarditis.

Up, up, and away

Atrial balloon septostomy may be done during cardiac catheterization to enlarge the patent foramen ovale, which improves oxygenation by allowing greater mixing of the pulmonary and systemic circulations.

Go with the flow

Corrective surgery may be performed to redirect blood flow by switching the positions of the major blood vessels. This procedure is typically performed in the first few weeks of life.

> In a child with transposition of the great arteries, the patent foramen ovale is sometimes enlarged with atrial balloon septostomy.

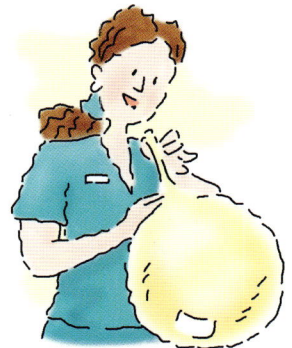

What to do

Nursing care begins with patient education. Teach the caregivers about the defect and answer any questions they may have. The child should be prepared for surgery and other invasive procedures.

- Monitor vital signs, pulse oximetry, and intake and output to assess kidney function and detect changes.
- Assess cardiovascular and respiratory status to detect early signs of decompensation.
- Monitor fluid status, enforcing fluid restrictions as appropriate to prevent fluid overload. Weigh the child daily.
- Offer the child high-calorie foods that are easy to ingest and digest.
- Encourage caregivers to help their child assume new activity levels and independence.

Congenital heart defects that decrease pulmonary blood flow

Tetralogy of Fallot

Tetralogy of Fallot is a combination of four cardiac defects:

- VSD
- Right ventricular outflow obstruction (pulmonic stenosis)
- Right ventricular hypertrophy
- Overriding aorta (aorta positioned above the VSD)

Blood shunts from right to left through the VSD, allowing unoxygenated blood to mix with oxygenated blood, which results in cyanosis. This heart defect accounts for about 10% of all congenital defects and occurs equally in males and females. (See *Looking at tetralogy of Fallot.*)

Looking at tetralogy of Fallot

Tetralogy of Fallot is a combination of four defects:

- VSD
- Right ventricular outflow obstruction (pulmonic stenosis)
- Right ventricular hypertrophy
- Overriding aorta (aorta positioned over the VSD)

Looking at tetralogy of Fallot (*continued*)

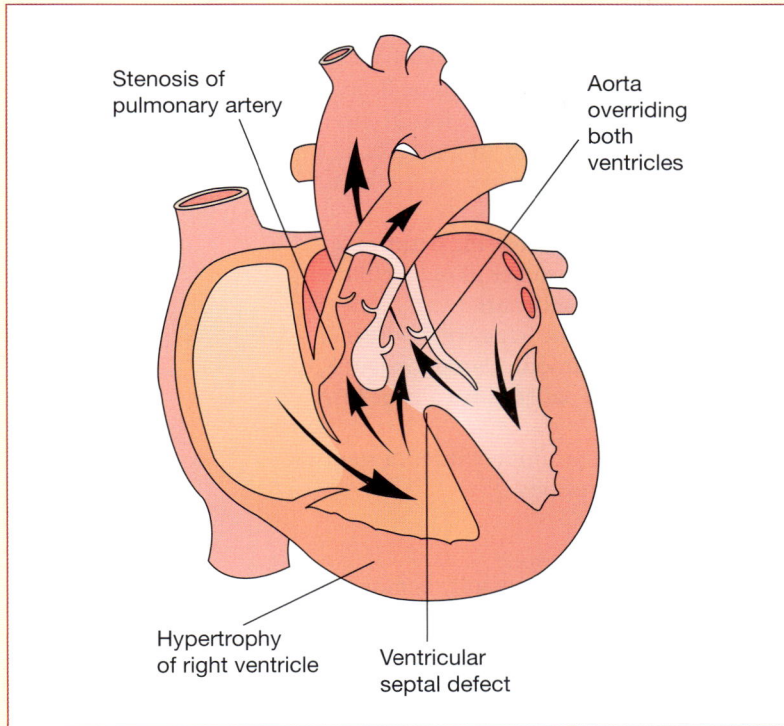

Stenosis of pulmonary artery

Aorta overriding both ventricles

Hypertrophy of right ventricle

Ventricular septal defect

What causes it

The cause of tetralogy of Fallot is unknown, but it is thought to be due to multifactorial causes including environmental and genetic factors. It is associated with chromosome 22 deletions and DiGeorge syndrome.

How it happens

In tetralogy of Fallot, unoxygenated venous blood returning to the right side of the heart may pass through the VSD to the left ventricle, bypassing the lungs, or it may enter the pulmonary artery, depending on the extent of the pulmonic stenosis. Rather than originating from the left ventricle, the aorta overrides both ventricles.

VSD usually lies in the outflow tract of the right ventricle. Severe obstruction of right ventricular outflow produces a right-to-left shunt, causing decreased systemic arterial oxygen saturation, cyanosis, reduced pulmonary blood flow, and hypoplasia of the entire pulmonary vasculature. Right ventricular hypertrophy develops in response to the extra force needed to push blood into the stenotic pulmonary artery.

What to look for

Cyanosis is the hallmark of tetralogy of Fallot. Children may have cyanotic or "blue" spells ("tet" spells), characterized by dyspnea; deep, sighing respirations; bradycardia; fainting; seizures; and loss of consciousness after exercise, crying, straining, infection, or fever. Not all children are cyanotic, and these children may be referred to as "pink tets."

Other signs and symptoms include:
- clubbing, diminished exercise tolerance, increasing dyspnea on exertion, stunted growth, and eating difficulties in older children
- squatting during episodes of shortness of breath
- loud systolic murmur best heard along the left sternal border, which may diminish or obscure the pulmonic component of S_2
- continuous murmur of the ductus in a patient with a large PDA
- thrill at the left sternal border
- obvious right ventricular impulse and prominent inferior sternum associated with right ventricular hypertrophy.

What tests tell you

Findings from chest x-rays, ECG, and echocardiography demonstrate the defects:
- Chest x-ray may demonstrate cardiomegaly and a boot-shaped cardiac silhouette.
- MRI is the gold standard for assessing right ventricular function. It can also be used to measure intracardiac pressures and blood flows.
- Echocardiography provides information on the overall cardiac function and the status of the valves. Cardiac catheterization provides visualization of the defects when the anatomy cannot be completely defined by echocardiography. It can also help to rule out coronary artery abnormalities.

Complications

Complications of tetralogy of Fallot may include hypercyanotic tet spells, right ventricular dysfunction, infective endocarditis, polycythemia, and death.

How it's treated

Tetralogy of Fallot may be managed by:
- knee–chest position and administration of oxygen and morphine to improve oxygenation
- beta-blockers, such as propranolol, to prevent tet spells (in severe cases) and prophylactic antibiotics to prevent infective endocarditis

- palliative surgery to reduce hypoxia during tet spells (involving the Blalock–Taussig procedure, which joins the subclavian artery to the pulmonary artery)
- complete surgical closure to relieve pulmonic stenosis and close the VSD, directing left ventricular outflow to the aorta (Brock procedure).

What to do

Educating the caregivers (and the child, if old enough) is a major part of nursing care:

- Explain tetralogy of Fallot to the caregivers; explain that their child will set their own exercise limits and will know when to rest.
- Teach the caregivers how to recognize tet spells, which can cause dramatically increased cyanosis; deep, sighing respirations; and syncope (tell them to place the child in the knee–chest position and to report such spells immediately; emergency treatment may be necessary). Older children may often squat during a tet spell.
- During hospitalization, alert the staff to the child's condition.
- Because of the right-to-left shunt through the VSD, treat IV lines like arterial lines and remember that a clot dislodged from a catheter tip in a vein can cross the VSD and cause cerebral embolism (which can also happen if air enters the venous lines).
- If the child requires medical attention for an unrelated problem, advise the caregivers to inform the doctor immediately of the child's history of tetralogy of Fallot; any treatment must take this serious heart defect into consideration.

Other cardiovascular disorders

Other cardiovascular disorders that are common among children and adolescents include endocarditis and Kawasaki disease (KD).

Endocarditis

Endocarditis (also known as *infective* or *bacterial endocarditis*) is an infection of the endocardium, heart valves, or cardiac prosthesis resulting from bacterial or fungal invasion.

Untreated endocarditis is usually fatal, but, with proper treatment, 70% of patients recover. The prognosis is worst when endocarditis causes severe valvular damage, leading to insufficiency and heart failure, or when it involves a prosthetic valve.

What causes it

Most cases of endocarditis in children occur in patients with:

- abnormal heart valves

- prosthetic heart valves
- congenital heart defects (especially VSD, PDA, and tetralogy of Fallot)
- rheumatic heart disease.

Other predisposing conditions include Marfan syndrome, degenerative heart disease, IV drug use, and, rarely, a syphilitic aortic valve.

The root of the problem

Some patients with endocarditis have no underlying heart disease. Infecting organisms differ among these groups. In patients with native valve endocarditis who do not use injection drugs, causative organisms usually include streptococci (especially *Streptococcus viridans*), staphylococci, and enterococci. Fungal causes are rare in this group. The mitral valve is involved most commonly, followed by the aortic valve.

In those who use injection drugs, *Staphylococcus aureus* is the most common infecting organism. Less commonly, streptococci, enterococci, gram-negative bacilli, or fungi cause the disorder. The tricuspid valve is involved most commonly, followed by the aortic valve, and then the mitral valve.

Postprosthesis predicament

In patients with prosthetic valve endocarditis, early cases (those that develop within 60 days of valve insertion) are usually due to staphylococcal infection. However, gram-negative aerobic organisms, fungi, streptococci, enterococci, or diphtheroids may also cause the disorder.

The course is usually fulminant and is associated with a high mortality rate. In late cases (occurring after 60 days), patients show signs and symptoms similar to those of native valve endocarditis.

How it happens

In endocarditis, bacteremia—even transient bacteremia following dental or urogenital procedures—introduces the pathogen into the bloodstream. This infection causes fibrin and platelets to aggregate on the valve tissue and engulf circulating bacteria or fungi. These organisms then flourish and form friable wartlike vegetative growths on the heart valves, endocardial lining of a heart chamber, or epithelium of a blood vessel. (See *Degenerative changes in endocarditis*.)

It's a cover up

Such growths may cover the valve surfaces, causing ulceration and necrosis, or extend to the chordae tendineae, leading to rupture and subsequent valvular insufficiency. Ultimately, they may embolize to the spleen, kidneys, central nervous system, and lungs.

What to look for

Early clinical features of endocarditis are usually nonspecific and include malaise, weakness, fatigue, weight loss, anorexia, arthralgia,

Degenerative changes in endocarditis

This illustration shows typical growths on the endocardium produced by fibrin and platelet deposits on infection sites.

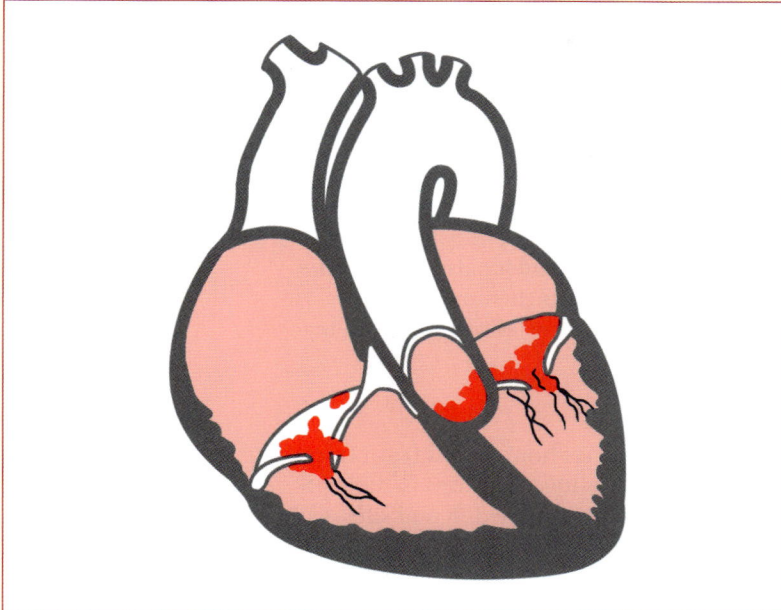

night sweats, chills, valvular insufficiency, and, in 90% of patients, an intermittent fever that may recur for weeks. A more acute onset is associated with organisms of high pathogenicity such as *S. aureus*.

Murmur by megaphone

Endocarditis commonly causes a loud, regurgitant murmur typical of the underlying heart lesion. A sudden change in the murmur or the discovery of a new murmur in the presence of fever is a classic physical sign of endocarditis.

In about 30% of patients, embolization from growing lesions or diseased valvular tissue may produce:

- splenic infarction—pain in the left upper quadrant, radiating to the left shoulder, and abdominal rigidity
- kidney infarction—hematuria, pyuria, flank pain, and decreased urine output
- pulmonary infarction—cough, pleuritic pain, pleural friction rub, dyspnea, and hemoptysis (most common in right-sided

endocarditis, which commonly occurs among injection drug users and after cardiac surgery)
- cerebral infarction—hemiparesis, aphasia, or other neurologic deficits
- peripheral vascular occlusion—numbness and tingling in an arm, leg, finger, or toe or signs of impending peripheral gangrene.

Pinpoint spots

Other signs of endocarditis may include splenomegaly; petechiae of the skin (especially common on the upper anterior trunk) or buccal, pharyngeal, or conjunctival mucosa; and splinter hemorrhages under the nails.

Osler, Roth, and Janeway

Rarely, endocarditis produces Osler nodes (tender, raised, subcutaneous lesions on the fingers or toes), Roth spots (hemorrhagic areas with white centers on the retina), and Janeway lesions (purplish macules on the palms or soles).

What tests tell you

Three or more blood cultures in a 24- to 48-hour period (each from a separate venipuncture) identify the causative organism in most patients. Blood cultures should be drawn from three different sites, with 1 hour between each venipuncture.

Nearly 14% of patients may have negative blood cultures due to previous antibiotic therapy or infections with *Mycoplasma*, *Chlamydia*, or a fungus.

Other abnormal but nonspecific laboratory test results may include:
- normal or elevated white blood cell (WBC) count
- abnormal histiocytes (macrophages)
- elevated erythrocyte sedimentation rate (ESR)
- normocytic, normochromic anemia (in 70% to 90% of patients)
- proteinuria and microscopic hematuria (in about 50% of patients)
- positive serum rheumatoid factor (in about 50% of all patients after endocarditis is present for 3 to 6 weeks)
- valvular damage, identified by echocardiography
- atrial fibrillation and other dysrhythmia that accompany valvular disease, identified by ECG.

Complications

Complications of endocarditis may include heart failure, aortic root abscesses, myocardial abscesses, pericarditis, cardiac dysrhythmia, meningitis, cerebral emboli, brain abscesses, septic pulmonary infarcts, arthritis, glomerulonephritis, acute kidney failure, and death.

How it's treated

The goal of treatment is to eradicate the infecting organism. Initial antibiotic therapy is usually a combination of vancomycin and gentamicin. The remaining therapeutic regimen will be decided based on identification of the infecting organism and on sensitivity studies. IV antimicrobial therapy should start promptly and continue up to 6 weeks.

Supportive treatment includes bed rest, acetaminophen for fever and aches, and sufficient fluid intake. Severe valvular damage, especially aortic or mitral insufficiency, may require corrective surgery if refractory heart failure develops or in cases requiring that an infected prosthetic valve be replaced.

What to do

Provide reassurance by teaching the patient and their family about this disease and the need for prolonged treatment. In addition, follow these steps:
- Before giving antibiotics, obtain the patient's history of allergies. Administer antibiotics on time to maintain consistent antibiotic blood levels.

Monitoring marathon
- Observe for signs of infiltration or inflammation at the venipuncture site—possible complications of long-term IV drug administration. To reduce the risk of these complications, rotate venous access sites at least every 3 days (72 hours).
- Watch for signs of embolization (hematuria, pleuritic chest pain, left upper quadrant pain, or paresis), a common occurrence during the first 3 months of treatment. Tell the caregivers—and the child, if old enough—to watch for and report these signs, which may indicate impending peripheral vascular occlusion or splenic, kidney, cerebral, or pulmonary infarction.
- Monitor the patient's kidney status (blood urea nitrogen [BUN] levels, creatinine clearance, and urine output) to check for signs of renal emboli or evidence of drug toxicity.
- Observe for signs of heart failure, such as dyspnea, tachypnea, tachycardia, crackles, jugular vein distention, edema, and weight gain.

The education edge
- Instruct the caregivers to watch closely for fever, anorexia, and other signs of relapse after treatment stops. Suggest quiet diversionary activities to prevent excessive physical exertion.
- Make sure that the patient who is susceptible to endocarditis (and their caregivers) understands the need for prophylactic antibiotics before, during, and after dental work and genitourinary, gynecologic, or GI procedures.

- Teach the patient how to recognize symptoms of endocarditis and to notify the doctor immediately if such symptoms occur.
- Teach the child and their caregivers the importance of meticulous oral care when the child is susceptible to endocarditis.

Kawasaki disease

KD, also known as *mucocutaneous lymph node syndrome,* is an acute systemic vasculitis. It has become a leading cause of acquired heart disease in children in the United States. Most cases occur in children younger than age 5 years, with 1.5 times the incidence in boys than in girls.

Although KD is a self-limiting disorder, cardiac sequelae may develop in about 20% of children who are not treated. These sequelae may include damage to the coronary arteries and myocardium.

What causes it

The cause of KD is unknown. It has geographic or seasonal outbreaks in late winter or early spring, suggesting an infectious process. However, it isn't spread person to person.

How it happens

In KD, inflammation of the small to medium blood vessels occurs throughout the body. However, the coronary arteries and, subsequently, the myocardium are most vulnerable to damage. Later progression of the vasculitis may damage the walls of medium-sized vessels, possibly leading to coronary artery aneurysms. Systemic vasculitis usually begins to subside in 6 to 8 weeks.

What to look for

The three phases of KD are acute, subacute, and convalescent.

Acute phase

The acute phase of KD involves abrupt onset of high fever that doesn't respond to antipyretics and antibiotic therapy. Signs and symptoms during this phase include:

- fever
- irritability (possibly inconsolable)
- cervical lymphadenopathy
- congested conjunctivae and dry eyes
- erythema of the oral cavity, lips, and tongue, leading to the characteristic "strawberry tongue"
- desquamation of the palms of the hands and soles of the feet
- myocarditis
- intermittent signs of heart failure
- transient arthritis of the small joints. (See *Clinical criteria for KD.*)

Clinical criteria for KD

To be diagnosed with KD, a child must have a fever that lasts for more than 5 days and show four of the following five signs and symptoms:
1. bilateral conjunctivitis without discharge
2. strawberry tongue and mucous membrane dryness with possible fissures
3. erythema of the palms or soles with peeling (usually at week 2 or 3) and peripheral edema
4. polymorphous rash
5. cervical lymph node swelling (one node >1.5 cm).

Subacute phase

The subacute phase begins as fever subsides and continues until all clinical signs have resolved. Because the damaged coronary arteries will stretch to their maximum diameter during this phase, the child is at risk for coronary thrombosis and aneurysms. Signs and symptoms that may occur during this phase include:

- irritability
- periungual desquamation (peeling that occurs around the nails of the fingers and toes)
- arthritis of larger, weight-bearing joints.

Convalescent phase

By the convalescent phase, all the clinical signs of KD have resolved. Laboratory results may, however, still be abnormal, and this phase will end when those results are normal. This phase usually occurs 6 to 8 weeks after the onset of fever, and the child usually seems to be "back to normal" by the end of the convalescent phase.

What tests tell you

Along with the clinical findings, diagnostic tests may show:

- elevated ESR
- tissue biopsy showing initial proliferation of the adventitia and intima of vessels and thickening of vessel walls
- echocardiogram showing changes to the myocardium or coronary arteries.

Complications

Cardiac complications of KD include myocarditis, mitral regurgitation, dysrhythmias, and vasculitis—usually the coronary arteries that supply blood to the heart. Inflammation of the coronary arteries can lead to an aneurysm. Aneurysms increase the risk of blood clots forming and blocking the artery, which could lead to a heart attack or cause life-threatening internal bleeding.

How it's treated

High-dose IV immunoglobulin (IVIG) may reduce the duration of fever as well as coronary artery involvement (if given in the first 10 days of the disease course). Aspirin therapy is used to reduce fever and inflammation. Kawasaki treatment is a rare exception to the rule against aspirin use in children. For the occurrence of giant aneurysms, anticoagulation therapy may be instituted.

Most children recover completely following treatment, but cardiovascular involvement may lead to serious morbidity, usually due to coronary thrombosis.

What to do

Monitor cardiovascular status and intake and output carefully, including daily weights. Observe the child for fluid volume overload due to myocarditis and assess them frequently for signs of heart failure. In addition, follow these steps:

- Administer IVIG as you would a blood product, obtaining vital signs during and immediately following the infusion and being alert for signs of allergic reaction (the single infusion is usually given over 10 to 12 hours).

Soft and soothing

- Decrease skin inflammation with cool compresses, unscented lotions, and the use of soft clothing.
- Provide gentle mouth care during the acute phase of the illness along with a diet of clear, nonirritating liquids and soft foods.
- Maintain a quiet environment to promote rest and reduce irritability. Teach caregivers that irritability is a hallmark symptom of KD (because caregivers are, at times, surprised by their child's uncharacteristic behavior).

Hush little baby, don't you cry

- Support the caregivers' efforts to console their crying child and reassure them that irritability usually subsides during the convalescent phase.
- Because antibody development may be suppressed, do not administer live immunizations (such as the measles-mumps-rubella or varicella vaccines) until 7 to 11 months after IVIG administration.

Come on in—the water's fine

- Because arthritis symptoms may persist for several weeks in weight-bearing joints, provide warm baths and passive range of motion exercises to maintain joint function and reduce stiffness.
- Teach the caregivers signs and symptoms of MI in children, such as abdominal pain, vomiting, restlessness, inconsolable crying, and pallor (possibly chest pain in older children). Instruct the caregivers in cardiopulmonary resuscitation of the child.

Quick quiz

1. Which sign best indicates the presence of coarctation of the aorta?
    A. Clubbing of fingers and toes
    B. Generalized cyanosis, especially with crying
    C. Rapid and irregular apical heartbeat
    D. Bounding brachial pulses with weak femoral pulses

Answer: D. The child with coarctation of the aorta has bounding pulses in the upper extremities and weak pulses in the lower extremities because the narrowed aorta causes higher blood pressure in the upper extremities.

2.   Which nursing intervention is most important to perform before administering digoxin (Lanoxin) to a child?
    A.   Checking apical pulse for 1 full minute
    B.   Positioning the child with the head slightly elevated
    C.   Counting the child's respiratory rate for 1 full minute
    D.   Calculating the child's urine output

Answer: A. The child's apical heart rate should be counted for 1 full minute before digoxin administration. If the heart rate is below the rate specified in the order (typically, 90 to 110 beats/min for infants and young children or <70 beats/min in older children), the dose should be withheld and the doctor notified.

3.   An infant is diagnosed with PDA. Which drug may be administered to achieve pharmacologic closure of the defect?
    A.   Digoxin (Lanoxin)
    B.   Prednisone (Deltasone)
    C.   Furosemide (Lasix)
    D.   Indomethacin (Indocin)

Answer: D. Indomethacin is administered to an infant with PDA in an effort to close the defect.

4.   Which cardiac defect is associated with VSD, right ventricular hypertrophy, right ventricular outflow obstruction, and an overriding aorta?
    A.   Tricuspid atresia
    B.   Hypoplastic left heart syndrome
    C.   PDA
    D.   Tetralogy of Fallot

Answer: D. Tetralogy of Fallot has four cardiac defects: VSD, right ventricular outflow obstruction, right ventricular hypertrophy, and an overriding aorta.

5.   In a child with KD, the greatest concern is:
    A.   avoiding aspirin because of the risk of Reye syndrome.
    B.   monitoring the child for any signs of heart failure.
    C.   meticulously bathing the child with soap and water.
    D.   ensuring that the child drinks plenty of orange juice daily.

Answer: B. With KD, the child has problems with the skin, mucous membranes, lymph nodes, joints, and heart and circulatory system. By far, the most serious, and therefore of greatest concern, is the cardiovascular system, with the risk of heart failure.

Scoring

☆☆☆ If you answered all five items correctly, fabulous! You've gone straight to the heart of cardiac problems.

☆☆ If you answered three or four items correctly, good work! Your knowledge of cardiac problems is heartfelt.

☆ If you answered fewer than three items correctly, don't take it to heart! A quick review will get your knowledge pumping.

Suggested References

American Dental Association. (2024). *Antibiotic prophylaxis prior to dental procedures.* https://www.ada.org/en/member-center/oral-health-topics/antibiotic-prophylaxis

Bouchlarhem, A., Boulouiz, S., Bazid, Z., Ismaili, N., & El Ouafi, N. (2024). Is there a causal link between acute myocarditis and COVID-19 vaccination: An umbrella review of published systematic reviews and meta-analyses. *Clinical Medicine Insights: Cardiology, 18,* 11795468231221406. https://doi.org/10.1177/11795468231221406

Carr, M. R. (2019). *Pediatric atrial septal defects.* https://emedicine.medscape.com/article/889394-overview

Collins, M. S. (2022). *Patent ductus arteriosus imaging.* https://emedicine.medscape.com/article/350577-overview

Linnard-Palmer, L. (2019). Cardiovascular: Perfusion. In L. Linnard-Palmer (Ed.), *Pediatric nursing care: A concept-based approach* (pp. 267–283). Jones & Bartlett Learning.

Mayo Clinic. (2023). *Cardiac catheterization.* https://www.mayoclinic.org/tests-procedures/cardiac-catheterization/about/pac-20384695

Wilson, W. R., Gewitz, M., Lockhart, P. B., Bolger, A. F., DeSimone, D. C., Kazi, D. S., Couper, D. J., Beaton, A., Kilmartin, C., Miro, J. M., Sable, C., Jackson, M. A., Baddour, L. M., & American Heart Association Young Hearts Rheumatic Fever, Endocarditis and Kawasaki Disease Committee of the Council on Lifelong Congenital Heart Disease and Heart Health in the Young; Council on Cardiovascular and Stroke Nursing; and the Council on Quality of Care and Outcomes Research. (2021). Prevention of viridans group streptococcal infective endocarditis: A scientific statement from the American Heart Association. *Circulation, 143*(20), e963–e978. https://doi.org/10.1161/CIR.0000000000000969

Chapter 17

Respiratory problems

Just the facts

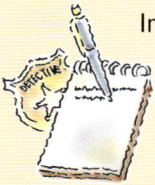

In this chapter, you'll learn:

♦ respiratory anatomy and physiology

♦ tests used to diagnose respiratory disorders in children

♦ treatments and procedures used for children with respiratory problems

♦ respiratory disorders that affect children and nursing interventions for each.

Anatomy and physiology

The structures of the respiratory system are responsible for oxygen distribution and gas exchange. A child's respiratory tract is constantly growing and changing for the first 12 years of life. It differs anatomically from an adult's respiratory system in ways that predispose the child to respiratory difficulties, making respiratory problems common during childhood. (See *Structures of the respiratory system.*)

Chest and lungs

The *lungs* are the main component of the respiratory system. They inspire air, extract oxygen, and exhale the waste product carbon dioxide.

Totally lobular

The right lung has three lobes; the left has two. The mediastinum is the space between the two lungs. The lungs are surrounded by a framework of ribs, vertebrae (posteriorly), and the sternum (anteriorly), creating the *chest*.

Roll out the barrel

At birth, the chest is relatively round shaped. It will gradually develop into a flattened shape across the front and back as the child grows. However, certain respiratory diseases can alter the shape of the chest. For example, obstructive diseases such as asthma and cystic fibrosis (CF) can produce a barrel-shaped chest when they become severe.

Structures of the respiratory system

This illustration shows the structures of the respiratory system.

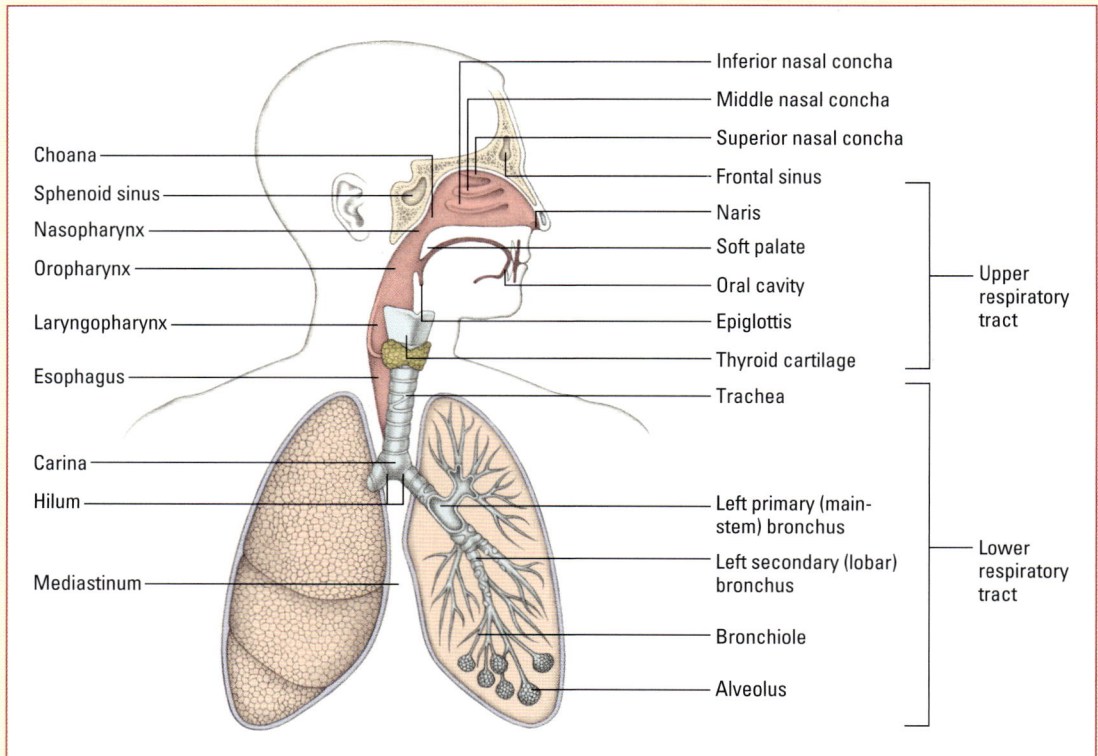

Choana

Sphenoid sinus

Nasopharynx

Oropharynx

Laryngopharynx

Esophagus

Carina

Hilum

Mediastinum

Inferior nasal concha

Middle nasal concha

Superior nasal concha

Frontal sinus

Naris

Soft palate

Oral cavity

Epiglottis

Thyroid cartilage

Upper respiratory tract

Trachea

Left primary (main-stem) bronchus

Left secondary (lobar) bronchus

Bronchiole

Alveolus

Lower respiratory tract

Upper respiratory tract

The upper respiratory tract consists of the:
* nose and nasal passages
* mouth and oropharynx
* pharynx
* larynx.

Nose and nasal passages

The nose and nasal passages serve as a conduit for air to and from the lungs. They're lined with ciliated mucous membranes that filter, warm, and moisten the air.

Nasal for 4 weeks

Infants and young children have smaller nares and narrow nasal passages, making them prone to airway occlusion. Because neonates prefer to breathe through their noses, nasal patency is essential for life-sustaining activities such as breathing and feeding. The neurologic pathways that will coordinate mouth breathing will not develop until age 4 weeks.

Mouth and oropharynx

After about age 4 weeks, air may also enter the respiratory system via the mouth and oropharynx. The child's small oral cavity and large tongue leave the child prone to airway occlusion.

Pharynx

The pharynx, or throat, serves as a conduit for the respiratory and digestive tracts. It is composed of smooth muscle and mucous membranes. The tonsils and adenoids, located in the pharynx, grow rapidly in early childhood and can leave the child prone to occlusion if they become inflamed. The tonsils and adenoids may decrease in size after age 12 years. (See *Locating the tonsils and adenoids*.)

Locating the tonsils and adenoids

These illustrations show the locations of the tonsils and adenoids. Inflammation of these structures can cause airway occlusion because of their locations.

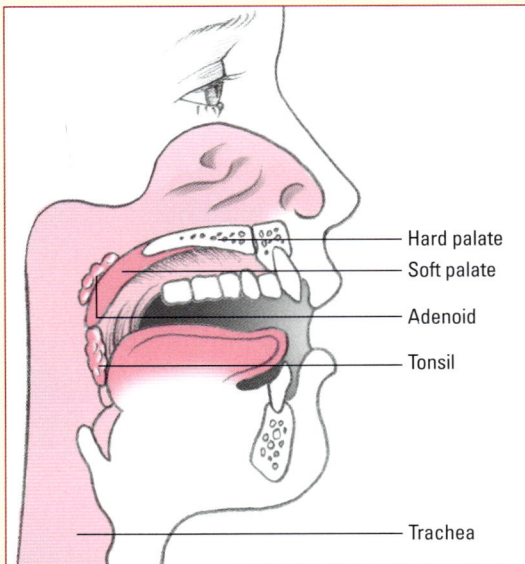

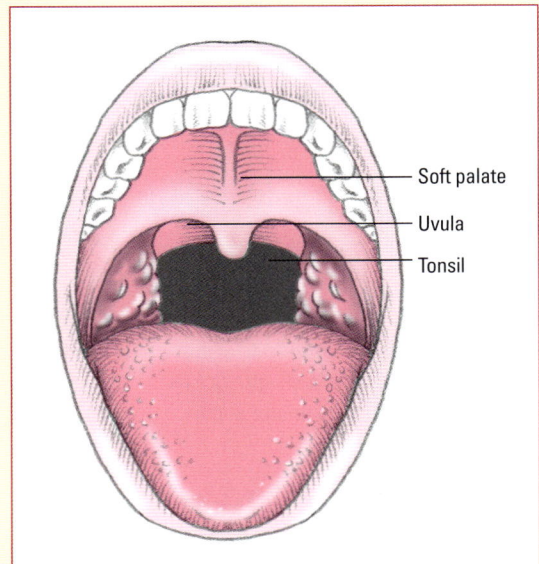

Larynx

The larynx, or the upper end of the trachea, consists of a rigid frame-work of cartilage. It contains the epiglottis, a flaplike structure that overhangs the entrance to the trachea, and the glottis, the opening to the trachea.

No solids or fluids beyond this point

The epiglottis and glottis prevent solids and fluids from entering the air passages during swallowing. The glottis contains the vocal cords, which produce vocal sounds when they vibrate. The child's long, floppy epiglottis is vulnerable to swelling that may lead to obstruction.

Lower respiratory tract

The lower respiratory tract is composed of the:
- trachea
- bronchi
- alveoli.

Trachea

The trachea acts as a passageway for air into the lungs. It's made up of C-shaped rings of cartilage and is supported by smooth muscle. In infants, the cartilage is soft, making the airway more easily collaps-ible when the neck is flexed. A child's trachea is higher than an adult's and gives rise to two major bronchi: the right and the left. The right bronchus is shorter, wider, and situated more vertically than the left. Because of this, aspirated foreign bodies are more likely to become lodged in the right bronchus. (See *Estimating tracheal diameter*.)

Advice from the experts

Estimating tracheal diameter

One way to estimate the size of a child's trachea is to remember the "rule of the finger." The diameter of a child's trachea is roughly equal to the diameter of their little (or pinky) finger. This rule may come in handy when selecting the appropriate size of endotracheal (ET) tube if intuba-tion becomes necessary.

Bronchi

The bronchi, the larger air passages of the lungs, are composed of the same cartilaginous rings and smooth muscle as the trachea. The bron-chi divide into progressively smaller passages called *bronchioles*.

As a child grows taller in stature, there's increased branching of the bronchioles, leading to greater lung surface area. The cartilaginous rings disappear as the bronchioles get smaller, leaving the smallest divisions with a lining of a single layer of cells. The bronchioles terminate in alveoli.

Alveoli

Alveoli are the small, saclike structures in which the exchange of oxygen for carbon dioxide takes place. Each alveolus is surrounded by many capillaries.

Throughout the first 12 years of life, the alveoli change in size and shape and increase in number, resulting in an increased area available for gas exchange as the child grows. A neonate's lung tissue contains about 25 million alveoli; this number increases to about 300 million by age 8 years.

No confusion—it's diffusion

The alveoli promote gas exchange by diffusion (the passage of gas molecules through the respiratory membranes). By diffusion, oxygen from the alveoli passes to the blood, and carbon dioxide, a byproduct of cellular metabolism, passes out of the blood into the alveoli, where it's channeled away during exhalation.

Airway resistance

Airway resistance (the effort or force required to move air into the lungs) is greater in children than in adults because children's airways are narrower than those of adults. In infants, airway resistance is about 15 times that of an adult. When there's edema or swelling in the airway due to an irritant or infectious process, the airway is further narrowed, increasing the airway resistance even more. Increased airway resistance makes the child work harder to breathe. This is indicated by:

- increased respiratory rate
- retractions
- nasal flaring
- use of accessory muscles.

Pulmonary circulation

In pulmonary circulation, blood passes through the lungs to obtain oxygen to distribute to the cells and tissues of the body in a four-step process:

1. Oxygen-depleted blood enters the lungs from the pulmonary artery that arises from the heart's right ventricle.

2. Blood then flows through the main pulmonary arteries into the smaller vessels of the main bronchi, through the arterioles, and, eventually, into the capillary networks that surround the alveoli.
3. There, oxygen diffuses from the alveoli into the capillaries, and the oxygenated blood flows through progressively larger vessels, enters the main pulmonary vein, and flows into the left atrium.
4. From there, the oxygenated blood passes into the left ventricle and exits the heart through the aorta for distribution throughout the body.

Inspiration and expiration

An infant's ribs are primarily cartilage and are very flexible, making them inefficient in ventilating. Infants primarily engage in diaphragm breathing, also known as *abdominal breathing*. As the diaphragm moves downward during inspiration, a negative pressure is created, allowing the lungs to expand to draw air in.

Muscles to stabilize, muscles to breathe

The intercostal muscles of the chest are used for stabilization. However, after age 6 years, a child will begin to use the intercostal muscles for breathing. Then, contraction and relaxation of these respiratory muscles move air into and out of the lungs. Normally, expiration is passive. (See *Normal pediatric respiratory rates*.)

Normal pediatric respiratory rates

This chart shows the normal respiratory rates from birth to age 18.

Age	Breaths/min
Birth–6 months	30–60
6 months–2 years	20–30
2–10 years	20–28
10–18 years	12–20

Retractions reveal distress

When an infant or a child is having difficulty breathing, retractions of the respiratory muscles will occur. The depth and location of the retractions will indicate the severity of the respiratory distress:
- In mild distress, there are isolated intercostal retractions.
- In moderate distress, there are subcostal, suprasternal, and supraclavicular retractions.
- In severe distress, there are all the retractions mentioned above along with accessory muscle use. (See *Looking for retractions*.)

Looking for retractions

This illustration shows you where to look for retractions. The types of retractions you see in a child can indicate the severity of their respiratory distress.

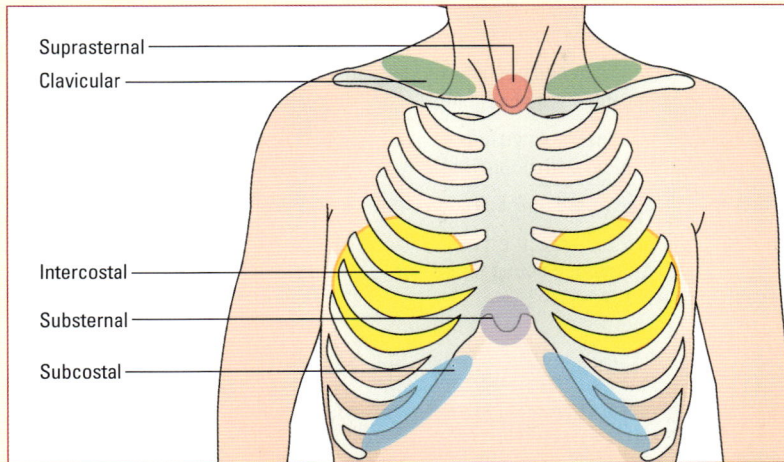

- Suprasternal
- Clavicular
- Intercostal
- Substernal
- Subcostal

Adventitious breath sounds

Adventitious breath sounds are sounds not normally heard on auscultation of the lungs. Due to the thinness of the chest wall, breath sounds seem louder and harsher in infants and young children, and adventitious breath sounds may transmit over larger areas.

Ventriloquist lungs

Sounds may seem to originate in the lungs when they are actually referred sounds from the upper airway, such as when there's mucus in the nose or throat. Auscultating in the axillae of infants and small children is a good way to hear adventitious breath sounds if they are present. (See *Types of adventitious breath sounds*.)

Blown away

When assessing breath sounds, follow these steps:
- Encourage small children to breathe deeply by asking them to pretend they're blowing out candles or have them blow away a tissue.
- Listen with the bell of the stethoscope for low-pitched sounds.
- Listen with the diaphragm for higher pitched sounds.

Types of adventitious breath sounds

This chart describes the types of adventitious breath sounds you might hear in a pediatric patient.

Breath sound	Characteristics	Causes
Wheezing	• Continuous, musical, high-pitched sounds heard in mid- to late expiration (may be audible without a stethoscope)	• Indicative of edema and obstruction in small airways
Crackles	• Intermittent, medium- to high-pitched popping sounds heard during inspiration (may clear with coughing)	• Caused by fluid in the alveoli, bronchioles, or bronchi
Rhonchi	• Continuous, snoring, low-pitched sounds heard throughout respiration (may clear with coughing)	• Due to secretions, edema, or obstruction in large bronchi and the trachea
Stridor	• High-pitched crowing sound heard on inspiration	• Caused by upper airway obstruction at or above the vocal cords
Pleural friction rub	• Grating, rubbing, loud, high-pitched sound heard during inspiration and expiration	• Due to inflamed pleural surfaces

Diagnostic tests and monitoring techniques

Children with suspected or diagnosed respiratory problems may need to undergo invasive or noninvasive diagnostic tests as well as monitoring procedures.

Chest x-ray

A chest x-ray is used to visualize internal structures on film. On a chest x-ray, soft tissues, such as organs and muscles, appear as gray forms.

Dense tissue such as bone appears white and clearly defined. The chest x-ray is used to rule out foreign body aspiration, determine infectious process, and gain information on cardiac size and contour, vessel and cardiac chamber size, and status of pulmonary blood flow.

Inspiration, expiration, front and back

Inspiratory and forced expiratory films are best to rule out foreign body aspiration. Anterior–posterior and lateral films are best to view internal structures for diagnosis of disease processes in the chest.

Nursing considerations

Explain the procedure to the child, assuring them that there are no "hurting parts" to the test. If possible, show the child an actual x-ray film to illustrate what the x-ray can and cannot show. (Young children may think an x-ray machine will be able to tell what they are thinking and feeling.)

You'd be surprised what a child can aspirate! On a chest x-ray, an aspirated foreign body will appear white.

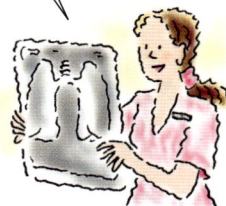

- Protect the child from radiation exposure by covering their gonads and thyroid gland with lead shields during the test.
- Make sure the child holds still during the test and tell them that doing so is their special job. (You may need to assist the child to do so.)

Pulmonary function tests

Pulmonary function tests (PFTs) are a series of measurements used to evaluate ventilatory function. They aid in the assessment of lung function in children with acute or chronic respiratory disorders. (See *Understanding PFT results*.)

Understanding PFT results

You may need to interpret PFT results in your assessment of a patient's respiratory status. Use this chart as a guide to common PFTs.

Restrictive and obstructive

The chart mentions restrictive and obstructive defects.

- A restrictive defect is one in which a person cannot inhale a normal amount of air; it may occur with chest wall deformities, neuromuscular diseases, or acute respiratory tract infections.
- An obstructive defect is one in which something obstructs the flow of air into or out of the lungs; it may occur with disorders such as asthma, chronic bronchitis, emphysema, and CF.

Test	Implications
Tidal volume (VT): amount of air inhaled or exhaled during normal breathing	Decreased V_T may indicate restrictive defect and suggests the need for further tests such as full chest x-rays.
Minute volume (MV): amount of air breathed per minute	Normal MV can occur in emphysema. Decreased MV may indicate other diseases such as pulmonary edema.
Inspiratory reserve volume (IRV): amount of air inhaled after normal inspiration	Abnormal IRV alone doesn't indicate respiratory dysfunction. IRV decreases during normal exercise.
Expiratory reserve volume (ERV): amount of air that can be exhaled after normal expiration	ERV varies, even in healthy people.
Vital capacity (VC): amount of air that can be exhaled after maximum inspiration	Normal or increased VC with decreased flow rates may indicate reduction in functional pulmonary tissue. Decreased VC with normal or increased flow rates may indicate respiratory effort, decreased thoracic expansion, or limited movement of the diaphragm.
Inspiratory capacity (IC): amount of air that can be inhaled after normal expiration	Decreased IC indicates restrictive defect.
Forced vital capacity (FVC): amount of air that can be exhaled after maximum inspiration	Decreased FVC indicates flow resistance in the respiratory system from obstructive disorders, such as chronic bronchitis, emphysema, and asthma.
Forced expiratory volume (FEV): volume of air exhaled in the first (FEV_1), second (FEV_2), or third (FEV_3) FVC maneuver	Decreased FEV_1 and increased FEV_2 and FEV_3 may indicate obstructive disease. Decreased or normal FEV_1 may indicate restrictive defect.

Serial testing

Normal values can change dramatically with growth. For this reason, serial determination of pulmonary function is more informative than a single PFT, especially when evaluating a disorder for severity or progression or when evaluating the effects of treatment.

Breathing on cue

PFTs require the child to cooperate and understand instructions. Most children are not able to perform the testing until about age 5 years because it requires manipulating equipment, holding their breath, and exhaling on cue with directions.

Nursing considerations

Explain the test to the child and their caregivers, stressing that there's no pain involved. Tell the child that their job will be to follow instructions related to handling equipment, holding their breath, and inhaling on cue. Have them practice doing these things before the actual test. In addition, follow these steps:

- Note that results may not be accurate because the young child may have difficulty following the necessary directions.
- Instruct the child and their caregivers that they should have only a light meal before the test.
- Withhold bronchodilators and intermittent positive-pressure breathing therapy before the test.

Pulse oximetry

Pulse oximetry is a noninvasive monitoring technique used to estimate arterial oxygen saturation through a probe that measures the absorption of red and infrared light as it passes through tissue. It reads the amount of light that passes through a vascular bed and converts the amount of light absorbed by the oxygen-carrying hemoglobin, which gives a saturation value.

Sensing saturation

The sensor can be located on an extremity, a digit, a palm, or an earlobe, or for an infant, wrapped around the foot. It works best when there's adequate peripheral perfusion. A reading of 95% or greater is ideal for most children.

Nursing considerations

Explain this type of monitoring to the child and their caregivers and put the probe on a caregiver or nurse so the child can see that it is painless. Reassure them that even though it is used to measure oxygen in the blood, no needles are needed. In addition, follow these steps:

- Place the probe on a site with good perfusion, such as the finger, foot, or toe.
- Periodically rotate sites for probe placement to prevent skin breakdown under the probe.
- To ensure that the value is accurate, make sure the pulse reading on the pulse oximeter matches the child's heart rate.

Treatments and procedures

Respiratory treatments and procedures commonly used for the pediatric patient include aerosol therapy, assisted ventilation, chest physiotherapy (CPT), ET intubation, oxygen administration, and tracheotomy.

Aerosol therapy

Metered-dose inhalers (MDIs) are used to administer medications such as bronchodilators and inhaled corticosteroids to children.

Spaced out

Children need to use a spacer with a valve if they cannot coordinate inspiration with medication release or if they are younger than age 5 years. The spacer is a tube that captures the aerosol released, allowing the child to breathe it in over a couple of minutes. It may be beneficial even for children older than 5 years to use a spacer to ensure that medication delivery is optimized.

Underage aerosol

Nebulizer therapy is sometimes used for infants or when children are sick and have difficulty using an MDI. A nebulizer aerosolizes the medication, releasing it into a small mask that is placed over the child's face. The child can then breathe in the medication through their mouth by taking deep, slow breaths.

Liquid to vapor

Vaporizers are used to create vapor from a liquid. They vaporize cool water to increase the humidity in a room for the benefit of children with swollen, reactive airways. They can relieve many symptoms of upper airway irritation and congestion in young children.

Nursing considerations

Before beginning treatment, show the child the MDI with a spacer or nebulizer mask. Let the child place the MDI/spacer to their mouth or the mask to their face before the medication has been added.

- To determine the effectiveness of aerosol therapy, assess the patient's breath sounds before and after treatment.
- Monitor the patient's tolerance of the procedure. An infant or young child may fight the MDI with a spacer mask or the mask over their face during nebulizer therapy. (Calming techniques such as swaddling may be necessary.)
- After teaching the child and their caregivers how to use the device correctly (which is necessary for optimal effectiveness), observe while they demonstrate their technique; provide support and correct technique as needed. (See *Using an MDI*.)

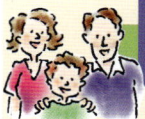

It's all relative

Using an MDI

To optimize treatment, make sure your patient (and their caregivers) knows how to use an MDI properly by providing them with the following instructions:

1. Shake the canister while taking a deep breath in and out.
2. Use a spacer with each use of the MDI.
3. Depress the button on the canister at the beginning of the next inhalation.
4. Breathe the mist in deeply, hold your breath for the count of 10, and then exhale.
5. Repeat as needed to complete the dosage. (Dosages are usually set in numbers of puffs or inhalations.)

Oxygen administration

Some children require more than the 21% oxygen that is present in room air to maintain an adequate oxygenation status. Oxygen is usually required for children who have a partial pressure of arterial oxygen (PaO_2) less than 60 mm Hg or an oxygen saturation range of 89% to 92% on pulse oximetry.

When oxygen therapy is used, the goal is usually to keep oxygen saturation above 92%. Because oxygen is a drug, it should be administered only in the prescribed dosage. It is usually administered in liters per minute (if via nasal cannula) or as a percentage (if via mechanical ventilation or an oxygen hood or tent). Oxygen can be drying, so it must be humidified before it is delivered to the patient.

Oxygen can be administered through an ET or tracheostomy tube during mechanical ventilation or via an anesthesia bag and mask. For children breathing on their own, oxygen can be delivered via a nasal cannula, an oxygen hood or tent, or a mask.

Nursing considerations

Explain to the caregivers (and the child, if they are old enough) why oxygen is being administered and how it will help the child's condition. If an ET tube must be used, prepare the child for its insertion, explaining what they will feel and reassuring them that they will get used to the tube quickly. In addition, follow these steps:

- Monitor the effectiveness of oxygen therapy by assessing the child's color, pulse oximetry, and PaO_2 using ABG analysis.
- Make sure that the patient is receiving the appropriate concentration of oxygen; also make sure that the oxygen is being humidified before delivery to the patient.

Indoor camping

- For infants in an oxygen tent, keep the flaps of the tent closed snugly around the patient; openings in the tent will allow oxygen to rapidly escape, so the tent must be kept fully enclosed.
- Try to cluster care and procedures to avoid frequently opening the tent.
- Check the infant's clothes and bed linens frequently for moisture and change as necessary to keep them dry.

Respiratory disorders

Disorders of the respiratory system that can occur during childhood include asthma, bronchiolitis, croup, CF, and pneumonia.

Asthma

Asthma is a chronic, inflammatory airway disorder that causes episodic airway obstruction and hyperresponsiveness of the airway to multiple stimuli. It results from bronchospasms, increased mucus secretion, and mucosal edema. It is characterized by:

- recurrent cough
- wheezing
- shortness of breath
- reduced expiratory flow
- exercise intolerance
- respiratory distress.

What causes it

Asthma exacerbations or attacks are caused by inflammation of the lungs, including the protective mechanisms of mucus formation, swelling, and airway muscle contraction.

Overreacting

The lungs react excessively in response to a stimulus (trigger), increasing anxiety and physical responses, in addition to releasing histamine and intracellular chemical mediators that result in bronchospasm. The result is a vicious cycle of anxiety and the physiologic response to anxiety.

Choose your triggers

Common asthma triggers include:

- exercise
- viral or bacterial agents
- allergens, such as mold, dust, and pollen
- pollutants
- changes in weather
- food additives
- animal dander.

Many people with asthma, especially children, have extrinsic and intrinsic asthma.

Outside and sensitive

Extrinsic, or *atopic*, asthma begins in childhood. Patients are typically sensitive to specific external (extrinsic) allergens and have a family history of asthma or other allergies. Extrinsic allergens that can trigger an asthma attack include elements such as pollen, animal dander, house dust or mold, kapok or feather pillows, food additives containing sulfites, and other sensitizing substances. Extrinsic asthma in childhood is commonly accompanied by other hereditary allergies, such as eczema and allergic rhinitis.

A look within

Patients with *intrinsic*, or *nonatopic*, asthma react to internal, nonallergenic factors. Intrinsic factors that can trigger an asthma attack include irritants, emotional stress, fatigue, endocrine changes, temperature variations, humidity variations, exposure to noxious fumes, anxiety, coughing or laughing, and genetic factors. Most episodes occur after a severe respiratory tract infection, especially in adults.

Exercise-induced asthma is a narrowing of the airways that makes it difficult to move air out of the lungs triggered by physical activity. Symptoms include coughing; wheezing; chest tightness; and prolonged, unexpected shortness of breath after 5 to 20 minutes of exercise. These symptoms are commonly worse in cold, dry air.

A potent mix

Environmental factors interact with inherited factors to cause asthmatic reactions with associated bronchospasms.

How it happens

Asthma attacks follow a predictable course of bronchospasm, inflammation, and airway narrowing. Here's how asthma develops:
1. The tracheal and bronchial linings overreact to various stimuli, causing episodic smooth muscle spasms that severely constrict the airways.
2. Mucosal edema and thickened secretions also block the airways.
3. Immunoglobulin E (IgE) antibodies, attached to histamine-containing mast cells and receptors on cell membranes, initiate intrinsic asthma attacks.
4. When exposed to an antigen such as pollen, the IgE antibody combines with the antigen.
5. On subsequent exposure to the antigen, mast cells degranulate and release mediators. These mediators cause the bronchoconstriction and edema of an asthma attack.

Ready, set, spasm!
1. As a result of an attack, expiratory airflow decreases, trapping gas in the airways and causing alveolar hyperinflation.
2. Atelectasis may develop in some lung regions. The increased airway resistance initiates labored breathing.

Repeat and damage
With repeated episodes of bronchospasm, swelling airways, and mucus plugging, cells that line the airways suffer damage, leaving a chronically irritated and scarred lining that results in air trapping or hyperinflation.

What to look for

An acute asthma attack may begin dramatically, with simultaneous onset of multiple, severe symptoms, or insidiously, with gradually increasing respiratory distress. Look for these signs and symptoms:
- Sudden onset of breathing difficulty
- Frequent coughing or frequent respiratory infections such as pneumonia or bronchitis (which may be an indication that the child's airway is overly sensitive to stimuli)
- Rapid and labored respirations and a tired appearance due to the ongoing exertion of breathing
- Nasal flaring and intercostal retractions
- Productive cough and expiratory wheezing
- Use of accessory muscles, decreased air movement, and respiratory fatigue
- Barrel chest and use of accessory muscles after repeated acute exacerbations (See *Four levels of asthma severity.*)

Four levels of asthma severity

There are four major classifications of asthma severity based on the frequency of symptoms and exacerbations, effects on activity level, and lung function study results. The four levels are mild intermittent, mild persistent, moderate persistent, and severe persistent.

Level of severity	Clinical findings
Intermittent	• Symptoms occur less than two times per week. • The patient is with no symptoms and normal peak expiratory flow (PEF) between exacerbations. • No interference with normal activity • Nighttime symptoms occur less than two times per month. • Short-acting beta-agonist 2 days/week • Lung function studies show FEV_1 or PEF 80% of normal values; PEF may vary by 20%.
Mild persistent	• Symptoms occur more than two times per week but less than once per day; exacerbations may affect activity. • Nighttime symptoms occur more than one to four times per month. • Short-acting beta-agonist 2 days/week but not daily • Minor limitations in normal activity • Lung function studies show FEV_1 or PEF 80% of normal values; PEF may vary by 20%–30%.
Moderate persistent	• Symptoms occur daily. • Exacerbations occur more than two times per week and may last for days; exacerbations affect activity. • Bronchodilator therapy is used daily. • Nighttime symptoms occur three to four times per month or more than once weekly but not nightly. • Daily use of short-acting beta-agonist • Some limitation in normal activity • Lung function studies show FEV_1 or PEF 60%–80% of normal values; PEF may vary by 30%.
Severe persistent	• Symptoms occur throughout the day. • Exacerbations occur frequently and limit physical activity. • Nighttime symptoms occur more than once per week. • Use short-acting beta-agonist several times a day. • Extremely limited normal activity • Lung function studies show FEV_1 60%.

What tests tell you

Several tests are used to diagnose asthma, assess its severity, and identify allergens:

- PaO_2 and partial pressure of arterial carbon dioxide ($PaCO_2$) are usually decreased, except in severe asthma, when $PaCO_2$ may be normal or increased, indicating severe bronchial obstruction.

Function or obstruction?

- PFTs reveal signs of airway obstructive disease, low-normal or decreased VC, and increased total lung and residual capacities. (Pulmonary function may be normal between attacks.)
- Serum IgE levels may increase from an allergic reaction.
- Sputum analysis may indicate the presence of Curschmann spirals (casts of airways), Charcot–Leyden crystals, and eosinophils.
- Chest x-rays can be used to diagnose or monitor the progress of asthma and may show hyperinflation with areas of atelectasis.
- ABG analysis detects hypoxemia (decreased PaO_2; decreased, normal, or increasing $PaCO_2$) and guides treatment.
- Skin testing may identify specific allergens.

Up to the challenge?

- Bronchial challenge testing evaluates the clinical significance of allergens identified by skin testing.
- Electrocardiogram shows sinus tachycardia during an attack; during a severe attack, this test may show signs of cor pulmonale (right-axis deviation, peaked P wave) that resolve after the attack.

Complications

Status asthmaticus, unrelenting, severe respiratory distress, and bronchospasm may occur despite pharmacologic and supportive interventions. Mechanical ventilation may be needed due to respiratory failure. Death may occur if a child in acute exacerbation isn't treated in a timely manner and proceeds to respiratory failure without intubation.

How it's treated

The best treatment for asthma is prevention of exacerbations. Management includes medications, environmental management of asthma triggers, and education and support of the child and caregivers. Choice of medications to promote optimal respiratory function is typically based on the asthma's level of control and severity.

Antiinflammatory agents

Antiinflammatory medications to reduce mucosal edema in airways include inhaled corticosteroids, such as fluticasone (Flovent) and budesonide (Pulmicort). These drugs are preventive medications, usually taken daily to stop the release of chemicals such as histamine during the inflammatory process.

Antiinflammatory drugs must be taken consistently to be effective. These medications are not effective after wheezing starts but may help gain control and speed the resolution of an asthma attack.

Cortico-reactions

Adverse reactions of corticosteroids include glucose metabolism abnormalities, increased appetite, fluid retention, weight gain, moon face, mood alteration, growth suppression, and hypertension, all of which may be severe if used daily for long-term therapy.

Bronchodilators

Bronchodilators are used to relax smooth muscle in the airway for moderate-to-severe symptoms resulting in rapid bronchodilation within 5 to 10 minutes. Short-acting beta-agonists are the first-line of treatment for quick relief of acute symptoms and for prevention of exercise-induced bronchospasm. These medications include albuterol (Proair, Proventil) and levalbuterol (Xopenex).

Open wide

Bronchodilators relax the muscle bundles that constrict airways for airway dilation and relaxation and are used for acute or daily therapy, nocturnal symptoms, and exercise-induced bronchospasm. When used for long-term control, they work best when a specific amount is maintained in the bloodstream, so serum level checks and dosage adjustments may be required. Adverse effects include tachycardia, nervousness, nausea and vomiting, and headaches.

Leukotriene modifiers

Leukotriene modifiers such as montelukast (Singulair) may be used as a steroid-sparing adjunct for the prevention of bronchospasm. They improve pulmonary function and enhance the effect of corticosteroids, allowing for lower dosages of corticosteroids. They are often helpful for patients with asthma, seasonal allergies, and respiratory symptoms with physical activity. Adverse reactions include diarrhea, laryngitis, pharyngitis, nausea, otitis media, sinusitis, or headache. Behavioral side effects include nightmares or mood changes. Administering leukotriene modifiers daily, at bedtime, may promote adherence.

Allergy shots and oxygen

The use of allergy shots for hyposensitization—to reduce sensitivity to environmental allergens that may be unavoidable, such as mold or pollen—is controversial because their actual effect is questionable.

Oxygen is administered by nasal cannula or facemask for the child exhibiting difficulty breathing. The oxygen must be humidified to decrease drying and thickening of mucus secretions.

What to do

Nursing interventions are focused on maintaining airway patency and fluid status, promoting rest, and decreasing stress for the child and their caregivers.

- Upon arrival at the clinic or hospital setting, evaluate the child's current respiratory status, remembering the ABCs (airway, breathing, and circulation); move on to other activities only after establishing that the child does not need immediate intervention to promote oxygenation.
- If the child is not moving air or is unable to talk, take emergency action.
- Continue to assess the quality of the child's breathing; obtain oxygen saturation via pulse oximeter and PEF rate in an older child (the frequency of assessment is based on the severity of symptoms).

Top to bottom, looking for problems

- Assess skin, intake and output, and perform a head-to-toe assessment to identify associated problems contributing to the asthma exacerbation.
- Assess the child's psychosocial status, looking for indications of anxiety or fear, and promote comfort for the child and their family. (Encouraging the caregivers' presence can be reassuring for the child and can decrease their anxiety and fear.)
- Place the child in a sitting (semi-Fowler) position to facilitate respiratory effort.
- Administer fluids, to restore and maintain fluid balance because adequate hydration helps break up trapped mucus plugs in a narrowed airway. (Intravenous [IV] fluids may be necessary if adequate fluid intake is not possible due to compromised respiratory status and risk of aspiration with tachypnea.)

Please do not disturb

- Promote rest and stress reduction by grouping nursing tasks and avoiding repeated disturbances.
- Support the family by encouraging them to rest and giving them the opportunity to assist with the child's treatments as they wish; update them frequently on the child's condition.
- Provide discharge planning and home care teaching that gives the caregivers a thorough understanding of the disease, how to prevent attacks, and maintain the child's health to avoid illness that leads to hospitalization. (Include education on medication therapy and stress the need for follow-up care.)

Smoke provokes

- Teach caregivers about the dangers of smoking around a child with asthma. Encourage them to quit or, at the very least, never smoke indoors, even if the child is not in the home at the time. If caregivers smoke outside, they should be encouraged to wear a smoking jacket so that the child does not inhale smoke residue from the caregiver's clothing.
- Teach the older child signs of early respiratory distress, so they can seek treatment before the signs get more serious. (A plan should be communicated to the child's school to ensure that medications are given as needed and school officials can recognize respiratory distress.)

Bronchiolitis

Bronchiolitis is an illness that usually occurs after an upper respiratory infection causes inflammation and obstruction of the small airways (bronchioles)—either early in life as a single episode or with multiple occurrences in the first year of life. It most commonly affects toddlers and preschoolers but can become severe in infants younger than 6 months old, causing life-threatening respiratory distress that requires hospitalization.

What causes it

RSV is the leading cause of bronchiolitis. However, other causes exist including viruses, bacteria, and mycoplasmal organisms. Premature infants and those with bronchopulmonary dysplasia, immunodeficiency, or congenital heart disease are at especially high risk.

How it happens

Bronchiolitis occurs when viruses or other infectious agents invade the mucosal cells lining the bronchi and bronchioles, causing the cells to die. Cell death results in cell debris that clogs and obstructs the bronchioles and irritates the airway. The airway lining responds by swelling and producing excessive mucus resulting in partial airway obstruction and bronchospasm. The process continues as both lungs are invaded and the obstructed airways allow air in, but the swollen airways and mucus buildup do not allow for expulsion of the air, creating wheezing and crackles in the airways.

Diminishing returns

Air trapped below the obstructed airways interferes with gas exchange, leading to decreased oxygen and increased carbon dioxide levels. Airflow continues to decrease, and breath sounds diminish.

What to look for

The diagnosis of bronchiolitis is based on clinical findings and the child's age. Clinical findings may include:

- recent history of upper respiratory symptoms, including nasal stuffiness or serous nasal discharge accompanied by mild fever and a cough in older toddlers and preschoolers
- wheezing, deep and frequent cough, and labored breathing
- rapid, shallow respirations accompanied by nasal flaring and retractions
- tachypnea, paroxysmal cough, and increasing irritability with increasing respiratory distress.

The child commonly appears ill, is less playful, and has little interest in eating or has a history of spitting up food with thick, clear mucus.

What tests tell you

Bronchiolitis is diagnosed primarily by history and physical examination.

- Chest x-rays usually show nonspecific findings of inflammation but may show areas of consolidation that are difficult to differentiate from bacterial pneumonia.
- Viral cultures or antigen testing by nasal swab or a direct aspiration of nasal secretions or nasopharyngeal washings may indicate RSV.
- If the bronchiolitis is severe and advanced, there may be a rise in $PaCO_2$, leading to respiratory acidosis and hypoxemia.

Complications

Some children with more severe cases require intubation and assisted ventilation if they become too fatigued to breathe effectively and if they progress to respiratory failure. Death may result due to severe RSV bronchiolitis in children with preexisting cardiopulmonary disease. Bronchiolitis in infancy may increase the chances of childhood wheezing and asthma.

How it's treated

Usually, supportive management with high humidity, adequate fluid intake, and rest is all that is needed when the bronchiolitis is mild to moderate in severity. The child with more severe bronchiolitis will need:
- monitoring with pulse oximetry.

Hydrate and humidify
- Humidified oxygen therapy via nasal cannula or an oxygen hood or tent to alleviate dyspnea and hypoxia
- IV hydration if the child is tachypneic and unable to maintain hydration status (due to decreased intake with respiratory distress or insensible fluid loss due to fever and increased respiratory rate)

Drugs to the rescue
Pharmacologic therapy includes:
- aerosol medications, such as bronchodilators (research is mixed regarding effectiveness of bronchodilators), steroids, and beta-adrenergic agonists to act directly on inflamed and obstructed airways

- antipyretics to reduce fever
- antibiotics (only if a secondary bacterial infection such as otitis media is present)
- antivirals, which have limited success when treating infants and young children with RSV. Ribavirin (Virazole) is the only antiviral approved to treat children with RSV. It is typically used in conjunction with other clinical approaches for high-risk cases of RSV.

'Tis the season

There are two approved RSV monoclonal antibody products that help prevent severe RSV disease in infants and young children: nirsevimab (Beyfortus) and palivizumab (Synagis). A single-dose injection of nirsevimab is recommended during an RSV season for the following pediatric patients:

- Infants younger than 8 months of age born during RSV season or entering their first RSV season. Many infants younger than 8 months of age do not need nirsevimab if they were born 14 or more days after their birthing parent received the RSV vaccine.
- Some infants and young children aged 8 through 19 months who are at increased risk for severe RSV disease:
  - Children who were born prematurely and have chronic lung disease
  - Children with severe immunocompromise
  - Children with CF who have severe disease
  - Native American and Alaska Native children

Palivizumab (Synagis) use is limited to children younger than 24 months of age with certain conditions that place them at increased risk for severe RSV disease (children with congenital heart disease, bronchopulmonary dysplasia, chronic lung problems, CF, or prematurity). Palivizumab (Synagis) is given for 5 consecutive months during RSV season (November to April).

RSV vaccine

An RSV vaccine (Abrysvo) is recommended during weeks 32 through 36 of pregnancy to prevent severe RSV disease in infants. This vaccine should typically be given September through January.

Preventive therapy may be indicated for RSV bronchiolitis in high-risk infants or children with congenital heart disease, bronchopulmonary dysplasia, chronic lung problems, CF, or prematurity.

What to do

Nursing care focuses on careful attention to respiratory function:

- Assess airway and respiratory function carefully and frequently because it is important to intervene in a timely manner for worsening respiratory symptoms to prevent respiratory distress.
- Maintain respiratory function by administering oxygen and pulmonary care therapies.

Head's up

- Elevate the head of the bed to ease the work of breathing and assist mucus to drain from upper airways.
- Use oxygen saturation level as an indicator of the severity of the disease and to spot early signs of deterioration.
- Maintain isolation in a separate room or cohort room for RSV infection and use meticulous handwashing and contact precautions such as gowns and gloves to prevent spreading infection. (RSV is highly contagious and has the potential to spread during close contact.)

Assess and destress

- Perform psychosocial assessment by observing the child and their caregivers for signs of fear and anxiety, which can worsen respiratory distress.
- Help reduce anxiety by providing thorough explanations and updates, and encourage caregivers to participate in the child's care as able (to promote emotional security).
- Cluster nursing activities to promote rest and decrease stress because rest is required to improve the child's breathing and healing.
- Administer antipyretics to control temperature and promote comfort as needed.
- Assist in hydrating the child by encouraging oral fluid intake if possible or maintaining IV infusion.
- Assist in discharge planning and home care teaching when the child is able to go home. Supportive therapies may be needed at home until the resolution of all symptoms, which may take weeks.

Croup

Croup, also known as *acute laryngotracheobronchitis,* is a self-limiting upper airway obstructive disease that affects young children (usually younger than age 5 years). It involves severe inflammation and obstruction of the upper airway and is most common from the late fall to early spring, although it may occur throughout the year.

What causes it

Croup usually results from viral infection with common causative organisms, typically parainfluenza, RSV, *H. influenzae,* or *Mycoplasma pneumoniae.* It also may be of bacterial origin (diphtheria or pertussis). It affects more males than females and is typically seen in children between ages 6 months and 3 years.

How it happens

Croup is usually preceded by an upper respiratory infection that proceeds to laryngitis and then descends into the trachea (and sometimes the bronchi), causing inflammation of the mucosal lining and subsequent narrowing of the airway. Profound airway edema may lead to obstruction and seriously compromised ventilation. (See *How croup affects the upper airway.*)

How croup affects the upper airway

In croup, inflammatory swelling and spasms constrict the larynx, reducing airflow. This cross-sectional drawing (from chin to chest) shows the upper airway changes caused by croup. Inflammatory changes obstruct the larynx (which includes the epiglottis) almost completely and significantly narrow the trachea.

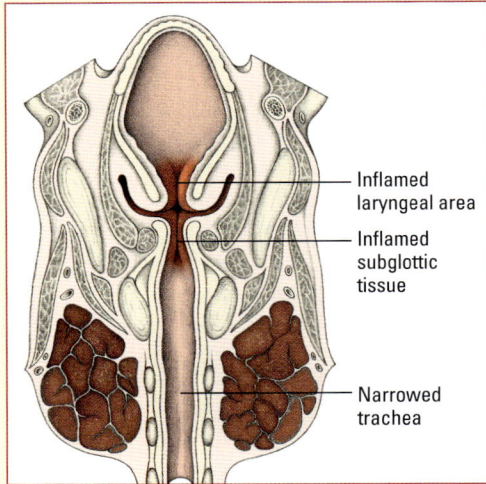

- Inflamed laryngeal area
- Inflamed subglottic tissue
- Narrowed trachea

If it barks like a seal . . .

The flexible larynx of a young child is particularly susceptible to spasm, which may cause complete airway obstruction. When the child's airway is significantly narrowed, they struggle to inhale air past the obstruction and into the lungs, producing the characteristic inspiratory stridor and suprasternal retractions and the classic barking or seal-like cough.

It's always darkest before the dawn

Croup is characterized by gradual onset of a low-grade fever. Worsening of symptoms at night and a cough are common. The airway obstruction increases, leading to retractions, restlessness, anxiety, tachycardia, and tachypnea. Severe obstruction leads to respiratory exhaustion, hypoxemia, carbon dioxide accumulation, and respiratory acidosis.

What to look for

History and physical examinations typically reveal:
- upper respiratory infection
- inspiratory stridor and substernal and suprasternal retractions
- barking cough and hoarseness
- pallor or cyanosis

- restlessness and irritability
- low-grade fever
- crackles, rhonchi, expiratory wheezing, and localized areas of diminished or absent breath sounds
- retractions, wheezing, and cyanosis (in severe cases).

What tests tell you

The diagnosis of croup is based primarily on history and clinical findings. Croup is differentiated from epiglottitis by a lateral neck radiograph that shows a normal epiglottis. X-rays show symmetrical narrowing of the subglottic space ("steeple sign").

Complications

If the child experiences obstruction that is severe enough to prevent adequate exhalation of carbon dioxide, respiratory acidosis results and the child eventually experiences respiratory failure.

How it's treated

Most children with croup do not require hospitalization. The mainstays of at-home treatment are vaporizers, oral fluids, and antipyretics. The major objectives of treatment are to maintain an airway and provide for adequate respiratory exchange. High humidity with cool mist provides relief for most children and can be accomplished using a cool air vaporizer or a steamy bathroom at home. In the hospital, hoods for infants or mist tents for toddlers are sometimes used to increase humidity and provide supplemental oxygen if needed.

Reading the signs

Caregivers must learn the signs of respiratory distress so they can seek medical attention if symptoms progress. Indications for hospitalization include:
- dusky or cyanotic skin color
- severe stridor
- significant retractions
- agitation, restlessness, or obtundation (mental dullness).

Epi for edema

These medications are used to treat croup:
- Nebulized racemic epinephrine is used for its alpha-adrenergic properties, which decrease subglottic inflammation and edema by causing mucosal vasoconstriction. This drug acts quickly—within 10 to 15 minutes—lasts about 2 hours, and can be administered as a nebulization every 20 to 30 minutes for severe croup and every 4 to 6 hours for moderate croup.

- Corticosteroids reduce subglottic edema and inflammation. Dexamethasone (Decadron) given one time early in the course of croup results in a shorter hospital stay and reduces cough, dyspnea, and, commonly, the need for intubation.
- Acetaminophen or ibuprofen reduces fever and oxygen consumption in the febrile child with croup.

What to do

The most important nursing intervention for the child with croup is continuous observation and accurate assessment of respiratory status, including careful monitoring of color, respiratory effort, evidence of fatigue, and vital signs to assess for worsening of symptoms that would require further management.

- Continually assess for possible respiratory failure and have intubation equipment readily accessible at the bedside.
- Assess for airway obstruction by evaluating respiratory status.
- Administer prescribed medications as ordered, which may include racemic epinephrine via nebulizer, antibiotics if croup is bacterial in origin, and corticosteroids to reduce inflammation.

I get misty

- Provide humidified air via a cool mist vaporizer or mist tent and oxygen as necessary. The caregivers may need to stay with the child in the mist tent to decrease crying or apprehension that would contribute to more respiratory distress and hypoxia.
- Because oral hydration is essential to help loosen secretions, encourage the child to drink unless their respiratory rate is greater than 60 breaths/min, putting them at risk for aspiration. If aspiration risk exists, fluids may need to be administered IV.
- Help the child find the most comfortable position for the best oxygenation. Most infants and small children prefer sitting upright and many want to be held.

A friend from home

- Help reduce the child's anxiety by maintaining a quiet environment, promoting rest and relaxation, and minimizing intrusive procedures. Encourage the caregivers to bring a favorite toy for the child.
- Support the caregivers, who may be frightened by the rapid progression of croup and the alarming sound of the cough and stridor, by answering questions and explaining treatments and procedures. Encourage them to be present and participate in their child's care as appropriate.
- Educate the caregivers about caring for the child at home. (See *Croup class*.)

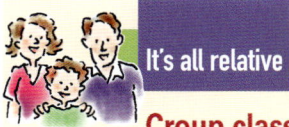

Croup class

Teach caregivers how to care for their child with croup at home by telling them:
- medication dosages, administration techniques, and possible adverse reactions
- symptoms of croup to watch for and report
- how to manage home vaporizer or mist treatments
- how to alleviate symptoms (such as awakening with a seal-like barking cough) by putting the child in the bathroom and running hot water to produce steam (always with constant adult supervision).

Cystic fibrosis

CF is a chronic, autosomal recessive, inherited disorder of the exocrine glands that affects multiple organ systems. It is characterized by chronic airway infection that leads to bronchiectasis, bronchiolectasis, exocrine pancreatic insufficiency, intestinal dysfunction, abnormal sweat gland function, and reproductive dysfunction. CF is accompanied by many complications. All 50 states and the District of Columbia screen for CF soon after birth. This early screening can delay or prevent serious, lifelong health problems related to CF. Life expectancy for the person with this disease averaged 56 years for patients born between 2018 and 2022 based on the CF Foundation Patient Registry data, but there continues to be advances in treatment and technology.

What causes it

The gene responsible for CF is located on chromosome 7q. It encodes a membrane-associated protein called the *cystic fibrosis transmembrane conductance regulator* (*CFTR*). The exact function of CFTR remains unknown, but it appears to help regulate chloride and sodium transport across epithelial membranes. Causes of CF include abnormal coding found on as many as 350 CFTR alleles and autosomal recessive inheritance.

How it happens

Abnormally thick secretions affect the normal function of multiple organ systems, including the:
- bronchi, resulting in chronic bronchial pneumonia and obstructive emphysema
- small intestine, causing intestinal obstruction and failure of the neonate to pass meconium (meconium ileus)

- pancreatic ducts, leading to malabsorption syndromes
- bile ducts, leading to biliary cirrhosis and portal hypertension
- salivary and sweat glands, leading to increased sodium and chloride excretion
- autonomic nervous system, which may lead to hyperactivity.

What to look for

Clinical manifestations may appear at birth or may take years to develop and can vary in severity. Respiratory assessment findings may include:

- dyspnea
- dry, nonproductive cough
- wheezing
- atelectasis and generalized obstructive emphysema due to mucoid obstruction as the disease progresses with the characteristic features of barrel-shaped chest, cyanosis, and clubbing of fingers and toes
- chronic sinusitis
- bronchitis
- bronchopneumonia.

Eye on the gastrointestinal

Gastrointestinal (GI) assessment findings include:
- meconium ileus in a neonate
- weight loss despite increased appetite
- malnourishment and vitamin deficiency
- obstruction of pancreatic ducts and absence of pancreatic enzymes, leading to malabsorption syndrome with chronic diarrhea and large, frothy, foul-smelling stools
- abdominal cramping and distention and foul-smelling flatus
- cirrhosis leading to possible portal hypertension with resultant splenomegaly and esophageal varices.

Heritage

Reproductive system assessment findings include:
- decreased fertility due to increased viscosity of cervical mucus, blocking the entry of sperm in females
- sterility in males due to blockage of the vas deferens with abnormal secretions, preventing sperm formation.

To the heart of it all

Cardiovascular system assessment findings include:
- right-sided heart enlargement (cor pulmonale) and heart failure resulting from obstruction of pulmonary blood flow
- hyponatremia, which may lead to circulatory collapse if sodium is not replaced.

What tests tell you

Elevated sodium and chloride levels detected on a sweat test are used to establish a diagnosis. Stool analysis reveals steatorrhea (fat in the stool). Chest x-rays show evidence of generalized obstructive emphysema.

Complications

One complication of CF is pneumothorax, which is most commonly caused by rupture of subpleural blebs through the visceral pleura. This condition occurs most commonly in children with more advanced disease. Other complications include bronchiectasis, intestinal obstruction, rectal prolapse, cor pulmonale, diabetes mellitus, and nasal polyps.

How it's treated

Pulmonary treatment of CF is aimed at prevention and treatment of pulmonary infection by improving aeration, removing mucopurulent secretions, and administering antimicrobial agents.

Twice per day keeps infection away

Prevention of infection is maintained with good pulmonary hygiene with a daily routine of CPT, which is usually performed twice daily and more often if needed during pulmonary infections. Some children can use a flutter mucus clearance device, a handheld device that facilitates removal of mucus by increasing sputum expectoration. The child blows into the plastic pipe that contains a stainless steel ball on the inside.

Dilate and stimulate

Bronchodilators delivered in an aerosol help open the bronchi for easier expectoration and are administered before CPT if the child has reactive airway disease or wheezing. Recombinant human deoxyribonuclease, known generically as *dornase alfa* (Pulmozyme), is used to decrease the viscosity of mucus. Physical exercise is also an important adjunct to daily CPT because it stimulates mucus secretion and provides a sense of well-being. Oxygen is administered to children with acute episodes, as needed, but is used cautiously because many of these children have chronic carbon dioxide retention.

What to do

Nursing care will vary depending on where a child is in the disease process and whether they are being treated for an acute exacerbation of pulmonary infection or are simply undergoing routine care.

Oil change not included

When PFTs are low or when children have difficulty breathing or experience a flare-up of infection, they may need to be hospitalized for a "pulmonary tune-up." This type of treatment may include:

- IV antibiotic therapy for *Pseudomonas* infection when it interferes with daily functioning
- rigorous CPT
- inhalation therapy.

The deluxe treatment

Nursing care also involves:

- encouraging pulmonary hygiene (such as CPT, postural drainage, aerosol treatments with bronchodilators, and breathing exercises) to aid in sputum expectoration
- monitoring respiratory status by evaluating breathing patterns and vital signs.

No dieting here

- Promoting adequate nutrition by providing a diet high in calories and high in protein, with fats as tolerated and increased salt intake during hot weather or febrile periods
- Maintaining calorie counts, monitoring intake and output, and recording daily weights
- Administering medications as ordered, including aminoglycosides to prevent or treat infection, bronchodilators, and pancreatic enzymes
- Administering vitamin supplements and iron and medium-chain triglycerides as dietary supplements

Infection-free zone

- Monitoring for signs of infection and limiting exposure to people with respiratory infections
- Promoting adequate rest by clustering nursing interventions and scheduling regular rest periods
- Providing and encouraging activities according to the child's developmental level and physical capabilities and arranging for a school tutor or help with schoolwork if a school-age child is hospitalized
- Providing family support through education and referrals for counseling, support groups, and other resources, such as a dietitian, social worker, physical therapist, tutor, or religious leader

Pneumonia

Pneumonia is an acute inflammation or infection of the respiratory bronchioles, alveolar ducts and sacs, and alveoli (the parenchyma) of the lungs that impairs gas exchange.

What causes it

Infection can result from viruses, bacteria, mycoplasma, or aspiration of foreign substances. Viral pneumonia is the most common type, commonly caused by RSV. Other viral causes include severe acute respiratory syndrome coronavirus 2019 (SARS-COVID-19), influenza and parainfluenza viruses, rhinovirus, and adenovirus.

Major causative organisms in bacterial pneumonia include pneumococci, streptococci, and staphylococci. Children with bacterial pneumonia appear more ill than those with viral pneumonia and have more localized physical findings.

How it happens

Bacterial and viral pneumonia begin as upper respiratory infections:
- Bacterial pneumonia typically begins as a mild upper respiratory infection in which bacteria circulate through the bloodstream to the lungs, leading to cell damage throughout one or more lobes of a single lung.
- Viral, or mycoplasma, pneumonia begins as an upper respiratory tract infection. The virus infiltrates the alveoli near the bronchi of one or both lungs, where they replicate and burst out to kill cells and send out cell debris.

Invasion of the cell snatchers

Invasion of the virus, bacteria, or mycoplasma results in exudate from cell death. This exudate fills the alveolar spaces, with pooling and clumping in dependent areas of the lung to create areas of consolidation. Bacterial pneumonia most commonly causes lobular involvement and sometimes consolidation. Viral pneumonia most commonly results in inflammation of interstitial tissue. (See *Types of pneumonia*.)

Types of pneumonia

Pneumonia is classified according to the location and extent of involvement:
- *Lobar pneumonia* involves a large segment of one or more lung lobes; if it involves both lungs, it's known as *bilateral* or *double pneumonia*.
- *Bronchopneumonia* begins in the terminal bronchioles and involves nearby lobules, which become clogged to form consolidated patches.
- *Interstitial pneumonia* is confined to the alveolar walls and peribronchial and interlobular tissues.
- *Aspiration pneumonia* is caused by aspiration of fluid or food substance in a child who has difficulty swallowing; who is unable to swallow due to paralysis, weakness, or congenital anomalies; or who has an absent cough reflex. It can also occur if the child is fed while crying or breathing rapidly.

What to look for

Regardless of the causative agent, symptoms of pneumonia may include:
- elevated temperature
- rhonchi
- crackles
- wheezes
- dyspnea
- tachypnea
- restlessness
- decreased breath sounds if consolidation exists.

Fretful and feverish

Infants may also demonstrate vomiting, seizures, poor feeding, fretfulness, fever, stiff neck, bulging anterior fontanel, circumoral cyanosis, respiratory distress, diminished breath sounds and crackles, and pleural friction rub.

Headache and hacking

Older children usually experience headache, abdominal or chest pain, high fever with chills, intermittent drowsiness and restlessness, tachycardia, tachypnea, hacking nonproductive cough, expiratory grunting, circumoral cyanosis, diminished breath sounds and disappearance of crackles (indicating consolidation), and moist crackles and cough that produce copious, blood-tinged mucus (as the disease resolves).

What tests tell you

Diagnosis of pneumonia is made by chest x-ray, which shows abnormal density of tissue such as lobar consolidation. Other tests include the following:
- Sputum specimen, Gram stain and culture, and sensitivity tests help differentiate the type of infection and the drugs that are effective against it.
- Blood cultures reflect bacteremia and are used to determine the causative organism.
- WBC count reveals leukocytosis in bacterial pneumonia; the WBC count is normal or low in viral or mycoplasmal pneumonia.
- ABG levels vary, depending on the severity of pneumonia and the underlying lung state.
- Bronchoscopy or transtracheal aspiration enables collection of material for culture.
- Pulse oximetry may show a reduced oxygen saturation level.

Complications

Hospitalization is reserved for seriously ill children. Complications of pneumonia include pleural effusion, empyema, and tension pneumothorax. Some effusions require surgical drainage.

How it's treated

Treatment for all types of pneumonia consists mainly of symptomatic therapy, such as pain and fever control, supportive care of the airway and hydration status, and rest promotion.

- Bacterial pneumonias are treated with organism-sensitive antibiotics; mycoplasma pneumonias may also be treated with antibiotics to prevent secondary bacterial infection.
- Some children may also be treated with antiinflammatory medications.
- To help prevent pneumonia, immunization with pneumococcal conjugate vaccine (PCV20) is recommended for all children in the United States beginning at 2 months of age. In addition, pneumococcal polysaccharide vaccine (PPSV or PPV23) is recommended for children older than age 2 years who are immunosuppressed or have chronic diseases, such as asthma and sickle cell disease.

What to do

The goal of nursing care is to restore optimal respiratory function:

- Ease respiratory effort by administering oxygen therapy as ordered.
- Perform ongoing respiratory assessment, watching for respiratory distress by monitoring vital signs and respiratory status.
- Use a humidifier or mist tent to create a high-humidity atmosphere.
- Perform CPT, postural drainage, and suctioning as needed to remove mucus from airways.
- Reposition the child frequently and elevate the head of the bed to prevent pooling of secretions and ease respirations.
- Provide relief from pain when coughing and deep breathing with medications such as acetaminophen and ibuprofen; antitussives may sometimes be used before periods of rest and before eating.
- Administer prescribed medications as ordered, including antibiotics and antipyretics.

What goes in must come out

- Monitor intake and output and weigh the child daily.
- Encourage adequate oral intake or administer IV fluids to prevent dehydration.
- Promote rest by clustering nursing care to minimize disturbances and maintain bed rest as necessary to conserve energy.
- Provide a diet of high-calorie foods in small amounts in a relaxed atmosphere.

Keeping caregivers in the loop

- Provide support to the child and their family by answering questions, providing updates, and encouraging the caregivers to participate in the child's care.

- Begin discharge planning early, providing teaching on medications, especially antibiotics that must be taken at prescribed intervals for the full course.

Quick quiz

1. In which anatomic structure does gas exchange take place?
   A. Nasopharynx
   B. Trachea
   C. Bronchioles
   D. Alveoli

Answer: D. The exchange of oxygen for carbon dioxide occurs in the alveoli.

2. Which of the following respiratory rates is concerning for an 18-month-old?
   A. 22 breaths/min
   B. 35 breaths/min
   C. 30 breaths/min
   D. 25 breaths/min

Answer: B. Normal pediatric respiratory rate for a child aged 6 months to 2 years is 20 to 30 breaths/min.

3. Which of the following breath sounds is characterized by continuous high-pitched sounds heard in mid- to late expiration?
   A. Crackles
   B. Pleural rub
   C. Wheezing
   D. Stridor

Answer: C. Wheezing, which is indicative of edema and obstruction in the small airways, has a continuous musical quality in the mid- to late expiratory phase of respiration.

4. All of the following are important parts of the management of a child with bronchiolitis **except**:
   A. antipyretics.
   B. adequate hydration and nutrition.
   C. humidified oxygen.
   D. antihistamines.

Answer: D. Antihistamines are not a mainstay of bronchiolitis treatment; however, children with RSV are at risk for dehydration and difficulty breathing. Antipyretics, adequate hydration, and nutrition as well as humidified oxygen can be helpful at alleviated symptoms and maintaining the comfort of the child.

Scoring

⭐⭐⭐ If you answered all four items correctly, excellent work! You can breathe easy about your knowledge of respiratory problems.

⭐⭐ If you answered three items correctly, good job! Your knowledge of respiratory problems in children is unobstructed.

⭐ If you answered fewer than three items correctly, don't hyperventilate! Take a deep breath, review the chapter, and move on.

Suggested References

Chang, Y. (2023). Best practices for pediatricians in diagnosing and treating asthma. *Contemporary Pediatrics, 4*, 18–19. https://www.contemporarypediatrics.com/view/best-practices-for-pediatricians-in-diagnosing-and-treating-asthma

Dowdy, R. A. E., & Cornelius, B. W. (2020). Medical management of epiglottitis. *Anesthesia Progress, 67(2)*, 90–97. https://doi.org/10.2344/anpr-66-04-08

Frost, H. M., Keith, A., Fletcher, D. R., Sebastian, T., Dominguez, S. R., Kurtz, M., Parker, S. K., Wilson, M. L., & Jenkins, T. C. (2024). Clinical outcomes associated with amoxicillin treatment for acute otitis media in children. *Journal of the Pediatric Infectious Diseases Society, 13(3)*, 203–210. https://doi.org/10.1093/jpids/piae010

Glasper, E. A. (2023). Can respiratory syncytial virus (RSV) infection in children be eliminated through immunization? *Comprehensive Child & Adolescent Nursing, 46(1)*, 5–7. https://doi.org/10.1080/24694193.2023.2182593

Haghighi, M. (2024). Watchful waiting strategy in the treatment of acute otitis media in children. *Journal of Comprehensive Pediatrics, 15(1)*, e141136. https://doi.org/10.5812/jcp-141136

Hawk, H. (2023). *Croup: A common pediatric respiratory illness. Nursing Made Incredibly Easy, 21*, 27–33. https://doi.org/10.1097/01.NME.0000884100.58583.fe

Kenyon, C. C., Maltenfort, M. G., Hubbard, R. A., Schinasi, L. H., De Roos, A. J., Henrickson, S. E., Bryant-Stephens, T. C., & Forrest, C. B. (2020). Variability in diagnosed asthma in young children in a large pediatric primary care network. *Academic Pediatrics, 20(7)*, 958–966. https://doi.org/10.1016/j.acap.2020.02.003

Owens, G. (2023). Best practices in the treatment and management of cystic fibrosis: Managed care perspectives on the role of new therapies. *Journal of Managed Care Medicine, 26*, 31–35. http://jmcmpub.org/wp-content/uploads/2024/01/26.3_JMCM_Aug2023_web.pdf

Yang, S., Lu, S., Wang, Y., Guo, Y., Zhang, Z., Wang, W., & Wang, L. (2024). Respiratory syncytial virus subtypes in children with bronchiolitis: Does it correlate with clinical severity? *BMC Infectious Diseases, 24(1)*, 263. https://doi.org/10.1186/s12879-024-09129-y

Chapter 18

Urinary problems

Just the facts

In this chapter, you'll learn:

♦ anatomy and physiology of the urinary tract

♦ tests used to diagnose urinary problems and disorders

♦ treatments and procedures used for children with urinary problems

♦ specific acquired and congenital urinary disorders.

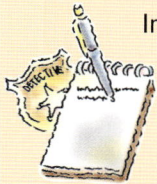

Anatomy and physiology

The key structures of the urinary system are the kidneys and urinary tract.

Kidneys

The kidneys are bean-shaped organs located near the middle of the back. Their primary functions are to filter waste products from the blood, form urine, and send it to the bladder through the ureters. Other functions of the kidneys include regulation of volume, electrolyte concentration, acid–base balance of body fluids, and blood pressure and support of red blood cell (RBC) production (erythropoiesis).

The kidney is divided into two distinct areas:

1. *Renal cortex*—the outside, superficial area of the kidney
2. *Renal medulla*—the internal portion of the kidney in which the nephrons are located

Nephrons

Nephrons are the kidney's functional units. These microscopic structures form urine. (See *A closer look at a nephron*.)

A child acquires the adult number of nephrons shortly after birth, although these structures continue to mature throughout early childhood. The renal corpuscle within the nephron filters blood plasma. The renal tubules within the nephron allow the filtered fluid to pass through on its way to the bladder.

A closer look at a nephron

The nephron is the kidney's basic functional unit and the site of urine formation:

1. The renal artery, a large branch of the abdominal aorta, carries blood to each kidney.

2. Blood flows through the interlobular artery (running between the lobes of the kidneys) to the afferent arteriole, which conveys blood to the glomerulus.

3. Blood passes through the glomerulus into the efferent arteriole and into the peritubular capillaries, venules, and the interlobular vein.

4. The peritubular capillary network of vessels then supplies blood to the tubules of the nephron.

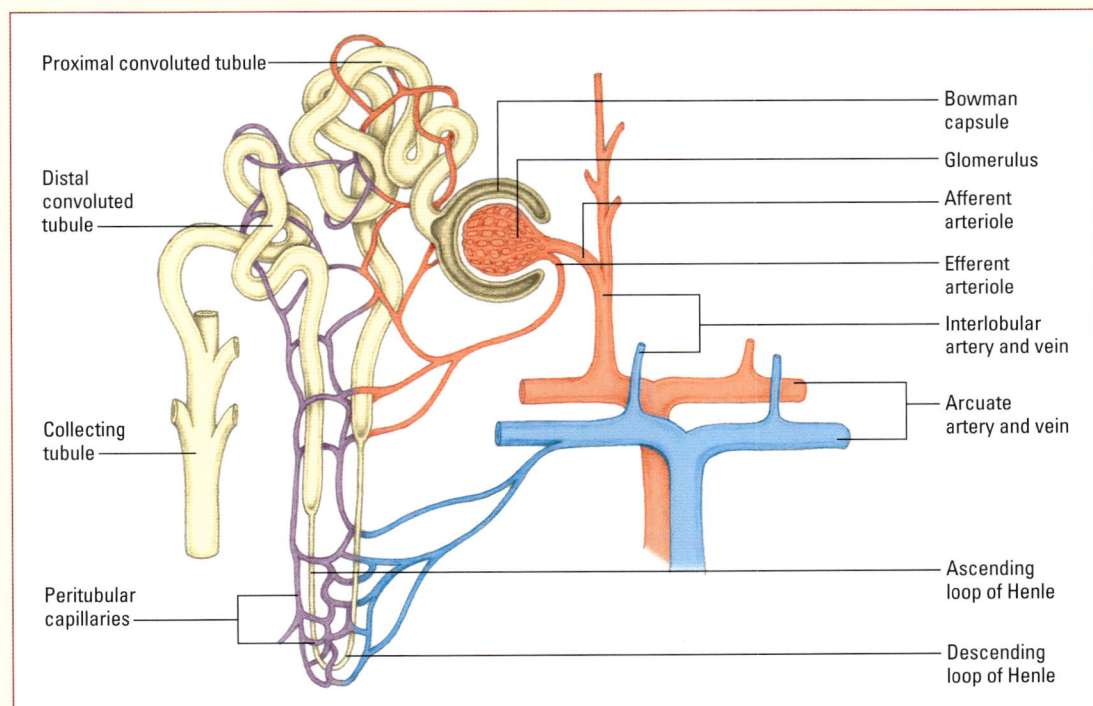

Multitasking kidneys

To produce urine, the various parts of the kidney perform three basic functions:

1. Glomerular filtration (the process of filtering blood as it flows through the kidneys)
2. Tubular resorption
3. Tubular secretion

   While waste products and excess fluids are filtered out of the blood for elimination, necessary fluids, electrolytes, proteins, and blood cells are retained (resorbed) into the bloodstream.

Urinary tract

The urinary tract consists of the bladder, urethra, and ureters. The bladder is a balloon-shaped pouch of a thin, flexible muscle in which urine is temporarily stored before being eliminated from the body through the urethra. Urine is produced by the kidneys and passed into the bladder through two ureters, one from each kidney.

A friendly nudge

Peristaltic contractions within the ureters push urine from the kidneys toward the urinary bladder. A valve mechanism prevents urine from backing up into the kidneys as the bladder fills. When the bladder is full, the following occur:

- The micturition reflex is triggered, and nervous innervation causes relaxation of the internal sphincter muscle.
- Relaxation of the internal sphincter muscle sends a message to the brain to indicate the need to void.
- The person then releases the external sphincter, and urine passes through the urethra and out of the body.

Any volunteers?

Voluntary control of these urethral sphincters usually occurs in a child between ages 18 and 24 months. However, the psychological readiness to initiate toilet training may develop much later.

Urine

Urine is a liquid waste product that's filtered out of the blood by the kidneys, stored in the bladder, and expelled from the body through the urethra during urination. About 96% of urine is water, and the other 4% is waste product.

A child's bladder can hold 1 to 1.5 oz (30 to 45 mL) of urine for every year of age. Average urine output will vary according to age. (See *Urine output in children.*)

Urine output in children

This chart shows the average volume of urine output per 24 hours for children according to age.

Age group	Urine output (mL/day)
Neonate	50–300
Infant	300–550
Preschool	500–800
School age	600–1,400
Adolescent	1,000–1,500

Diagnostic tests

Diagnostic tests commonly used to assess urinary system problems in the pediatric population include:

- urinalysis and urine culture
- blood urea nitrogen (BUN) and creatinine levels
- x-ray of the kidneys, ureters, and bladder (KUB)
- excretory urography
- voiding cystourethrogram (VCUG)
- kidney ultrasound
- kidney biopsy.

Urinalysis and urine culture

Urinalysis determines urine characteristics, such as specific gravity, pH, and physical properties (color, clarity, odor), and detects the presence of RBCs, white blood cells (WBCs), casts, and bacteria.

Culture on a plate

In a urine culture, the urine specimen is placed on a medium and bacteria that may be present are allowed to grow and are then counted. As soon as bacteria are identified, sensitivity testing can determine which antibiotics would be most effective for treating the infection.

Catch 'em while you can

Specimens for urinalysis and urine culture are typically obtained as clean-catch specimens but may also be obtained from an infant's diaper (urinalysis only), a urine collection bag for infants and young children, bladder catheterization, or a suprapubic bladder tap.

Nursing considerations

Nursing considerations differ according to the child's age and gender. For male children, the head of the penis and the urinary meatus must be cleaned. For female children, the urinary meatus must be cleaned, carefully washing between the labia.

Lather up, rinse away

Soapy water, which is then rinsed away, is usually used for cleaning. If an antiseptic towelette is provided, it may be used without rinsing afterward. In addition, follow these steps:

- Instruct the child or caregivers on how to clean the penis or meatus.
- Instruct the child or caregivers to collect the urine specimen by first starting to urinate into the toilet bowl to clear the urethra of

contaminants and then catching 3 to 6 oz (90 to 180 mL) of urine in a sterile container.

- For neonates and infants, apply a urine bag to obtain a clean specimen; the bag fits over the perineum in female children and the penis (and perhaps the scrotum) in male children to catch urine as the infant voids (instruct the caregivers to inform you as soon as the child voids, so the container can be removed and fecal contamination can be avoided).
- When obtaining a urine specimen from a catheterized child, don't take the specimen from the collection bag; aspirate a specimen through the collection port in the catheter with a sterile needle and syringe.

Keep it clean

A clean-catch specimen may be needed to diagnose a urinary tract infection (UTI). In addition to the procedures used for routine urinalyses, follow these steps:

- It's useful to instruct the child or caregivers to use an antiseptic solution to clean the urethral meatus (with a prepared towelette or a cotton ball soaked in the solution); the urethral meatus should be cleaned at least three times, using a new towelette or cotton ball each time.
- It's useful to stress to the child and caregivers the importance of not touching the inside of the sterile container to maintain its sterility.

BUN and creatinine

Serum BUN and creatinine levels are obtained from blood samples drawn from venipuncture.

- BUN levels can provide a great deal of information about kidney function; they measure the blood nitrogen that's part of the urea resulting from catabolism of amino acids (proteins). When the glomerular filtration rate (GFR) reduces suddenly and severely, the BUN level rises suddenly.
- Plasma creatinine levels become elevated when there is catabolism of creatinine phosphate in skeletal muscles. An elevation in these levels indicates poor renal function.
- The ratio between BUN and creatinine may also be examined. The ratio is usually between 10:1 and 20:1. Results vary with muscle damage, as in the case of a crushing injury or degenerative muscle disease.

Nursing considerations

Nursing considerations are aimed at making venipuncture less stressful for the child.

- Use lidocaine and prilocaine (eutectic mixture of local anesthetics [EMLA]) cream or some other form of topical anesthetic to make it easier and less traumatic to draw blood from a child; remember to apply it at least 1 hour before drawing blood.
- Allow the parent or caregiver to be present and allow the child to hold a comfort object, such as a stuffed animal or blanket, during the venipuncture.
- Follow dietary orders as necessary; sometimes, when BUN levels are elevated, protein intake may need to be limited.

KUB radiography

KUB assesses the size, shape, position, and possible areas of calcification of the KUB. A KUB may be required as a first step if a problem with these structures is suspected.

Nursing considerations

The nurse should help the child remain quiet and lie still during the x-ray. Tell the child that this is their "job" and that there's no "hurting part" involved.

Depending on facility policy, parents and caregivers may be able to remain in the radiology room with the child. Instruct them that they must be shielded from radiation by wearing a lead apron.

Excretory urography

Excretory urography is an x-ray of the lower urinary tract, during which a dye is injected intravenously (IV). A series of x-rays is taken as the dye passes through the bloodstream, filters through the kidneys, passes through the ureters into the bladder, and then passes through the urethra to be eliminated from the body.

Nursing considerations

Begin by explaining the reason for the test to the child and caregivers and telling them what to expect.

- Prepare the child for insertion of the IV line and reassure them that it's the only needlestick they will experience.
- Assess for a history of allergies to dyes, iodine, or shellfish because of the use of an iodine-based contrast medium.
- Administer a bowel preparation as ordered; the colon must be emptied because a full bowel won't allow proper visualization of the urinary tract.
- Insert an IV line to allow for the injection of the dye.

- Explain to the child that they may feel warm or a bit woozy when the dye is injected; reassure them that this is normal and that the feeling will pass quickly.
- On the day of the test, allow only clear liquids to be consumed until after the test is completed.

Voiding cystourethrogram

VCUG is an x-ray of the bladder and the lower urinary tract. A catheter is inserted through the urethra into the bladder, and a water-soluble contrast medium is injected through the catheter. The catheter is then withdrawn, and x-ray images are taken as the bladder is emptied.

This test is performed to determine if there are abnormalities of the lower urinary tract, particularly vesicoureteral reflux, a condition that increases the risk of or prolongs a UTI. Sedation is rarely required or desirable because the child must urinate during the test.

Nursing considerations

VCUG can be a difficult test for children. Insertion of a catheter can be uncomfortable and embarrassing. The child will be asked to void during the test without going into the bathroom, which can be confusing to a child who has recently been toilet trained. In addition, the thought of voiding in the x-ray room in full view of the technician can be embarrassing. Reassure the child that the hospital staff realizes they know how to use the bathroom and that they will be urinating during the test only because they are being asked to do so.

In addition, follow these steps:
- Explain the reason for the test and prepare the child for insertion of the catheter.
- Before the test, make sure the child is dressed in comfortable clothing and is wearing no metal objects.
- Assess for a history of allergies to dyes, iodine, or shellfish because of the use of an iodine-based contrast medium.
- Tell the caregivers of infants and young children that the child may be wrapped tightly in a blanket to help them lie still during the procedure.
- Assure the caregivers that the amount of radiation received by the child is minimal.
- Inform the caregivers that a VCUG can't be performed while the child has an active UTI.

Behind closed doors
- Insert a urinary catheter just before the test; provide as much privacy as possible by closing the door or drawing curtains and allow

a parent or caregiver to remain in the room if the child desires (depending on the child's age and family preference, a nurse of the same gender may be the best person to insert the catheter).

- After the procedure, remove the urinary catheter and encourage the child to drink fluids to reduce burning on urination and to flush out residual dye; pouring a glass of very cold water over the genital area during the first few voids after catheter removal helps to minimize burning.

Kidney biopsy

Although kidney biopsy isn't performed routinely in children, it may be used to evaluate decreased kidney function, persistent blood in the urine, or protein in the urine. It may also be performed to evaluate the functioning of a newly transplanted kidney.

In kidney biopsy, a needle is inserted through the child's flank under ultrasound guidance. A small specimen of kidney tissue is withdrawn and sent for microscopic study.

Nursing considerations

Prepare the child and caregivers for the procedure, which can be frightening. Use a doll to show the child how it will be done. In addition, follow these steps:

- Reassure the caregivers that ultrasound will allow the doctor to see exactly where the doctor will be inserting the needle and will prevent damage to other organs.
- Provide analgesic agent as ordered.
- Assist with positioning and holding the child throughout the procedure.

Treatments and procedures

Common treatments and procedures used in the care of a child with a urinary disorder include bladder catheterization, hemodialysis, kidney transplantation, and peritoneal dialysis.

Always prepare children for treatments and procedures with an age-appropriate explanation of what to expect. When treatments and procedures involve surgery, preparation should include an explanation of the anesthesia and what to expect postoperatively.

Bladder catheterization

Bladder catheterization may be performed for diagnostic or treatment purposes. In this procedure, the urethral meatus is thoroughly cleaned and an appropriate-sized catheter is inserted through the urethra into the bladder.

Insert and drain

In intermittent catheterization, a straight catheter is inserted and a urine specimen may be taken; the catheter is removed after the bladder is drained.

Insert and inflate

If the catheter is to remain in place, an indwelling catheter, also called a *Foley catheter*, may be used and attached to a drainage bag for urine collection. An indwelling catheter has an inflatable balloon near its tip to hold the catheter in place in the bladder.

Nursing considerations

Remember that catheterization can be uncomfortable and embarrassing for a child. The older child may feel more comfortable when a nurse of the same gender inserts the catheter. The younger child may be confused and fearful if they have been told it's wrong for anyone to touch their "private parts." Have the caregivers explain to the child that this situation is different.

To minimize trauma, follow these steps:

- Educate the child and caregivers about the purpose of the catheterization; if it's being done to obtain a sterile specimen, explain why this is preferable to a clean-catch specimen.
- Prepare the child to facilitate the procedure and ease the child's fears; use a doll to show them what will happen.
- Obtain consent prior to performing the procedure.
- Be sure to choose the appropriate-sized catheter. For a premature neonate, a size 5-Fr feeding tube may be used; for a larger infant or a small toddler, use a size 8-Fr feeding tube; for children aged 4 years and above, use a size 8- to 14-Fr catheter.
- Provide as much privacy as possible; close the door, draw the room divider curtain, and allow the child to keep on as much clothing as possible.
- Allow the caregiver to be present if the child desires.
- Give the child coping mechanisms to deal with discomfort (such as "Squeeze your parent's hand if it hurts" or "Count to 10 and the hurting part will be over").
- Use distraction techniques to help keep the child's mind off what is happening. This can be accomplished with toys with which the child likes to play or with bubbles. Just be sure to keep everything clear of the sterile field that has been set up.

Generous and gentle

When inserting the catheter, follow these steps:

- Clean the urethral meatus three times with an antiseptic swab, using a different swab each time.

- Generously lubricate the tip of the catheter and gently insert it through the urethra into the bladder until urine returns and is collected in the sterile specimen container.
- If the catheter doesn't easily enter the meatus, use a smaller catheter; never force it into the urethral meatus.
- If performing an intermittent catheterization, gently remove the catheter after the bladder is drained; clean off the antiseptic and lubricant with water.
- If inserting an indwelling urinary catheter, insert the inflatable balloon with sterile water and gently pull on the catheter to make sure it is inflated; next, connect the catheter to the closed drainage system.

Hemodialysis

Hemodialysis involves the use of a machine to clean waste products from the bloodstream when the kidneys are severely damaged or have failed. The blood travels through tubes to an artificial kidney in the machine, and waste products and excess fluid are removed from the body. The purified blood then flows back to the body through another set of tubes. Ideally, this would be done in a pediatric dialysis center.

To stick or not to stick

The child on hemodialysis may have a double-lumen central catheter in place in their chest to serve as a site for blood removal. Children needing long-term dialysis may have a subcutaneous graft, anastomosing a vein and an artery. This graft reduces the risk of infection but means the child will need two venipunctures each time dialysis is performed. EMLA cream should be used to reduce discomfort.

Nursing considerations

Provide diversional activities to prevent boredom, such as games, music, drawing or coloring materials, and videos; encourage a family member to stay with the child. In addition, follow these steps:
- Weigh the child before beginning hemodialysis.
- If the child has a subcutaneous graft, check the blood access site every 2 hours for patency and signs of clotting; don't use the arm with this site for taking blood pressure or drawing blood.
- During dialysis, monitor vital signs, clotting times, blood flow, the function of the vascular access site, and arterial and venous pressures.

Look out for losses
- Watch for complications, such as septicemia, embolism, hepatitis, and rapid fluid and electrolyte loss.
- After dialysis, monitor vital signs and the vascular access site; weigh the child and watch for signs of fluid and electrolyte imbalances.
- Use standard precautions when handling blood and body fluids.

Kidney transplantation

Kidney transplantation involves replacing a person's diseased kidney with a healthy kidney from another person. The donor kidney may come from a living donor or a cadaver donor. Although hemodialysis and peritoneal dialysis are life-preserving procedures and may even be carried out in the home, kidney transplantation is the preferred method of renal replacement therapy in the pediatric population because it offers the opportunity for a normal life.

Nursing considerations

By the time a child undergoes kidney transplantation, they most likely have a long history of procedures and hospitalizations. The child should be given as many choices as possible; a choice as simple as which arm to use for a blood draw can help to give the child a sense of control.

In addition, follow these steps:
- Provide emotional support and guidance to the child and caregivers; prepare them for the procedure, including what will occur preoperatively, during the procedure, and postoperatively.
- Arrange for the child and their caregivers to tour the intensive care unit and meet the nursing staff before the transplantation.
- Administer immunosuppressive medications as ordered; a child who will have or has had a kidney transplant will be taking immunosuppressive medications to decrease the risk of organ rejection.
- Monitor for signs and symptoms of infection; while immunosuppressed, the child is at increased risk for infection.

You sneeze, you leave
- Make sure that no one with obvious infection takes care of the child.
- Prepare the child and caregivers for the possibility of continuing to need hemodialysis temporarily after the transplantation because the transplanted kidney might not work effectively right away.

Peritoneal dialysis

In peritoneal dialysis, the blood is cleaned of waste products and excess fluids using the lining of the abdomen as a filter. Peritoneal dialysis is especially useful for children who are candidates whose incomes are below the federal poverty threshold for vascular access and for those who live far from a medical center. This procedure includes these steps:
- A peritoneal dialysis catheter is inserted through a small abdominal incision or a puncture hole into the peritoneal cavity. The catheter is then connected to fluid bags and tubing.

- A cleaning solution is drained from a bag into the abdomen.
- Fluids and waste products flow through the lining and are "caught" by the dialysis fluid.
- This fluid is then drained from the abdomen, taking the extra fluids and waste products with it.

Nursing considerations

Prepare the child and caregivers for the insertion of the catheter into the abdominal cavity. Make sure a valid informed consent form has been signed and included in the child's chart. In addition, follow these steps:

- Monitor the child's reaction to the sedation, anesthesia, and pain management regimen.
- Make sure strict sterile technique is used at all times during catheter placement and peritoneal dialysis.
- Monitor the child's response to the therapy.
- Make the child as comfortable as possible and provide sufficient rest periods.
- Assess for bleeding from the catheter insertion site.
- Maintain patency of the peritoneal dialysis catheter; keep it in place, without kinks or pulling, and with the fluid bags at the correct level.
- Monitor for signs of infection at the insertion site.

Urinary disorders

Urinary disorders that may affect children include acute poststreptococcal glomerulonephritis, chronic glomerulonephritis, congenital urologic anomalies, hemolytic uremic syndrome (HUS), nephrotic syndrome, kidney failure (acute and chronic), and Wilms tumor.

Acute poststreptococcal glomerulonephritis

Glomerulonephritis is an inflammation of the tubules of the kidneys (glomeruli), which filter waste products from the blood. When this inflammation follows an infection with streptococcal bacteria (most commonly via strep throat), it's called *acute poststreptococcal glomerulonephritis*. It's most commonly seen in male children between ages 3 and 7 years but can occur at any age. Up to 95% of children recover fully; the rest may progress to chronic kidney failure.

An interesting point: The relationship between acute glomerulonephritis and scarlet fever was first recognized as early as the 18th century. Its relationship with hemolytic streptococcus was identified later in the 1950s.

What causes it

Acute poststreptococcal glomerulonephritis typically follows a group A beta-hemolytic streptococcal infection of the respiratory tract. Less commonly, it may follow a skin infection such as impetigo.

How it happens

The disease usually begins about 1 to 6 weeks after a streptococcal infection, although 2 weeks is the most common time of onset.

Clumping with the enemy

In this immunologic disorder, antigens from streptococci clump together with the antibodies that killed them and become trapped in the tubules of the kidneys. The tubules become inflamed, and edema of the capillary walls decreases the amount of glomerular perfusion. The kidneys then become incapable of filtering and eliminating body wastes.

What to look for

Edema may initially appear on the face, especially around the eyes. Later, edema may occur in the legs. Changes in urination may include low urine output (oliguria), blood in the urine (hematuria), protein in the urine (proteinuria), and cola-colored (smoky) urine. Other signs and symptoms may include:

- high blood pressure
- mild anemia, pallor
- joint pain and stiffness
- malaise, lethargy
- anorexia
- fever
- headache.

What tests tell you

Urinalysis reveals the presence of protein, RBCs, and WBCs in the urine. Blood studies show elevated levels of urea and creatinine.

- Antistreptolysin-O test confirms that the child has had a streptococcal infection.
- Throat culture, if performed during an acute infection, confirms the presence of group A beta-hemolytic streptococci.
- Kidney ultrasound shows slightly enlarged kidneys bilaterally.
- Kidney biopsy may be performed to assess the renal tissue or confirm the diagnosis.

Complications

No complications are typically associated with acute poststreptococcal glomerulonephritis. Generally, a full recovery can be expected within a matter of weeks to months. If complications occur, they may include:

- hypertensive encephalopathy
- chronic or progressive problems of kidney function
- kidney failure (in rare instances)
- pulmonary edema and heart failure (occasionally).

How it's treated

Treatment may involve antibiotics for 7 to 10 days to treat infections contributing to the ongoing antigen–antibody response. Other medications may include:

- antihypertensive agents to control high blood pressure
- diuretics to reduce fluid retention and edema
- corticosteroids to decrease antibody synthesis and suppress the inflammatory response.

Lay low

The child may be placed on bed rest to reduce their metabolic demands. In the acute phase, a low-sodium, low-protein diet may be ordered to prevent fluid retention, and fluid restrictions may be ordered to decrease edema. In rare instances, dialysis may be necessary.

What to do

Nursing care of the child with acute poststreptococcal glomerulonephritis focuses on monitoring and education.

- Check vital signs and electrolyte values; monitor intake and output and measure the child's weight daily.
- Assess renal function daily through serum creatinine, BUN, and urine creatinine clearance levels; watch for and immediately report signs of acute kidney failure (oliguria, azotemia, and acidosis) and monitor for ascites and edema.

Battle the boredom

- Provide quiet, age-appropriate activities that the child can enjoy while on bed rest; allow them to gradually resume normal activities as symptoms subside.
- Monitor for signs of complications, such as sudden major changes in vital signs, a change in the amount or appearance of urine output, significant weight gain, changes in vision, changes in motor abilities, seizure activity, severe pain, or behavioral changes.

Medication education

- Teach the child and caregivers about medications the child will be taking; tell them that the child should continue taking the prescribed medications even if they are feeling better and to report adverse effects.

- Teach the child and caregivers about necessary dietary restrictions. Most commonly, this would include limited water and sodium intake.

Strep alert

- Advise the child and caregivers to immediately report signs of a streptococcal throat infection, such as sore throat and fever.
- Teach the caregivers to monitor the child's weight and blood pressure on a regular basis; instruct them to report changes in the child's condition, such as increased edema, changes in appetite, signs of infection, abdominal pain, headaches, lethargy, or changes in urine output.

Congenital anomalies of the ureter, bladder, and urethra

Congenital anomalies of the ureter, bladder, and urethra are among the most common birth defects, occurring in about 5% of births. Some of these abnormalities are obvious at birth; others are recognized only after they produce symptoms.

What causes it

Causes of these congenital anomalies are unknown.

How it happens

The most common malformations include duplicated ureter, retrocaval ureter, ectopic orifice of the ureter, stricture or stenosis of the ureter, ureterocele, bladder exstrophy, congenital bladder diverticulum, hypospadias, and epispadias. Their pathophysiology, signs and symptoms, diagnosis, and treatments vary. (See *Congenital urologic anomalies*.)

What to look for

Signs and symptoms will vary. (See *Congenital urologic anomalies*.)

What tests tell you

With the exception of bladder exstrophy, hypospadias, and epispadias (which can be diagnosed on clinical examination), diagnostic tests are used to visualize the defect.

Complications

Complications will vary according to the specific anomaly but may include UTI, vesicoureteral reflux, voiding dysfunction, and hydronephrosis.

Congenital urologic anomalies

Three congenital urologic anomalies are described here, along with their pathophysiology, clinical features, and diagnosis and treatment.

Duplicated ureter

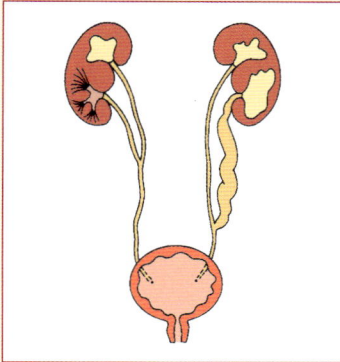

Pathophysiology
- Most common ureteral anomaly
- Complete—double-collecting system with two separate pelvises, each with its own ureter and orifice
- Incomplete—two separate ureters that join before entering the bladder

Clinical features
- Persistent or recurrent infection
- Frequency, urgency, or burning on urination
- Diminished urine output
- Flank pain, fever, and chills

Diagnosis and treatment
- Excretory urography
- Voiding cystoscopy
- Cystoureterography
- Retrograde pyelography
- Surgery for obstruction, reflux, or severe kidney damage

Retrocaval ureter (preureteral vena cava)

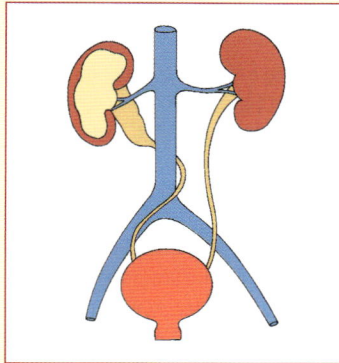

Pathophysiology
- Right ureter that passes behind the inferior vena cava before entering the bladder (with compression of the ureter between the vena cava and the spine that causes dilation and elongation of the pelvis, hydroureter, hydronephrosis, and fibrosis and stenosis of the ureter in the compressed area)
- Relatively uncommon; higher incidence in children assigned male at birth

Clinical features
- Right flank pain
- Recurrent UTI
- Renal calculi
- Hematuria

Diagnosis and treatment
- Excretory urography demonstrating superior ureteral enlargement with spiral appearance

(*continued*)

Congenital urologic anomalies *(continued)*

• Surgical resection and anastomosis of the ureter with the renal pelvis or reimplantation into the bladder

Ectopic orifice of ureter

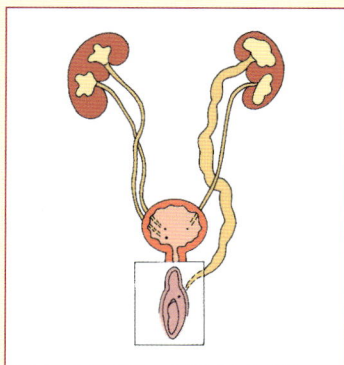

Pathophysiology
• Ureters single or duplicated in female children (ureteral orifice usually inserting in the urethra or vaginal vestibule, beyond external urethral sphincter)
• In male children, in prostatic urethra, seminal vesicles, or vas deferens

Clinical features
• Symptoms rare if ureteral orifice opening between trigone and bladder neck
• Obstruction, reflux, and incontinence (dribbling) in 50% of females
• In males, flank pain, frequency, and urgency

Diagnosis and treatment
• Excretory urography
• Urethroscopy, vaginoscopy
• VCUG
• Resection and ureteral reimplantation into the bladder for incontinence

How it's treated

Surgical repair is needed. The specific procedure will depend on the anomaly. (See *Congenital urologic anomalies*.)

What to do

Because these anomalies aren't always obvious at birth, carefully evaluate the neonate's urogenital function. Document the amount and color of urine, voiding pattern, strength of stream, and indications of infection, such as fever and urine odor.

Neighborhood watch

Tell caregivers to watch for these signs at home. In all children, watch for signs of obstruction, such as dribbling, oliguria or anuria, abdominal mass, hypertension, fever, bacteriuria, or pyuria.

When caring for the hospitalized child, follow these steps:
• Monitor renal function daily; record intake and output accurately; weigh diapers if necessary.

- Follow strict sterile technique in handling cystostomy tubes or indwelling urinary catheters.
- Make sure that ureteral, suprapubic, or urethral catheters remain in place and don't become contaminated; document type, color, and amount of drainage.
- Apply transparent adhesive dressing (Tegaderm) to protect the exposed mucosa of the neonate with bladder exstrophy; don't use heavy clamps on the umbilical cord and avoid dressing or diapering the infant.

Sensitive skin care

- For the infant with exstrophy, use warm water and mild soap to keep the surrounding skin clean. Rinse well and keep the area as dry as possible to prevent excoriation. Apply barrier cream to the surrounding skin as needed.
- Provide reassurance and emotional support to the caregivers and, when possible, allow them to participate in their child's care to promote normal bonding.
- As appropriate, suggest or arrange for genetic counseling.

Hemolytic uremic syndrome

HUS is a complex of symptoms that includes acute kidney failure, hemolytic anemia, and thrombocytopenia. It's an acute kidney disease that occurs mostly in infants and children from age 6 months to 3 years. It's one of the main causes of acute kidney failure in the young child, with the severity of symptoms ranging anywhere from subclinical to life threatening.

What causes it

In pediatrics, the most common cause of HUS is an infection with a specific strain of Shiga toxin–producing *Escherichia coli*, usually the strain known as O157:H7. Such *E. coli* may be found in contaminated meat or produce and in swimming pools or lakes contaminated with feces.

The usual suspects

HUS usually follows an attack of infectious bacterial diarrhea caused by *E. coli*, *Shigella*, *Salmonella*, *Yersinia*, or *Campylobacter*. Viral infections, such as varicella, echovirus, and coxsackie A and B viruses, may also cause it. Occasionally, HUS can appear with no associated diarrhea. HUS may follow an upper respiratory infection and may be associated with long-term illnesses such as acquired immunodeficiency syndrome (AIDS) and cancer.

How it happens

The bacterial infection causes endothelial cell injury in the lining of the small glomerular arterioles. The endothelial cell damage triggers microvascular lesions with platelet–fibrin microthrombi that occlude the arterioles and capillaries. This platelet aggregation results in thrombocytopenia, and the kidneys become swollen and pale.

Although damage occurs mainly in the endothelial lining of the glomerular arterioles, other organs may be involved. Cardiac involvement may include heart failure and dysrhythmia. Pancreatitis or type 1 diabetes mellitus may occur from pancreatic involvement. Ocular involvement may include retinal or vitreous hemorrhage.

What to look for

The child's history typically shows a recent episode of diarrhea. Less commonly, there may be a history of upper respiratory tract infection or viral infection. Signs and symptoms may include:
- irritability, weakness, and lethargy
- pallor
- fatigue
- dehydration
- edema
- ecchymosis, petechiae, and purpura
- decreased or absent urine output (oliguria or anuria)
- hypertension
- gastrointestinal (GI) bleeding with blood in stool
- seizures
- heart failure.

What tests tell you

A urinalysis shows the presence of protein and RBCs, hemosiderin, WBCs, and casts.

In the blood

Blood studies show:
- microangiopathic hemolytic anemia (severe) and mild-to-moderate thrombocytopenia
- prothrombin time, activated partial thromboplastin time, and fibrinogen levels within normal ranges
- elevated lactate dehydrogenase and indirect bilirubin levels
- markedly elevated BUN and creatinine levels
- increased reticulocyte count
- negative Coombs test

- moderately elevated WBC count
- plasma containing free hemoglobin, the concentration of which coincides with the degree of the anemia.

I got culture

Other studies may include a stool culture, which may be positive for a specific type of *E. coli*. Bone marrow biopsy shows hyperplasia. Kidney biopsy would clinically establish the diagnosis but is rarely required.

Complications

Complications of HUS may include:
- hypertension
- acute kidney failure
- chronic kidney failure
- need for hemodialysis
- neurologic deficits with seizures and coma
- stroke
- bleeding complications such as disseminated intravascular coagulation (DIC).

How it's treated

Antibiotics aren't effective in treating HUS, except when caused by *Shigella dysenteriae*. Treatment of HUS may include:
- daily plasma exchange until remission is achieved (in severe cases)
- maintenance of adequate fluid and electrolyte balance and correction of acidosis to prevent seizures and azotemia (In the early stages, the child should be given fluids *without* potassium.)
- corticosteroids
- early dialysis if fluid overload, hyperkalemia, hyponatremia, or other signs of acute kidney failure occur
- management of hypertension with antihypertensive medications and, if needed, fluid and salt restriction
- eculizumab (Soliris) for atypical HUS cases
- maintenance of optimal nutritional status.

What to do

Monitoring and maintaining fluid and electrolyte balance is impor-tant. Intake and output should be accurately recorded, and the child's weight should be recorded once or twice daily during the acute phase.
- Monitor blood pressure and pulse pressure at least every 4 hours.
- Assess hydration status at least every 4 to 6 hours.
- Monitor the child's nutritional status.

- Observe and report signs and symptoms of complications, such as seizures, shock, infection, and DIC.
- Prepare the child and their family for the possibility of hemodialysis or peritoneal dialysis.
- Teach the parents or caregivers and child to avoid eating raw or partially cooked meat or drinking untreated water to decrease the risk of infection with *E. coli*.

Nephrotic syndrome

Nephrotic syndrome is a condition in which the kidneys lose a significant amount of protein in the urine, resulting in low blood levels of protein. The syndrome is characterized by proteinuria, hypoalbuminemia, hyperlipidemia, and edema. The prognosis is highly variable depending on the underlying cause.

Preschool predominance

Primary nephrotic syndrome occurs predominantly in preschool children; the incidence peaks between ages 2 and 3 years, and the syndrome is rare after the age of 8 years. It's more common in male children than in female children. Some forms of nephrotic syndrome may eventually progress to end-stage kidney disease.

What causes it

Causes of nephrotic syndrome include:
- lipid nephrosis
- glomerulonephritis
- metabolic diseases such as diabetes mellitus
- collagen–vascular disorders such as SLE
- circulatory diseases, such as heart failure, sickle cell anemia, and renal vein thrombosis
- nephrotoxins, such as mercury, gold, and bismuth
- allergic reactions.

How it happens

In nephrotic syndrome, the injured glomerular filtration membrane allows the loss of plasma proteins, especially albumin and immunoglobulin, resulting in decreased levels of serum albumin (hypoalbuminemia). Hypoalbuminemia results in decreased colloidal osmotic pressure and fluid accumulation in the interstitial spaces. Edema subsequently results from sodium and water retention. (See *What happens in nephrotic syndrome*.)

What happens in nephrotic syndrome

This flowchart illustrates the pathophysiology of nephrotic syndrome.

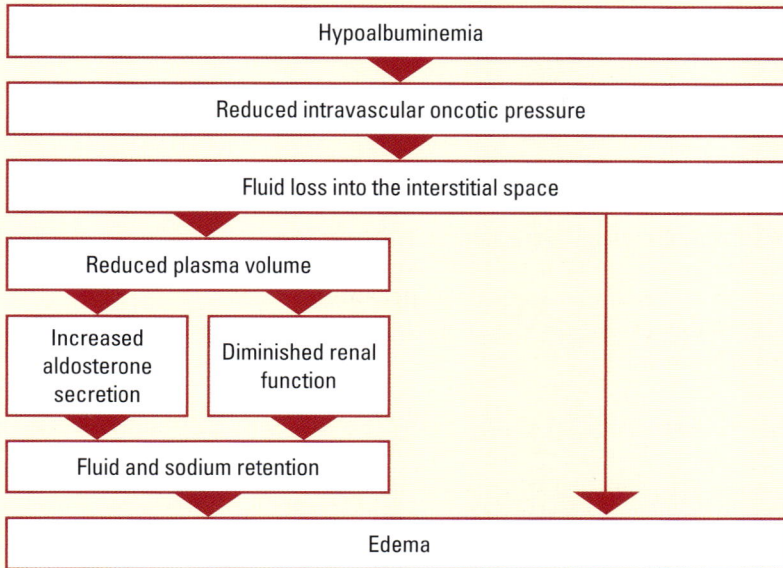

```
┌─────────────────────────────────────────────────────┐
│                  Hypoalbuminemia                     │
└─────────────────────────────────────────────────────┘
                         ▼
┌─────────────────────────────────────────────────────┐
│          Reduced intravascular oncotic pressure      │
└─────────────────────────────────────────────────────┘
                         ▼
┌─────────────────────────────────────────────────────┐
│            Fluid loss into the interstitial space    │
└─────────────────────────────────────────────────────┘
                         ▼
┌───────────────────────────────┐
│     Reduced plasma volume      │
└───────────────────────────────┘
        ▼                ▼
┌──────────────┐  ┌──────────────┐
│  Increased   │  │ Diminished   │
│  aldosterone │  │ renal        │
│  secretion   │  │ function     │
└──────────────┘  └──────────────┘
        ▼                ▼
┌───────────────────────────────┐
│   Fluid and sodium retention   │
└───────────────────────────────┘
        ▼                              ▼
┌─────────────────────────────────────────────────────┐
│                       Edema                          │
└─────────────────────────────────────────────────────┘
```

What to look for

Signs and symptoms of nephrotic syndrome include:
- oliguria with dark, concentrated urine
- edema starting around the eyes (periorbital) and then becoming more generalized
- weight gain
- abdominal distention, which may be so severe that it causes respiratory difficulty, abdominal pain, anorexia, and diarrhea
- irritability
- lethargy, easy fatigability, and activity intolerance
- pallor
- hypertension (in later stages).

What tests tell you

Urinalysis shows severe proteinuria, hematuria, and casts; it also shows an elevated specific gravity because of the proteinuria. When performed, kidney biopsy identifies the type of nephrotic syndrome the child has and can be used to monitor response to medical management.

Highs and lows

Blood studies show:
- high levels of lipids, especially cholesterol (hypercholesterolemia)

- low levels of protein, especially albumin
- normal to high hematocrit and hemoglobin level
- high platelet levels.

Complications

Complications of nephrotic syndrome may include:
- hypovolemic shock
- venous thrombosis
- respiratory difficulties
- impaired skin integrity from severe edema
- infection
- loss of proteins required to fight infections, resulting in increased risk of infections
- loss of proteins that prevent blood from clotting, resulting in clot formation within the blood vessels
- adverse effects of steroid therapy.

How it's treated

Prednisone commonly produces a rapid improvement in symptoms (remission). IV administration of albumin may be used, followed by IV furosemide (Lasix), to induce diuresis. If marked hypertension exists, antihypertensive medications may be used. Other medications may include:
- pain medication to lessen discomfort
- prophylactic antibiotics to control and prevent infection
- immunosuppressive medications for children who don't respond to steroids.

Hold the salt

Dietary changes may include some restriction of salt intake. Bed rest may be required during the acute phase, especially when the child is hypertensive.

What to do

The child with nephrotic syndrome is likely to require multiple hospitalizations. Because these hospitalizations interrupt the child's normal routine, it's important to provide them with activities that support their continued development and simply allow them to have fun.

A delicate balance

Other interventions focus on monitoring and assessment:
- Maintain fluid balance and monitor for signs of fluid volume excess, such as edema, ascites, weight gain, decreased and concentrated urine, and pulmonary congestion.
- Assess for signs of electrolyte imbalance—cardiovascular, neurologic, GI, and skin changes—and work with the health care providers to correct imbalances that may exist.
- Assess general nutritional status and work to improve it by providing a diet the child will eat (with sufficient protein and other

nutrients and without excess sodium). Caregivers can help with this, too, by bringing in food from home that the child likes, as long as it fits within the child's dietary restrictions.
- Assess for adverse effects of medications and report them to the health care provider as soon as possible.

Protection from infection
- Assess for signs of infection and work to prevent it; if infection occurs, report it as soon as possible.
- Monitor for pain and provide appropriate pain relief measures.
- Provide emotional support and education to the child and parents or caregivers.

Kidney failure, acute

Kidney failure is a general term used to describe what happens when the kidneys aren't functioning at an optimum level. In *acute* kidney failure, the kidneys suddenly stop filtering waste products from the blood.

What causes it

Most commonly, acute kidney failure in children is a temporary condition resulting from dehydration or other condition that causes poor renal perfusion (which can be resolved by increasing the child's fluid volume). The causes of acute kidney failure may be classified as prerenal, intrarenal, or postrenal. (See *Causes of acute kidney failure*.)

Causes of acute kidney failure

The causes of acute kidney failure may be classified as prerenal, intrarenal, or postrenal.

Prerenal
Prerenal causes, which are most common in children, may include:
- dysrhythmia that cause reduced cardiac output
- heart failure
- burns
- dehydration
- diuretic overuse, hemorrhage, hypovolemic shock
- DIC
- sepsis.

Intrarenal
Intrarenal causes of acute kidney failure include:
- poorly treated prerenal failure
- nephrotoxins
- transfusion reaction
- acute glomerulonephritis, acute interstitial nephritis, or acute pyelonephritis
- sickle cell anemia
- SLE.

Postrenal
Postrenal causes of kidney failure are uncommon in children older than age 1 year. They may include:
- bladder obstruction
- ureteral obstruction
- urethral obstruction.

How it happens

The pathophysiology of acute kidney failure varies depending on whether the cause is prerenal, intrarenal, or postrenal.

Prerenal failure

Prerenal failure ensues when a condition that diminishes blood flow to the kidneys leads to hypoperfusion.

It's rude to interrupt

When renal blood flow is interrupted, so is oxygen delivery. The ensuing hypoxemia and ischemia can rapidly and irreversibly damage the kidney. The renal tubules are most susceptible to hypoxemia's effects.

Azotemia (excess nitrogenous waste products in the blood) develops in 40% to 80% of people with acute kidney failure and is also a consequence of renal hypoperfusion. The impaired blood flow results in a decreased GFR and increased tubular resorption of sodium and water. Usually, restoring renal blood flow and glomerular filtration reverses azotemia.

Intrarenal failure

Intrarenal failure, also called *intrinsic* or *parenchymal kidney failure*, results from damage to the filtering structures of the kidneys. Causes of intrarenal failure are classified as *nephrotoxic, inflammatory*, or *ischemic*.

Damage in the basement

When the damage is caused by nephrotoxicity or inflammation, the delicate layer under the epithelium (the basement membrane) becomes irreparably damaged, typically leading to chronic kidney failure.

Severe or prolonged lack of blood flow caused by ischemia may lead to kidney damage (ischemic parenchymal injury) and excess nitrogen in the blood (intrinsic renal azotemia).

Totally radical

Acute tubular necrosis is the precursor of intrarenal failure; it can result from ischemic damage to renal parenchyma during unrecognized or poorly treated prerenal failure. The ischemic tissue generates toxic, oxygen-free radicals, which cause swelling, injury, and necrosis.

Postrenal failure

Bilateral obstruction of urine outflow leads to postrenal failure. The obstruction may be in the bladder, ureters, or urethra.

What to look for

Acute kidney failure is a critical illness in children. Its early signs are oliguria, azotemia, and, rarely, anuria.

System alert

Electrolyte imbalance, metabolic acidosis, and other severe effects follow as the person becomes increasingly uremic and kidney dysfunction disrupts other body systems:

- *GI*—anorexia, nausea, vomiting, diarrhea or constipation, stomatitis, bleeding, hematemesis, dry mucous membranes, uremic breath
- *Central nervous system*—headache, drowsiness, irritability, confusion, peripheral neuropathy, seizures, coma
- *Cutaneous*—dryness, pruritus, pallor, purpura, and, rarely, uremic frost
- *Cardiovascular*—hypotension (early in the course of the disease), hypertension (later in the course of the disease), dysrhythmia, fluid overload, heart failure, systemic edema, anemia, altered clotting mechanisms
- *Respiratory*—pulmonary edema, Kussmaul respirations

What tests tell you

- Blood studies show elevated BUN, serum creatinine, and potassium levels; decreased sodium, calcium, bicarbonate, and hemoglobin levels; decreased hematocrit; and low blood pH.
- Urine studies show casts, cellular debris, and decreased specific gravity; in glomerular diseases, it shows proteinuria and increased urine osmolality.
- ECG shows changes associated with electrolyte imbalance and heart failure.
- Ultrasound of the kidney shows the size of the kidneys and may reveal the presence of a tumor, cyst, or urinary tract obstruction.
- Excretory urography demonstrates the appearance of the kidney structure and, possibly, the presence of obstruction.

Complications

Kidney failure affects many body processes. Complications may include fluid volume overload, dysrhythmia or seizures from electrolyte imbalance, heart failure, hypertension or hypotension, tachypnea, pulmonary edema, infection, skin breakdown, malnutrition, or development of chronic kidney failure.

How it's treated

The key to managing acute kidney failure is prevention. For children with dehydration or any type of fluid loss, fluid volume should be restored as soon as possible to prevent disruption of perfusion to the kidneys. Caution should be exercised whenever nephrotoxic drugs are used in the pediatric population. Treatment of acute kidney failure may include:

- diet high in carbohydrates and fats and low in protein, sodium, and potassium to meet metabolic needs

- fluid restriction
- careful monitoring of electrolytes and fluid status; IV therapy to maintain and correct fluid and electrolyte balance
- diuretic therapy with Lasix or mannitol (Osmitrol) to treat oliguria
- Kayexalate by mouth or enema to reverse hyperkalemia with mild symptoms (malaise, loss of appetite, muscle weakness); hypertonic glucose, insulin, and sodium bicarbonate IV for more severe hyperkalemic symptoms (numbness and tingling and ECG changes)
- antihypertensive agents to control elevated blood pressure
- blood products as needed to control anemia or reverse effects of bleeding
- hemodialysis or peritoneal dialysis (occasionally required).

What to do

Care of the child with acute kidney failure includes careful monitoring and dietary education. The child and caregivers will need emotional support and reassurance, with clear explanations of all procedures.

No fluid shall go unmeasured

Measure and record intake and output, including body fluids, such as wound drainage, nasogastric output, and diarrhea; weigh the child daily. Monitor vital signs; watch for and report signs of inadequate renal perfusion (hypotension) and acidosis.

Maintain proper electrolyte balance by:
- strictly monitoring potassium levels
- watching for symptoms of hyperkalemia (malaise, anorexia, paresthesia, or muscle weakness)
- monitoring for and immediately reporting ECG changes (tall, peaked T waves; widening QRS segment; and disappearing P waves)
- avoiding administering medications containing potassium.

Monitor and maintain

Other interventions focus on monitoring and maintaining nutritional status and preventing infection:
- Maintain nutritional status; provide a high-calorie, low-protein, low-sodium, and low-potassium diet with vitamin supplements. (Give the anorexic child small, frequent meals.)
- Use sterile technique because the child with acute kidney failure is highly susceptible to infection; don't allow personnel with upper respiratory tract infections to care for the child and limit visitors who have symptoms of infection.
- Use guaiac tests to monitor stools for blood, a sign of GI bleeding.

Wilms tumor

Wilms tumor, also called *nephroblastoma*, is the most common form of kidney cancer in children as well as the most common intra-abdominal tumor in children. The average age at diagnosis is 2 to 4 years. The tumor favors the left kidney and is usually unilateral. It can remain encapsulated for a long time, and prognosis is excellent if metastasis hasn't occurred.

What causes it

Studies have shown an increased risk in children with specific chromosomal abnormalities. Wilms tumor has also been associated with several congenital anomalies, including hypospadias and cryptorchidism.

How it happens

Wilms tumor is an embryonal cancer of the kidney originating during fetal life. In the early stages, the tumor is well encapsulated, but it may later spread into the lymph nodes, renal vein, or vena cava; metastasis to the lungs or other sites may occur.

Life is but a stage

The tumor is staged to determine the best treatment:
- *Stage I*—The tumor is limited to one kidney.
- *Stage II*—The tumor extends beyond the kidney but can be completely excised.
- *Stage III*—The tumor has spread but is confined to the abdomen and lymph nodes.
- *Stage IV*—The tumor has metastasized to the lung, liver, bone, and brain.
- *Stage V*—The tumor involves both kidneys.

What to look for

The child usually has a nontender abdominal mass, commonly first identified by the caregivers during bathing or dressing or by a pediatrician during a routine physical examination. The mass can be palpated in the region of the lower abdomen and is usually confined to one side. Other signs and symptoms may include an enlarged abdomen, hypertension, vomiting, hematuria, anemia, and constipation.

What tests tell you

- Ultrasound will determine if the mass originated within the kidney and if the mass is a solid tumor.
- CT scan or magnetic resonance imaging will determine the extent of the tumor and whether it has spread to other organs.
- Excretory urography assesses function of the unaffected kidney.

- Chest x-ray and CT scan of the chest will determine if the tumor has metastasized to the lungs.

Complications

Recurrence of Wilms tumor may occur in several sites, such as the lungs, liver, and the surgical area. Other complications may include:
- musculoskeletal defects from radiation therapy
- possible development of other (metastatic) cancers in the bones, breast, and thyroid
- decreased fertility, especially after radiation therapy
- kidney failure.

How it's treated

Most commonly, treatment involves surgical removal of the entire affected kidney (radical nephrectomy). Exploratory surgery of the lymph nodes and the liver may be performed at the same time to determine if the tumor has spread outside the kidney.

Keep the kidney

If the tumor is bilateral, neither kidney is removed during the initial surgery. Rather, a biopsy of the tumor is taken to help determine the tumor type. Chemotherapy will reduce the size of bilateral tumors. Later, with bilateral tumors, the child has further surgery, removing just the tumors and a portion of the kidneys, saving most of both kidneys to maintain kidney function.

Chemotherapy is typically administered after nephrectomy. In addition, radiation therapy may be used because it has been found to improve survival rates.

What to do

A great deal of emotional support is needed for the child and caregivers dealing with this diagnosis. The child should be thoroughly prepared for treatments and procedures, including surgeries, chemotherapy, and radiation and their adverse effects. The nurse should serve as an advocate for the child and their caregivers, making certain that questions are answered and concerns are addressed in a timely manner.

In addition, follow these steps:
- Keep in mind that a Wilms tumor is very soft, and the capsule can easily rupture before or during surgery; if this happens, there can be rapid metastasis to other organs.
- Make sure that after the diagnosis is suspected or confirmed, there's absolutely no further palpation of the abdomen because this can cause rupture of the capsule.
- Tell the caregivers and the child that they may need frequent imaging of the remaining kidney to detect recurrence of the tumor.

Quick quiz

1. The main functioning unit of the kidney is the:
    A. renal cortex.
    B. renal medulla.
    C. nephron.
    D. ureter.

Answer: C. The nephron, located within the renal medulla, is the main functional unit of the kidney; it filters out waste products and excess water, forming urine.

2. An x-ray done with IV contrast media to show the structure of the urinary system is called:
    A. KUB.
    B. excretory urography.
    C. VCUG.
    D. kidney biopsy.

Answer: B. In excretory urography, IV contrast medium is injected and then x-rays are taken to visualize the structures of the entire urinary elimination system.

3. A child has decreased output of pink-tinged urine, facial edema, and a history of a sore throat "a little while ago." The nurse anticipates the doctor will be evaluating the child for:
    A. cryptorchidism.
    B. adverse effects of hemodialysis.
    C. HUS.
    D. acute poststreptococcal glomerulonephritis.

Answer: D. Pink-tinged urine, facial edema, and a history of a sore throat are the typical signs and symptoms of acute poststreptococcal glomerulonephritis.

4. A child is admitted to the pediatric unit with a new diagnosis of nephrotic syndrome. Which set of symptoms would the nurse expect to see?
    A. Periorbital edema, polyuria, proteinuria, and hyperproteinemia
    B. Hypercholesterolemia, hypoproteinemia, proteinuria, and periorbital edema
    C. Pedal edema, hypolipidemia, hematuria, and oliguria
    D. Hyperlipidemia, glycosuria, hyperproteinemia, and generalized edema

Answer: B. The four classic signs and symptoms of early stages of nephrotic syndrome are hypercholesterolemia, hypoproteinemia, proteinuria, and periorbital edema.

5. A child on the pediatric unit has a Wilms tumor. One of the most important nursing functions for this child is to:
- A. prepare the parents or caregivers for the possible loss of the child.
- B. maintain the child's fluid volume.
- C. ensure the child's nutritional status.
- D. make sure that no abdominal palpation is performed.

Answer: D. Remember that a Wilms tumor is very soft and the capsule surrounding it can rupture easily, causing distant and potentially devastating metastasis to other organs.

Scoring

⭐⭐⭐ If you answered all five items correctly, bravo! Your knowledge of urinary problems flows unobstructed.

⭐⭐ If you answered three or four items correctly, good for you! Take a potty break and read on.

⭐ If you answered fewer than three items correctly, go with the flow! You'll breeze through the rest of your work.

Suggested References

American Cancer Society. (2018). *What are Wilms tumors?* https://www.cancer.org/cancer/wilms-tumor/about/what-is-wilms-tumor.html

Banasiak, N., Moriarty-Daley, A., Mackey, W., & Meadows-Oliver, M. (2016). Genitourinary disorders. In N. Banasiak, A. Moriarty-Daley, W. Mackey, & M. Meadows-Oliver (Eds.), *Pediatric primary care nurse practitioner review and resource manual* (pp. 391–416). American Nurses Association.

Centers for Disease Control and Prevention. (n.d.). *Group A Strep Infection.* https://www.cdc.gov/group-a-strep/

Cowen, K., Wisely, L., Dawson, R., Ball, J., & McGillis Bindler, R. (2022). The child with alternations in genitourinary function. In K. Cowen, L. Wisely, R. Dawson, J. Ball, & R. McGillis Bindler (Eds.), *Principles of pediatric nursing: Caring for children* (8th ed., pp. 667–700). Pearson.

Gallo, P. (2020). Nephrology. In K. Kleinman, L. McDaniel, & M. Molloy (Eds.), *The Harriet Lane handbook* (22nd ed., pp. 472–501). Elsevier.

Gillespie, R. S. (2022). *Pediatric hemolytic uremic syndrome.* https://emedicine.medscape.com/article/982025-overview

Kallen, R. J. (2023). *Pediatric nephrotic syndrome.* https://emedicine.medscape.com/article/982920-overview

King, S. (2022). Genitourinary disorders. In B. Richardson (Ed.), *Pediatric primary care: Practice guidelines for nurses* (5th ed., pp. 393–416). Jones & Bartlett Learning.

Linnard-Palmer, L. (2024). Genitourinary elimination. In L. Linnard-Palmer (Ed.), *Pediatric nursing care: A concept-based approach* (2nd ed., pp. 385–400). Jones & Bartlett Learning.

Weatherington, A. (2020). Genitourinary disorders. In D. Maaks, N. Starr, M. Brady, N. Gaylord, M. Driessnack, & K. Duderstadt (Eds.), *Burns' pediatric primary care* (7th ed., pp. 819–850). Elsevier.

Chapter 19

Musculoskeletal problems

Just the facts

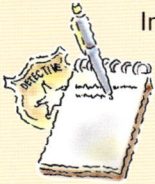

In this chapter, you'll learn:

◆ basic anatomy and physiology of the musculoskeletal system

◆ common diagnostic tests for musculoskeletal problems

◆ orthopedic treatments and procedures

◆ selected musculoskeletal disorders in the pediatric population.

Anatomy and physiology

The musculoskeletal system is one of the most complex systems within the body. The muscles and bones allow the body to move and function. If a problem occurs in the musculoskeletal system, mobility and general activities of daily living may be impaired.

Bones

The body's form and function are supported by the skeletal system. The mature human skeleton is made up of 206 bones that are shaped according to their function. Newborn infants have over 300 bones, a number of which fuse together by the time a child is around 9 years old. The skeletal system:
- enables movement of the body by supporting soft tissues
- provides support and allows a person to stand erect
- protects underlying organs
- serves as a reservoir for storing minerals such as calcium and phosphorus
- serves as a site for red blood cell formation.

The long and short of it

Long bones are found in the upper and lower extremities. They are responsible for carrying the body's weight and helping make ambulation possible. Short bones, found in the hands and feet, are shaped to provide strength in a compact area. Some bones, such as the ribs and sternum, are flat and thin; they provide structure. Other bones are large and irregularly shaped (e.g., the pelvic bone).

Universal coverage

The composition of bone differs depending on the type of bone, but all are covered by a double layer of connective tissue, called the *periosteum*, which helps provide nourishment to the bone. In children, the periosteum is thick and vascular, so a child's bone tends to heal faster than that of an adult with the same injury.

Bone growth and formation

The epiphysis is the growth end of the long bones. The epiphyseal plate, or *growth plate*, is located in the epiphysis.

A plate of cartilage

The epiphyseal plate is composed of cartilage cells that grow and develop, thereby causing the bone to lengthen. The growth plate is gradually replaced by bone until only the epiphyseal line remains. When the plate is completely replaced by bone, the bones can no longer lengthen; they can only increase in breadth. Injury to the growth plate may seriously impede bone growth. Children are particularly susceptible to growth plate injuries.

Cartilage serves as a smooth surface for articulating bones. Because young children have a more cartilaginous skeleton, they may be less prone to severe fractures than adults.

Salty framework

Ossification is the process of developing new bones from tissue. Osteoblasts form bone cells that lay down a framework for the new bone. Calcium and phosphorus combine to form salts, which are then deposited into the framework. The thyroid and parathyroid glands regulate this deposition. (See *Bone growth and remodeling*.)

Bone growth and remodeling

The ossification of cartilage into bone, or *osteogenesis*, begins at about week 9 of fetal development. The diaphyses (shaft) of long bones are formed by birth, and the epiphyses (growth end) begin to ossify around that time. The stages of growth and remodeling of the epiphyses of a long bone are shown in these illustrations.

Creation of an ossification center

At about the ninth month of fetal development, an ossification center develops in the epiphysis. Some cartilage cells enlarge and stimulate ossification of surrounding cells. The enlarged cells die, leaving small cavities. New cartilage continues to develop.

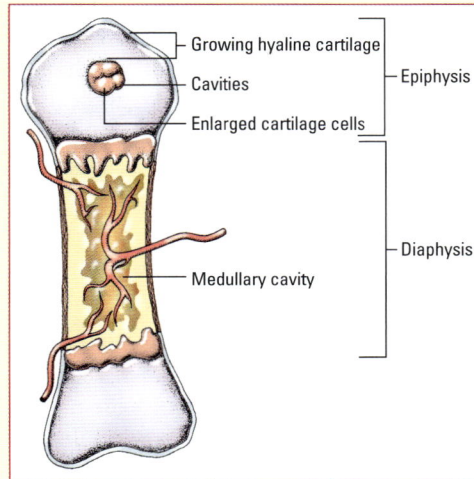

Osteoblasts form bone

Osteoblasts (bone-forming cells) begin to form bone on the remaining cartilage, creating the scaffolding or trabeculae network of cancellous (spongy) bone. Cartilage continues to form on the outer surfaces of the epiphysis and along the upper surface of the epiphyseal plate.

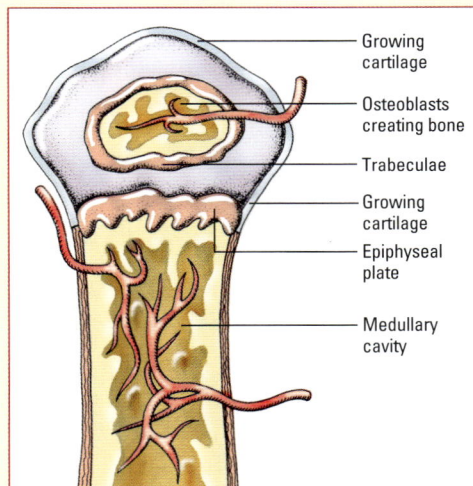

(*continued*)

Bone growth and remodeling (*continued*)

Bone growth

Cartilage is replaced by compact bone near the outer surfaces of the epiphysis. Only cartilage cells on the upper surface of the diaphyseal plate continue to multiply rapidly, pushing the epiphysis away from the diaphysis. This new cartilage ossifies, creating trabeculae on the inner or medullary side of the epiphyseal plate.

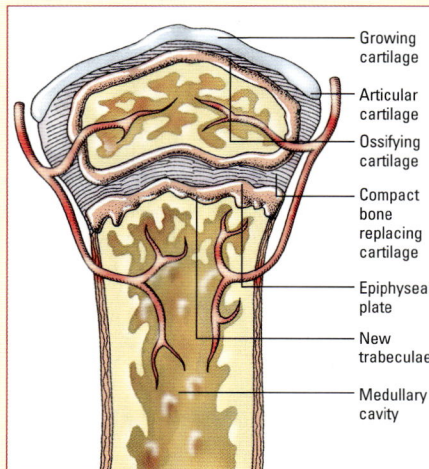

Remodeling

Osteoclasts (cells associated with bone resorption) produce enzymes and acids that reduce trabeculae created by the epiphyseal plate, thus enlarging the medullary (bone marrow) cavity. In the epiphysis, osteoclasts reduce bone, making its calcium available for new osteoblasts that give the epiphysis its adult shape and proportion. In young adults, the epiphyseal plate completely ossifies (closes) and becomes the epiphyseal line; longitudinal growth of bone then ceases.

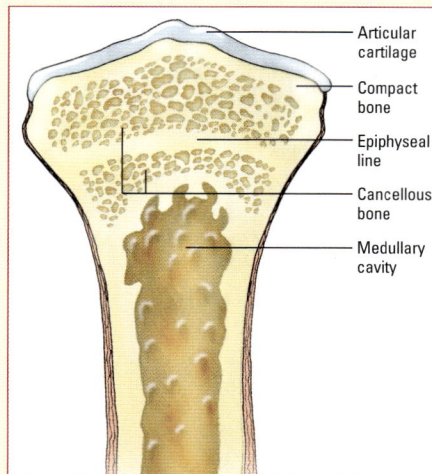

Bone bank deposit

To maintain equilibrium, bone is deposited where it's needed within the skeletal system. If increased stress is placed on a certain bone, more bone is deposited. If there is no stress on the bone, part of the bone mass is reabsorbed.

Resorption is the process by which old bone is dissolved. The bone cells known as *osteocytes* and *osteoclasts* are responsible for the resorption of bone in this framework. This process can release calcium into the circulation.

Muscles

Muscles are the major organs that enable movement. They are fibrous bundles covered with thin connective tissue. They also serve as repositories for some metabolites. Muscles are attached at each end directly to the bone or to a tendon, ligament, or fascia:

- *Tendons* hold muscles to bones and are formed by strong, nonelastic collagen cords.
- *Ligaments* hold bones to other bones; they encircle the joints and add strength and stability.
- The *fascia* is a fibrous membrane of supporting, connective tissue.

Muscles in opposition

The movement enabled by muscles occurs through the contracting and lengthening of opposing muscle groups. As a muscle shortens on contraction, it pulls the bones to which it is attached, bringing the bones closer together. Most muscles are attached to two bones that *articulate* (join or work together as a single unit) at an intervening joint.

Taking turns

For the most part, movement happens when one bone moves while the other is held stable. The body of the muscle that produces movement of the extremity usually lies proximal (closest) to the bone that's moved.

600 volunteers

There are more than 600 *voluntary muscles* (muscles we control) in the body. These muscles are called *striated* or *skeletal muscles*. Other types of muscles include visceral muscles (also called *smooth* or *involuntary muscles*) and the cardiac muscle.

Joints

Joints are formed when two surfaces of bones come together and articulate.

Joints on the move

There are three types of joints, classified by the degree of movement:
- *Synarthrodial* (immovable) joints separate bone by a thin layer of cartilage—for example, the skull and various bones of the cranium.
- *Amphidiarthrodial* (semi-movable) joints separate bone with cartilage or a fibrocartilaginous disk—for example, the joints between the vertebral bodies.
- *Diarthrodial* (freely movable) joints are commonly called *synovial joints*. Most joints in the body are synovial joints. They are lined with a membrane that secretes and lubricates the joint with synovial fluid—for example, the knees, shoulders, and hips. They are encased by the joint capsule, which is strengthened by ligaments that surround the capsule.

Flex or extend

Muscles are categorized according to the type of joint movement produced when the muscle is contracted. They are designated as flexor or extensor muscles depending on whether the joint is flexed or extended. Range of motion (ROM) is determined by the degree of movement in a joint. (See *Types of joint movement*.)

Types of joint movement

There are seven types of joint movement:
- *Flexion* is a bending forward of the joint; this decreases the angle between the bones that are connected.
- *Extension* is an increase of the joint angle that occurs with straightening of the limb.
- *Abduction* is the movement of the limb away from the midline, or *central axis*, of the body.
- *Adduction* is the movement of the limb toward or beyond the midline, or *central axis*, of the body.
- *Internal rotation* is the turning of the body part inward, toward the midline, or *central axis*, of the body.
- *External rotation* is the turning of the body part away from the midline, or *central axis*, of the body.
- *Circumduction* is the movement of the body part in a circular motion.

Diagnostic tests

Tests used to assess the musculoskeletal system and guide treatment include muscle and bone marrow biopsy, and x-rays.

Muscle and bone marrow biopsy

Biopsy of the muscles and bones involves the removal of a small specimen of muscle or bone marrow for analysis. It is usually performed at the bedside and takes about 20 minutes. Local anesthetics or systemic analgesic agents are used to help alleviate the pain. The puncture site may remain tender for a few weeks. For bone marrow biopsy, the proximal tibia is the most commonly used site in young children. In older children, the vertebral bodies T10 to L4 are preferred.

Nursing considerations

Biopsy can be an extremely frightening procedure for a child (and their family). Thoroughly prepare the child and their family. Allowing the child to "perform" the procedure on a doll (using correct positioning, a syringe, and a bandage) will enhance their understanding of the procedure and may help ease their fears. This is another great time to involve the child's life.

In addition, follow these steps:

- Clarify the meaning of *biopsy* in context; many caregivers (and older children) automatically think of cancer when they hear the word *biopsy*.
- Provide analgesic agents as ordered.
- Assist the child into the desired position depending on the site to be used. If necessary, assist in holding the child still during the procedure. (Allow a caregiver to be present in a comforting capacity only, leaving the positioning and restraint of the child to the health care professionals.)
- When the specimen is obtained, apply direct pressure to the site for 5 to 10 minutes.
- Cover the site and make sure the child remains still for approximately 30 minutes after the procedure.

X-rays

Radiography is the most widely used diagnostic test in the assessment of children with bone abnormalities or other conditions affecting the bones. X-rays can show pathology, such as a fracture, and can show bone density and irregularities. X-rays are used not only for initial evaluation but also for monitoring and evaluating the effectiveness of treatment.

Invisible bone

Normally, the calcium deposits in bones will make skeletal structures appear radiopaque, or white, on x-rays. However, in the infant and young child (whose skeleton is composed mostly of growth cartilage), structures are radiolucent and may not appear on x-ray. Thus, x-rays are less reliable in this population. High-resolution ultrasound may provide a more accurate picture.

Nursing considerations

Always explain to the child the reason for obtaining an x-ray. Explain that an x-ray simply takes pictures (of whatever part of the body is being radiographed). Reassure the child that the x-ray itself does not hurt, but keep in mind that a child with an injury may experience discomfort during positioning for the x-ray.

It is common to allow the caregivers to remain with the child during the procedure as long as appropriate precautions are taken. In addition, follow these steps:

- Tell the child that it is their job to remain still during the procedure.
- Obtain previous x-rays if possible, which may be useful for comparison.
- If an adolescent is sexually active, assess for possible pregnancy, a contraindication for radiography.
- Remove metallic objects, such as jewelry or snaps on gowns, before the x-ray because metallic objects may be mistaken for pathology.

Treatments and procedures

Children may experience dysfunction in any part of the musculoskeletal system. Treatment depends on a thorough assessment and appropriate interventions based on findings. These interventions are typically designed to promote healing and lessen the impact of the condition on mobility. Principles of body mechanics are used to maintain the integrity of the musculoskeletal system.

Prevent and restore

Nursing care of orthopedic conditions involves the correction of alterations in the musculoskeletal system. These preventive and restorative measures include:

- casting or splinting and traction, which are used to help correct, maintain, and support the body part in a functional position
- surgical repairs such as tendon release
- limb amputations, which may be necessary in some circumstances.

Casting or splints

Casts or splints may be required when a child has a fractured bone, weakness, paralysis, or spasticity. They are also used following corrective orthopedic surgery.

The cast may be made of plaster or, more commonly, of synthetic material, such as fiberglass or plastic. Polyester and cotton impregnated with water-activated polyurethane resin may also be used. (See *Types of casts for children.*)

Types of casts for children

These illustrations show the types of casts commonly used for children.

Full spica cast

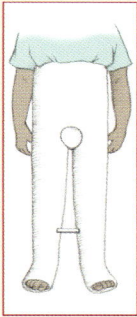

Long leg cast

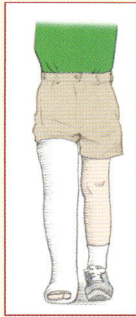

Bootie cast

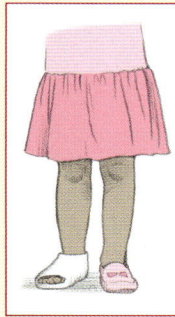

Long arm cast

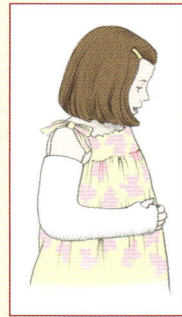

1½ spica cast

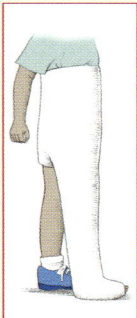

Cylinder cast

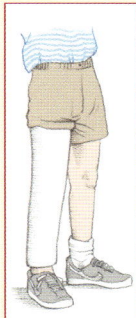

Bilateral long leg cast

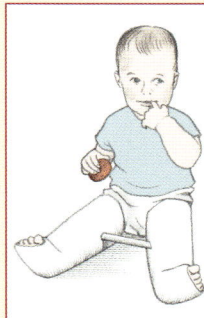

Short arm cast

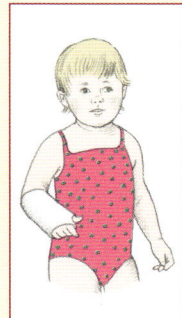

Single spica cast

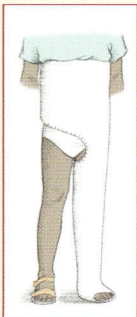

Short leg cast

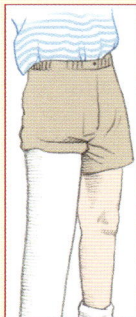

Shoulder spica cast

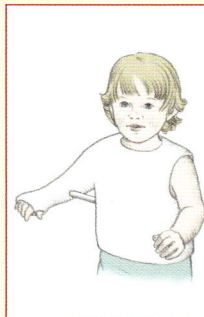

Depending on the type of material that is used, drying time for the cast may be as little as 7 minutes or as much as 48 hours. Weight bearing on the affected part of the body is typically avoided until the cast has dried.

Splints

Splints are "half-casts" and offer a bit more flexibility than a standard cast. They also do not offer quite as much support as a cast. Splints may be custom formed to the child or may be ready to wear. Most splints have Velcro straps to adjust to the child's body. Instruct the child and their family to keep the splint on as much as possible and to avoid excess activities that would further compromise the injury.

A wash and a blow-dry
Some synthetic casts may be waterproof. Double-check that the inner lining of the cast is waterproof as well before allowing the child to get the cast wet. If appropriate, instruct the patient and family to dry the cast after bathing or immersion by using a blow-dryer in a cool setting.

Nursing considerations

Explain each step of the procedure to the child before the procedure and again as the cast is being applied. If plaster will be used, explain that the child will experience a sensation of warmth when it's first applied. As it dries, the cast—and the child—will feel cold.

In addition, follow these steps:
- If a closed reduction is necessary, explain to the child that there will be some pain. Allow the caregivers to remain close to the child and hold their hand to help lessen anxiety.
- Assess the casted area every 30 minutes for the first few hours, then every hour for 24 hours, and then every 4 hours for an additional 48 hours. Drainage from a wound under the cast should be noted.
- If there are signs and symptoms of compromise in the affected area, notify the provider immediately. Also notify the provider if cracks are noted in the cast.
- Assess for signs of skin breakdown, a common occurrence. The area around the cast edges will typically become pink and warm, and swelling may also occur. (Provide skin care to prevent further breakdown.)

Cast scratch fever
- Because cool air can relieve the itchiness that accompanies casting, instruct the caregivers to blow cool air down into the cast using a blow-dryer in a cool setting. Also advise against putting an object down the cast in an attempt to scratch.

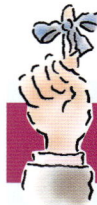

> **Memory jogger**
>
> Remember the five "Ps" when checking for signs of compromised blood supply in a child with a cast.
> **P**ain
> **P**allor
> **P**aresthesia
> **P**aralysis
> **P**ulselessness

May I have your autograph?

- Ask the child if they would like their care team to sign their cast to help them cheer up, feel important to the medical staff, and view the staff as friends.
- Explain to the child and their family that the cast must be worn as recommended. It should not be removed, and overly rigorous activities should be discouraged (to prevent dislodgment or malalignment of a fracture).

The cut stops here—promise!

- When the fracture is healed, prepare the child for cast removal with the cast cutter. Let them hear the noise and feel the vibrations and show them (on your body) how the cutter stops when it touches skin and will not, therefore, cut anything except the cast.
- Inform the child that their skin will look different after cast removal, especially if it has been in the cast for weeks. Reassure them that this is temporary. Apply baby oil and then gently wash the area to remove the dead skin. (See *Cast care*.)

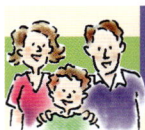

It's all relative

Cast care

Be sure to include these points in your teaching plan for the child with a cast and their family:

- Mechanism of bone healing and necessity for casting
- Cast care, including air exposure, elevation, and movement
- Measures to protect the cast
- Measures for skin care
- Methods to relieve itching
- Measures to keep the cast dry
- Ways to test for sensation, movement, and circulation
- Measures for coping with swelling
- Ways to relieve skin irritation
- Monitoring for wound drainage
- Exercises for the casted extremity

- Instruct the child and their family in an exercise regimen to help regain muscle strength and function following the injury.

Traction

Although it is not as widely used now, traction is still used in some circumstances. Traction can be continuous or intermittent. It is used to:

- stabilize or immobilize a certain body part
- reduce muscle spasms

- relieve pressure on spinal nerves
- realign fractures or joint dislocations.

Just hanging out

Traction uses weights and pulleys to exert a pulling force and maintain the body part in correct alignment. Weights must hang freely, and the ropes should not have knots that could interfere with free movement.

Serial x-rays are taken while the child is in traction in order to monitor progress and determine the need for changes in the direction and amount of traction pull.

Central location

The child should be kept in the center of the bed to maintain countertraction and prevent complications. Traction can cause muscle spasms that may require analgesic agents or muscle relaxants. The child is in bed for extended periods; therefore, circulatory and skin assessment is vital.

Traction in twos

There are two basic types of traction:
1. Skin
2. Skeletal

Skin traction

Skin traction is a noninvasive traction that is especially useful for a child who may not require continuous traction. It is applied by placing foam rubber straps against the affected part and then securing the straps with elastic bandages.

Sometimes, the straps have an adhesive backing. If this type of strap is used, protect the skin by first applying compound benzoin tincture or other skin protectant. Traction should be removed by two people. (See *Types of skin traction*.)

Types of skin traction

This chart describes the various types of skin traction.

Traction	Purpose	Patient positioning
Buck extension	Used for a fractured hip to prevent muscle spasms and dislocation	• Child lies flat on bed. • Head of the bed is elevated only for activities of daily living.
Cervical traction	Used for neck strain and arthritic or degenerative conditions of the cervical vertebrae	• Child lies flat on bed or with the head of the bed elevated 15–20 degrees.

Types of skin traction (*continued*)

Traction	Purpose	Patient positioning
Dunlop traction	Used for a fractured humerus	• Child lies flat on bed. • Arm is suspended horizontally.
Pelvic girdle	Used for muscle spasms, lower back pain, or a herniated disk	• Child lies with head and knees raised to keep the hips flexed at a 45-degree angle.
Russell traction	Used for adolescents with a femur fracture or certain knee injuries	• Child lies with the head of the bed elevated 30–45 degrees.
Bryant traction	Used for children with a fractured femur who are younger than age 2 years and weigh < 31 lb (14 kg)	• Hips are flexed at a 90-degree angle. • Buttocks are raised 1″ (2.5 cm) above the mattress.

Skeletal traction

Skeletal traction exerts a greater force than skin traction by using wires or pins inserted into the bone. They are usually placed under anesthesia. Skeletal traction is continuous. (See *Types of skeletal traction.*)

Types of skeletal traction

This chart describes the different types of skeletal traction.

Traction	Purpose	Special considerations
Thomas leg splint with Pearson attachment	Used for bone alignment and as a more effective line of pull	• Child is placed in the supine position with the knee flexed.
External fixation devices (Ilizarov)	Used to manage open fractures that have soft tissue damage or to provide stability for severe comminuted fractures	• Child is on bed rest (however, early mobility and active exercise of other joints are necessary).
Halo	Used to provide immobilization of the cervical spine and to support the neck following injury	• Early ambulation is recommended. • The anterior metal bars maintain traction. • The posterior bars can be used to position the patient.
Skeletal tongs (Crutchfield, Vinke, Gardner-Wells)	Used to maintain alignment of the cervical spine, for immobilization, and for reduction of cervical roll fractures	• Child is on bed rest. • Special frames may be used for turning.

Nursing considerations

The sight and idea of a body part in skeletal traction can be frightening to a child (and their family). Explain what the child will see and feel before the traction is applied. Use dolls and toy traction devices to show the child what's about to happen and help familiarize them with the equipment and reduce fear.

In addition, follow these steps:

- Involve the family as much as possible to reduce anxiety, alleviate boredom, encourage cooperation with the recommended treatment, and minimize disruption of the family structure.
- Maintain the traction system and frequently check the ropes, pulleys, and weights for proper function.
- Maintain correct alignment of the affected body part.

Don't fall behind

- Provide age-appropriate activities to help maintain the child's developmental level, prevent developmental delay, and alleviate boredom.
- Frequently assess for signs of skin breakdown. Place sheepskin under the affected extremity to help alleviate pressure.
- Provide footplates for the affected side to prevent footdrop.

Pin and skin

- For the child in skeletal traction, assess the pin insertion sites for signs of infection or *tenting* (new skin that has attached to the insertion site, creating a tentlike configuration); tenting may cause the skin to tear, which can promote infection.
- Clean the area around the pin insertion sites frequently and cover the tips of the pins to prevent injury to the skin or other parts of the child's body. Notify the provider immediately if the pins become loose and keep the child immobilized until skeletal traction is assessed.

Musculoskeletal disorders

Musculoskeletal disorders that may occur in children include congenital clubfoot, developmental dysplasia of the hip (DDH), Ewing sarcoma, fractures, juvenile idiopathic arthritis (JIA) (formerly *juvenile rheumatoid arthritis*), Legg-Calvé-Perthes disease, slipped capital femoral epiphysis (SCFE), Osgood-Schlatter disease, and scoliosis.

Congenital clubfoot

Congenital clubfoot is a deformity that occurs in utero in approximately 1 of every 1,000 births.

Male children are twice as likely to be affected as female children. If a family has one child with a clubfoot, the chances of having another affected child increase markedly.

Although talipes equinovarus is the most commonly occurring type of clubfoot, other variations may be present and are identified according to the orientation of the deformity. (See *Recognizing clubfoot.*)

Recognizing clubfoot

Clubfoot (talipes) may have various names, depending on the orientation of the deformity, as shown in these illustrations.

Talipes equinus

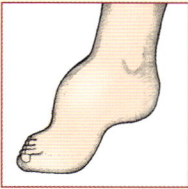

Talipes varus

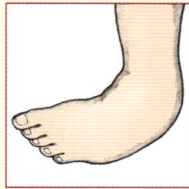

Talipes calcaneovalgus

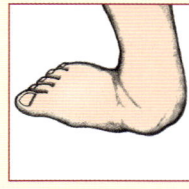

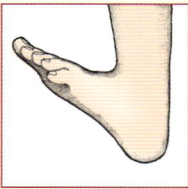

Talipes calcaneus

Talipes equinovarus

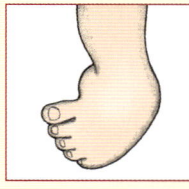

Talipes equinovalgus

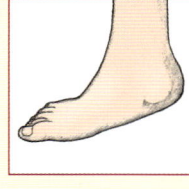

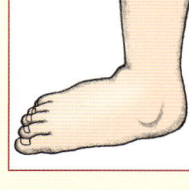

Talipes cavus

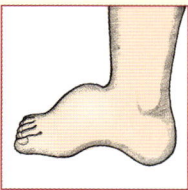

Talipes calcaneovarus

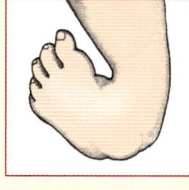

Talipes valgus

What causes it

Clubfoot may be caused by a mechanical force (the position in utero), through prenatal exposure to drugs or infections, or by an inherited factor. It can be a singular birth defect or associated with certain syndromes. An infant with a clubfoot should be carefully examined for additional anomalies.

How it happens

Regardless of the cause of the clubfoot, the result is a nonfunctional position of the foot and ankle due to abnormal muscles and joints and contracture of soft tissue. The position of the foot determines the classification of the clubfoot.

The classic definition of talipes equinovarus requires the following three components:

1. Plantar flexion of the foot at the ankle joint
2. Inversion deformity of the heel
3. Turning in of the forefoot

What to look for

The deformity is usually obvious at birth. The foot is usually inverted (turned in), also known as a *varus* position. An everted (turned outward) foot is known as a *valgus position*. A single foot or both feet may be affected. The deformity may be mild with some flexibility noted or severe with the foot completely rigid. In the most severe form, the foot has a club-like appearance.

What tests tell you

Early diagnosis of clubfoot is usually relatively simple because the deformity is obvious. However, x-rays may show superimposition of the talus and calcaneus bones and a ladder-like appearance of the metatarsals.

Complications

If identification and treatment of clubfoot is not instituted early on, chronic impairment may result. The prognosis is good, however, for infants who receive treatment.

How it's treated

Treatment of clubfoot consists of manipulation of the foot to stretch the contracted tissues. Splinting is then applied to maintain that correction. If treatment is begun shortly after birth, the correction is fairly rapid. If treatment is delayed for any reason, the foot quickly becomes more rigid, which can occur in a matter of days. Treatment is typically begun in the neonatal nursery. Straps and splints are applied and are quite effective until formal casting can be done.

Casting call

Casts are applied sequentially by first correcting the forefoot adduction, then the heel inversion, and then the flexion of the ankle. Casts are usually changed at 1- to 2-week intervals to allow the infant's foot to grow and to manipulate the foot gradually. Treatment lasts for several months depending on the severity of the deformation. To maintain the long-term correction, exercises and a night brace are commonly prescribed.

Release me

In approximately one-half of patients with clubfoot, corrective surgery is required to release the tightened structures around the foot. The outcome of this surgery is usually good; the foot appears normal and is adequate for normal footwear and sports. For infants, surgery is usually limited to soft tissue to prevent interference with bone growth.

From designer wedges . . .

For the older child or the child with severe clubfoot, the bones of the foot may need to be realigned by using bone wedges. Casts are worn for months following surgery. A specialized splint called the *Denis Browne boots* or *splint* may sometimes be used.

. . . to designer shoes

This splint consists of specially made shoes attached to an adjustable bar that provides the eversion, rotation, and dorsiflexion needed to achieve a slight overcorrection. It is worn for several weeks and then worn only at night to help maintain this position. Compliance in using this orthosis can be an issue. Make sure you teach the caregivers the importance of using it regularly.

What to do

The primary concern related to clubfoot is the need for early recognition, preferably during the neonatal period. Look for exaggerated appearances in the infant's feet. Apparent clubfoot (resulting from positioning in utero) can be differentiated from true clubfoot because an apparent clubfoot will easily move back to normal position.

When caring for a child with clubfoot, follow these steps:
- Do not use excessive force when assessing a clubfoot.
- Stress to the child's family the importance of prompt treatment; clubfoot demands immediate therapy and orthopedic supervision until growth is completed.

Put up your feet and relax

- After casting, elevate the child's feet with pillows; check the toes every 1 to 2 hours for temperature, color, sensation, motion, and capillary refill time and watch for edema.

- Before discharge, teach caregivers to recognize signs of circulatory impairment, such as numbness or tingling of the toes, coldness in the toes, or lack of capillary refill.
- Emphasize the need for long-term orthopedic care to maintain the correction.

The agony of the feet

- Help the caregivers (and child) deal with grief or other emotional issues that arise from this problem.
- Teach caregivers the prescribed exercises that the child should do at home.
- Urge caregivers to make sure the child wears their corrective shoes and splints during naps and at night. Make sure they understand that treatment for clubfoot continues throughout the entire growth period.

Developmental dysplasia of the hip

The hip joint develops early in utero. By the end of the first trimester, the shape of the joint is recognizable and the cartilage, ligaments, capsule, and vascular pattern are formed.

Relationship problems

DDH is a spectrum of conditions in which there's an abnormal relationship between the proximal femur and the acetabulum. It occurs in approximately 3 to 5 of every 1,000 live births. Females are six times more likely to be affected as males. A positive family history of DDH increases the risk fivefold.

Frankly breech

Another important risk factor for DDH is a breech presentation at birth. Children who present in a frank breech position have a risk of DDH almost 20 times higher than children who have a cephalic presentation. The way infants are carried in some cultures may also contribute to the development of DDH. (See *Carried away with DDH*.)

Other associated abnormalities include oligohydramnios (decreased amniotic fluid in utero), torticollis, and metatarsus adductus (a form of clubfoot).

What causes it

Dislocation of the hip is usually a developmental problem in an otherwise normal child. It is not always clear when it occurs. A child who develops a deformity in utero is usually more severely affected than the child who has a hip that dislocates after birth.

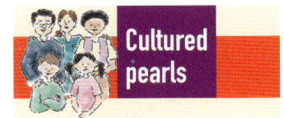

Cultured pearls

Carried away with DDH

Some experts suggest that the infant-carrying practices of certain cultures may influence the development of DDH. For instance, the rate of DDH increases by 25 to 50 times among Native Americans, who traditionally carry their infants tightly swaddled, sometimes strapped to a cradleboard, which keeps the legs in an extended position. On the other hand, DDH is rarely seen in certain African populations in which the infant is carried with their front side bound to their caregiver's back. This position keeps the infant's legs flexed and abducted, which may prevent the development of DDH.

What's in a name?

Although *congenital dislocation of the hip* is a common term for DDH, it implies that the dislocation occurs at birth. However, the problem may occur over several months after birth. Therefore, *DDH* is a more accurate description of the hip pathology that exists in this disorder.

How it happens

There are three typical forms of DDH:

- Dysplasia is a result of the femoral head failing to exert appropriate pressure against the acetabulum. As a result, the femoral head becomes small and flattened, and the acetabulum becomes shallow and eventually flat. A dysplastic hip may progress to a subluxated or dislocated hip. The abductor muscles of the hip will also shorten and contract.
- The hip is considered *subluxated* when the femoral head (the ball) is in contact with the acetabulum (the socket), but not deeply centered within it.
- *Dislocation* occurs when the femoral head (the ball) is no longer in contact with the acetabulum (the socket). (See *Forms of DDH.*)

Forms of DDH

These illustrations show a normal hip and the three presentations of DDH.

Normal hip

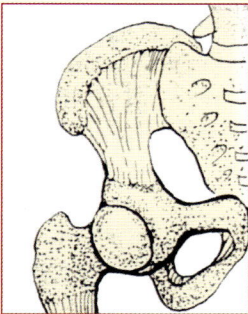

Dysplasia
The acetabulum is more flattened than cup shaped.

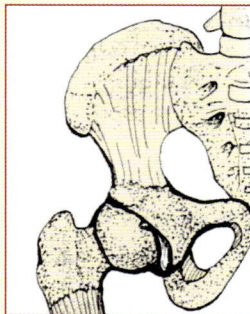

(*continued*)

Forms of DDH (*continued*)

Subluxation
The femoral head is in contact with the acetabulum but isn't deeply centered within it.

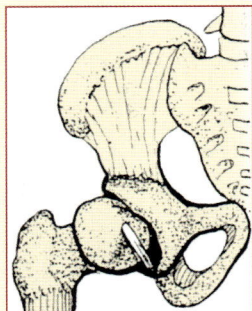

Dislocation
The femoral head is no longer in contact with the acetabulum.

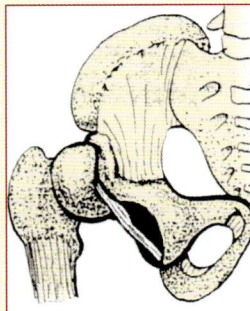

What to look for

A dislocation diagnosed in the first few weeks of life can be treated conservatively. If the diagnosis is delayed until walking age, reconstructive surgery is usually required for correction, which greatly increases the likelihood of complications.

It is important for nurses to be aware of risk factors for DDH and to assess the infant and child carefully for signs of a hip problem. Physical signs of DDH include asymmetrical skin folds, Galeazzi sign, limited hip abduction, and hip instability.

Asymmetrical skin folds
When the infant is lying on their back with their hips and knees flexed at a 90-degree angle, the same number of skin folds should appear in the medial (inner) aspect of both thighs. If a hip is dislocated, the soft tissues of the thigh may fold down on each other like an accordion, producing a larger number of skin folds on the affected side.

Galeazzi sign
If there is a dislocation, the femoral head may be placed superior to the acetabulum when the hips and knees are flexed at 90 degrees. This malpositioning will cause the knee on the affected side to be significantly lower than the other knee, a sign known as *Galeazzi sign*.

Limited hip abduction
The normal range of hip abduction in an infant is from 0 (with thighs perpendicular to the table) to almost 90 degrees (with thighs resting on the table). In DDH, a shortening of the adductor muscle on the

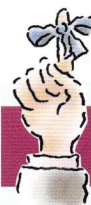

Memory jogger

Here's an easy way to keep adduction and abduction straight.

Adduction is moving a limb toward the body's midline; think of it as adding two things together.

Abduction is moving a limb away from the body's midline; think of it as taking something away like abducting, or kidnapping.

medial aspect of the thigh while the femoral head is displaced supe-
riorly causes the thigh to be limited in its range. This sign may not
be apparent in the neonate because, at this age, there has not been
enough time for muscle spasms and contractures to develop.

Hip instability

Testing hip stability is important in the diagnosis of DDH. In neonates, this test is usually the only clue to a problem.

A clunky diagnosis

Barlow test and Ortolani test are used to evaluate hip stability.
- A positive Barlow test is noted when a clunk is heard as the examiner adducts the thigh toward the midline while trying to displace
  or dislocate the femoral head posteriorly.
- A positive Ortolani test occurs when a clunk is felt as the examiner
  abducts the thigh to the table from the midline while lifting up
  the greater trochanter with the finger.

What tests tell you

A *Trendelenburg test* can be used to assess for hip dislocation in children who are old enough to stand and bear weight. When the child
stands on the affected leg, the opposite hip slants downward instead
of remaining level.

A limp or a waddle

As the child walks, there's a characteristic limp known as the *Trendelenburg gait*. This limp is due to a weakness of the hip abductor
muscles. If both hips are dislocated, the child will have lordosis and a
waddling gait.

X-rays will show the location of the femoral head and a shallow acetabulum. X-rays are also used to monitor treatment or
deterioration.

Complications

For children who do not receive treatment before age 7 years, treatment is very unsatisfactory. Delayed treatment may have lifelong
implications for walking, development of back problems, and
self-esteem. DDH may cause:
- degenerative hip changes
- abnormal acetabular development
- lordosis (abnormally increased concave curvature of the lumbar
  and cervical spine)
- joint malformation
- sciatic nerve injury (paralysis)
- avascular necrosis of the femoral head
- soft tissue damage
- permanent disability.

How it's treated

Treatment of DDH depends on the severity of the dysplasia, how quickly the diagnosis is made, and the child's age and includes a Pavlik harness, spica cast, and surgical correction.

Pavlik harness

If treatment is instituted early, the success of treatment with a Pavlik harness is greater than 90%. As the child ages and treatment is delayed, the prognosis worsens. (See *Two views of the Pavlik harness.*) In some cases, a Pavlik harness cannot be used. If the family cannot consistently and correctly use the harness, another form of treatment should be used.

Two views of the Pavlik harness

These illustrations show an infant in a Pavlik harness. The Pavlik harness maintains the hip in abduction, with the femoral head in the acetabulum.

Front view

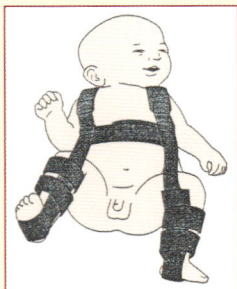

Back view

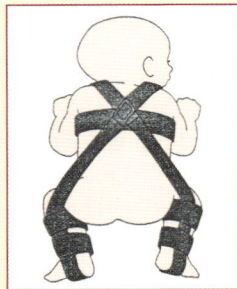

Whoa, Nellie!

In the child younger than age 6 months, careful positioning to maintain the hip in abduction with the head of the femur in the acetabulum is achieved with a Pavlik harness. This harness is worn at all times, except for bathing until the hips are stable on examination. When the hips are stable, usually in 1 to 3 weeks, the harness is then used during sleep for 6 additional weeks.

Harness hip hooray!

If DDH is diagnosed during the neonatal period, the harness may be needed for only 2 to 3 months. The older infant may need to wear it for 4 or 5 months.

Don't double up

Caregivers should be taught how to apply the harness correctly and to avoid double and triple diapering (which can cause extreme abduction, leading to avascular necrosis). The harness doesn't interfere with the child's ability to receive immunizations as the thighs remain exposed.

Spica cast

For the child older than age 6 months, a Pavlik harness cannot reliably treat the dysplasia. These children require a spica cast to hold the hips in a flexed and abducted position. Traction is commonly used before the application of the cast to gently stretch out the soft tissues around the hip that have contracted. Traction is usually used for 2 to 3 weeks before placement of the cast. Sometimes, the traction can be done at home.

A temporary setback

When the cast has been applied, it usually remains on for several months and is removed and reapplied to accommodate growth. It may delay walking for a few months, but the child usually learns quickly how to walk when the cast is removed.

Hold and turn

Care for a child in a spica cast is essentially the same as that for a child in a Pavlik harness. Caregivers should be encouraged to hold the child as much as possible. The infant should be turned frequently to prevent skin breakdown.

Surgical correction

For the child older than age 18 months, surgical correction is usually required. Surgery enables the removal of tissues that block reduction and positioning of the femoral head into the acetabulum under direct visualization. Occasionally, a bone graft is required.

What to do

Listen sympathetically to the family's expression of anxiety and fear. Explain possible causes of DDH and reassure them that early, prompt treatment will probably result in complete correction.

You'd be cranky too

During the child's first few days in a cast or harness, they may be prone to irritability due to the unaccustomed restriction of movement. Encourage the child's caregivers to stay with them as much as possible and to calm and reassure them. Ensure caregivers that the child will adjust to this restriction and return to normal sleeping, eating, and playing behavior in a few days.

   If treatment requires a spica cast, follow these steps:
- Position the child on a Bradford frame (a rectangular frame of pipe with attached sheeting used for immobile patients) elevated on blocks with a bedpan under the frame or on pillows to

support the child's legs. Be sure to keep the cast dry and change the child's diapers often.

- Turn the child every 2 hours during the day and every 4 hours at night. Check color, sensation, and motion of the infant's legs and feet. (Be sure to examine their toes and notify the provider of dusky, cool, or numb toes.)

Investigate the itch

- If the child complains of itching, they may benefit from an over-the-counter antihistamine, or you may aim a blow-dryer set on cool at the cast edges to relieve itching. (Don't scratch or probe under the cast; investigate persistent itching.)
- Provide adequate stimuli to promote growth and development. If the child's hips are abducted in a frog-like position, tell caregivers that the child may be able to fit on a tricycle that they can push (if the child cannot pedal) or an electric child's car.

A change of scenery

- Encourage caregivers to let the child sit at a table (by sitting them on pillows on a chair), sit on the floor for short periods of play, and play with other children of their age.
- Tell caregivers to watch for signs that the child is needing an adjustment of the cast and to notify the provider if any of the following are seen: skin breakdown, cyanosis, cool extremities, pain, or an ill-fitting or broken cast.

Fractures

Bones are designed to withstand stress. However, when increased stress and traumatic force are exerted on the bone, a fracture will occur. Fractures can occur in almost any bone, but the long bones are the most commonly fractured. Other common sites of fracture include the wrists, fingers, toes, and skull.

What causes it

Fractures commonly occur during athletic activities and accidents. They may also result from child abuse (suspected in the case of infants without a known cause for a weakened bone, multiple or repeated episodes of fractures), bone tumors, or metabolic disease.

How it happens

Fractures occur when traumatic forces are exerted on the bone. Because children are more flexible than adults, they may not be as prone to fractures.

Sticks and stones may bend my bones

Rather than fracturing completely, children's bones tend to simply bend, buckle, or sustain an incomplete fracture.

A stressful situation

Stress fractures are associated with unusually strong physical stress and are commonly seen in children who suddenly begin a vigorous training program. (See *Common fractures in children*.)

Common fractures in children

Bends, buckle fractures, greenstick fractures, and complete fractures commonly occur during childhood. Each of these fractures is described and illustrated below.

Bends

Bends are common in childhood because of the flexibility of children's bones. Children's bones can be bent up to 45 degrees, or possibly more, before breaking.

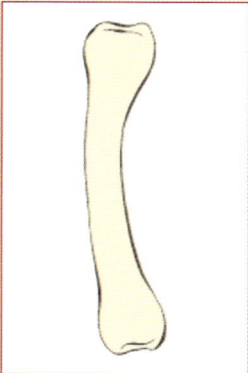

Greenstick fractures

Greenstick fractures occur when the bone is bent beyond its limits, causing an incomplete fracture.

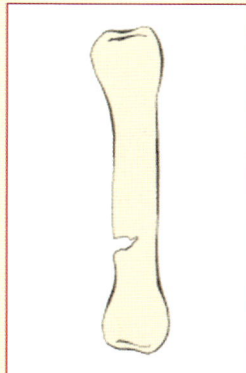

Buckle fractures

Buckle fractures occur due to compression of the porous bone, causing a raised area or bulge at the fracture site.

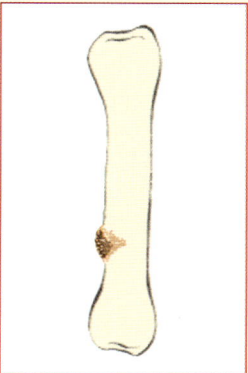

Complete fractures

Complete fractures occur when the bone is broken into separate pieces.

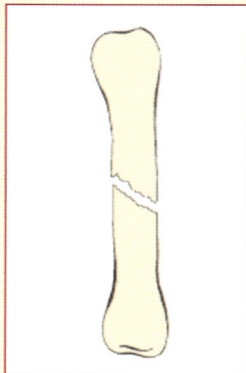

The remodeling team

After a fracture occurs, the body quickly begins a repairing process. A blood clot is formed at the site of the fracture. Osteoblasts and fibroblasts then converge on the site and begin to lay down an organic matrix. This forms a callus into which calcium salts are deposited, evolving into bone tissue that connects the pieces of the original bone. After that happens, the callus is remodeled into a strong, permanent bone.

What to look for

Bone fractures are classified according to:
- type of injury to the bone or surrounding tissue
- whether they are *open* (in which the skin has been broken due to penetration of bone fragment or external trauma) or *closed* (in which the fracture is contained under the skin's surface)
- whether there's involvement of the epiphyseal (growth) plate.

Sudden and sharp

Fractures usually cause sudden, sharp pain at the fracture site. Pain increases with movement and limits motion in the affected part. Swelling, bruising, or discoloration around the site may occur. There may be obvious deformity or abnormal positioning of the affected part.

What tests tell you

X-rays provide the definitive diagnosis for a fracture. Occasionally, an incomplete fracture is not seen initially on the x-ray and appears only after the film has dried after several hours. Serial x-rays are taken to monitor healing and check the alignment of the bone.

Complications

Complications of fractures include infection, particularly in open fracture. A fracture that affects the growth plate can interrupt and alter growth. The impact of this alteration depends on the area of the epiphyseal plate that's affected.

The *Salter-Harris classification system* is used to determine the severity of the injury on the epiphyseal plate. Type I injuries typically do not affect growth. Type III injuries and above require intervention to prevent future dysfunction in the bone and affected body part. (See *Salter-Harris classification system*.)

Salter-Harris classification system

The Salter-Harris classification system divides growth plate fractures into five categories. These categories are based on the type of damage to the growth plate.

Type I

The epiphysis is completely separated from the metaphysis or end of bone. Although a type I fracture generally requires casting, it rarely requires manipulation. Growth disturbance is not common unless the blood supply has been injured.

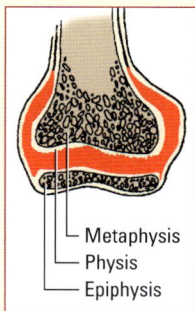

- Metaphysis
- Physis
- Epiphysis

Type II

Type II is the most common type of fracture. The epiphysis and the growth plate are separated from the cracked metaphysis. This type of fracture must be manipulated and casted for normal growth to continue. Minimal shortening of the bone may occur but usually does not result in functional limitations.

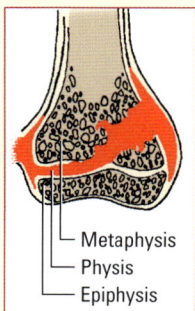

- Metaphysis
- Physis
- Epiphysis

Type III

Type III is a rare fracture that usually involves the lower tibia or a long bone of the lower leg. It occurs when the fracture runs completely through the epiphysis and separates part of the epiphysis and the growth plate from the metaphysis. Surgery may be necessary. Growth usually is not affected as long as the blood supply to the bone is intact.

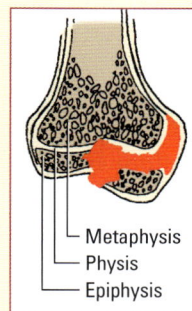

- Metaphysis
- Physis
- Epiphysis

Type IV

A type IV fracture runs through the epiphysis, across the growth plate, and into the metaphysis. It occurs most commonly in the humerus near the elbow. Perfect alignment must be achieved for normal growth to occur.

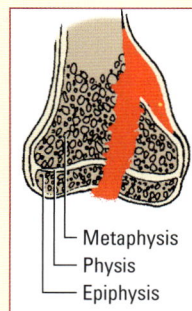

- Metaphysis
- Physis
- Epiphysis

(*continued*)

Salter-Harris classification system (*continued*)

Type V
A crush or compression injury, a type V fracture most likely occurs in the knee or ankle. It is an uncommon injury. Stunting of growth is possible, and prognosis is poor. Surgery is required as well as future reconstructive or corrective surgery.

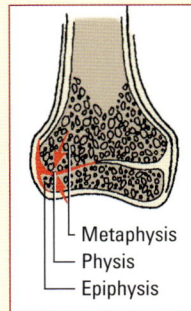

- Metaphysis
- Physis
- Epiphysis

From bone to lung
Fat embolism is a major, life-threatening complication of a fracture. Fat globules are released into the circulation and can become lodged in the capillaries of the lung, thereby decreasing the exchange of oxygen and carbon dioxide. Signs of an embolism are increasing blood pressure, dyspnea, and other signs of respiratory compromise.

How it's treated
Reducing or realigning the bone into proper placement and allowing it to heal is the treatment required for a fracture. The reduction may be closed (through external manipulation of the body part) or open (done through surgery).

Closed reductions are usually treated with casting. Surgical repair of a fracture involves the use of either internal or external fixation devices.

Permanent hardware
Internal devices (rods, pins, or wires) are permanent; they remain in the child unless a problem develops. External devices are pins or wires that are inserted through the bone and then attached to an external frame. When the bone heals, the devices are removed. Follow-up evaluation is essential to prevent and quickly treat complications that may arise.

What to do
Fractures are usually treated in an emergency setting. Formal preparation for treatments and procedures may not be possible.

Prepare on the go
Tell the child (and their family) everything that's being done as it's happening and provide as much support as possible to help ease the child's fears and enhance cooperation.

- Provide emergency care to the child with a fracture; steps should be taken to quickly assess the injury, prevent further damage, and promote comfort.
- Frequently check for neurologic and circulatory compromise to the affected area.

Cast caution

- After the cast or splint has been applied, continue to assess the area around the cast.
- When a fracture requires long-term immobilization with traction, reposition the patient often to increase comfort and prevent pressure injuries, assist with active ROM exercises to prevent muscle atrophy, and encourage deep breathing and coughing to prevent pneumonia.

Are you shocked?

- Watch for signs of shock in the child with a severe open fracture of a large bone, such as the femur.
- Assist the child to regain normal function as quickly as possible; encourage the child to start moving around as soon as they can, help them walk, and demonstrate how to use crutches properly.
- Help the family deal with the fracture and help the child understand what's happening.

Postscript

- Encourage the child to talk about the experience and express their feelings after the emergency is over; use this time to answer questions and clear up misconceptions (as would usually be done before treatment).

Slipped capital femoral epiphysis

As the name implies, a child with SCFE has a portion of the femoral head distal to the growth plate (physis) that slips out of the socket, causing pain and a limp. In many cases, the pain is referred to the knee. The SCFE can occur in one or both hips. Depending on how severe the slip is and how long it has occurred, the treatment and prognosis can be short and sweet or long and complex.

What causes it

It is not fully understood what causes SCFE, but it is seen more commonly in younger teens who are obese. There may be a genetic predisposition. Kids with endocrine disorders such as diabetes, hypothyroidism, or growth hormone deficiencies are more prone to having an SCFE. This may be due to the abnormal cartilage growth and mineralization that occurs with these disorders.

How it happens

Any time the force placed on the femoral head exceeds that of the growth plate (the capital femoral physis), an SCFE is bound to happen. No one is quite sure what causes a weakening of the growth plate, but some factors include the normal thinning and widening of the growth plate during growth spurts or trauma. Other conditions that affect normal bone health such as cancer or certain medications may also predispose a child to SCFE.

What to look for

The biggest symptom of SCFE is pain in the knee, groin, thigh, or hip. The pain may be mild or severe depending on the severity of the slip. Some children with a mild slip may experience stiffness. A limp is often noticed. Increased activity frequently brings increased pain. SCFE is often classified according to the time of presentation.

Preslip—Children with preslip SCFE have pain but no overt signs of displacement. A widening of the proximal femoral physis may be seen on x-ray.

Acute—Children presenting with acute SCFE have pain that is recent (<2 to 3 weeks). It is commonly seen with traumatic injuries such as a fall and accounts for only 10% to 15% of cases. These children are in severe pain and may show a visible deformity. The child may refuse to bear weight. Children with an acute form of SCFE are at significant risk of further joint damage. They should be kept non–weight bearing until treatment is started.

Chronic—Chronic SCFE is the most common presentation of all types of SCFE. Pain can be vague and intermittent over a long period of time. The pain is commonly found in the knee, hip, groin, or thigh. On occasion, a diagnosis is missed or delayed because there is no actual hip pain. A limp is usually present with the foot of the affected side turning outward. ROM is decreased and painful in all directions. The upper thigh and gluteal muscles may begin to atrophy.

Acute on chronic—Children with chronic SCFE who suddenly have increased pain and symptoms are classified as acute on chronic presentation. Joint changes and effusion are typically seen. SCFE is also classified as stable or unstable or, according to severity, as mild, moderate, or severe.

What tests tell you

X-rays are the most common test used for the diagnosis of SCFE. A widening or irregularity of the physis is seen. If the slip is very mild, an MRI or bone scan may be used. Ultrasounds or CT scans have not been shown to be any more effective in the diagnosis of SCFE than regular x-rays. Other lab tests may be used to identify additional causes of SCFE (such as hypothyroidism).

Complications

Complications of SCFE can cause permanent joint damage or a discrepancy in leg length. Osteonecrosis or avascular necrosis is essentially the death of the bone. It can occur with severe slips, a delay in treatment, or due to a complication of the treatment itself. Chondrolysis is a narrowing of the joint itself and a loss of cartilage often due to untreated SCFE. It can also be seen in children with severe SCFE that requires a prolonged period of bed rest. Children with SCFE are at higher risk of developing osteoarthritis.

How it's treated

Surgery is the treatment for SCFE. The orthopedic surgeon places a screw through the growth plate and femoral head to stabilize the joint. In many cases, the surgeon will also stabilize the opposite hip due to the high risk of slippage bilaterally. Postoperative care includes teaching the child how to use crutches or a walker and the gradual return to normal activities.

What to do

SCFE can be a frightening diagnosis for a teen (or child) and their family. Reassure the family that with proper treatment, the outcomes are generally very good. Allow the child to express their fears and answer any questions they may have. Explain the importance of following the recommended treatment in order to prevent any long-term consequences.

Osgood-Schlatter disease

Osgood-Schlatter disease is not exactly a disease. It is an overuse injury of the knee in a growing adolescent. The patellar tendon becomes inflamed at the tibial junction, eventually leading to pain and swelling at the tibial tuberosity. It usually will go away as the child matures.

What causes it

Osgood-Schlatter disease happens when the repeated strain from activities puts stress on the patellar tendon. Athletic kids are more likely to develop Osgood-Schlatter disease than nonathletes. One-quarter to one-half of teens will have both knees affected.

How it happens

Active children are often involved in sports or other activities that require a lot of stress and contraction of the quadriceps. This contraction exerts a pull on the developing patellar tendon. Repeated strain leads to inflammation of the tendon (apophysitis), thus causing a slight tear. As the body tries to repair the tear, a callus is formed. The result is pain and swelling at the tibial tuberosity—the bony protrusion on the tibia just below the kneecap.

What to look for

Knee pain is the hallmark symptom of Osgood-Schlatter disease. It starts out as a dull ache, then increases with continued use. It is exacerbated by activities that require a lot of knee use (running, climbing stairs, kneeling, etc.). The pain goes away with rest. Other symptoms include tenderness and swelling at the tibial tuberosity and tight hamstrings and quads.

What tests tell you

The diagnosis of Osgood-Schlatter disease is made by clinical examination. Unless there are unusual signs and symptoms such as redness, warmth, nighttime pain, or an acute onset of severe pain, x-rays are not needed.

Complications

Complications of this process are rare. The most common complication is continued chronic pain. A persistent prominence of the tibial tubercle may occur. Very rarely, Osgood-Schlatter disease may cause a hyperextension of the knee known as *genu recurvatum* (backward-bending knee).

How it's treated

Treatment includes pain control, continuing physical activity, and PT. NSAIDs such as ibuprofen (Motrin/Advil) or naproxen (Naprosyn/Aleve) may be used for 4 to 7 days to decrease the inflammation and provide pain control. Applying ice after physical activity may also be helpful. Children and adolescents can continue to play as long as the pain is tolerable. Once pain is controlled, they should participate in PT to help strengthen their quadriceps and hamstring muscles. On rare occasions, surgery is needed to resect the ossicle that has developed or to remove the prominent tuberosity.

What to do

The name Osgood-Schlatter disease can frighten a child and the family. Reassurance that this is not a disease and will usually resolve within 6 to 18 months. In addition, follow these steps:

- Encourage the child, however, to be active as long as the pain is tolerable and resolves within 24 hours.
- Educate the child and family on strengthening and stretching exercises of the quadriceps and hamstrings.
- Encourage the use of a protective pad to prevent direct trauma to the tibial tubercle.

Scoliosis

Scoliosis is a spinal deformity, defined as a lateral curvature of the spine that's greater than 10 degrees and is always associated with some rotation of the involved vertebrae. Posterior curvature of the spine is known as *kyphosis*, and anterior curvature is known as *lordosis*. Although some curvature is normal, excessive curvature becomes pathologic. Scoliosis is classified as either nonstructural (functional) or structural. (See *Looking at scoliosis*.)

Looking at scoliosis

The spinal deformity that occurs in scoliosis is shown in this illustration.

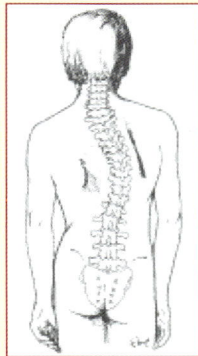

Scoliosis can occur at any age, but idiopathic scoliosis is seen in greatest numbers in children after age 8 years. Female children are four to five times more likely to be affected than males, and the incidence is higher if another family member is affected. The deformity progresses during growth periods and stabilizes when vertebral growth is complete.

What causes it

In nonstructural scoliosis, the spine is structurally normal and the disorder never progresses to structural scoliosis. Nonstructural scoliosis may be caused by poor posture, leg-length discrepancies, an irritated sciatic nerve, or an infectious process such as appendicitis. A very rare psychological scoliosis is known as *hysterical scoliosis*.

Not sure about structure

Structural scoliosis can be categorized by its major causes: neuromuscular, congenital, syndromic, or idiopathic. Neuromuscular disorders such as cerebral palsy, poliomyelitis, or muscular dystrophy can cause scoliosis. Birth defects, injuries, certain infections, tumors, and metabolic factors are also identified causes. Connective tissue disorders leading to Marfan syndrome, neurofibromatosis, osteogenesis imperfecta, or rheumatic disease may also cause structural abnormalities. The cause of *idiopathic scoliosis*, the most common type of structural scoliosis, is currently unknown. There may be a genetic component as some studies of identical twins show a higher incidence of idiopathic scoliosis than that of fraternal twins. Children also have a higher incidence of acquiring scoliosis if a biological parent had it.

How it happens

The spine is normally curved in order to maintain proper balance, with the muscles on either side of the spine supporting it. If a lateral curve has developed, a convex rotation of the spine and ribs will eventually cause the vertebrae to become rotated or wedge shaped. Muscles become contracted, and a compensatory curve develops so that the body can maintain balance and posture. The curve either stabilizes on its own or progresses. The amount of progression depends on the child's sex, the initial severity of the curve, and the remaining growth potential. The curve will naturally worsen as the spine continues to grow.

What to look for

Examination of the child usually begins with a general inspection of the back with the child in a standing position. Obvious asymmetries can be seen, including:
- one shoulder higher than the other
- prominent scapula
- uneven waistline
- rib hump.

Over for obvious

When the child bends over, these asymmetries become even more obvious. The shoulder and hip levels become uneven. The head should normally align directly over the sacrum, but in persons with a spinal deformity, there may be deviation from the midline. These differences disappear in nonstructural scoliosis.

Something suspicious

Scoliosis classically produces no symptoms. If the child has pain, the scoliosis is likely due to some other disorder, such as a bone or spinal cord tumor. Neurologic symptoms, wasting of the hands or lower extremities, and an age of onset younger than 10 years suggest a different cause. These secondary causes must be ruled out. In cases of secondary scoliosis, the curvature often will resolve when the underlying cause is treated.

What tests tell you

X-rays are used to evaluate the entire spine in the standing position, looking at both the anteroposterior and lateral planes.

- Measurement of skeletal maturity and shoulder and hip levels determines the degree of scoliosis.
- An abnormal forward-bending test, in which the patient bends forward 90 degrees with the hands joined at the midline, demonstrates asymmetry of the shoulders and height of the ribs.
- Two types of measurement devices—A level plane ruler, used for measurement while the patient is bending over, and a scoliometer, designed to assess the angle of trunk rotation—can be used to help determine the severity of the curve and guide management decisions. It can also be used to help reassure the child and their family.

Complications

Generally, scoliosis is mild and there are few problems. Few children with scoliosis will continue with back pain throughout adulthood. Complications can sometimes lead to serious, debilitating, or even life-threatening sequelae. The curve can cause the thoracic area to become smaller, thus crowding the heart and lungs. This can lead to pulmonary and cardiac compromise.

Negotiating the curves

The severity of complications increases with the severity of the curvature:

- Severe curves can affect vital lung capacity, causing tachypnea or even hypoxia; severe restrictive lung disease and even death from cor pulmonale may occur if scoliosis is left untreated.
- Large thoracic curves greater than 60 degrees are associated with a shortened lifespan.
- Large lumbar curvatures may lead to subluxation of the vertebrae and arthritic changes in the spine; disabling pain in adulthood may result because of these changes.
- Neurologic sequelae and paralysis may be a complication if the vertebral column is manipulated during surgery.
- Infection is always a risk after surgery.

How it's treated

Treatment of scoliosis depends on the magnitude of the curve, skeletal maturity, and the risk of progression. No treatment is necessary in children with functional scoliosis or in whom the curve is less than 20 degrees. Structural scoliosis is treated as early as possible in order to lessen or prevent progression. Stretching and strengthening the back muscles improve posture and maintain flexibility.

Brace yourself

Bracing is used in skeletally immature children with curves between 20 and 40 degrees. A silastic, thoracolumbosacral brace is molded to the child and exerts gentle pressure on the spine. This brace is worn 23 hours per day until growth is complete, usually for several years. It is removed only for hygiene and skin care. This brace, also known as an *underarm brace*, can be fairly well concealed under clothing. A more cumbersome under-chin brace is sometimes needed with more complex curvatures. This brace is less likely to be concealed under clothes and may not be tolerated by the child. Bracing usually does not cure scoliosis but does prevent it from progressing further and may even decrease the amount of curvature noted at the end of treatment.

No confusion, it's spinal fusion

Spinal fusion surgery, rod placement, and bone grafting may be required to correct curves greater than 45 degrees. Activities are restricted for several months until the fusion is solid.

What to do

It is essential to assess continually for compliance because noncompliance with recommended treatment measures may be detrimental. In addition, follow these steps:

- Teach the prescribed treatment routines to the child and their family and explain the consequences of not following these recommendations (to help ensure the best possible outcome).
- Emphasize activity restrictions; provide alternative exercises and activities that are beneficial.

Stealth brace

- Help the child find clothing that minimizes the appearance of the brace to enhance their self-image; teach them to wear a light T-shirt or jersey underneath the brace and to place a smooth cloth over the chin pad (to minimize skin breakdown and promote skin integrity).

A strange new world

- For children requiring surgical correction, preoperative teaching is essential. Prepare the child for the presence of various catheters, a special bed (Stryker frame), and the use of certain body mechanics in order to restrict bending at the fusion site. Peer support groups may also be helpful when the child can return home.

Quick quiz

1. The growth plate of the bone is known as:
   A. the epiphyseal plate.
   B. the metaphyseal plate.
   C. the diaphyseal plate.
   D. the medullary plate.

Answer: A. The diaphysis is the shaft of the long bone. The metaphysis is the wider portion of the long bone next to the epiphysis. The medullary cavity is where the bone marrow is found.

2. When teaching families about treatment for their baby's clubfoot, educate the family that the casts will be:
   A. placed on the affected foot for 2 weeks only.
   B. placed on both feet for 6 weeks.
   C. placed on the affected foot initially and then changed every 2 to 3 weeks as the baby's foot grows and is manipulated.
   D. placed on both feet initially and then changed every 4 to 5 weeks as the baby's feet grow and are manipulated.

Answer: C. Serial casting is done on the affected foot (or both feet if affected) and changed every 2 to 3 weeks as the baby's foot grows and is manipulated. Treatment lasts for several months depending on the severity of the deformation.

3. A nurse is caring for a child with SCFE. What findings would they expect on examination?
   A. Pain in the affected hip only and a noticeable limp
   B. Pain in the knee, hip, groin, or thigh; possible complaints of stiffness; and perhaps a limp
   C. Pain and swelling of the affected hip and a severe limp
   D. Redness, swelling, and pain above the knee of the affected side

Answer: B. SCFE often will refer pain to the knee, groin, or thigh. A mild slip may only cause stiffness. The severity of the limp depends on the severity of the slip. Redness and swelling would suggest a different cause.

4. Educating patients and families about Osgood-Schlatter disease should include teaching that:
   A. the disease progresses to a point that the child can no longer participate in any activity.
   B. the disease name is a misnomer and it is really an overuse injury.
   C. the disease means the child must be on bed rest until the injury resolves.
   D. the disease means the child will require surgery.

Answer: B. Osgood-Schlatter disease is not really a disease but an overuse injury to the patellar tendon. It will heal with rest and maturity of the muscles and tendons. Children should be encouraged to stay active. Icing and short-term use of NSAIDs may help the pain.

Scoring

☆☆☆   If you answered all four items correctly, hip hooray! You've earned the right to flex your muscles.

☆☆   If you answered three items correctly, fine work! Now you're ready to bone up for the next quiz.

☆   If you answered fewer than three items correctly, don't let it rattle your bones! There are still four quizzes in your future—no bones about it.

Suggested References

American Academy of Orthopaedic Surgeons. (2019). *Ewing's sarcoma*. https://orthoinfo.aaos.org/en/diseases--conditions/ewings-sarcoma/

American Academy of Orthopaedic Surgeons. (2022). *Developmental dislocation (dysplasia) of the hip (DDH)*. https://orthoinfo.aaos.org/en/diseases--conditions/developmental-dislocation-dysplasia-of-the-hip-ddh/

American Academy of Orthopaedic Surgeons. (2023a). *Perthes disease*. https://orthoinfo.aaos.org/en/diseases--conditions/perthes-disease/

American Academy of Orthopaedic Surgeons. (2023b). *Juvenile arthritis*. https://orthoinfo.aaos.org/en/diseases--conditions/juvenile-arthritis/

Claytor, C. (2020). Musculoskeletal disorders. In D. Maaks, N. Starr, M. Brady, N. Gaylord, M. Driessnack, & K. Duderstadt (Eds.), *Burns' pediatric primary care* (7th ed., pp. 885–918). Elsevier.

Cowen, K., Wisely, L., Dawson, R., Ball, J., & McGillis Bindler, R. (2023). The child with alternations in musculoskeletal function. In K. Cowen, L. Wisely, R. Dawson, J. Ball, & R. McGillis Bindler (Eds.), *Principles of pediatric nursing: Caring for children* (8th ed., pp. 813–848). Pearson.

Linnard-Palmer, L. (2024). Mobility. In L. Linnard-Palmer (Ed.), *Pediatric nursing care: A concept-based approach* (2nd ed., pp. 401–416). Jones & Bartlett Learning.

Mayo Clinic. (2019). *Clubfoot*. https://www.mayoclinic.org/diseases-conditions/clubfoot/symptoms-causes/syc-20350860

Mayo Clinic. (2023). *Scoliosis*. https://www.mayoclinic.org/diseases-conditions/scoliosis/symptoms-causes/syc-20350716

Patterson, M. (2023). Musculoskeletal disorders. In B. Richardson (Ed.), *Pediatric primary care: Practice guidelines for nurses* (5th ed., pp. 459–486). Jones & Bartlett Learning.

Walter, K. (2023). *Slipped capital femoral epiphysis*. https://emedicine.medscape.com/article/91596-overview

Chapter 20

Gastrointestinal problems

Just the facts

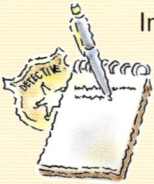

In this chapter, you'll learn:

♦ anatomy and physiology of the gastrointestinal (GI) system
♦ diagnostic tests for children with GI disorders
♦ treatments and procedures used for children with GI disorders
♦ GI disorders that affect infants and children.

Anatomy and physiology

The functions of the gastrointestinal (GI) tract enable ingestion and propulsion of food, digestion and absorption of food and nutrients needed by the body, and elimination of waste products.

Structures of the GI system

The GI system consists of two major components:
1. Alimentary canal
2. Accessory organs of digestion

It's alimentary, my dear Watson

The alimentary canal of the GI tract consists of a hollow, muscular tube that begins in the mouth and ends at the anus. It includes the:
- oral cavity
- pharynx
- esophagus
- stomach
- small intestine
- large intestine.

Accessories make the system

Accessory glands and organs that aid GI function include the:
- salivary glands
- liver
- biliary duct system (gallbladder and bile ducts)
- pancreas.

Digestion

Digestion starts in the oral cavity, where chewing (mastication), salivation (the beginning of starch digestion), and swallowing (deglutition) take place. (See *The growing GI system*.)

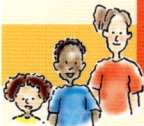

The growing GI system

Here are some highlights of the developing GI system during the first few years of life.

Salivary assistance
• Saliva production begins at age 4 months and aids in the process of digestion. Saliva contains mucus to protect oral mucosa and to coat food. Food breakdown begins in the mouth with the enzymes ptyalin and amylase.
• The sucking and extrusion reflex (a reflex that protects the infant from food substances their system is too immature to digest) persists until ages 3 to 4 months.

Stomach
• The stomach capacity of the neonate is 30 to 60 mL and gradually increases to 200 to 300 mL by age 12 months and to 1,500 mL in the adolescent.
• Up until ages 4 to 8 weeks, the neonatal abdomen is larger than the chest and the musculature is poorly developed.
• Spit-ups are frequent in the neonate because of the immature muscle tone of the lower esophageal sphincter and the low-volume capacity of the stomach.
• Peristalsis occurs within 2½ to 3 hours in the neonate and extends to 3 to 6 hours in older infants and children.
• Digestive enzymes are deficient until at least ages 4 to 6 months; gas, diarrhea, sensitization for food allergies, and microscopic hemorrhages can develop if solid foods are introduced before this time.

Intestinal
• From ages 1 to 3 years, the composition of intestinal flora becomes more adultlike and stomach acidity increases, reducing the number of GI infections.
• Exposure to breast milk increases intestinal flora early on and provides some protection against viruses and pathologic flora.
• Increased myelination of nerves to the anal sphincter allows for physiologic control of bowel function, usually at about age 2 years; psychological readiness for toilet training may occur at a later age.

Liver
• The liver is immature at birth, resulting in inefficient detoxifying of substances and medications. Medication dosages may need to be adjusted.
• The liver's slow development of glycogen storage capacity makes the infant prone to hypoglycemia.
• Infants are more prone to dehydration and fluid and electrolyte imbalances due to greater body surface area, high rate of metabolism, and immature kidney function.

The rise and fall of hormones

Hunger is controlled by the lateral hypothalamus in the brain. A fall in blood nutrients, a rise or fall in hormones governing metabolism, hunger contractions from the stomach, and emotional input signal the hypothalamus to stimulate hunger. Fullness of the stomach, blood levels of nutrients and hormones, and emotions or habits stimulate the satiety center in the ventromedial area of the hypothalamus to decrease hunger.

The tasteful tongue

The tongue provides the sense of taste and is the strongest muscle in the body. Saliva secreted from the salivary glands moistens the mouth and lubricates the food bolus to ease swallowing.

Look out stomach, here it comes!

When a person swallows a food bolus, the following occur:
1. The upper esophageal sphincter relaxes, allowing food to enter the esophagus.
2. The epiglottis closes with swallowing to prevent food from being aspirated into the trachea.
3. As food moves through the esophagus, glands in the esophageal mucosal layer secrete mucus, which lubricates the food and protects the esophageal mucosal layer from being damaged by poorly chewed foods. (See *Choking hazards*.)

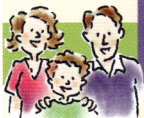

It's all relative

Choking hazards

Foods that are round and less than 1¼″ (3.2 cm) in diameter can obstruct the airway of a child when swallowed whole. Teach caregivers to cut foods into small pieces to prevent obstruction of the airway. Common foods that may cause choking include:
- hot dogs
- Vienna sausages
- nuts
- popcorn
- marshmallows
- grapes
- hard candy
- fruits with pits
- dried beans.

---

4. Lower esophageal contractions (called *peristalsis*) gradually push the food down the esophagus and through the lower esophageal sphincter into the stomach.

Stomach

Until the child is approximately age 2 years, the stomach is round. It will gradually elongate and take the adult shape and position in the abdomen by age 7 years.

The stomach lies in the left upper quadrant of the abdomen and is made up of three parts:

1. The *fundus* is an enlarged portion above and to the left of the esophageal opening in the stomach; the *cardiac sphincter* is at the opening of the esophagus to the stomach.
2. The *body* is the middle portion of the stomach.
3. The *pylorus* is the lower portion of the stomach, lying near the junction of the stomach and the duodenum. The pyloric sphincter is at the opening of the stomach to the duodenum.

A gastric response

The secretory cells in the lining of the stomach are believed to be functional at birth. The lining of the stomach secretes gastrin in response to stomach wall distention. In turn, gastrin stimulates the release of highly acidic digestive secretions consisting mainly of pepsinogen, which is converted to pepsin, hydrochloric acid, intrinsic factor, and proteolytic enzymes. Limited amounts of water, alcohol, and some drugs are absorbed in the stomach. Intrinsic factor is necessary for vitamin B_{12} absorption.

Triple overtime

The stomach's three functions are to store food, mix food with gastric juices via peristaltic contractions, and slowly distribute this food (now called *chyme*) into the small intestine through the pyloric opening for further digestion and absorption.

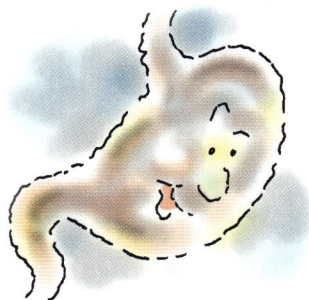

Small intestine

Nearly all digestion and absorption take place in the small intestine. The small intestine lies coiled in the abdomen and consists of three major sections:

1. Duodenum
2. Jejunum
3. Ileum

Contractions and secretions

Peristaltic contractions and various digestive secretions break down carbohydrates, proteins, and fats, enabling the intestinal mucosa to absorb these nutrients, along with water and electrolytes. *Secretin* and *cholecystokinin* are the hormones that affect intestinal secretions and gastric motility.

Distribution center

The surface area of the small intestine is increased by millions of villi in the mucous membrane lining. Digested food is absorbed through the mucosal walls and into the blood for distribution throughout the body. Failure to feed, malnutrition, ischemia, and infections affect the small intestine's ability to absorb nutrients, resulting in growth delays.

Large intestine

The ileocecal valve is the sphincter between the ileum of the small intestine and the cecum of the large intestine. It prevents secretions from returning to the ileum. By the time chyme passes through the small intestine and enters the ascending colon of the large intestine, it has been reduced to mostly indigestible substances.

Downward spiral

From the ascending colon, chyme passes through the transverse colon and descending colon to the rectum, and finally into the anal canal, where it is expelled. The anal sphincter voluntarily controls defecation, except in infants and patients with spinal cord injuries.

A large job description

The large intestine does not produce hormones or digestive enzymes; it is, however, the site of water and sodium and potassium absorption. The mucosa produces alkaline secretions that lubricate the intestinal wall as chyme pushes through and protect the mucosa from acidic bacterial actions. The large intestine also harbors bacteria, such as *Escherichia coli* and *Enterobacter aerogenes*, which help to break down cellulose into usable carbohydrates and synthesize vitamin K. Vitamin K is needed by humans for blood clotting. Older children and adults get most of their vitamin K from bacteria in the gut and some from their diet. Babies have very little vitamin K in their bodies at birth. Vitamin K does not cross the placenta to the developing baby, and the gut does not have any bacteria to make vitamin K before birth. After birth, there is little vitamin K in breast milk, and breast-fed babies can be low in vitamin K for several weeks until the normal gut bacteria start making it. Infant formula has added vitamin K, but even formula-fed babies have very low levels of vitamin K for several days. With low levels of vitamin K, some babies can have very severe bleeding—sometimes into the brain, causing significant brain damage. This bleeding is called *hemorrhagic disease of the newborn* (HDN). As a preventive measure, babies are routinely given vitamin K injections at birth.

Accessory glands and organs

Allied with the GI tract are the liver, biliary duct system, and pancreas, which contribute the hormones, enzymes, and bile that are vital to digestion.

Liver

The liver is in the right upper quadrant (RUQ) of the abdomen and is the body's largest gland. It plays an important role in carbohydrate metabolism, detoxifies various endogenous and exogenous toxins in plasma, and synthesizes plasma proteins, nonessential amino acids, and vitamin A.

Essential storage

The liver also stores essential nutrients, such as iron and vitamins K, D, and B_{12}. It secretes bile and removes ammonia from body fluids, converting it to urea for excretion in urine.

Biliary duct system

Bile is a greenish fluid that helps the small intestine emulsify and absorb fats and fat-soluble vitamins and neutralize stomach acids. Bile exits through bile ducts that merge into the right and left hepatic ducts to form the common hepatic duct. This common duct joins the cystic duct from the gallbladder to form the common bile duct to the duodenum.

Gallbladder

The gallbladder, located beneath the liver, stores and concentrates bile produced by the liver. Secretion of the hormone cholecystokinin causes the gallbladder to contract and relax the ampulla of Vater, releasing bile into the common bile duct for delivery to the duodenum.

Pancreas

The pancreas is a large gland located behind the stomach and attached to the duodenum. The pancreas performs exocrine and endocrine functions. Its exocrine function involves cells that secrete digestive enzymes, bicarbonate, and hormones into the small intestine to aid in digestion.

Alpha beta Langerhans

The endocrine function of the pancreas involves the islets of Langerhans, which house alpha and beta cells. Alpha cells secrete glucagon, which stimulates glycogenolysis in the liver. Beta cells secrete insulin to promote carbohydrate metabolism.

Diagnostic tests

Tests used to diagnose GI disorders include air or barium enema, barium swallow, endoscopic retrograde cholangiopancreatography (ERCP), endoscopy, and stool specimen testing.

Air or barium enema

An air or barium enema, also called a *lower GI series*, allows x-ray visualization of the colon. Air or barium is introduced into the rectum after insertion of a rectal tube, and a series of fluoroscopy and x-rays are taken as the air or barium passes through the lower GI tract.

Nursing considerations

Explain the procedure to the child and their caregivers. Prepare the child for insertion of the rectal tube and air or barium and explain that they may be slightly uncomfortable as they change positions on the x-ray table. Also explain that the child will have to wait until the test is over to expel air or to go to the bathroom and that their bowel movements may look whitish until the barium has passed through their system.

- Usually, the child will be on a liquid diet for 24 hours before the test.

An interesting way to start the day

- Bowel preparations are administered before the examination; an enema the night before the test, the morning of the test, or both may be used for children and infants. (Prepare the child for the enema and provide as much privacy as possible.)
- Tell the child that x-rays will be taken on a test table and that they must hold still (even though they will feel like they have to go to the bathroom).
- Cover the genital area with a lead apron during the x-rays.

Exit the barium

- Hydrate the child well with electrolyte-containing fluids after the procedure to prevent dehydration and to help expel the barium to prevent barium impaction.

Barium swallow

A barium or diatrizoate meglumine (Gastrografin) swallow, also called an *upper GI series*, provides imaging of the upper GI tract. It is used primarily to examine the esophagus.

Follow the swallow

A series of x-rays is taken while the swallowed barium or Gastrografin moves into the esophagus, stomach, and duodenum to reveal abnormalities. The barium outlines the stomach walls and delineates ulcer craters and filling defects. Gastrografin and barium facilitate imaging through x-rays, but Gastrografin is less toxic if it escapes from the GI tract.

Seeking the ileocecal valve

A small bowel series is an extension of the upper GI series; additional imaging is done as the barium or Gastrografin flows farther down the GI tract through the small intestine to the ileocecal valve.

Nursing considerations

- Explain the procedure to the child and their caregivers. Tell the child that they will need to take big swallows of a thick drink that looks like a milkshake but does not taste as good. Explain that pictures will be taken while they are drinking and afterward and that they will need to hold still during the x-rays.
- Maintain the child on a nothing by mouth (NPO) status beginning at midnight before the test.
- After the test, monitor bowel movements for excretion of barium and monitor GI function.

Endoscopy

Endoscopy allows visualization of the GI system (and, when needed, biopsy of tissue) with a fiberoptic scope.

The direct approach

Fiberoptic testing allows direct visualization of the GI tract. Different types of fiberoptic testing are used to examine different portions of the GI tract:

- *Esophagogastroduodenoscopy* allows visual inspection of the esophagus, stomach, and duodenum.
- *Colonoscopy* allows direct visualization of the descending, transverse, and ascending colon.
- *Proctosigmoidoscopy* allows inspection of the anus, rectum, and distal sigmoid colon.

Nursing considerations

- Explain the procedure to the child and their caregivers and make sure that written, informed consent has been obtained.
- Oral and tongue piercings must be removed. They may accidently dislodge and enter airway as foreign bodies.
- Prepare the child for sedation by explaining that it will make them sleepy and will keep them from hurting during the procedure.
- A mild sedative may be administered before the examination; prepare the child for insertion of an intravenous (IV) line for sedation during this procedure.
- The child may be kept on NPO status beginning at midnight before the test for an upper GI series.
- The child may be placed on a liquid diet for 24 hours before the examination or require enemas and laxatives until the bowel is clear for a lower GI series.
- After the procedure, assess vital signs for dyspnea and fever with a decrease in blood pressure and an increase in pulse, indicating the possibility of bleeding from perforation.

Stool specimen

Stool specimens are obtained to examine the stool for suspected GI bleeding, infection, or malabsorption. Tests include the guaiac test for occult blood and microscopic tests for ova, parasites, and fat.

Nursing considerations

Nursing interventions focus on proper collection and handling of the specimen.

- Obtain the specimen in the correct container (the container may need to be sterile or contain a preservative).
- Be aware that the specimen may need to be transported to the laboratory immediately or placed in the refrigerator.
- For infants, stool specimens may be obtained from the diaper. However, apply a urine bag to prevent urine from contaminating the stool.

Treatments and procedures

Treatments and procedures for children with GI disorders include alternative feeding methods, and GI intubation.

Alternative feeding methods

Children who are unable to take nutrients by mouth (e.g., premature neonates with a poor sucking reflex, children who cannot take in enough calories, or children with disorders of the mouth and esophagus, such as atresia and fistulas) are fed by alternative feeding methods. These methods include nasogastric (NG) gavage, orogastric (OG) gavage, duodenum and jejunum gavage, gastrostomy feedings, and jejunostomy feedings. These feedings may be administered intermittently or continuously.

Nursing considerations

Explain to the child and their caregivers why the alternative feeding method is needed and prepare the child for insertion of the feeding tube.

NG and OG feedings

In NG and OG feedings, a tube is inserted into the stomach by way of one of the nares (NG) or the mouth (OG). Follow these steps:
* To determine the correct length of the feeding tube, measure from the tip of the child's nose to their ear and add to that amount the length from their ear to their xiphoid process.

Cold coil in a cup
* Lubricate the tube with sterile water or a water-soluble lubricant before administration.
* Facilitate insertion of the NG tube by having the child take large swallows of water as the tube is being inserted; allow the child to practice first. When the feeding tube is secured, check placement immediately by checking the pH of aspirate from the NG tube or by requesting a chest radiograph. A pH of between 0 and 5 confirms placement of an NG tube.
* Placement of the NG tube should be checked regularly—at the start of intermittent feedings and at least every 4 hours thereafter.

Recycle the residual
* Check the residual amount of formula by aspirating stomach contents into a syringe. Record the amount of residual formula and the color, odor, and consistency of the gastric contents before refeeding the contents.
* Administer feeding by gravity or feeding pump.

Clear the clogs
* Irrigate the feeding tube with 10 mL of sterile water after each feeding to prevent stagnant formula from clogging the tube.
* Record the total amount of formula administered and describe how well it was tolerated. Observe for signs of aspiration and

intolerance, including low oxygen saturation, difficulty breathing, increased crying or discomfort, and vomiting.

Pinch and position
- If the feeding tube will be removed after feeding, pinch the tube while withdrawing it to prevent aspirating fluid left in the tube.
- Position the child with their head elevated during the feeding and for 1 hour afterward to prevent aspiration.

Sucking for satiation
- When feeding infants by NG or OG tube, nonnutritive sucking is essential for oral stimulation. It helps the infant to relate a full stomach with oral sucking and fulfills the developmental need to suck.

Duodenum and jejunum gavage feedings
Duodenum and jejunum gavage feedings are administered with indwelling feeding tubes in the duodenum or jejunum.

Feedings are administered as they are with NG and OG feedings; however, the residual gastric contents and tube placement do not need to be checked. Duodenum and jejunum feeding tubes are not removed after each feeding.

Gastrostomy and jejunostomy feedings
Gastrostomy and jejunostomy feedings are administered with a surgically placed feeding tube. The tube has one exit site on the abdomen but is composed of two separate chambers, each with a unique entry port. One side of the tube ends in the stomach and is typically used for medication administration. The other side of the tube ends in the jejunum and is typically used for formula administration.

It wouldn't work in outer space
In gastrostomy and jejunostomy feedings:
- Boluses of formula or water are administered by gravity or by feeding pump.
- The feeding tube must be flushed with sterile water after each feeding to prevent clogs.
- The child should be positioned with their head elevated at a 30-degree angle after feeding to prevent aspiration and encourage gastric emptying.
- Long-term gastrostomy tubes have a button closure that allows for the removal of the gastrostomy tube between feedings.
- As with NG or OG tubes, infants fed by gastrostomy tube should engage in nonnutritive sucking for oral stimulation. It helps the infant to relate a full stomach with oral sucking and fulfills the developmental need to suck.

GI intubation

GI intubation is the insertion of an NG tube for diagnostic and therapeutic purposes. It is used to:

- empty the stomach and intestine
- aid in diagnosis and treatment of stomach and upper GI tract disorders
- decompress obstructed areas
- detect and treat GI bleeding
- administer medications or feedings.

Nursing considerations

Prepare the child for insertion of the NG tube with a simple, age-appropriate explanation. Because many children panic at the sight of the tube, it is important to maintain a calm and reassuring manner and provide emotional support.

In addition, follow these steps:

- When inserting the tube, instruct the child to take swallows of water to ease insertion, which also gives the child a job to do and provides a degree of distraction.

What goes in must come out

- Maintain accurate intake and output records.
- Record the amount, color, odor, and consistency of gastric drainage every 4 hours. Coffee-ground–like contents may indicate GI bleeding.
- When irrigating the tube, note the amount of normal saline solution instilled and aspirated.
- Check for fluid and electrolyte imbalances.
- Provide good oral and nasal care. Make sure the tube is secure and does not put pressure on the nostrils.
- Medications are given in liquid form. Clamp the tube for 30 to 45 minutes to ensure medication absorption before reconnecting suction.

Anchors away

- To support the tube's weight and prevent its unintentional removal, anchor the tube to the child's clothing.
- After removing the tube from a child with GI bleeding, watch for signs and symptoms of recurrent bleeding.

GI disorders

GI disorders that may affect children include appendicitis, celiac disease, Hirschsprung disease, intussusception, pyloric stenosis, intussusception, and pyloric stenosis.

Appendicitis

Appendicitis is an inflammation and obstruction of the blind sac (vermiform appendix) at the end of the cecum. It is one of the most common major surgical diseases in school-aged children, and its peak incidence occurs in children between ages 10 and 12 years. Although the appendix has no known function, it does regularly fill and empty itself with food.

What causes it

The appendiceal lumen becomes obstructed with fecal matter, calculi, tumors, or strictures from trauma or infection due to bacteria, viruses, or parasites.

How it happens

The obstruction of the appendiceal lumen sets off an inflammatory process that can lead to infection, thrombosis, necrosis, and perforation. If the appendix ruptures or perforates, the infected contents spill into the abdominal cavity, causing peritonitis.

What to look for

At first, midabdominal cramps and tenderness are diffuse; eventually, they localize in the right lower quadrant (RLQ) at McBurney point. The child will guard against anyone trying to examine the abdomen. (See *Abdomen assessment tips*.)

Advice from the experts

Abdomen assessment tips

Keep these tips in mind when assessing a child's abdomen:
- Warm your hands before beginning the assessment.
- Note guarding of the abdomen and the child's ability to move around on the examination table.
- Flex the child's knees to decrease muscle tightening in the abdomen.
- Have the child use deep breathing or distraction during the examination; a parent can help divert the child's attention.

- Have the child "help" with the examination. Place your hand over the child's hand on the abdomen and extend your fingers beyond the child's fingers to decrease ticklishness of palpating the abdomen.
- Before palpation, auscultate the abdomen as palpation can produce erratic bowel sounds; lightly palpate tender areas last.

The child may experience nausea and vomiting and have a low-grade fever. Later complaints include lethargy, irritability, constipation, and, rarely, diarrhea.

Much ado about the RLQ

Auscultation reveals normal bowel sounds. As the inflammation increases, constant pain is noted in the RLQ with rebound tenderness; the pain is exacerbated by coughing and deep breathing.

Calm before the storm

If peritonitis occurs, abdominal distention and rigidity progress. Sudden cessation of abdominal pain signals perforation or infarction.

What tests tell you

Diagnosis of appendicitis is based on physical findings and characteristic clinical symptoms. A moderately elevated white blood cell (WBC) count with increased numbers of immature cells supports the diagnosis. C-reactive protein may be elevated. Computed tomography (CT) scan may be used to confirm diagnosis.

Complications

The most common complication of appendicitis is peritonitis from appendix rupture, which is a clinical emergency. Signs and symptoms of peritonitis include fever, abdominal distention and rigidity, sudden relief of pain, decreased bowel sounds, nausea, and vomiting. Other possible complications include ischemic bowel and postoperative wound infection.

How it's treated

Appendectomy is an effective treatment for appendicitis. Laparoscopic appendectomies decrease recovery time and hospital stay. If peritonitis develops, treatment involves GI intubation, parenteral replacement of fluids and electrolytes, and administration of antibiotics. Non-perforated appendicitis is increasingly being treated with antibiotics instead of surgery.

What to do

Because appendectomies are usually performed on an emergency basis, there may not be time to formally prepare the child for surgery.

Seize the day

Seize the opportunities that nursing care provides (bedside care, transporting the child, administering medications) to provide brief explanations and answer the child's questions. At the very least, tell the child that they will be given a special medicine and will not feel anything during surgery.

Tell them where they will be when they wake up and when they will see their caregivers. Tell the child what to expect when they awaken (IV line, NG tube, level of discomfort, and what will be done to make them feel better). In addition, follow these steps:

- Position the child preoperatively in a semi-Fowler or right-side–lying position with knees bent to decrease pain.
- Administer IV fluids to prevent dehydration and keep the patient on NPO status until surgery is performed.
- Never apply heat to the right lower abdomen; this may cause the appendix to rupture.

Postoperative care

- Be aware that the child with a ruptured appendix may have a drain and an NG tube attached to low intermittent suction.
- Keep the incision site clean and dry; change dressings when soiled.

A malodorous sign

- Document the return of bowel sounds, the passing of flatus, and bowel movements—all signs of peristalsis.
- Administer antibiotics and pain medication as ordered.

Infection detection

- Instruct the caregivers in care of incision and the signs and symptoms of infection.

Celiac disease

Celiac disease is an immune reaction to eating gluten, a protein found in wheat, barley, and rye. The disease may become apparent between ages 6 and 18 months, after gluten-containing foods are introduced into the diet. Family history increases the risk of developing celiac disease. In the United States, about 3 to 13 per 1,000 children have celiac disease, although the disease often goes undiagnosed. It is more common in people who have type 1 diabetes and a family member with celiac disease or dermatitis herpetiformis, Down syndrome or Turner syndrome, autoimmune thyroid disease, Sjögren syndrome, or microscopic colitis.

What causes it

This disorder probably results from environmental factors and a genetic predisposition, but the exact mechanism is unknown. Some genetic mutations appear to increase the risk of developing the disease.

How it happens

When the body's immune system overreacts to gluten in food, the immune reaction damages the villi that line the small intestine.

Villi absorb vitamins, minerals, and other nutrients from food. The damage resulting from celiac disease makes the inner surface of the small intestine unable to absorb nutrients necessary for health and growth. As a result, children with celiac disease may become malnourished if the condition remains undiagnosed.

What to look for

Symptoms vary but typically include recurrent attacks of diarrhea or constipation, steatorrhea (fatty, foul-smelling stools), abdominal pain and distention, vomiting, anorexia, irritability, and coagulation difficulties from the malabsorption of fat-soluble vitamins. Inspection reveals signs of generalized malnutrition and failure to thrive, such as a potbelly or muscle wasting in buttocks and legs.

What tests tell you

- Histologic changes seen on small bowel biopsy specimens confirm the diagnosis.
- A glucose tolerance test shows poor glucose absorption.
- Serum laboratory tests indicate decreases in levels of albumin, calcium, sodium, potassium, cholesterol, and phospholipids.
- Hemoglobin level, hematocrit, WBC counts, and platelet counts may also be decreased.
- Immunologic assay screen (immunoglobulin [Ig] A and IgG antibodies) is positive for celiac disease.
- Stool specimens reveal a high-fat content.
- Endoscopy is done to view the small intestine and to take a small tissue biopsy to analyze for damage to the villi.

Complications

If not detected and properly treated, celiac disease can cause malnutrition, loss of calcium and bone density, lactose intolerance, and cancer. People with celiac disease who do not maintain a gluten-free diet have a greater risk of developing several forms of cancer, including intestinal lymphoma and small bowel cancer.

How it's treated

Lifelong elimination of gluten from the child's diet is essential and is the only treatment for managing celiac disease. In addition to wheat, foods that contain gluten include barley, bulgur, durum, farina, graham flour, malt, rye, semolina, spelt (a form of wheat), triticale, and, sometimes, oats.

A high-protein, low-fat, high-calorie diet is required. Supportive treatment includes gluten-free vitamins to supplement folic acid, calcium, phosphorus, magnesium, vitamin B_{12}, and iron. Children may also receive administration of vitamins A, E, K, and D in water-soluble forms.

What to do

Because of the need for lifelong adherence to the diet, the child and their caregivers should be referred to a nutritionist who can help them make informed choices and plan a nutritious diet. (See *Teaching points for celiac disease.*)

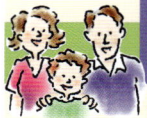

It's all relative

Teaching points for celiac disease

Nursing interventions for a child with celiac disease focus primarily on educating the caregivers about caring for the child at home, with an emphasis on dietary needs:

• Eliminate gluten from the diet.
• Replace vitamins and calories; give small, frequent meals.
• Monitor for steatorrhea; its disappearance is a good indicator that the child's ability to absorb nutrients is improving.
• Read nutritional labels for sources of gluten. Packaged foods should be avoided unless they are labeled as gluten free or have no gluten-containing ingredients. In addition to cereals, pastas, and baked goods—such as breads, cakes, pies, and cookies—other packaged foods that may contain gluten include beer; candies; gravies; imitation meats or seafood; processed luncheon meats; salad dressings and sauces, including soy sauce; self-basting poultry; and soups. Some hair products and skin products also contain gluten.

Hirschsprung disease

Hirschsprung disease (congenital aganglionic megacolon) is the absence of parasympathetic ganglionic cells in a segment of the colon, usually at the distal end of the large intestine. The lack of nerve innervation causes an absence of or alteration in peristalsis in the affected part of the colon. (See *A look at Hirschsprung disease.*)

A look at Hirschsprung disease

Hirschsprung disease is a congenital disorder of the large intestine characterized by the absence or marked reduction of parasympathetic ganglion cells in the colorectal wall.

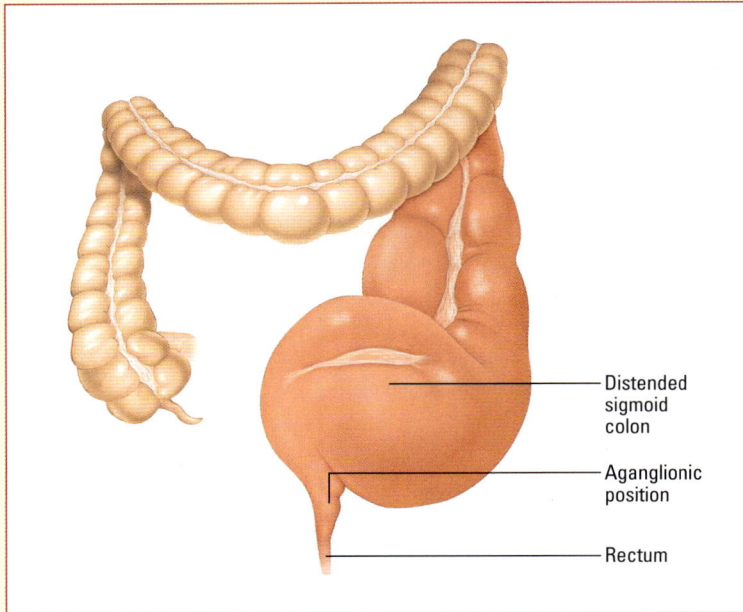

- Distended sigmoid colon
- Aganglionic position
- Rectum

What causes it

Hirschsprung disease is a congenital condition in which nerves fail to develop in all or part of the large intestine. Waste cannot pass through the portion of the colon that lacks nerve tissue. The disease may coexist with other congenital anomalies, particularly Down syndrome, and anomalies of the urinary tract. According to the National Institute of Diabetes and Digestive and Kidney Diseases, 1 in 5,000 children are affected, but 1 in 100 children with Down syndrome have Hirschsprung disease.

How it happens

As stool enters the affected part of the colon, because of the lack of nerve tissue, it remains there until additional stool pushes it through. This affected part of the colon dilates, and a mechanical obstruction may result.

What to look for

In a neonate, history commonly reveals a failure to pass meconium and stool within the first 24 to 48 hours after birth. On inspection, the infant may have abdominal distention and easily palpable stool masses. When stool does pass through, it is liquid or ribbon-like. The child may experience bile stained or fecal vomiting, irritability, lethargy, and weight loss. They may exhibit signs of dehydration, including pallor, dry mucous membranes, and sunken eyes.

What tests tell you

- Rectal biopsy provides definitive diagnosis by showing the absence of ganglion cells.
- Rectal manometry reveals failure of the internal anal sphincter to relax and contract.
- Abdominal x-rays, using contrast dye, show distention of the colon.

Complications

Disease progression causes the most complications, including severe diarrhea, bowel perforation, sepsis, incontinence, stricture formation, enterocolitis, and hypovolemic shock.

How it's treated

Surgery to remove or bypass the affected part of the colon is the treatment of choice in these children. Surgery should be performed as soon as the child's fluid and electrolyte imbalances are stabilized.

Out with the bad

Laparoscopic surgery involves pulling the ganglionic segment of bowel through to the anus to remove the affected portion. This is sometimes called a "pull-through surgery." If a total obstruction is present, surgery may be done in two steps. A temporary colostomy or ileostomy may be necessary to decompress the colon. Next, a second surgery is performed to remove the affected segment of bowel and close the ostomy.

What to do

The infant's caregivers will need a great deal of emotional support. Prepare them for each procedure, including surgeries, by offering thorough explanations and making sure that their questions are answered. Encourage them to express their feelings and concerns and encourage their participation in the infant's care to the extent possible.

Preoperative care

- Administer IV fluids to maintain fluid and electrolyte balance and prevent dehydration and shock.
- Maintain NPO status and insert an NG tube for gastric decompression.

Forced evacuation

- Administer isotonic enemas (normal saline solution) to evacuate the bowels and prevent enterocolitis before surgery; do not administer tap water due to the risk of water intoxication.
- Administer antibiotics and other medications as ordered.

Postoperative care

After colostomy or ileostomy, follow these steps:

- Monitor fluid intake and output; an ileostomy is especially likely to cause excessive electrolyte loss.
- Keep the area around the stoma clean and dry; use colostomy or ileostomy appliances to collect drainage.
- Monitor for return of bowel sounds to begin diet.
  After corrective surgery, follow these steps:
- Keep the wound clean and dry to prevent infection.
- Do not use a rectal thermometer or suppositories.

Bowel sounds = dinner bell

- Begin oral feedings when active bowel sounds begin and NG drainage decreases.
- Educate the caregivers about suture line care.
- Teach the caregivers how to recognize the beginning signs of constipation, such as straining during defecation and a distended abdomen, fluid loss and dehydration (decreased urine output, sunken eyes, poor skin turgor), enterocolitis (vomiting, diarrhea, fever, lethargy, sudden marked abdominal distention), and strictures (abdominal distention, constipation, vomiting).

Expert advice

- Before discharge (if possible), arrange for a consultation with an enterostomal therapist who can provide the caregivers with valuable tips on colostomy or ileostomy care.
- Teach the caregivers which foods increase the number of stools (raisins, prunes, plums) and tell them to avoid offering these foods.

Patience is a virtue

- Caution the caregivers that complete continence of stool can take years to develop and that constipation may occur.

Intussusception

Intussusception is a telescoping or invagination of a bowel segment into itself, the most common site being the ileocecal valve. It usually occurs at about age 6 months but can occur in children up to age 3 years and, rarely, in older children. It's almost equal in males and females until age 4 years, then more common in males, and is more likely to occur in children with cystic fibrosis.

Intussusception can be fatal, especially if treatment is delayed for more than 24 hours. (See *Understanding intussusception*.)

Understanding intussusception

In intussusception, a bowel section invaginates and is propelled along by peristalsis, pulling in more bowel. In this illustration, a portion of the cecum invaginates and is propelled into the large intestine. Intussusception typically produces edema, hemorrhage from venous engorgement, incarceration, and obstruction.

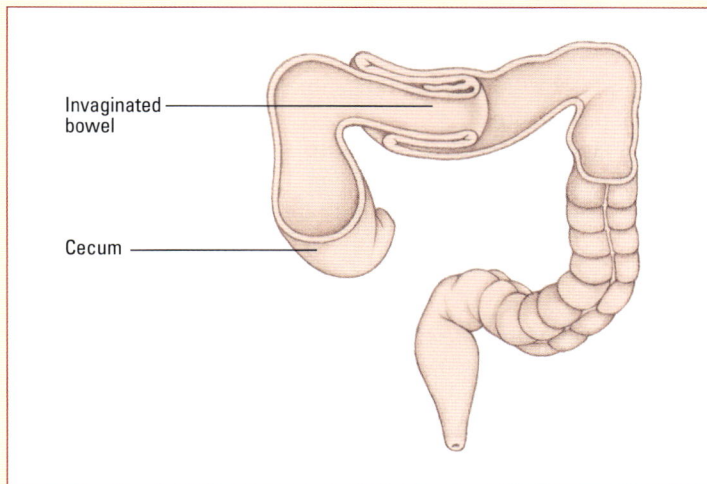

Invaginated bowel

Cecum

What causes it

The cause of intussusception is unknown in most cases. It may result from polyps, hyperactive peristalsis, or an abnormal bowel lining. It may also be linked to viral infections because seasonal peaks are noted (spring and summer).

How it happens

When a bowel segment invaginates, peristalsis propels it along the bowel, pulling more bowel along with it. Invagination causes inflammation and swelling at the affected site. Edema eventually causes obstruction and necrosis from occlusion of the blood supply to the bowel.

What to look for

The medical history may reveal intermittent attacks of colicky abdominal pain characterized by screaming, drawing knees to the chest, sweating, and grunting. Caregivers report vomitus-containing bile or fecal material, which can lead to dehydration, fluid and electrolyte imbalance, and metabolic alkalosis. They also describe the passage of red, "currant jelly–like" stool containing mucus and blood. Passage of "currant jelly–like" stool is a late sign.

Tender to the touch

Inspection and palpation may reveal a distended and tender abdomen with a palpable, sausage-shaped abdominal mass. Other clinical signs include fever, increased pulse, shallow respirations, and decreased blood pressure (shock-like state).

What tests tell you

- Abdominal x-rays and ultrasound or CT show a soft tissue mass and signs of complete or partial obstruction.
- Barium or air contrast enemas may be used to help diagnose intussusception. Barium should be used with caution as the barium may leak through an unsuspected perforation and cause peritonitis.

Complications

Without proper treatment, strangulation of the intestine may occur, with gangrene, shock, perforation, and peritonitis. These complications can be fatal.

How it's treated

An NG tube is inserted to decompress the intestine and minimize vomiting. Ten percent of children with intussusception may have a spontaneous reduction of the bowel. Therapy may include hydrostatic reduction or surgery.

Forceful introduction

During hydrostatic reduction, air pressure or water-soluble contrast medium is introduced into the rectum using fluoroscopy. The force from the fluid or air moves the invaginated bowel back into its original position.

If at first you don't succeed . . . reduce or resect

Surgery is indicated when hydrostatic reduction fails, intussusception recurs, or signs of shock or peritonitis are present. Manual reduction is attempted first by pulling the intussusception back through the bowel. If manual reduction fails, or if the bowel segment is gangrenous or strangulated, resection of the affected bowel segment is performed.

What to do

Intussusception is a painful condition; the onset of symptoms may be sudden and severe. The child may be inconsolable, and the caregivers are likely to be terrified and distressed from seeing their child in so much pain. Provide the caregivers with as much emotional support and reassurance as possible.

Explain on the go

Because intussusception is treated as an emergency, use caregiving opportunities (during bedside care, medication administration, transport to testing areas) to provide as much explanation as possible about tests and procedures and make sure the caregivers' questions are answered.

Music to soothe

To the extent possible, allow the caregivers to remain with the child to comfort them (by holding them, stroking the child's face and hands, singing a soothing song).

Better days ahead

For the child who is old enough to understand, provide simple explanations as procedures are being performed and reassure them that you are there to help them and they will feel better soon.

- Prepare for air enema insertion or water-soluble contrast medium to confirm the diagnosis and reduce the invagination by hydrostatic pressure.
- Monitor vital signs; a change in temperature may indicate sepsis.
- Monitor intake and output to prevent dehydration and administer IV fluids as ordered.
- Monitor NG tube output and replace volume lost as ordered.
- Administer pain medication as ordered.
- For the child who has undergone hydrostatic reduction, monitor for the passage of stool to determine the need for surgery.

Postoperative care

After surgery, encourage the caregivers to stay with the child as much as possible. In addition, follow these steps:

- Administer antibiotics as ordered to prevent infection.
- Monitor the incision site for signs of infection, such as inflammation, drainage, and suture separation.
- Monitor for the return of bowel sounds to allow advancement of the diet.
- Continue to offer emotional support and encouragement to the caregivers.

Pyloric stenosis

Pyloric stenosis is hyperplasia (increased mass) and hypertrophy (increased size) of the circular muscle at the pylorus, the lower opening of the stomach leading to the duodenum. The increased mass and size of the muscle narrows the pyloric canal, preventing the stomach from emptying normally. Pyloric obstruction leads to vomiting and gastritis from prolonged filling of the stomach. It's most commonly seen in males between ages 1 and 6 months. The incidence is 2 to 4 per 1,000 live births.

What causes it

The exact cause of pyloric stenosis is unknown. It is not an inherited disorder but may have a genetic component as it can occur in siblings and offspring of affected people. It occurs more often in male babies (especially first-born) and in infants born prematurely. There is an increased risk with birthing parent smoking during pregnancy. It may be associated with malrotation, esophageal atresia, and anorectal malformations.

How it happens

Spasms of the pylorus muscle cause the narrowing of the passageway between the stomach and the duodenum. Swelling and inflammation further reduce the size of the lumen and could result in complete obstruction. Normal emptying of the stomach is prevented, resulting in vomiting and gastritis.

What to look for

Palpation reveals an olive-shaped bulge below the right costal margin and a distended upper abdomen.

Waving and projecting

The child experiences projectile vomiting during or shortly after feedings. The vomiting is preceded by reverse peristaltic waves (left to right), but not by nausea. Vomitus is not bile stained but may be blood stained due to gastritis. Constipation and very little urine occur as very little food or fluid gets into the intestines.

Déjà lunch

The child will resume eating after vomiting and exhibits poor weight gain. Symptoms of malnutrition and dehydration are present despite the child's apparent adequate intake of food.

What tests tell you

- Vomitus may be positive for blood.

- Blood chemistry may reveal hypocalcemia, hyponatremia, hypokalemia, and hypochloremia.
- Arterial blood gas analysis may reveal metabolic alkalosis.
- Abdominal ultrasound reveals a hypertrophied sphincter and confirms the diagnosis of pyloric stenosis.

Complications

Complications of pyloric stenosis include malnutrition, dehydration, infection, metabolic alkalosis, and failure to thrive.

How it is treated

Surgery, a pyloromyotomy, is performed by laparoscopy to treat pyloric stenosis.

The child remains on NPO status before surgery. IV fluids are administered to correct fluid and electrolyte imbalances and prevent dehydration, and an NG tube is inserted and kept open for gastric decompression.

What to do

Provide the child with an age-appropriate explanation of all tests, procedures, and surgery. Make sure the caregivers' questions are answered. In addition, follow these steps:
- Monitor vital signs and intake and output to assess renal function and check for dehydration.
- Record the amount of vomitus as well as its frequency, characteristics, and relation to feedings.
- Perform daily weight measurements on the same scale to assess growth. Using the same scale every day ensures that the weight measurements are accurate.
- Assess abdominal and cardiovascular status to detect early signs of compromise.
- Position the child, preferably on their right side, to prevent aspiration of vomitus.

Postoperative care
- Feed the child small amounts of oral electrolyte solution and then increase the amount and concentration of food until normal feeding is achieved.

No need to say "excuse me"
- Hold the child upright and burp them frequently during feedings.
- Provide a pacifier to maintain comfort and satisfy the infant's sucking reflex.
- Monitor intake and output.
- Keep the incision area clean to prevent infection; clean with soap and water, and keep the diaper's contents away from the incision.

Going with the flow

- Position the child on their right side, allowing gravity to help the flow of fluid through the pyloric valve; elevate the child's head after feeding.
- Administer analgesic agents around the clock for pain management.
- Teach the caregivers proper incision site care and to monitor for signs and symptoms of infection and dehydration.
- When diapering the infant, gently slide the diaper under the buttocks rather than lifting the legs up; fold the front of the diaper to keep below the incision.

Quick quiz

1. A 2-month-old male infant is admitted with a diagnosis of pyloric stenosis. Due to the projectile vomiting he has had, which problem is he at risk for?
    A. Metabolic acidosis
    B. Metabolic alkalosis
    C. Hyperkalemia
    D. Hypernatremia

Answer: B. Projectile vomiting causes loss of hydrochloric acid, which results in metabolic alkalosis.

2. A 12-year-old male is admitted to the pediatric unit with complaints of RLQ abdominal pain and vomiting. When the nurse checks on the child 2 hours later, he states that the pain has stopped. The nurse should suspect that:
    A. he had indigestion, which has been relieved.
    B. he's afraid of going to surgery.
    C. his appendix has ruptured.
    D. he has irritable bowel syndrome.

Answer: C. Abdominal pain in the RLQ and vomiting are symptoms of appendicitis. When the appendix ruptures, a sudden relief of pain occurs, after which the pain resumes more severely. Indigestion would indicate epigastric pain. Irritable bowel syndrome may affect entire abdomen, not just RLQ. Fear of surgery does not suddenly stop pain.

3. An 18-month-old child is admitted to the pediatric unit with intussusception. As the nurse is preparing the child for an air enema reduction, they pass a soft brown stool. What should the nurse do?
    A. Notify the doctor in order to cancel the procedure.
    B. Prepare the child for emergency surgery.
    C. Take vital signs and monitor for abdominal sounds.
    D. Administer an enema to clear the rectal area for testing.

Answer: A. Passing a normal-looking brown stool indicates that the child no longer has an invaginated section of bowel. Passing a brown stool is a normal passage that does not indicate preparation for emergency surgery or administration of an enema. The nurse may obtain vital signs and monitor for abdominal sounds after notifying the doctor of the passage of a normal stool.

4. The nurse is completing discharge teaching for a child and their caregivers regarding the diet to treat celiac disease. Which meal selection would be appropriate for this child?
- A. A bologna sandwich on whole wheat bread, a chocolate chip cookie, and a glass of milk
- B. A vegetable pizza, an apple, and a diet cola
- C. A corn tortilla with hamburger and cooked vegetables and a glass of fruit juice
- D. A hot dog on a roll, celery and carrot sticks, and a chocolate milkshake

Answer: C. Celiac disease is intolerance to wheat, barley, rye, and oats. Some of these children also have lactose intolerance, especially when they have an acute episode of the disease. Wheat bread, pizza dough, and hot dog rolls contain grains, which the child is unable to eat. Milk and milkshakes contain lactose.

Scoring

☆☆☆ If you answered all four items correctly, congratulations! You've thoroughly digested the material in this chapter.

☆☆ If you answered three items correctly, good job! Your knowledge of GI disorders is unobstructed.

☆ If you answered fewer than three items correctly, don't give yourself an ulcer! Swallow your pride and prepare for the last three quizzes.

Suggested References

Centers for Disease Control and Prevention. (2024). *Immunization schedules*. https://www.cdc.gov/vaccines/hcp/imz-schedules/index.html.

Cochran, W. J. (2022a). Hypertrophic pyloric stenosis. In J. Belkind-Gerson (Ed.), *Merck manual professional version*. Merck & Co. Inc. https://www.merckmanuals.com/professional/pediatrics/gastrointestinal-disorders-in-neonates-and-infants/hypertrophic-pyloric-stenosis

Cochran, W. J. (2022b). Intussusception. In J. Belkind-Gerson (Ed.), *Merck manual professional version*. Merck & Co. Inc. https://www.merckmanuals.com/professional/pediatrics/gastrointestinal-disorders-in-neonates-and-infants/intussusception

Goday, P. S. (2021). Gastrointestinal disorders: Red flags and best treatments. *Contemporary PEDS Journal, 38*, 16–19.

Hatfield, N. T., & Kincheloe, C. A. (2022). Gastrointestinal disorders. In N. T. Hatfield & C. A. Kincheloe (Eds.), *Introductory maternity & pediatric nursing* (5th ed., pp. 797–821). Wolters Kluwer.

Linnard-Palmer, L. (2019). Gastrointestinal elimination. In L. Linnard-Palmer (Ed.), *Pediatric nursing care: A concept-based approach* (pp. 177–193). Jones & Bartlett Learning.

Lipsett, S. C., Monuteaux, M. C., Shanahan, K. H., & Bachur, R. G. (2022). Nonoperative management of uncomplicated appendicitis. *Pediatrics, 149*(5), e2021054693.

Radiological Society of North America, Inc. (2022). *Therapeutic enema for intussusception.* https://www.radiologyinfo.org/en/info/intussusception

-

Chapter 21

Endocrine and metabolic problems

Just the facts

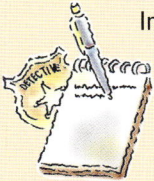

In this chapter, you'll learn:

◆ function of the glands of the endocrine system

◆ tests used to diagnose endocrine and metabolic problems

◆ treatments for children with endocrine and metabolic problems

◆ disorders of the endocrine system and metabolic function.

Anatomy and physiology

The endocrine system is composed of glands that secrete hormones necessary for normal metabolic function. Along with the nervous system, the endocrine system regulates and integrates the body's metabolic activities. (See *Endocrine system components*.)

Too little, too much

Altered endocrine function involves a hyposecretion or hypersecretion of hormones, which affects the body's metabolic processes and function. Nursing care involves measures to support hormonal secretion, such as hormone replacement, or curtail secretion, such as radiation therapy. Inborn errors of metabolism involve a biochemical alteration that affects metabolism.

Glands

The major glands of the endocrine system are:
- pituitary gland
- thyroid gland
- parathyroid glands
- adrenal glands
- pancreas
- ovaries and testes.

Endocrine system components

Endocrine glands secrete hormones directly into the bloodstream to regulate body function. This illustration shows the locations of the major endocrine glands (except the gonads).

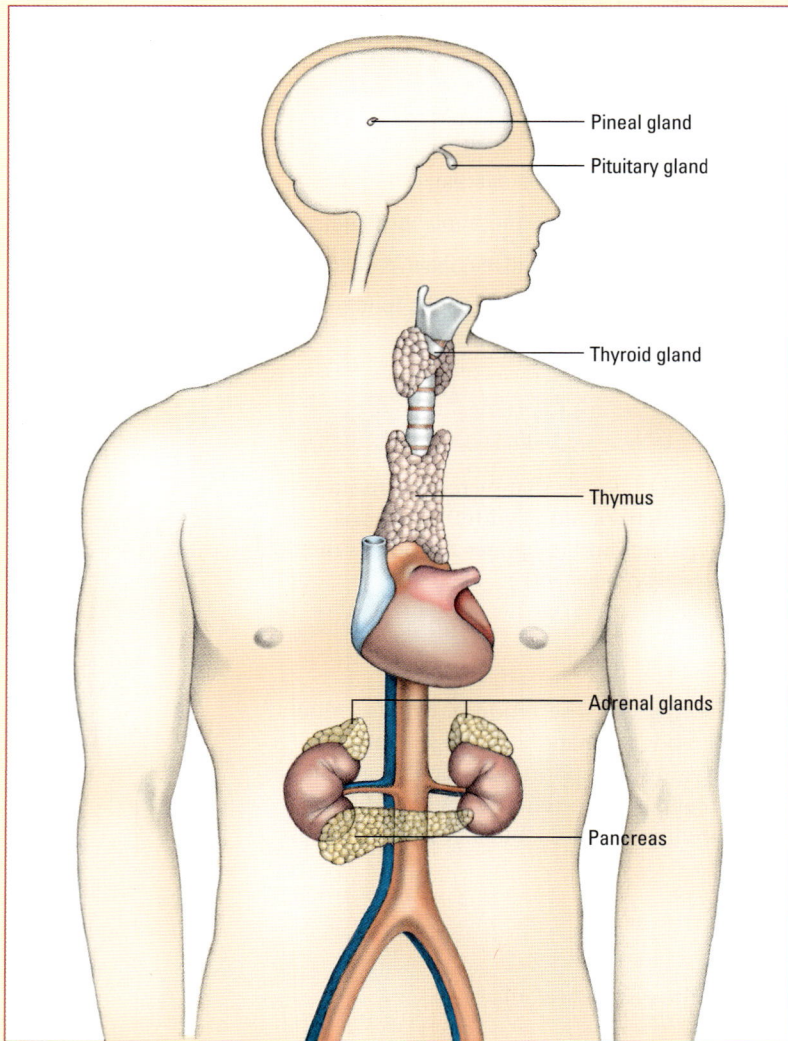

Pituitary gland

The pituitary gland (also called the *hypophysis* or *master gland*) rests in the sella turcica, a depression in the sphenoid bone at the base of the brain.

Small but mighty

This pea-sized gland connects with the hypothalamus via the infundibulum, from which it receives chemical and nervous stimulation. The pituitary has two main regions:

1. Anterior pituitary
2. Posterior pituitary

Prolific producer

The anterior pituitary, also called the *adenohypophysis*, makes up 80% of the pituitary gland. It produces seven hormones:

1. Growth hormone (GH) or *somatotropin*
2. Thyroid-stimulating hormone (TSH) or *thyrotropin*
3. Corticotropin
4. Follicle-stimulating hormone (FSH)
5. Luteinizing hormone (LH)
6. Prolactin
7. Melanocyte-stimulating hormone

Hormones in storage

The posterior pituitary, or *neurohypophysis*, makes up about 20% of the pituitary gland. It serves as a storage area for antidiuretic hormone (ADH) or *vasopressin*, and oxytocin, which are produced by the hypothalamus.

Thyroid gland

The thyroid gland lies directly below the larynx, partially in front of the trachea. Its two lateral lobes—one on either side of the trachea—join with a narrow tissue bridge, called the *isthmus*, to give the gland its butterfly shape.

Thyroid lobe duo

The two lobes of the thyroid gland function as one unit to produce the hormones triiodothyronine (T_3), thyroxine (T_4), and calcitonin. T_3 and T_4 are collectively referred to as thyroid hormones (THs), the body's major metabolic hormones. They regulate metabolism by speeding up cellular respiration.

The calcitonin–calcium connection

Calcitonin maintains the blood calcium level by inhibiting the release of calcium from bone. Secretion of calcitonin is controlled by the calcium concentration of the fluid surrounding the thyroid cells.

Parathyroid glands

The parathyroid glands are the body's smallest known endocrine glands. These glands are embedded on the posterior surface of the thyroid, one in each corner.

Parathyroid hormone: a parathyroid production

Working together as a single gland, the parathyroid glands produce parathyroid hormone (PTH). The main function of PTH is to help regulate the blood's calcium balance. This hormone adjusts the rate at which calcium and magnesium ions are removed from urine. PTH also increases the movement of phosphate ions from the blood to urine for excretion.

Adrenal glands

There are two adrenal glands in the body; each gland is situated on top of a kidney. These almond-shaped glands contain two distinct structures—the adrenal cortex and the adrenal medulla—that function as separate endocrine glands.

Adrenal cortex

The adrenal cortex is the large outer layer of the adrenal gland and forms the bulk of the gland. It has three zones or cell layers:
1. *Zona glomerulosa*, the outermost zone, which produces mineralo-corticoids, primarily aldosterone
2. *Zona fasciculata*, the middle and largest zone, which produces the glucocorticoids cortisol (hydrocortisone), cortisone, and corticosterone as well as small amounts of the sex hormones androgen and estrogen
3. *Zona reticularis*, the innermost zone, which produces mainly glucocorticoids and some sex hormones

Adrenal medulla

The adrenal medulla, or inner layer of the adrenal gland, functions as part of the sympathetic nervous system and produces two catecholamines:
1. Epinephrine
2. Norepinephrine

A leading role

Because catecholamines play an important role in the autonomic nervous system, the adrenal medulla is considered a neuroendocrine structure.

Pancreas

The pancreas, a triangular gland, is nestled in the curve of the duodenum, stretching horizontally behind the stomach and extending to the spleen. The pancreas performs endocrine and exocrine functions.

Acinar cells make up most of the gland and regulate pancreatic exocrine function.

Clusters of islets

The endocrine cells of the pancreas are called the *islet cells* or *islets of Langerhans*. These cells exist in clusters and are found scattered among the acinar cells. The islets contain alpha, beta, and delta cells that produce important hormones:

- Alpha cells produce glucagon.
- Beta cells produce insulin.
- Delta cells produce somatostatin.

Gonads

The gonads include the ovaries in the female and the testes in the male.

Ovaries

The ovaries are oval-shaped glands in females located on either side of the uterus. They produce ova (eggs) as well as estrogen and progesterone.

It's hormonal

Estrogen and progesterone are responsible for:

- promoting the development and maintenance of female sex characteristics
- regulating the menstrual cycle
- maintaining the uterus for pregnancy
- preparing the mammary glands for lactation.

Testes

The testes are located in the scrotum. They produce the male hormone testosterone, which stimulates and maintains male sex characteristics. They also produce spermatozoa.

Hormones

Hormones are complex chemical substances that trigger or regulate the activity of an organ or a group of cells. They include pituitary hormones, THs, adrenal hormones, androgens, and estrogens. (See *Effects of altered hormonal function.*)

Pituitary hormones

Pituitary hormones include the anterior pituitary hormones (GH, TSH, FSH, LH, and prolactin) and the posterior pituitary hormones

Effects of altered hormonal function

This chart shows the effects that may result from excessive or deficient secretion of select hormones.

Hormone	Hypofunction	Hyperfunction
Anterior pituitary hormones		
GH	• Epiphyseal fusion with cessation of growth • Prepubertal dwarfism • Pituitary cachexia (Simmonds disease) • Generalized delayed growth • Hypoglycemia	• Prepubertal gigantism • Acromegaly (after full growth is attained) • Diabetes • Postpubertal hypoproteinemia
TSH	• Hypothyroidism • Marked delay of puberty • Juvenile myxedema	• Hyperthyroidism • Thyrotoxicosis • Graves disease
Corticotropin	• Acute adrenocortical insufficiency (Addison disease) • Hypoglycemia • Increased skin pigmentation	• Cushing syndrome
Gonadotropins	• Absent or incomplete spontaneous puberty	• Precocious puberty • Early epiphyseal closure
FSH	• Hypogonadism • Sterility • Absence or loss of secondary sex characteristics • Amenorrhea	• Precocious puberty • Primary gonadal failure • Hirsutism • Polycystic ovary • Early epiphyseal closure
LH	• Hypogonadism • Sterility • Impotence • Absence or loss of secondary sex characteristics • Ovarian failure	• Precocious puberty • Primary gonadal failure • Hirsutism • Polycystic ovary • Early epiphyseal closure
Prolactin	• Inability to lactate • Amenorrhea	• Galactorrhea • Functional hypogonadism
Melanocyte-stimulating hormone	• Diminished or absent skin pigmentation	• Increased skin pigmentation
Posterior pituitary hormone		
ADH or vasopressin	• Diabetes insipidus	• Syndrome of inappropriate ADH secretion • Fluid retention • Hyponatremia

Effects of altered hormonal function (*continued*)

TH hormones

T_4 and T_3	• Hypothyroidism • Myxedema • Hashimoto thyroiditis • Greatly reduced general growth (Extent depends on age at which deficiency occurs.) • Cognitive impairment (in infants)	• Exophthalmic goiter (Graves disease) • Accelerated linear growth • Early epiphyseal closure

Parathyroid gland hormone

PTH	• Hypocalcemia (tetany)	• Hypercalcemia (bone demineralization) • Hypophosphatemia

Adrenal hormones

Aldosterone	• Adrenocortical insufficiency	• Electrolyte imbalance • Hyperaldosteronism
Gluco-corticoids (cortisol and corticosterone)	• Addison disease • Acute adrenocortical insufficiency • Impaired growth and sexual function	• Cushing syndrome • Severe impairment of growth with slowing in skeletal maturation

(ADH and oxytocin). Each of these hormones has a particular function:

- GH, secreted by the anterior pituitary gland, affects most body tissues. It triggers growth by increasing protein synthesis and fat mobilization and decreases carbohydrate use.
- TSH is secreted by the anterior pituitary gland and stimulates the thyroid.
- FSH, secreted by the anterior pituitary gland, stimulates the graafian follicles to mature and secrete estrogen in the female. In males, it stimulates development of the seminiferous tubules.
- LH, secreted by the anterior pituitary gland, produces the rupture of the follicle, which results in the discharge of a mature ovum in the female. In the male, it stimulates the production of androgens, particularly testosterone.
- Prolactin is secreted by the anterior pituitary gland and stimulates milk secretion.

- ADH is secreted by the posterior pituitary gland. It controls the concentration of body fluids by altering the permeability of the distal convoluted tubules and collecting ducts of the kidneys to conserve water.
- Oxytocin, secreted by the posterior pituitary gland, stimulates the contraction of the uterus and the letdown reflex in lactating women.

TH hormones

The THs are T_3 and T_4. These hormones are necessary for normal growth and development and act on many tissues to increase metabolic activity and protein synthesis.

Adrenal hormones

The adrenal hormones are cortisol, aldosterone, androgens, and estrogen:

- Cortisol is a glucocorticoid that stimulates glucogenesis and increases protein breakdown and free fatty acid mobilization; it also suppresses the immune response and provides for an appropriate response to stress.
- Aldosterone, a mineralocorticoid, regulates the resorption of sodium and the excretion of potassium by the kidneys; it is affected by corticotropin and is regulated by angiotensin II, which, in turn, is regulated by renin. Together, aldosterone, angiotensin II, and renin are involved in the pathogenesis of hypertension.
- Androgens are male sex hormones; they promote male traits, especially secondary sex characteristics, such as facial hair and a low-pitched voice.
- Estrogens are responsible for the development of secondary female sex characteristics.

Pancreatic hormones

The islets of Langerhans are small clusters of endocrine cells in the pancreas. These structures contain cells that produce insulin, glucagon, and somatostatin:

- Insulin: a hormone that raises the blood glucose level by triggering the breakdown of glycogen to glucose
- Glucagon: lowers the blood glucose level by stimulating the conversion of glucose to glycogen
- Somatostatin: inhibits the release of GH, corticotropin, and certain other hormones

Hormone release and transport

Although all hormone release results from endocrine gland stimulation, release patterns of hormones vary greatly.

- Secretion of PTH (by the parathyroid gland) and prolactin (by the anterior pituitary) occurs fairly evenly throughout the day.
- Corticotropin (secreted by the anterior pituitary) and cortisol (secreted by the adrenal cortex) are released in spurts in response to body rhythm cycles; levels of these hormones peak in the morning.
- Secretion of insulin by the pancreas has both steady and sporadic release patterns.

Hormonal action

When a hormone reaches its target site, it binds to a specific receptor on the cell membrane or within the cell. Polypeptides and some amines bind to membrane receptor sites. The smaller, more lipid-soluble steroids and THs diffuse through the cell membrane and bind to intracellular receptors.

Right on target!

After binding occurs, each hormone produces unique physiologic changes, depending on its target site and its specific action at that site. A particular hormone may have different effects at different target sites.

Hormonal regulation

To maintain the body's delicate equilibrium, a feedback mechanism regulates hormone production and secretion. The mechanism involves hormones, blood chemicals and metabolites, and the nervous system. The feedback mechanism may be simple or complex.

For normal function, each gland must contain enough appropriately programmed secretory cells to release active hormones on demand.

Unsupervised cells

Secretory cells need supervision. A secretory cell can't sense on its own when to release the hormone or how much to release. It gets this information from sensing and signaling systems that integrate many messages. Together, stimulatory and inhibitory signals actively control the rate and duration of hormone release.

It's nice to be recognized

When released, the hormone travels to target cells, where a receptor molecule recognizes it and binds to it. The sensitivity of a target cell depends on how many receptors it has for a particular site. The more receptor sites, the more sensitive the target cell.

Diagnostic tests

Diagnostic tests are used to assess endocrine system problems and metabolic function in the pediatric population:

- *Blood glucose tests* are used to diagnose type 1 and type 2 diabetes. Blood glucose tests commonly used for pediatric patients include the fasting blood glucose test.
- *GH tests* are used to determine pituitary function. The human growth hormone (hGH) test helps detect hypopituitarism, whereas the GH suppression test is used to diagnose pituitary hyperfunction.
- *Neonatal screening*, which began in the 1960s, is now performed in every state and may consist of tests for a variety of diseases. Typically, neonatal screens are performed for commonly occurring diseases that may cause severe cognitive impairment or death without early detection and treatment. These tests are typically done by dried filter paper blood spots. A very small amount of blood is required and is usually obtained by a heel stick. Examples of endocrine and metabolic tests that may be screened for during newborn screening include phenylketonuria (PKU), and congenital hypothyroidism.
- *Thyroid function tests* are used to determine thyroid function and include T_4 and T_3 studies.
- Radioimmunoassay is a test used to measure minute quantities of hormones.

Glucose, fasting plasma

The fasting plasma glucose test (also known as the *fasting blood sugar test*) is commonly used to screen for diabetes. It measures plasma glucose levels after an 8-hour fast.

To fast or not to fast

In the fasting state, plasma glucose levels decrease, stimulating the release of the hormone glucagon. Glucagon then acts to raise plasma glucose by accelerating glycogenolysis, stimulating glyconeogenesis, and inhibiting glycogen synthesis. Normally, secretion of insulin checks this rise in glucose levels. In diabetes, however, the absence or deficiency of insulin allows for persistently high glucose levels.

And the level is . . .

The normal range for fasting plasma glucose varies according to the laboratory procedure. Normal values after a fast of at least 8 hours differ according to the age of the child:

- Premature neonates—40 to 65 mg/dL (SI [Système International d'Unités], 2.2 to 3.6 mmol/L)
- Young children (birth to age 2 years)—60 to 110 mg/dL (SI, 3.3 to 6.1 mmol/L)
- Children (ages 2 to 18 years)—60 to 100 mg/dL (SI, 3.3 to 5.6 mmol/L)

Glucose tells all

A fasting plasma glucose level of 126 mg/dL or higher obtained on two or more occasions confirms provisional diabetes. An impaired blood glucose level is 125 mg/dL. A borderline or transiently elevated level requires a 2-hour postprandial plasma glucose test or an OGTT to confirm the diagnosis. A hemoglobin A_{1C} test may also be conducted to provide the average plasma glucose level over the past 3 months. A level of less than 5.7% is considered normal. Type 2 diabetes is diagnosed when there is a level greater than or equal to 6.5%.

Nursing considerations

- Explain the procedure to the caregivers and the child and encourage the caregivers to stay with the child.
- Determine how long the child must fast.
- Determine if the timing of the patient's medication will interfere with the test results and withhold medication if indicated.

Backup plan

- Apply a topical anesthetic (when possible) to two spots so an alternate puncture site will be available if the first one is not successful.
- Specify on the laboratory request the time the patient last ate, the sample collection time, and the time they received the last pretest dose of insulin (if applicable).

GH, human

The hGH test is used to detect hypopituitarism. Also known as *growth hormone* and *somatotropin*, hGH is a protein secreted by the anterior pituitary and is the primary regulator of human growth. Children generally have higher hGH levels than adults; these levels can range from undetectable to 16 ng/mL (SI, 16 mcg/L).

The hGH test, a quantitative analysis of plasma hGH levels, is usually performed as part of an anterior pituitary stimulation or suppression test.

The lowdown on levels

Increased hGH levels may indicate a pituitary or hypothalamic tumor (commonly an adenoma), which causes gigantism in children and acromegaly in adults and adolescents.

The highs . . .

Patients with diabetes sometimes have elevated hGH levels without acromegaly. Suppression testing is necessary to confirm the diagnosis.

. . . and the lows

Pituitary infarction, metastatic disease, and tumors may reduce hGH levels. Dwarfism may be caused by low hGH levels, but confirmation of the diagnosis requires stimulation testing with arginine or insulin.

Nursing considerations

Prepare the child for the test with a simple, developmentally appropriate explanation. Tell the child and their caregivers that another sample may have to be drawn the following day for comparison. Explain to the caregivers that the laboratory requires at least 2 days of samples for analysis.

In addition, follow these steps:
- Withhold all medications that affect hGH levels, such as pituitary-based steroids, as ordered. If these medications must be continued, note this on the laboratory request.
- Make sure the patient is relaxed and recumbent for 30 minutes before the test because stress and physical activity elevate hGH levels. Explain that the child must fast and limit physical activity for 10 to 12 hours before the test.
- Between 6 a.m. and 8 a.m. on 2 consecutive days, or as ordered, draw venous blood and send it to the laboratory.

GH, suppression

The GH suppression test, also known as the *glucose loading test*, is used to diagnose pituitary hyperfunction. It evaluates excessive baseline levels of hGH from the anterior pituitary by measuring the secretory response to a loading dose of glucose.

Failure to suppress

Normally, hGH raises plasma glucose and fatty acid concentrations; in response, insulin secretion increases to counteract these effects. A glucose load should suppress hGH secretion. In a patient with excessive hGH levels, the failure to suppress hGH indicates anterior pituitary dysfunction and confirms a diagnosis of acromegaly or gigantism.

Glucose normally suppresses hGH to levels ranging from undetectable to 3 ng/mL (SI, 3 mcg/L) in 30 minutes to 2 hours. In a patient with active acromegaly, basal hGH levels are elevated to 75 ng/mL (SI, 75 mcg/L) and aren't suppressed to less than 5 ng/mL (SI, 5 mcg/L) during the test. In children, rebound stimulation may occur after 2 to 5 hours.

Rest and repeat

When the hGH levels are unchanged or increased in response to glucose loading, hGH hypersecretion is indicated and may confirm suspected acromegaly or gigantism. This response may be verified by repeating the test after a 1-day rest.

Nursing considerations

Explain the test to the child and their caregivers. Tell the child that they may experience nausea after drinking the glucose solution and prepare them for the needlesticks. In addition, follow these steps:
- Withhold all steroids; if these or other medications must be continued, note this on the laboratory request.
- Administer up to 75 g of glucose solution by mouth; to prevent nausea, tell the child to drink the glucose slowly.

Neonatal T4 and TSH blood-spot test

Mandatory in all 50 states, a T_4 test is performed as part of the neonatal screening with the sample placed as a blood spot on filter paper. A low T_4 level (less than 6 mg/dL) must be followed by a TSH level, which may be performed on the same blood sample or from a separate sample. (See *Collecting a filter paper sample.*)

The birth surge

Also known as the *neonatal thyrotropin test*, the neonatal TSH test confirms congenital hypothyroidism. TSH levels normally surge after birth and trigger a rise in TH, which is essential for neurologic development. At age 1 to 2 days, TSH levels are normally 25 to 30 mcIU/mL (SI, 25 to 30 mU/L). Thereafter, levels are normally less than 25 mcIU/mL (SI, 25 mU/L).

Failure to respond

In primary congenital hypothyroidism, the thyroid gland doesn't respond to TSH stimulation, which results in lower TH levels and higher TSH levels. Early detection and treatment of congenital hypothyroidism are critical to prevent cognitive impairment and cretinism.

Collecting a filter paper sample

To collect a specimen for neonatal TSH testing using the filter paper method, gather the following equipment and follow the easy steps provided later.

Equipment
- Alcohol swabs
- Sterile lancet
- Specially marked filter paper
- Sterile 2 in × 2 in gauze pads
- Adhesive bandage
- Labels
- Gloves

Steps
- Assemble the necessary equipment, wash your hands thoroughly, and put on gloves.
- Wipe the infant's heel with an alcohol swab and then dry it thoroughly with a gauze pad.
- Perform a heel stick and squeeze the infant's heel gently, filling the circles on the filter paper with blood, while making sure the blood saturates the paper.
- Gently apply pressure with a gauze pad to stop the bleeding and ensure hemostasis at the puncture site.
- Allow the filter paper to dry, label it appropriately, and send it to the laboratory.

Neonatal TSH levels must be interpreted in light of T_4 concentrations. Elevated TSH that's accompanied by decreased T_4 indicates primary congenital hypothyroidism. Depressed TSH and depressed T_4 may be present in secondary congenital hypothyroidism. When TSH is normal and is accompanied by depressed T_4, hypothyroidism due to a congenital defect or transient congenital hypothyroidism due to prematurity or prenatal hypoxia may be the cause. A complete thyroid workup must be done to confirm the cause of hypothyroidism before treatment can begin. (See *Neonatal TSH interference.*)

Neonatal TSH interference

Several factors may alter TSH levels or the results of tests used to measure TSH levels in the neonate:
- Corticosteroids, T_3, and T_4 lower TSH levels.
- Lithium carbonate, potassium iodide, excessive topical resorcinol, and TSH injection raise TSH levels.
- Failure to let a filter paper sample dry completely may alter results.
- Rough handling of a serum sample may cause hemolysis, which may alter results.

Nursing considerations

Explain the test to the caregivers. A sample is sent for T_4 and TSH levels. Perform a venipuncture or heel stick, collect and label the sample, and send it to the laboratory immediately.

T_4 test

T_4 is an amine secreted by the thyroid gland in response to TSH from the pituitary and, indirectly, to thyrotropin-releasing hormone (TRH) from the hypothalamus.

Cons, pros, and suspects

The rate of secretion is normally regulated by a complex system of negative and positive feedback involving the thyroid, the anterior pituitary, and the hypothalamus. T_4 is the suspected precursor (or prohormone) of T_3 and is converted to T_3 mainly in the liver and kidneys.

The T_4 that binds

Only a fraction of T_4 (about 0.3%) circulates freely in the blood; the rest binds strongly to plasma proteins, primarily to T_4-binding globulin (TBG). This minute fraction of free-circulating T_4 is responsible for the clinical effects of TH. TBG binds so tenaciously that T_4 survives in the plasma for a relatively long time, with a half-life of about 6 days. This test measures the total circulating T_4 level when TBG is normal.

More testing ahead

Serum T_4 testing is performed to evaluate thyroid function and to monitor thyroid replacement therapy.

Abnormally elevated levels of T_4 are consistent with primary and secondary hyperthyroidism, including excessive T_4 (levothyroxine [Synthroid]) replacement therapy. Overt signs of hyperthyroidism require further testing, and, in doubtful patients of hypothyroidism, the TSH or TRH test may be indicated. (See *T_4 levels in children.*)

T_4 levels in children

T_4 levels change as the child grows:
- Cord blood—7.4 to 13 mcg/dL (SI, 95 to 168 nmol/L)
- Younger than age 1 month—7 to 22.6 mcg/dL (SI, 90 to 292 nmol/L)
- Ages 1 month to 1 year—7.2 to 16.5 mcg/dL (SI, 93 to 213 nmol/L)
- Ages 1 to 5 years—7.3 to 15 mcg/dL (SI, 94 to 194 nmol/L)
- Ages 5 to 10 years—6.4 to 13.3 mcg/dL (SI, 83 to 192 nmol/L)
- Ages 10 to 15 years—5.6 to 11.7 mcg/dL (SI, 72 to 151 nmol/L)

Nursing considerations

Explain the test to the child and their caregivers. In addition, follow these steps:

- As ordered, withhold medications that may interfere with test results. If these medications must be continued, note this on the laboratory request. (If the test is being performed to monitor thyroid therapy, the patient should continue to receive daily thyroid supplements.)
- Perform a venipuncture, collect a sample, and send the sample to the laboratory immediately.

T_3 test (serum)

The T_3 test is a highly specific immunoassay that measures total serum content of T_3 to investigate clinical indications of thyroid dysfunction. It helps diagnose T_3 toxicosis, hypothyroidism, or hyperthyroidism and helps monitor the course of thyroid replacement therapy.

T_3 is the more potent TH. At least 50% and as much as 90% of T_3 is thought to be derived from T_4. The remaining 10% or more is secreted directly by the thyroid gland. Like T_4 secretion, T_3 secretion occurs in response to TSH released by the pituitary and, secondarily, to TRH from the hypothalamus.

A little T_3 goes a long way

Although T_3 is present in the bloodstream in minute quantities and is metabolically active for only a short time, its impact on body metabolism dominates that of T_4. T_3 binds less firmly to TBG, so it persists in the bloodstream for a short time; half of it disappears in about 1 day, whereas half of T_4 remains for 6 days.

It's all on the level

Normally, serum T_3 levels in children are:
- neonate—70 to 260 ng/dL (SI, 1.16 to 4 nmol/L)
- children ages 1 to 5 years—100 to 260 ng/dL (SI, 1.54 to 4 nmol/L)
- children ages 5 to 10 years—90 to 240 ng/dL (SI, 1.39 to 3.7 nmol/L)
- children ages 10 to 15 years—80 to 210 ng/dL (SI, 1.23 to 3.23 nmol/L).

A tandem rise

Serum T_3 and T_4 levels usually rise and fall in tandem. However, in T_3 toxicosis, only T_3 levels rise, whereas total and free T_4 levels remain normal. T_3 toxicosis occurs in patients with Graves disease, toxic adenoma, or toxic nodular goiter. T_3 levels also surpass T_4 levels in patients receiving thyroid replacement containing more T_3 than T_4. In iodine-deficient areas, the thyroid may produce larger amounts of the more cellularly active T_3 than T_4 in an effort to maintain the euthyroid state.

Nursing considerations

Explain the test to the child and their caregivers and allow a caregiver to be present during the venipuncture. In addition, follow these steps:

- As ordered, withhold medications that may influence thyroid function, such as steroids and propranolol (Inderal). If such medications must be continued, record this information on the laboratory request.
- Perform a venipuncture, collect the sample, and send it to the laboratory immediately.
- If a patient must receive thyroid preparations, such as T_3 (liothyronine [Triostat]), note the time of drug administration on the laboratory request.

Treatments and procedures

Common treatments and procedures used in the care of a child with an endocrine and metabolic system disorder include radioactive iodine (^{131}I) therapy and thyroidectomy.

^{131}I therapy

^{131}I therapy, a form of radiation therapy, is used to treat hyperthyroidism in children, particularly Graves disease. It shrinks functioning thyroid tissue, decreasing circulating TH levels.

After oral ingestion, ^{131}I is rapidly absorbed and concentrated in the thyroid as if it were normal iodine, resulting in acute radiation thyroiditis and gradual thyroid atrophy. ^{131}I causes symptoms to subside after about 3 weeks and exerts its full effect only after 3 to 6 months.

Nursing considerations

Explain the procedure and check the patient's history for allergies to iodine.

Expecting a glow

The idea of ingesting a radioactive material may be frightening to the child and their caregivers, especially when they hear about the precautions that must be taken. Reassure the child and their caregivers that this treatment will affect only the thyroid and that all the radioactive material will be excreted from the body.

In addition, follow these steps:

- Unless contraindicated, instruct the patient to stop TH antagonists 4 to 7 days before ^{131}I administration because these drugs reduce the sensitivity of thyroid cells to radiation.
- Tell the child to fast overnight because food may delay ^{131}I absorption.
- If the patient received an unusually large dose of ^{131}I or if treatment was for cancer, they may stay in the hospital for monitoring. In such cases, observe radiation precautions for 3 days.
- Do not allow pregnant nurses to care for the child.
- Encourage the patient to drink plenty of fluids for 48 hours to speed excretion of ^{131}I.

At home with radioactive iodine

If the child will be discharged after treatment, instruct the caregivers about observing radiation precautions at home:

- Tell the caregivers that the child must urinate into a lead-lined container for 48 hours.
- Tell the caregivers that the child must use disposable eating utensils and avoid close contact with young children and pregnant people for 7 days after therapy.
- Advise the caregivers to dispose of urine, saliva, and vomitus properly; urine and saliva will be slightly radioactive for 24 hours, and vomitus will be highly radioactive for 6 to 8 hours after therapy.

Thyroidectomy

Thyroidectomy (removal of all or part of the thyroid gland) is performed to treat hyperthyroidism and respiratory obstruction from goiter. *Subtotal thyroidectomy*, which reduces secretion of TH, is used to correct hyperthyroidism when drug therapy fails or radiation therapy is contraindicated. After surgery, the remaining thyroid tissue usually supplies enough TH for normal function, although hypothyroidism may occur later.

Nursing considerations

Prepare the child for surgery with an age-appropriate explanation, including the postoperative appearance of the site of surgery. Tell the child that their throat may be sore for a few days after surgery and medication will be given to make them feel better. Keep in mind that the child may be fearful of having their "throat cut"; provide clarification and answer all questions.

In addition, follow these steps:

- Iodine preparations are typically administered before surgery; to improve the taste of the preparation, mix it with fruit juice.
- Check for laryngeal nerve damage by asking the child to speak as soon as they awaken from anesthesia.
- Watch for signs of respiratory distress. Tracheal collapse, mucus accumulation in the trachea, laryngeal edema, and vocal cord paralysis can all cause respiratory obstruction with sudden stridor and restlessness.

Just in case

- Keep a tracheostomy tray at the bedside for the first 24 hours after surgery and be prepared to assist with emergency tracheotomy if necessary.
- Assess for signs of hemorrhage, which may cause shock, tracheal compression, and respiratory distress.
- Check the patient's dressing and palpate the back of their neck (where drainage tends to flow).

Dribbling drainage patrol

- Expect only scant drainage after 24 hours.
- As ordered, administer a mild analgesic agent to relieve a sore neck or throat; reassure the child that their discomfort should resolve within a few days.
- Test for positive Chvostek and Trousseau signs, indicators of neuromuscular irritability from hypocalcemia; keep calcium gluconate available for emergency intravenous (IV) administration.

Storm's a'brewin'

- Be alert for signs of thyroid storm, a rare but serious complication in children, characterized by sudden and dangerous signs and symptoms, including severe tachycardia (increased heart rate), severe irritability, vomiting, diarrhea, hyperthermia, and hypertension.

Endocrine and metabolic disorders

Endocrine and metabolic disorders that may affect children include congenital hypothyroidism, diabetes, Graves disease, and PKU.

Congenital hypothyroidism

Congenital hypothyroidism is a deficiency of TH secretion during fetal development or early infancy. If left untreated, it will seriously affect mental development. Congenital hypothyroidism is three times more common in females than in males.

The early bird catches the best prognosis

Early diagnosis and treatment produce the best prognosis. Infants treated before age 3 months usually grow and develop normally. Athyroid children (born without a thyroid gland) who remain untreated beyond age 3 months and children with acquired hypothyroidism who remain untreated beyond age 2 years suffer irreversible cognitive impairment. Skeletal abnormalities are reversible with treatment.

What causes it

Congenital hypothyroidism is caused by defective embryonic development (the most common cause), causing congenital absence or underdevelopment of the thyroid gland. It can also occur as an inherited autosomal recessive defect in the synthesis of T_4 (the next most common cause). Congenital hypothyroidism in infants can result if the birthing parent took antithyroid drugs during pregnancy. Other causes include chronic autoimmune thyroiditis and iodine deficiency during pregnancy.

How it happens

Hypothyroidism in infants and children is related to decreased TH production or secretion, which may result from one of several causes:

- Loss of functional thyroid tissue can be caused by an autoimmune process.
- Defective thyroid synthesis may be related to congenital defects; thyroid dysgenesis (defective development) is the most common defect.
- Hypothyroidism may also be related to decreased TSH secretion or resistance to TSH.
- If left untreated, lack of adequate TH levels seriously affects the nervous system and bone growth.

What to look for

The signs of untreated hypothyroidism usually appear at age 6 weeks:

- The infant with hypothyroidism may sleep more than usual; older children may show signs of lethargy.
- They may have noisy respirations due to tongue enlargement. (The tongue may also be dry.)

Cold to the touch

- The extremities may be cold, and the overall body temperature may be lower due to decreased metabolism.
- The child's neck will be short and thick.
- The extremities appear short and fat; the legs appear shorter in relation to trunk size.

Constipation consternation

- The abdomen becomes enlarged because of intestinal obstruction from constipation (which results from hypotonia of the intestinal tract).
- Other signs include delayed dentition; dry, scaly skin; easy weight gain; and slow pulse.

Whoa, horsey

Infants may have a hoarse cry, persistent jaundice, and respiratory difficulties. Older children may exhibit bone and muscle dystrophy, cognitive impairment (which develops as the disorder progresses), and stunted growth or dwarfism (short stature with the persistence of infant proportions).

What tests tell you

Elevated TSH level associated with low T_3 and T_4 levels points to congenital hypothyroidism. Because early detection and treatment can minimize the effects of congenital hypothyroidism, all states require measurement of infant TH levels at birth through neonate screening tests:

- Thyroid scan and ^{131}I uptake tests show decreased uptake levels and confirm the absence of thyroid tissue in athyroid children.
- Increased gonadotropin levels accompany sexual precocity in older children and may coexist with hypothyroidism.
- An electrocardiogram shows bradycardia and flat or inverted T waves in untreated infants.
- Hip, knee, and thigh x-rays reveal the absence of the femoral or tibial epiphyseal line and delayed skeletal development that's markedly inappropriate for the child's chronologic age.

Complications

If hypothyroidism is not treated by age 3 months, skeletal malformations and irreversible cognitive impairment can occur; treatment helps to prevent impairment. Learning disabilities and accelerated or delayed sexual maturation may also occur.

How it's treated

The treatment for congenital hypothyroidism is lifelong therapy with synthetic TH (levothyroxine, liothyronine). Supplemental vitamin D may also be prescribed to prevent rickets resulting from rapid bone growth. Surgery may be performed for the underlying cause such as a pituitary tumor. The child should have routine monitoring of T_4 and TSH levels as well as periodic evaluation of growth to ensure that thyroid replacement is adequate.

What to do

The child and their caregivers will need ongoing support and encouragement. They should be encouraged to express their concerns and feelings and may need help to develop effective coping mechanisms. Referral to a support group may be extremely helpful. In addition, follow these steps:

- When caring for a neonate, make sure neonatal screening has been done to allow for early detection of the disorder.
- Stress to the caregivers the importance of lifelong treatment, including TH replacement therapy as well as routine blood work to adjust the medication as the child grows.
- Administer medications as ordered.
- Offer support and encouragement to the caregivers.

Too high, too low

- After initiation of treatment for infantile hypothyroidism, monitor blood pressure and pulse rate and report hypertension and tachycardia immediately. (Normal infant heart rate is approximately 120 beats/min.) These signs as well as fever, irritability, and sweating indicate that the dose of TH replacement medication is too high.
- Teach the caregivers to look for signs and symptoms of inadequate treatment (a dose that's too low), including fatigue, lethargy, decreased appetite, and constipation.

Plan ahead

- Adolescent females require future-oriented counseling that stresses the importance of adequate TH replacement during pregnancy.
- If the infant's tongue is unusually large, position the infant on their side and observe them frequently to prevent airway obstruction.

Don't delay

If treatment is delayed and signs and symptoms develop, follow these steps:

- Help the child and their caregivers develop effective coping skills.
- Provide meticulous skin and mucous membrane care.
- Check rectal temperature every 2 to 4 hours; keep the patient warm, as needed.

Diabetes

Diabetes is a chronic disease of absolute or relative insulin deficiency or resistance.

Absolutely insufficient

Type 1 diabetes (characterized by absolute insulin insufficiency) is the most common childhood endocrine disorder. No longer rare, the incidence of type 2 diabetes in childhood is rising dramatically because of the increase in childhood obesity and sedentary lifestyles. Obesity induces resistance to insulin-mediated peripheral glucose uptake. It is characterized by insulin resistance with varying degrees of insulin secretory defects.

Diabetes (types 1 and 2) can occur at any age, but type 1 has a peak incidence at ages 10 to 15 years.

What causes it

Diabetes is caused by genetic factors and autoimmune factors (type 1) and may also develop as a result of a viral infection.

Genetic factors

Type 1 diabetes is not inherited, but predisposition plays a part in its development. Type 2 diabetes has strong polygenic (caused by several genes) familial susceptibility. Children born to males who have type 1 diabetes are about three times more likely to develop diabetes than children born to females with type 1 diabetes.

Autoimmune factors

About 70% to 85% of patients newly diagnosed with type 1 diabetes are found to have pancreatic islet cell antibodies.

These antibodies disappear in most people after diagnosis. It is thought that the presence of these antibodies makes the immune system vulnerable to a trigger event that may contribute to the development of type 1 diabetes, such as a virus, bacteria, or chemical irritant.

Viral infection

Several viruses, including coxsackie B, mumps, and congenital rubella, have been associated with the development of type 1 diabetes.

Vulnerable to viruses

The pancreatic islet cells are susceptible to injury and change by these viruses. These alterations cause the body to have an autoimmune response. Therefore, the virus is considered a trigger to the development of type 1 diabetes.

How it happens

Diabetes is characterized by disturbances in carbohydrate, protein, and fat metabolism. Insulin allows glucose transport into the cells for use as energy or storage as glycogen.

Free the fatty acids!

Insulin stimulates protein synthesis and free fatty acid storage in adipose tissues. Deficiency of insulin or insulin resistance and secretory defects compromise the body tissues' access to essential nutrients for fuel and storage.

What to look for

The three cardinal signs of diabetes are polyuria, polydipsia, and polyphagia. Other general signs and symptoms may include:

- weakness and fatigue
- nocturia in a child who has already attained nighttime control
- dehydration (dry mucous membranes and poor skin turgor)
- weight loss and hunger
- vision changes (retinopathy or cataract formation)
- frequent skin and urinary tract infections
- skin changes (cool temperature and dry, itchy skin, especially on the hands and feet).

Type 1 in a hurry

A child with type 1 diabetes will have rapidly developing symptoms, muscle wasting, and loss of subcutaneous (SC) fat. A child with type 2 diabetes will have more subtle symptoms of polyuria, polydipsia, polyphagia, weight loss, weakness, fatigue, and frequent infections developing over time.

The pancreas' last stand

A onetime remission of symptoms may occur shortly after insulin treatment is started. It is a last-ditch effort by the pancreas to produce insulin. The child may not need insulin for up to 1 year but may need oral antidiabetic drugs. Symptoms of hyperglycemia will reappear, and the child with type 1 diabetes will be insulin dependent for life.

Vaguely type 2

In children with type 2 diabetes, vague, long-standing symptoms develop gradually. These include:

- severe viral infection
- other endocrine diseases
- recent stress or trauma
- use of drugs that increase blood glucose levels
- obesity, particularly in the abdominal area.

What tests tell you

Two fasting plasma glucose tests above 126 mg/dL or, with normal fasting glucose, two blood glucose levels above 200 mg/dL during a 2-hour glucose tolerance test confirm the diagnosis. Other findings include:

- 2-hour postprandial blood glucose level greater than 200 mg/dL
- increased glycosylated hemoglobin ($HgbA_{1C}$) level
- urinalysis that may show acetone or glucose
- diabetic retinopathy, which may be revealed by an ophthalmic examination.

Complications

Diabetic ketoacidosis (DKA) and hypoglycemia may occur as well as hyperosmolar hyperglycemic nonketotic syndrome (HHNS). Long-term complications of diabetes are nephropathy, retinopathy, and neuropathy.

If the diabetes is not well controlled, complications can occur as early as 2 to 3 years after diagnosis. Therefore, good control and adherence to treatment regimen are necessary to postpone or prevent complications.

How it's treated

Treating the child with diabetes takes a multidisciplinary approach.

Team diabetes

The child, caregivers, and health care professionals (including an endocrinologist, nutritionist, and a diabetes nurse educator) should all be involved in the treatment plan. It may also be necessary for a mental health professional to be included because the treatment plan can have an impact on the child's emotional and psychological health.

Meal planning, exercise, and, sometimes, insulin or oral antidiabetic agents are prescribed to normalize carbohydrate, fat, and protein metabolism and avert long-term complications while preventing hypoglycemia.

Type 1 diabetes

Patients with type 1 diabetes must take insulin daily to achieve blood glucose control because of their absolute insulin deficiency. Insulin needs change and is affected by emotions, nutritional intake, activity, illness, and events such as puberty. (See *Insulin injection sites in children.*)

Insulin dosages are based on home blood glucose monitoring. Insulin can be administered as one or two injections per day or by insulin pump (continuous SC administration).

Type 2 diabetes

Patients with type 2 diabetes may require insulin to control blood glucose levels unresponsive to diet and antidiabetic agents, or during periods of acute stress. (See *Insulin therapy.*) There are several medications approved for treatment of type 2 diabetes in children and adolescents ages 10 years and older. Metformin is an oral antidiabetic agent (taken daily as an adjunct to diet and exercise) to improve glycemic control in children and adolescents with type 2 diabetes. Metformin, if not contraindicated, should be considered first-line therapy for the management of type 2 diabetes. In 2019, liraglutide (a glucagonlike peptide-1 [GLP-1] agonist) injections were approved

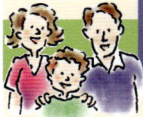

Insulin injection sites in children

Use the following illustration to instruct the child and their caregivers about the injection sites for insulin administration that are recommended by the American Diabetes Association.

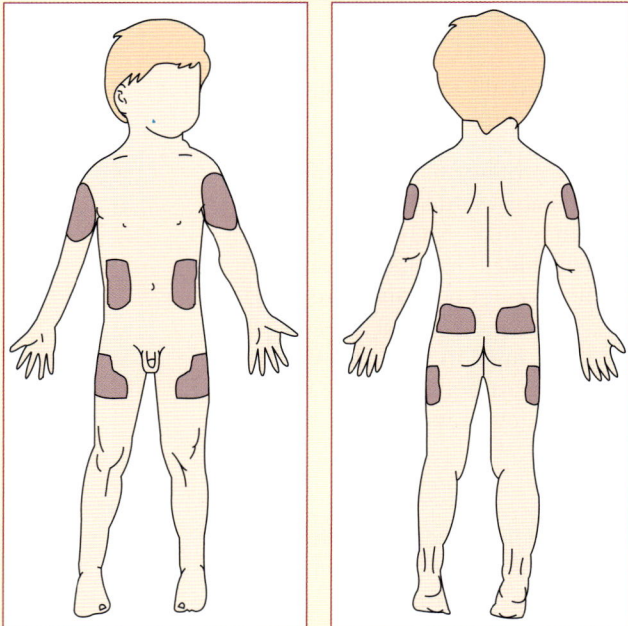

by the U.S. Food and Drug Administration (FDA) for the treatment of type 2 diabetes in children 10 years and older. It is sometimes used in combination with metformin, especially for those with an HgA$_{1C}$ of greater than 7.5%. Exenatide, another injectable GLP-1 agonist, was approved by the FDA in 2021 for the treatment of type 2 diabetes in children older than 10 years.

What to do

The child with diabetes may be facing lifelong treatment and restrictions, with the prospect of setbacks (until control is established) and serious complications. The child and their caregivers will need a great deal of ongoing support and assistance.

Insulin therapy

Insulin is administered as prescribed by the health care provider. There are several routes of administration and devices for injection.

SC route

Insulin is usually given by SC injection with a standard insulin syringe. SC insulin can also be given with a penlike injection device that uses a disposable needle and re-placeable insulin cartridges, eliminating the need to draw insulin into a syringe.

Jet propelled

Jet-injection devices are expensive and require special cleaning procedures, but they disperse insulin more rapidly and speed absorption. These devices draw up in-sulin from standard containers, which enable the patient to mix insulins, if necessary, but require a special procedure for drawing it up. After the insulin is drawn up, it is delivered into the SC tissue with a pressure jet.

Pump it up!

Multiple-dose regimens may use an insulin pump to deliver insulin continuously into SC tissue. The infusion rate selector automatically releases about half of the total daily insulin requirement evenly over 24 hours. The patient releases the remainder in bolus amounts before meals and snacks.

Ready, set, rotate!

When administering insulin injections SC, the injection sites should be rotated. Be-cause absorption rates differ at each site, rotating the injection site within a specific area such as the abdomen is recommended.

IV, intramuscular, and inhalation routes

Regular insulin or insulin lispro may also be administered intramuscularly (IM) or IV during severe episodes of hyperglycemia. These are the only types of insulin that should ever be administered by these routes. Inhaled insulin is taken using an oral inhaler to deliver ultra-rapid-acting insulin at the beginning of meals. Inhaled insulin is used in combination with an injectable long-acting insulin.

Rebel with restrictions

As the child grows, adherence may become an issue. A child or adolescent may simply become overwhelmed or tired of taking medication and adhering to dietary restrictions. These feelings should be recognized as normal. Referral to a support group will help the child and their caregivers cope with the diagnosis and its implications.

In addition, follow these steps:

- Emphasize that adherence to the treatment plan is essential; it is crucial to bring the child's blood glucose level within an acceptable range (usually 80 to 120 mg/dL) and alleviate or prevent DKA or hypoglycemia.

- For the child with unstable diabetes who is not experiencing DKA or HHNS, monitor blood glucose levels several times each day as prescribed until they stabilize.

Like a hawk!

- Monitor the child closely for signs and symptoms of DKA or HHNS. Suspect DKA or HHNS if the child exhibits Kussmaul respirations, develops a fruity odor to their breath, and shows signs and symptoms of severe dehydration. Notify the doctor immediately if these indications are evident.
- If the child has DKA or HHNS, treatment may include fluid and electrolyte replacement, increased insulin therapy, and therapy to reduce acidosis. Administer doses of IV insulin as prescribed. (Monitor blood glucose levels frequently during insulin infusion.)
- Monitor the child closely for signs and symptoms of hyperglycemia and hypoglycemia (caused by an excessively rapid change in blood glucose level). Teach these signs and symptoms to the child and their caregivers and provide specific instructions on how to handle each condition. (See *Hypo or hyper?*)

Hypo or hyper?

It is generally difficult to distinguish between hypoglycemia and hyperglycemia.

Too little . . .
Hypoglycemia symptoms include:
- lethargy
- hunger
- sweating
- pallor
- seizures
- coma.

. . . too much
Hyperglycemia symptoms include:
- sweet, fruity breath (acetone)
- dehydration
- decreased sodium, potassium, bicarbonate, chloride, and phosphate levels
- vomiting
- abdominal pain
- coma.

Make sure the child and their caregivers understand that the child should base their meal plan on a balanced diet that incorporates the six basic food groups.

Fitting in

Concentrated sweets are discouraged, so teach the child and their caregivers about alternative snack ideas to help the child feel more like their peers. (See *Diabetes teaching tips.*)

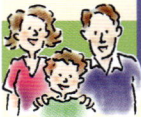

It's all relative

Diabetes teaching tips

Long-term management of diabetes requires extensive patient—and caregiver—education:

• Review the prescribed meal plan and teach the child (and their family) how to adjust their diet when engaged in extra activity.

• Advise the child and their caregivers about aerobic exercise programs; explain how exercise affects blood glucose levels and provide safety guidelines.

• Instruct the child on insulin administration, if prescribed, including type, peak times, dosage, drawing up the insulin, mixing (if applicable), administration technique, site rotation, sharps disposal, and storage.

• Teach the child and their caregivers how to perform blood glucose monitoring. Blood glucose monitoring can be done with a finger stick glucose or a continuous glucose monitor (CGM).

• Instruct the child on oral antidiabetic therapy, if prescribed, including dosage, frequency and time of administration, and potential adverse reactions.

   Tell the child and their caregivers about the American Diabetes Association website (www.diabetes.org) as a source of information. This site offers accurate information for the child with diabetes, their family, and health care professionals, along with general information about diabetes (advice on exercise, nutrition, and daily meal planning).

Show and tell

• Demonstrate to the child how to check their blood glucose; it is especially necessary for the child on a tightly controlled regimen.

Graves disease

Graves disease, also called *hyperthyroidism* in childhood, is associated with exophthalmos and an enlarged thyroid gland. Most cases occur in children between ages 6 and 15 years. The disease may be present in infants whose birthing parents were thyrotoxic during pregnancy.

What causes it

Graves disease is caused by an autoimmune response to TSH receptors. However, no specific etiology has been identified. There also seems to be a familial predisposition for the disease.

How it happens

In Graves disease, T_4 production is increased and the thyroid gland is enlarged (called a *goiter*). It is characterized by autoantibodies that attach to and then stimulate TSH receptors in the thyroid gland.

Stimulation overload

A goiter may be the result of increased stimulation of the thyroid gland or a response to increased metabolic demand. The latter occurs in iodine-deficient areas of the world, where the incidence of goiter increases during puberty (a time of increased metabolic demand). These goiters commonly regress to normal size after puberty in males but not in females.

What to look for

Symptoms of Graves disease begin gradually and develop on and off during a period of 6 to 12 months. Irritability and excessive motion are the most prominent symptoms. The child may also exhibit:
- hyperactivity
- short attention span
- insomnia
- tremors
- weight loss despite a tremendous appetite
- rapid, pounding pulse (even during sleep)
- warm and flushed skin
- widened pulse pressure
- cardiomegaly
- exophthalmos.

What tests tell you

- A thyroid scan reveals increased ^{131}I uptake.
- Immunometric assay shows suppressed sensitivity of TSH levels.
- Orbital sonography and CT scans show subclinical ophthalmopathy.
- Radioimmunoassay testing shows elevated T_4 levels.

Complications

Complications of Graves disease include muscle wasting, atrophy, and paralysis; vision loss or diplopia; and heart failure or cardiac dysrhythmia.

How it's treated

Graves disease is treated with antithyroid medications, such as propyl-thiouracil (PTU) and methimazole (Tapazole), to suppress the formation of T_4. Hypermetabolic symptoms will subside 4 to 8 weeks after therapy begins, but remission of Graves disease requires continued therapy for 6 months to 2 years. The child must be monitored closely for signs of leukopenia and thrombocytopenia. If these conditions occur, the medication is discontinued until the white blood cell and platelet counts return to normal levels.

Ablation to the rescue

If the child is unable or unwilling to comply with the medication regimen or if they have a toxic reaction to the medication, ablation therapy with ^{131}I is used to reduce the size of the thyroid gland.

When in doubt, take it out

Surgical removal of all or most of the thyroid may be necessary as a young adult. After ablation or surgical removal of the thyroid, the child must remain on lifelong thyroid replacement therapy.

What to do

Explain the disorder to the child and their caregivers and prepare them for all treatments and procedures:
- Teach the caregivers of a child being treated with antithyroid drugs or radioisotope therapy to identify and report symptoms of hypothyroidism.

Keep it cool

- Encourage a cool, quiet environment that's conducive to rest until there's a response to drug therapy; restrict physical activity.
- Advise the child with exophthalmos or other ophthalmopathy to wear sunglasses or eye patches to protect the eyes from light; moisten the conjunctiva frequently with isotonic eyedrops.
- Provide a balanced diet with six meals per day to meet the child's increased metabolic demand.

Cough with caution

- Tell the child who has had ^{131}I therapy not to expectorate or cough freely because their saliva is radioactive for 24 hours; stress the need for repeated measurement of serum T_4 levels and reassure the child and their caregivers who may be frightened by the term "radioactive."
- Educate the child and their caregivers to take PTU or methimazole with meals to minimize gastrointestinal (GI) distress and to avoid over-the-counter cough preparations because many contain iodine.

- Stress the importance of regular medical follow-up visits after discharge because hypothyroidism may develop 2 to 4 weeks postoperatively and after ^{131}I therapy.

Long-term commitment
- Explain that the child will need lifelong TH replacement. Encourage them to wear medical identification and to always carry their medication with them.

Phenylketonuria

PKU is an inborn error in amino acid (specifically phenylalanine) metabolism. It results in high serum levels of phenylalanine, increased urine concentrations of phenylalanine and its byproducts, cerebral damage, and cognitive impairment.

An error by any other name

PKU is also called *phenylalaninemia* and *phenylpyruvic oligophrenia*. The disorder occurs in 1 of approximately 14,000 births in the United States. About 1 person in 60 is a carrier without symptoms.

The case for early detection

Although blood phenylalanine levels approach normal at birth, they begin to increase within a few days. By the time they reach significant levels (about 30 mg/dL), cerebral damage has begun. Such irreversible damage is probably complete by age 2 or 3 years. Early detection and treatment can minimize cerebral damage.

What causes it

PKU is transmitted through an autosomal recessive gene.

How it happens

In PKU, an almost totally deficient activity of phenylalanine hydroxylase, an enzyme that acts as a catalyst in the conversion of phenylalanine to tyrosine, results in phenylalanine accumulation in the blood and urine. This accumulation leads to brain damage and cognitive impairment.

What to look for

The patient may have a family history of PKU. Typically, the history reveals no apparent abnormalities at birth.

Brain on hold

By age 4 months, the untreated child begins to show signs of arrested brain development, including cognitive impairment and, later, personality disturbances (schizoid and antisocial personality patterns and uncontrollable temper). About one third of patients have a history of seizures, which usually begin between ages 6 and 12 months. Many patients also show a precipitous decrease in IQ in their first year.

Got the blues?

On inspection, the patient typically has a lighter complexion than unaffected siblings and may have blue eyes. They may also exhibit macrocephaly, eczematous skin lesions, or dry, rough skin.

Hyper, irritable, and repetitive

The child is usually hyperactive and irritable. They may exhibit purposeless, repetitive motions, and have an awkward gait. A musty odor from the skin and urinary excretion of phenylacetic acid may also be noted.

What tests tell you

All 50 states require screening for PKU at birth. A tandem mass spectrometry screening or the Guthrie screening test on a capillary blood sample (bacterial inhibition assay) is a reliable indicator of the disorder. Because phenylalanine levels may be normal at birth, the infant should be evaluated after they start protein feedings. In infants with PKU, levels are usually abnormally high by day 4. More quantitative fluorometric or chromatographic assays provide additional diagnostic information.

Complications

Phenylalanine accumulation causes cognitive impairment.

How it's treated

To prevent or minimize brain damage, phenylalanine blood levels are kept between 3 and 9 mg/dL by restricting dietary intake of the amino acid phenylalanine.

The lowdown on phenylalanine

During the first month of life, a special, low-phenylalanine amino acid mixture is substituted for most of the protein in the diet, supplemented with a small amount of natural foods. An enzymatic hydrolysate of casein, such as Lofenalac powder or Pregestimil powder, is substituted for breast milk or cow's milk formula in the diets of affected infants. Dietary restrictions are required throughout life.

Don't overdo it!

Such a diet calls for close monitoring. The body does not make phenylalanine, so overzealous dietary restriction can induce phenylalanine deficiency, causing lethargy, anorexia, anemia, skin rashes, and diarrhea.

What to do

Teach the caregivers about PKU and provide emotional support and counseling. Psychological and emotional problems may result from the difficult dietary restrictions. In addition, follow these steps:
- If the child is experiencing seizures or has some mental dysfunction, implement safety measures to prevent injury.
- Refer the caregivers and child to appropriate community resources.

Just say "no" to chicken and cheese
- Teach the child and their caregivers about the critical importance of adhering to the child's diet; the child must avoid breads, cheese, eggs, flour, meat, poultry, fish, nuts, milk, legumes, and products with aspartame (reduced sugar condiments, diet sodas, sugar-free gums). Also, the child will need frequent tests for urine phenylpyruvic acid and blood phenylalanine levels to evaluate the effectiveness of the diet.
- Refer the family to a nutritionist.
- Teach the caregivers about normal physical and mental growth and development to help them recognize developmental delays from excessive phenylalanine intake.

Rebel with a cause
As the child grows older and is supervised less closely, their caregivers have less control over what they eat. As a result, deviation from the restricted diet becomes more likely, which increases the risk of further brain damage. Encourage the caregivers to allow the child some choices in the kinds of low-protein foods they eat to help make them feel trusted and more responsible, which will encourage adherence.

Quick quiz

1. The purpose of the endocrine system is to:
   A. deliver nutrients to the body's cells.
   B. regulate and integrate the body's metabolic activities.
   C. eliminate waste products from the body.
   D. stimulate secondary sex characteristics.

Answer: B. Along with the nervous system, the endocrine system regulates and integrates the body's metabolic activities.

2. The nurse draws blood from the heel of an infant for a Guthrie screening test. This test is used to diagnose which inborn error of metabolism?
   A. Absence of GALT
   B. PKU
   C. Galactosemia
   D. Hypothyroidism

Answer: B. The Guthrie screening test is a bacterial inhibition assay used to diagnose PKU. *B. subtilis*, present in the culture medium, grows if the blood contains an excessive amount of phenylalanine.

3. The gland that produces glucagon is the:
   A. pancreas.
   B. thymus.
   C. adrenal.
   D. pituitary.

Answer: A. The alpha cells of the pancreas produce glucagon, a hormone that raises the blood glucose level by triggering the breakdown of glycogen into glucose.

4. An infant with congenital hypothyroidism shows which sign or symptom?
   A. Shrill cry
   B. Diaphoresis
   C. Hypothermia
   D. Diarrhea

Answer: C. Hypothermia is one common finding in congenital hypothyroidism. Other common findings include lethargy, poor feeding, prolonged jaundice, vomiting, constipation, mottling, coarse facial features, hoarse cry, large fontanels, and hypotonia.

Scoring

☆☆☆ If you answered all five items correctly, astonishing! Your brain cells must be on steroids!

☆☆ If you answered three items correctly, wow! You've just won a trip to the islets of Langerhans! Bon voyage!

☆ If you answered fewer than three items correctly, don't moan over these hormones! Two more quick quizzes are ahead.

Suggested references

Atteih, S., & Ratner, J. (2021). Endocrinology. In K. Kleinman, L. McDaniel, M. Molloy (Eds.), *The Harriet Lane handbook* (22nd ed., pp. 228–260). Elsevier.

Bindler, R., Cowen, K., & Shaw, M. (2023). The child with alterations in endocrine function. In J. Ball, R. Bindler, K. Cowen, R. Dawson, & L. Wisely (Eds.), *Principles of pediatric nursing: Caring for children* (8th ed.). Pearson.

Gilman, L. (2020). Endocrine disorders. In B. Richardson (Ed.), *Pediatric primary care: Practice guidelines for nurses* (4th ed., pp. 497–522). Jones and Bartlett Learning.

Knoll, J., Forsyth, R., & Pryor, S. (2021). Genetics: Metabolisms and dysmorphology. In K. Kleinman, L. McDaniel, & M. Molloy (Eds.), *The Harriet Lane handbook* (22nd ed., pp. 300–327). Elsevier.

LaMothe, J. (2020). Pediatric obesity. In B. Richardson (Ed.), *Pediatric primary care: Practice guidelines for nurses* (4th ed., pp. 635–648). Jones & Bartlett Learning.

Linnard-Palmer, L. (2019). Metabolism. In L. Linnard-Palmer (Ed.), *Pediatric nursing care: A concept-based approach* (pp. 194–210). Jones & Bartlett Learning.

Schulz, A., Smaldone, A., & Whittemore, B. (2020). Endocrine and metabolic disorders. In D. Maaks, N. Starr, M. Brady, N. Gaylord, M. Driessnack, & K. Duderstadt (Eds.), *Pediatric primary care* (7th ed., pp. 940–970). Elsevier.

Chapter 22

Hematologic and immunologic problems

Just the facts

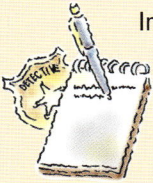

In this chapter, you'll learn:

♦ anatomy and physiology of the hematologic and immune systems
♦ normal function of blood cells and the role of genetics in the hematologic and immune systems
♦ tests used to diagnose hematologic and immunologic problems
♦ treatments and procedures for children with hematologic and immunologic problems
♦ hematologic and immunologic disorders that affect children.

Anatomy and physiology

The hematologic and immune systems are separate but interrelated. They help the body fight infection or invaders through different mechanisms but usually work together for the same goal. Both systems essentially arise from the *bone marrow* which, although housed within the bones, has little relationship to the skeletal system.

Hematologic system

Bone marrow contains the essential element in the hematologic system: the stem cell. The stem cell is sometimes referred to as the *pluripotential stem cell*, meaning it can transform into more than one type of blood cell. Every blood cell in the body arises from a stem cell.

Did you say organ system?

Although it is a fluid, blood is one of the body's major organ systems. It continually circulates through the heart and blood vessels, carrying vital elements to every part of the body.

Blood formation

Early in utero, the process of blood formation, called *hematopoiesis*, occurs in the liver and spleen. These organs retain some hematopoietic ability throughout life. After birth, the bone marrow becomes the main site of hematopoiesis.

Yellow with age

In infants and young children, all bones contain red bone marrow (red from the production of red blood cells [RBCs]) and are, therefore, capable of hematopoiesis. However, as the child approaches adolescence and bone growth ceases, the bone marrow in many bones transforms into yellow bone marrow (yellow from fat deposits) and does not produce blood cells. However, it can usually revert to red bone marrow during times of increased blood cell demand. Only the ribs, sternum, vertebrae, and pelvis continue to contain red bone marrow and produce blood cells.

Have a blast

The stem cells contained in the red bone marrow create primitive blood cells called *blast cells*. Blast cells are the least mature form of blood cells and are the precursors to RBCs, white blood cells (WBCs), and platelets. These cells are normal and should not be confused with the blast cells seen in leukemia and other cancers.

Like a fine wine

These blast cells then mature in the bone marrow. The maturation of blood cells, called *differentiation*, occurs in stages; thus, in normal bone marrow, you can see different forms of all the blood cell lines. (See *Human blood cell development.*) Mature blood cells travel by blood throughout the body to perform specific functions.

Human blood cell development

All blood cell types originate from the same stem cell. The following chart shows how this stem cell becomes differentiated, developing into each blood cell type.

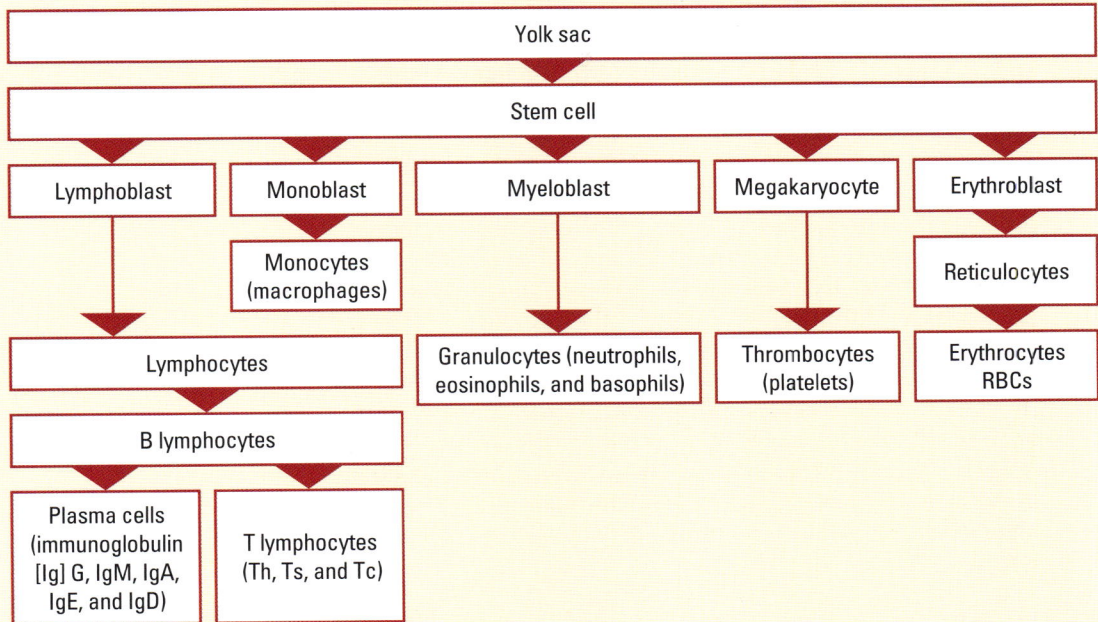

Yolk sac

Stem cell

Lymphoblast	Monoblast	Myeloblast	Megakaryocyte	Erythroblast

	Monocytes (macrophages)			Reticulocytes

Lymphocytes		Granulocytes (neutrophils, eosinophils, and basophils)	Thrombocytes (platelets)	Erythrocytes RBCs

B lymphocytes

Plasma cells (immunoglobulin [Ig] G, IgM, IgA, IgE, and IgD)	T lymphocytes (Th, Ts, and Tc)

Blood components

Blood is composed of plasma and cells. Plasma is the fluid portion of the blood. It's 90% water and 10% solutes, such as proteins, electrolytes, albumin, clotting factors, anticoagulants, antibodies, and dissolved nutrients. The three main cell types in the blood originate from blast cells and include:

1. RBCs or *erythrocytes*
2. WBCs or *leukocytes*
3. platelets or *thrombocytes*.

Red blood cells

In addition to the bone marrow, some RBCs are stored in the liver or spleen. RBCs carry oxygen to the tissues and carbon dioxide away from tissues. When tissue is low on oxygen (hypoxia), a hormone from the kidneys called *erythropoietin* stimulates the bone marrow to produce more RBCs. Synthetic forms of erythropoietin can be used to stimulate RBC production in premature neonates and patients receiving chemotherapy to help them maintain higher blood cell levels.

The cycle of life—RBC style

An RBC's lifespan is approximately 120 days, and an important waste product of RBC death is bilirubin. Bilirubin binds with albumin for transport to the liver and conjugates with glucuronide, forming direct bilirubin. Because unconjugated bilirubin is fat soluble and cannot be excreted in urine or bile, it may escape to extravascular tissue, especially fatty tissue and the brain, resulting in hyperbilirubinemia and skin that appears icteric (or jaundiced). Too much bilirubin may result in brain damage—a condition known as kernicterus. In newborns, the normal range of bilirubin levels is determined by the baby's age in hours. For instance, an infant who is 48 hours old will have a different range of acceptable levels than an infant who is 96 hours old. Other things that may place a newborn at risk for hyperbilirubinemia are being born premature, trauma at birth, having a sibling who has had hyperbilirubinemia, or having a blood group incompatibility with the birthing parent (such as the birthing parent having an O+ blood type and the baby having an A+ blood type).

Oxygen is carried in the cell in a protein (globin) and iron (heme) structure known as *hemoglobin* (Hgb). If adequate amounts of iron are not available, the protein structure cannot be formed and RBCs cannot carry their normal amount of oxygen. Lead can also replace iron in the molecule, causing lead toxicity which may result in developmental delays, neurologic abnormalities, and at extremely high levels, seizures and death.

White blood cells

WBCs fight different types of infection that occur in or on the body; each type of WBC has its own role in fighting infection. The two main categories of WBCs are granular leukocytes (granulocytes) and nongranular leukocytes (agranulocytes). (See *Two types of leukocytes*.)

Two types of leukocytes

Leukocytes vary in size, shape, and number and are characterized as granular and nongranular.

Granular
Granular leukocytes (granulocytes) are the most numerous. They include:
• *basophils*, which contain cytoplasmic granules that stain readily with alkaline dyes
• *neutrophils*, which are finely granular and recognizable by their multinucleated appearance
• *eosinophils*, which stain with acidic dyes.

Two types of leukocytes (*continued*)

Granular leukocytes

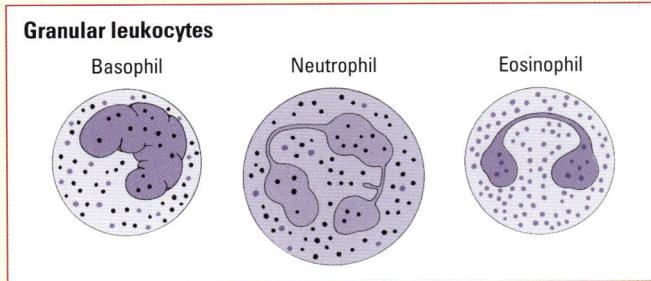

Granular leukocytes

Basophil   Neutrophil   Eosinophil

Nongranular

Nongranular leukocytes have few, if any, granulated particles in the cytoplasm. They include:

- lymphocytes
- monocytes.

Nongranular leukocytes

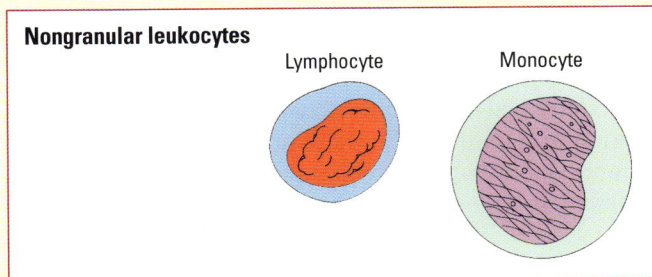

Nongranular leukocytes

Lymphocyte   Monocyte

Great granulocytes, batman!

Granulocytes include:

- *neutrophils*, which help devour invading microorganisms, such as bacteria, by phagocytosis
- *eosinophils*, which act in allergic reactions and may defend against large parasites and lung and skin infections
- *basophils*, which release heparin and histamine, are involved in inflammatory and infectious reactions, and are known as *mast cells* when they exist in body tissues.

Not a granule to be found

Agranulocytes include:

- *lymphocytes*, which are the main cells that fight infections and include natural killer (NK) cells, B cells, and T cells
- *monocytes*, which, along with neutrophils, help devour invading microorganisms by phagocytosis and also form macrophages in the body tissues.

Platelets

Platelets adhere to one another and plug holes in vessels or tissues where there's bleeding. This action is part of a larger coagulation (clotting) process. Platelets also release serotonin at injury sites. Serotonin, a vasoconstrictor, decreases blood flow to the injured area. Nonsteroidal antiinflammatory drugs (NSAIDs) such as aspirin, ibuprofen, and naproxen may affect platelet aggregation.

Hemostasis

Hemostasis is a complex process by which the body controls bleeding. When a blood vessel ruptures, local vasoconstriction and platelet clumping (aggregation) at the injury site initially help prevent hemorrhaging.

Like a waterfall

Activation of the coagulation system, called the *extrinsic cascade*, involves the release of thromboplastin from the damaged tissue cells. However, formation of a more stable clot requires initiation of the complex clotting mechanism known as the *intrinsic cascade system*.

When endothelial vessel injury or a foreign body in the bloodstream activates the intrinsic cascade, activating factor XII triggers clotting. Finally, prothrombin is converted to thrombin and fibrinogen to fibrin, which is necessary for creation of a fibrin clot.

Immune system

The body protects itself from foreign invaders, such as bacteria, viruses, parasites, and fungi, through the organs and cells of the immune system. The components of the immune system work together to differentiate "self" from "nonself" and to rid the body of those substances recognized as "nonself."

Immune system organs

Immune system organs and tissues are described as *lymphoid* because they are involved with the growth, development, and dissemination of lymphocytes. These organs and tissues include:
- lymph nodes
- thymus
- spleen
- tonsils
- Peyer patches in the intestine.

Lymph nodes

Lymph nodes are small, oval-shaped structures located along a network of lymph channels. Most abundant in the head, neck, axillae, abdomen, pelvis, and groin, they help remove and destroy antigens (substances capable of triggering an immune response) that circulate in the blood and lymph. Lymph nodes filter lymphatic fluid and return it to the bloodstream.

Lymphocytes in waiting

Lymph nodes filter foreign invaders, such as viruses and bacteria, and can store lymphocytes that might be needed in that area to fight infection.

Nodes of concern

In children, the lymphatic system grows rapidly between ages 3 and 6 years. At this age, slightly swollen (less than 0.5 cm) lymph nodes in the neck and groin areas are common. Lymph nodes that should cause concern are:
- enlarged (greater than 1 cm in diameter), firm, painless, and fixed to the skin (consistent with characteristics of malignancy)
- painful, soft, and producing heat (signs and symptoms of local inflammation or infection)
- nodes in the supraclavicular, infraclavicular, or axillary regions.

Thymus

The thymus is located in the mediastinal area of the chest and may look quite large on the chest x-ray of a neonate. The thymus is the largest in the preadolescent period. After adolescence, it begins to shrink in size.

The thymus uses hormones to enable the maturation of lymphocytes, produced by the bone marrow, into T lymphocytes (T cells). The mature T cells can then function normally.

Spleen

The spleen functions as a reservoir for blood and blood cells. It also acts like a screen to filter out unwanted invaders and help break up old RBCs that lose their elasticity with age and cannot squeeze through the fine mesh of the spleen. The spleen is particularly good at filtering out one specific bacterium called *Streptococcus pneumoniae*. Children without a spleen or with a nonfunctioning spleen (such as those with sickle cell disease) are more at risk for invasive streptococcal infections and should be put on prophylactic penicillin (until the age of at least 5 years). They also require immediate antibiotics if they have a fever.

Tonsils

The tonsils consist of lymphoid tissue that serves as a storage site for lymphocytes and can also produce some lymphocytes. In children, the tonsils may normally be slightly enlarged between ages 3 and 6 years while the immune system is at its peak of development.

Sounds of silence?

Caregivers of a 3- to 6-year-old child will commonly report that they snore. Snoring at this age is usually due to the enlarged tonsils partially obstructing the airway during sleep.

Immune system cells

All immune system cells are produced in bone marrow. The main cells of the immune system are B cells (B lymphocytes), phagocytes, and T cells (T lymphocytes).

B cells

B cells, which are involved in humoral immunity, produce antibodies. Each B cell is programmed to make a specific antibody. In humoral immunity, a B cell will divide and differentiate into plasma cells when it encounters its triggering antigen. The plasma cells will secrete antibodies to the antigen.

These antibodies then travel in the blood and lymph, which circulate throughout the body. When the antibodies find the antigen, they bind to it to tag it so that other immune system cells can destroy it.

Gobs of globulins

Some antibodies are proteins that perform special functions and are called *immunoglobulins* (Igs). There are five types of Igs produced by B cells:

1. Immunoglobulin A (*IgA*) defends external body surfaces and is present in colostrum, saliva, tears, and nasal fluids as well as

respiratory, gastrointestinal (GI), and genitourinary secretions (Neonates have small amounts of this Ig and are more susceptible to an overgrowth of organisms in mucous membranes such as oral *Candida*.).

2. Immunoglobulin D (*IgD*) is found on the surface of B cells and functions in controlling lymphocyte activation or suppression.
3. Immunoglobulin E (*IgE*) is the antibody responsible for hypersensitivity reactions; it has an immediate response to an antigen and stimulates the release of heparin and histamine from mast cells.
4. Immunoglobulin G (*IgG*) makes up the majority of plasma antibodies and is the main antibacterial and antiviral antibody; transfusions of IgG specific for viral diseases, such as varicella (chickenpox), are useful in treating children who are exposed but have decreased immune function (such as those on chemotherapy).
5. Immunoglobulin M (*IgM*) is the first Ig produced during an immune response; because it is very large, IgM is usually seen only in the blood and cannot pass into tissues to fight infections.

Phagocytes

Phagocytes are immune cells that engulf, kill, and digest particulate matter and foreign invaders. Phagocytes include neutrophils, monocytes, and macrophages. Macrophages are a type of monocyte; they are versatile scavenger cells found in tissues throughout the body. In addition to their phagocytic action, macrophages:

1. activate T cells
2. secrete various blood products, including clotting factors, enzymes, and regulatory molecules.

T cells

T cells are responsible for cell-mediated immunity. Lymphocytes derived from bone marrow migrate to the thymus, where they mature into T cells. In cell-mediated immunity, T cells directly attack antigens, including bacteria, viruses, and other pathogens. They have the ability to identify an antigen (target cell) and produce lymphokines that attack the target directly. Cell-mediated immunity is also responsible for tissue and transplant incompatibility rejections and delayed hypersensitivity reactions (such as a positive tuberculin test response).

There's definitely a T in team

Different types of T cells work together to create the best immune response possible. Helper T cells (CD4+ cells) stimulate B cells to mature into plasma cells, which produce Igs to fight antigens and also retain a memory of them for future encounters.

Search and destroy

The helper T cells also help the killer T cells (CD8+ cells) to more readily recognize the antigen and attack directly. Killer T cells bind to the surface of the invading antigen and disrupt the cell membrane, causing the antigen's destruction.

Complement system

The *complement system* is composed of several proteins that are important in the inflammatory process. It's activated by the antigen–antibody complexes (classic pathway) or toxins released by antigens (alternate pathway). The complement system is one of the body's primary defenses; it immediately assists in mast cell degradation, which enhances vascular permeability and assists in attracting neutrophils to the site.

Hypersensitivity

Hypersensitivity reactions are one of the body's immune responses to an antigen and may be immediate (occurring within minutes) or delayed (may take several hours). There are four types of hypersensitivity reactions, each serving a specific function.

Type I: atopy or anaphylaxis

In some people, certain antigens (allergens) induce B-cell production of IgE, which binds to receptors on mast cell surfaces. The mast cells degranulate and release various mediators, including heparin, histamine, and prostaglandins. These mediators cause vasodilation, bronchospasm, edema, and mucus secretion, leading to symptoms such as wheezing, hives, and rhinorrhea.

Second time around

IgE is produced in sufficient quantities only with repeated exposure and, therefore, may have little effect with occasional allergic reactions. Because severe reactions may not occur with the first exposure to a drug or allergen, the body may only produce antibodies, which will react with the second exposure. In severe reactions, anaphylaxis may occur, resulting in respiratory and cardiac arrest. Someone may not react to an antibiotic the first time—even if they are allergic—but may react upon subsequent exposures.

Type II: cytotoxic response

IgG and IgM are involved in tissue-specific hypersensitivity reactions (type II). The type II hypersensitivity response generally involves the destruction of a target cell by an antibody directed against cell-surface antigens.

Deadly complement

Binding of an antigen and an antibody activates the complement system, which ultimately disrupts the cellular membranes, causing cell death. Cytotoxic T cells and NK cells also contribute to tissue death in type II hypersensitivity. Examples of type II hypersensitivity include transfusion reactions and hemolytic disease in the neonate.

Type III: immune complex

Immune complex–mediated (type III) reactions are similar to type II in that the complex recognizes the same type of antigen. However, in type II, the antigen is found on the cell or organ surface, whereas in type III, the antigen is free floating and is attacked regardless of where it is located. If the antigens are left in the circulatory system, they may cause inflammatory reactions that can result in vessel wall damage and changes in permeability.

Attack first, ask questions later

Autoimmune disorders are caused by type III reactions in which the immune complexes have difficulty distinguishing between normal and abnormal tissue and may attack both. These disorders include systemic lupus erythematosus (SLE), juvenile rheumatoid arthritis, and glomerulonephritis.

Type IV: cell–mediated hypersensitivity

In type IV hypersensitivity, antigen is processed by macrophages and presented to T cells.

Release the lymphokines!

T cells function by releasing *lymphokines*, which recruit and activate other lymphocytes, monocytes, macrophages, and polymorphonuclear leukocytes. The coagulation (kinin) and complement pathways also contribute to tissue damage in this type of reaction. The most serious reactions occur with transplantation when the transplanted tissue is perceived as foreign and attacked. Type IV reactions also occur with exposure to plants or substances that trigger a response resulting in contact dermatitis.

Diagnostic tests

Tests used to diagnose hematologic and immunologic problems in children include allergy skin testing, bone marrow aspiration and biopsy, and complete blood count (CBC) with differential.

Allergy skin testing

Children commonly have short-term allergic problems that may disappear as the child grows older. A child older than 2 years with a history of chronic allergic symptoms, such as coughing rhinorrhea, watery eyes, and upper respiratory congestion, may need to be evaluated for allergies. Symptom management with medications (such as antihistamines) is recommended until the child reaches 4 years or older. If symptoms persist beyond this age, allergy testing may be warranted.

Radioallergosorbent test to the rescue

Allergy skin testing examines specific allergic antigens. The radioallergosorbent test (RAST) identifies antigens in the blood that are causing an immunologic reaction mediated by IgE. The quantity of circulating IgE correlates well with the clinical severity of the allergic symptoms.

The family tree of allergy

When testing is started, a pediatric allergist obtains a detailed history from the family and the child in an attempt to identify the specific antigen. Allergy skin testing entails injecting small amounts of common allergic antigens under the skin (intradermal) to assess for localized reaction. RAST is recommended when there is a strong suspicion that a specific substance is responsible for the allergy problem.

Nursing considerations

Allergy shots run the risk of causing an anaphylactic reaction, and the nurse should be prepared to provide emergency care. The child should remain in the facility for at least 15 minutes after the shot to be monitored for an injection site reaction and signs of an impending anaphylactic reaction.

A song and a wiggle

The child should be prepared for injections (for testing and treatment) and given a "job" to do such as holding very still. Distraction techniques (such as telling the child to wiggle their toes or sing a song) may help reduce the child's anxiety and enhance cooperation. A Child Life Specialist can help to educate, calm, and distract the child during procedures and medical interventions.

Bone marrow aspiration and biopsy

Bone marrow aspiration and bone marrow biopsy are slightly different tests that are usually done for the same reason. Both tests are done to visualize the components of the bone marrow and assess its physiology.

Bone bank withdrawal

In bone marrow aspiration, a specially designed needle with a stylet is inserted into the center of the bone to withdraw liquid bone marrow. The anterior and posterior crests of the iliac bone are most commonly sampled in children. In a bone marrow biopsy, a small section of bone (approximately the length of a fingernail) is taken, revealing the makeup of the bone and bone marrow.

To aspirate or biopsy—that is the question

Ideally, the marrow should show a wide variety of cell types in various stages of maturation. Primary, malignant, blast leukemic cells with few normal cells are seen in leukemia. When a solid tumor, such as neuroblastoma or rhabdomyosarcoma, has metastasized to the bone marrow, a biopsy may be more helpful in showing the clumps of tumor cells among normal cells. Both tests show whether the bone marrow is functioning normally.

Nursing considerations

Bone marrow aspiration or biopsy can be performed using a sedative, under light general anesthesia, or with a local injection to numb the area. Prepare the child for the test with an age-appropriate explanation and monitor for sedation or adverse effects of anesthesia.

In addition, follow these steps:
- Apply a pressure dressing after the procedure, which should be sufficient to stop blood loss.
- Be aware of the proper handling, labeling, and storage of the specimens to prevent the need to repeat the aspiration. Multiple tests may be performed on the specimens obtained.
- Provide analgesic agents as ordered. Postprocedure pain is short term after aspiration and consists of a dull ache for about 24 hours after biopsy.

CBC with differential

One of the most important tests for general screening for hematologic and immune problems is the CBC. An additional test that may be ordered is the *differential*, which is used to determine the percentage of each type of WBCs that are present.

Decrease = disorder

In general, the CBC reveals the numbers of the three main blood cells: WBCs, RBCs, and platelets. Decreased values in any cell line may be an indication of a disorder related to the bone marrow or the immune system or may be the result of infection.

WBC counts

WBC counts vary with age.

- A healthy neonate typically has higher counts of 15,000 to 20,000/mcL, with 60% to 70% being lymphocytes.
- The typical adult WBC count of 5,000 to 10,000/mcL is generally present in children after the age of 2 years.
- Counts over 15,000/mcL in children older than 6 months should be considered high and abnormal (although this does not necessarily indicate serious illness).

RBC counts

Although the RBC count is included in the CBC, the Hgb level and hematocrit are usually used as a gauge of the number of RBCs present:

- *Hgb* is a molecule responsible for carrying oxygen to the tissue and is somewhat affected by age. Higher levels of 15 to 20 g/dL are present in the neonate, but within 2 months, the normal range will be 12 to 15 g/dL.
- *Hematocrit* is approximately three times the level of Hgb, and normal ranges are 35% to 45%. This level is affected by hydration level and may be elevated with dehydration and decreased if the child has fluid overload.

Pediatric and parental platelets

Platelet counts should be between 150,000 and 500,000/mm^3, regardless of age.

Nursing considerations

Prior to drawing labs, prepare the child for venipuncture by answering questions and providing age-appropriate explanations. Allow the parent to be present to comfort the child. After the venipuncture, monitor the site for signs of continued bleeding.

Treatments and procedures

Treatments and procedures used for children with hematologic and immunologic problems include blood transfusion, medication (chemotherapy), radiation, and bone marrow transplantation.

Blood transfusion

Blood transfusion is necessary if levels of blood cells become too low or if the child is experiencing symptoms caused by a decrease in the number of available cells.

Pump up the vascular volume

Generally, transfusions are aimed at increasing volume within the vascular system, increasing RBCs to improve oxygenation, or increasing the number of platelets to reduce or correct bleeding problems:

- Whole blood is transfused if trauma with bleeding occurs and the risk of shock is present because of decreased intravascular volume. Blood loss from surgery may also require whole blood to replace cells and plasma.
- In children who have decreased levels of RBCs only, transfusion with packed RBCs is indicated. Because plasma is removed from these concentrated RBCs, transfusion increases intravascular volume only minimally (only small amounts of WBCs and platelets are contained in the transfused RBCs).
- Platelets are transfused when counts are below $10,000/mm^3$ due to the risk of spontaneous intracranial bleeding, which can lead to death. Transfusion may also be indicated at higher levels due to risk of bleeding, planned surgery or procedures, or symptoms of low platelets.

Nursing considerations

Prepare the child and their caregivers for the procedure by explaining transfusions in a developmentally appropriate manner. Reassure the caregivers (and the child, if old enough) about the measures that are taken to ensure the safety of transfused blood products.

In addition, follow these steps:

- Double-check the child's name, identification number, name bracelet, ABO group, and Rh status with another nurse to help prevent hemolytic transfusion reactions. If there is a discrepancy, do not administer the blood product and notify the blood bank immediately.
- Start the blood transfusion within 30 minutes after it arrives from the blood bank. If you cannot start the transfusion in this time frame, return the blood product to the blood bank.
- Take baseline vital signs just before the start of the transfusion and every 15 minutes during the transfusion. Specifically, monitor for signs of allergic reaction as well as fever.

Bone marrow transplantation

Bone marrow transplantation is used to treat diseases such as acute leukemia, aplastic anemia, and severe combined immunodeficiency disease. The hematopoietic stem cells may be malignant themselves or may have been destroyed by aggressive therapy for malignant disease. In the case of aplastic anemia, the stem cells are absent or just do not work.

Share and share alike

With transplantation, marrow or stem cells are transplanted from a human leukocyte antigen (HLA)-identical donor (usually a sibling) in the hope that the new stem cells will produce normal, healthy cells. Autologous bone marrow transplantation is another option for some patients. In this procedure, the patient's own marrow or stem cells are collected to help with bone marrow recovery after myeloablative chemotherapy.

A harvest of plenty

During bone marrow harvest, marrow is extracted from a donor through multiple bone marrow aspirations; 200 to 500 mL of marrow are collected, processed, and purified before being transfused into a waiting patient.

Getting ready to receive

The bone marrow recipient is given high-dose chemotherapy and, sometimes, radiation to destroy the malignant marrow and WBCs that might cause a reaction.

From harvest to seed

The collected donor marrow, which looks like a blood product, is then transfused through an intravenous (IV) or central line. If the transfusion is successful, in 7 to 14 days the transplanted stem cells will reseed the bone marrow and start producing normal blood cells.

Graft battles host

A great risk after bone marrow transplantation is that the new bone marrow may produce B cells that interpret the normal body tissue as being foreign and attack it. This is commonly seen in the skin, eyes, liver/GI, and other organs and is known as *graft-versus-host disease* (GVHD). The closer the HLA match of donated cells, the lower the chance of GVHD. Typically, this complication will start after the stem cells have engrafted, about 2 weeks after the transplantation.

Although some GVHD may not be harmful, if the stem cells continue to produce cells that attack tissue, the effect can be dramatic, with sloughing of skin, organ malfunction or failure, and eventual death.

Nursing considerations

The donor and the recipient should be prepared for the procedure with age-appropriate explanations. In addition, follow these steps:

- Administer immunosuppressants, such as steroids and cyclosporine, as ordered to control GVHD.
- Provide supportive care for mucositis, pain, fatigue, nausea/vomiting, and other post-chemotherapy symptoms such as WBC count recovers.
- Monitor the child for signs of GVHD, such as changes in skin color, appearance, or texture; hematuria; diarrhea, jaundice; and a change in mental status (even after they leave the facility).
- Because the child is at high risk for infection immediately after the transplantation, monitor closely for signs of illness.
- Prevent skin breakdown by using pressure-relieving or pressure-reducing beds or mattresses; turn the child frequently.
- Support the child and their family throughout this stressful time because the child will be critically ill with the potential for life-threatening complications.

Hematologic and immunologic disorders

Hematologic and immunologic disorders that may affect children include allergic rhinitis, aplastic anemia, atopic dermatitis, hemophilia, iron-deficiency anemia, leukemia, and Sickle cell anemia.

Allergic rhinitis

Inhaled airborne antigens, such as dust and pollen, may cause an immune response that results in watery eyes (allergic conjunctivitis) or an inflammation of the nasal mucosa (rhinitis). Depending on the allergen, allergic rhinitis may occur seasonally (e.g., hay fever) or year-round (perennial allergic rhinitis).

What causes it

Allergic rhinitis is a type I hypersensitivity reaction mediated by IgE. Hay fever occurs in the spring, summer, and fall and is usually induced by airborne pollens from trees, grass, and weeds. In the summer and fall, mold spores may also cause this hypersensitivity.

It may be difficult to identify the exact source of allergic rhinitis. Major perennial allergens and irritants include:

- house dust and dust mites
- feathers
- molds and fungi

- animal dander
- processed materials or industrial chemicals
- tobacco smoke, directly or from clothes worn while smoking (a major offender in children).

Children who have allergic symptoms beginning before the age of 2 years may outgrow them or may have reduced symptoms with time.

How it happens

Once the antigen is recognized by the immune system, a type I hypersensitivity reaction occurs. IgE is created by the conversion of B cells to plasma cells. Histamine release results in the swelling of the mucous membranes. Secondary sinus infections and middle ear infections may be triggered, and nasal polyps caused by edema and infection may increase nasal obstruction.

What to look for

Allergic rhinitis may produce symptoms that vary by age and may be difficult to distinguish from viral upper respiratory infections:

- The patient complains of sneezing attacks, rhinorrhea (profuse, watery nasal discharge), nasal obstruction or congestion, itching nose and eyes, and headache or sinus pain.
- Allergic rhinitis does not normally cause fever unless a secondary infection is present; fever with viral illnesses, such as an upper respiratory infection, is not uncommon.
- A family history of allergies, asthma, and atopic dermatitis (eczema) may indicate that symptoms are IgE mediated.
- Symptoms lasting longer than 2 weeks may indicate a more allergic than infective cause, especially if the child has not had a fever. (See *Allergic shiners*.)

Allergic shiners

In allergic shiners, blood circulation around the eye backs up around the orbit, resulting in dark circles under the eyes or *Dennie sign* (a peculiar horizontal line).

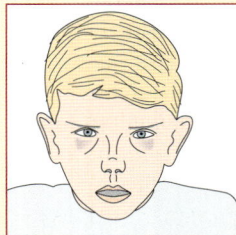

What tests tell you

Most laboratory tests aren't helpful in determining if a short-term illness is an allergy. A large number of eosinophils are seen in specimens of sputum and nasal secretions. The activity of the eosinophils is not completely understood, but they are known to destroy parasitic organisms and play a role in allergic reactions.

Sneezing in your sleep

CBC will be normal with either short- or long-term allergic problems but may be helpful in ruling out a more serious illness if fever is present. Skin testing for allergies, or *RAST*, is helpful after the symptoms are present for several weeks and begin to affect the quality of life, especially by causing sleep disturbances. Short-term or less severe allergic rhinitis remains primarily a clinical diagnosis in children.

Complications

Complications of allergic rhinitis are rarely serious but affect the quality of life of the child and their family. The child may have sleep disturbances from a runny nose, congestion, frequent sneezing, or coughing caused by postnasal drip.

The nose knows

Nosebleeds (epistaxis) may occur as a result of the allergic rhinitis itself or from overuse of medications, which dries mucous membranes. Children with allergic rhinitis are more susceptible to otitis media, sinusitis, bacterial conjunctivitis, and other infections of the upper respiratory tract.

How it's treated

Treatment of allergic rhinitis is aimed at controlling the symptoms and preventing infection. The most effective way to combat allergic rhinitis is to remove the environmental allergen. When exposed to allergens or if unable to remove the offending cause, administering drug therapy can help relieve symptoms. Antihistamines block histamine release and decrease the overall reaction and swelling of the tissue. This action reduces the inflammation of the mucous membranes and decreases nasal drainage. Overuse of antihistamines can dry out the mucous membranes to the point of causing sneezing and nosebleeds.

Timing is everything

One adverse effect of some antihistamines (e.g., diphenhydramine [Benadryl]) in children is sedation. Use of these types of antihistamines should be avoided before going to school and are usually more appropriate at bedtime or naptime. Other antihistamines, such as loratadine (Claritin) and cetirizine (Zyrtec), have been approved for use in children as young as 2 years and are much less sedating.

Up your nose with a nasal spray!

Topical nasal corticosteroids can also control allergy exacerbations. Long-term management may include immunotherapy or desensitization with injections of allergen extracts administered preseasonally, seasonally, or annually.

What to do

Stress the importance of taking daily antihistamines and teach the caregivers and child about their potential adverse effects and ways to reduce the child's exposure to the identified environmental allergen:

- Monitor a child who has received an allergy injection for at least 30 minutes to detect adverse reactions.
- Determine if family history is consistent with allergic problems and be aware that asthma is more common with a familial history of allergies.
- Because many of the allergy medications are over the counter, make sure the parent is giving the correct dose.

Atopic dermatitis

Atopic dermatitis, also called *eczema*, is a chronic condition of the skin characterized by superficial skin inflammation and intense itching. The skin does not hold moisture or oil and becomes dry, scaly, and itchy. Although this disorder may appear at any age, it typically begins during infancy or early childhood.

What causes it

The exact cause is unknown, but an allergic component is strongly suspected. A family history commonly reveals adults with childhood histories of atopic dermatitis, other forms of allergies, and asthma.

To make matters worse . . .

Exacerbating factors include irritants, skin infections (commonly caused by *Staphylococcus aureus*), and other allergens. Exposure to food allergens (such as milk proteins, soybeans, fish, or nuts) may coincide with flare-ups of atopic dermatitis.

How it happens

Scratching the skin causes vasoconstriction and intensifies itching, resulting in reddened, weeping lesions. Eventually, the lesions become scaly and lichenified. Usually, they are located in areas of flexion and extension, such as the neck, antecubital fossa, popliteal folds, and behind the ears. In infants, the lesions are also common on the cheeks and may look like a windburn.

What to look for

Atopic dermatitis begins with skin drying and then cracking which can lead to open sores with bleeding. These open sores are susceptible to secondary infections. Children commonly scratch in their sleep and can do most of the skin damage at that time if the itching is not controlled. Heat, sweating, dry skin, and clothing with wool or coarse materials tend to worsen the itching sensation. (See *Infant with atopic dermatitis.*)

Infant with atopic dermatitis

Children with atopic dermatitis have papular and vesicular skin eruptions with surrounding erythema. The vesicles rupture and discharge yellow, sticky exudate. The secretions form crusts on the skin as they dry.

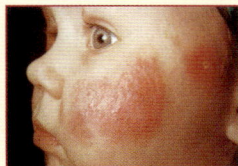

What tests tell you

Elevated levels of IgE and eosinophils are seen in this disorder, but routine laboratory values, such as CBC, are not affected. Allergy testing may be warranted in the older child, but avoiding the allergen may not affect the course of atopic dermatitis.

Complications

Atopic dermatitis may disrupt the family in general because it is a chronic condition that requires daily care. The child may have sleep difficulties from constant pruritus (itching).

From scratching to scarring

Skin damage from scratching leaves the child susceptible to secondary infection that may require either topical treatment with antibiotic ointment or systemic antibiotics. Scarring may occur due to excoriations from scratching.

How it's treated

Measures to ease this chronic disorder include meticulous skin care with moisturizers such as petroleum jelly, environmental control of offending allergens, and drug therapy (often topical steroids). The overall treatment plan is aimed at healing the skin, improving the itching, taming inflammation, and avoiding and treating infections. Moisturizing the skin is the most important part of management as it helps with itching and minimizing the risk for infection.

Too clean, too dry

Excessive bathing leads to further reduction of skin oils and worsens the dryness. Once-daily bathing in warm water with cream-based soaps, such as Tone, Dove, Caress, or Ivory cream, can relieve symptoms. Frequent application of nonirritating topical lubricants (lotions, creams, and ointments) is important, especially after bathing or showering.

Wash, then wear

Minimizing exposure to irritants, such as wool and harsh detergents, also helps control symptoms. New clothes should be washed before wearing to avoid exposure to irritating dyes or chemicals. Clothes washed with bleach should be double-rinsed to ensure that all bleach is removed (because it dries and irritates the skin). Hypoallergenic soaps should be used for all laundry, and starch should be avoided.

Down with itch and inflammation!

Drug therapy involves the use of topical corticosteroids and antipruritics. A mild steroid cream, such as hydrocortisone 1%, can relieve the inflammation and associated itching and may be massaged into the affected area two to three times per day for 1 week.

Diphenhydramine and hydroxyzine (Atarax) are effective antipruritics but may cause sedation. These medications are especially useful at bedtime to reduce nighttime scratching and resulting skin damage.

What to do

The nurse plays an important role in the management of atopic dermatitis and is commonly the key source of daily care plans for minimizing the impact of this condition on the child and their family:

- Instruct all caregivers about the management of the skin lesions.
- Make the family aware that atopic dermatitis is a chronic condition that is not usually related to an identifiable allergen.
- Make sure the caregivers are aware of serious complications such as infection and emphasize the need for evaluation of any open, draining areas.

Hemophilia

A hereditary bleeding disorder, hemophilia results from a deficiency of specific clotting factors. Hemophilia A (classic hemophilia) results from deficiency of factor VIII; hemophilia B (Christmas disease) results from deficiency of factor IX. There are two less common types of hemophilia. Hemophilia C is a deficiency of factor XI. von Willebrand disease includes a deficiency in von Willebrand factor, an important protein necessary for platelet adhesion.

What causes it

The inheritance pattern is X-linked recessive in about 80% of all patients with hemophilia. Hemophilia C is transmitted by an autosomal recessive trait in both sexes. von Willebrand disease is transmitted as an autosomal dominant disorder.

How it happens

Hemophilia produces mild to severe abnormal bleeding. After a platelet plug develops at a bleeding site, the lack of clotting factor prevents a stable fibrin clot from forming. Although hemorrhaging usually does not occur immediately, delayed bleeding is common.

A matter of degrees

Hemophilia may be severe, moderate, or mild, depending on the degree of normal clotting (factor VIII) activity:
- In severe disease, there is less than 1% normal clotting activity.
- In moderate disease, there is 1% to 5% normal clotting activity.
- In mild disease, there is 5% to 50% normal clotting activity.

Most children with hemophilia (60% to 70%) demonstrate the severe form.

What to look for

There is usually a family history of hemophilia or bleeding problems in males.

The circumcision clue

Bleeding can occur spontaneously, and the neonate may have prolonged bleeding times with routine blood collection for neonate tests. It's also common to diagnose hemophilia when the child has excessive and prolonged bleeding after circumcision.

Mountain out of a molehill

Later, spontaneous or disproportionately severe bleeding after minor trauma may produce large subcutaneous and deep intramuscular hematomas. Signs and symptoms of decreased tissue perfusion include restlessness, anxiety, confusion, pallor, cool and clammy skin, chest pain, decreased urine output, hypotension, and tachycardia.

What tests tell you

- A coagulation screen shows a normal prothrombin time (PT) with a prolonged partial thromboplastin time (PTT).
- Factor VIII coagulant activity is decreased in hemophilia A and is normal in hemophilia B.
- Factor IX is decreased in hemophilia B and normal in hemophilia A.
- Platelet aggregation and platelet count are normal in both hemophilia A and B.

Complications

Any type of hemophilia puts the child at risk for bleeding—even with normal activities—making it extremely important to take safety precautions during activities that could place the child at risk.

Head's up!

The greatest risk is with a head injury with intracranial bleeding or bleeding into joints. Joint mobility may be affected by repeated joint injury and may cause decreased range of motion. Any injury may cause bleeding into tissue that may require clotting factor transfusion and hospitalization for monitoring.

The incredible expanding spleen

Injury of the spleen with resulting bleeding may be life-threatening as the spleen expands with blood, causing hypovolemic shock. Historically, patients with hemophilia had higher rates of HIV and hepatitis C before screening for these viruses in blood products was started.

How it's treated

Hemophilia isn't curable, but treatment can prevent crippling deformities and prolong life. Increasing plasma levels of deficient clotting factors helps prevent disabling deformities caused by repeated bleeding into muscles, joints, and organs.

Everyone in the pool!

Hemophilia A or B can be treated with pooled factor obtained from blood products. Historically, these products ran a risk of transmitting viral illness, but current recombinant factors VIII and IX are safe and free from viral infection. Desmopressin acetate (DDAVP) is a synthetic vasopressin analogue. It has a minimal antidiuretic effect but does increase the factor VIII level up to fourfold. It has no effect on factor IX. Hemophilia C and von Willebrand disease are treated with DDAVP, and factor VIII replenishment may also help in von Willebrand disease.

What to do

The nurse's role involves educating the caregivers about safety issues while monitoring the child for acute problems. The child must become accustomed to restrictions in activities and precautions that may make their feel different from their peers. While this might be more easily accepted for the younger child, adolescents may struggle against restrictions and accommodations that highlight differences from their peers. Counseling may be needed to help the child deal with these issues and to help ensure adherence. In addition, follow these steps:

- Observe for evidence of bruising, bleeding, or change in mental status.
- If transfusions are ordered, monitor for blood product reactions, such as fever, chills, or irritability.

Do try this at home

- Because home infusions are commonly done (minimizing the need for hospitalization), educate the caregivers about the process and refer them to a home care infusion agency.
- Teach the family about age-appropriate safety measures, including padding hard surfaces and, later, wearing a bicycle helmet and other protective gear during sports activities.
- Teach the caregivers to recognize signs of bleeding by monitoring for nosebleeds and color of stool. Fresh blood in stool or black, tarry stools are signs of gastric bleeding; excessive swallowing during sleep may be a sign of bleeding and swallowing the blood.

Quash the rebellion

- As the child grows older, assess their participation in new activities and reinforce the need for safety measures. Include the child in these discussions and allow input into decisions as much choice as possible.
- Make families aware of support groups such as the National Hemophilia Foundation and inform them about any local support sources.

Iron-deficiency anemia

Iron-deficiency anemia is a disorder of oxygen transport in which the amount of Hgb circulating in the blood is inadequate. Without sufficient iron, the body cannot produce the Hgb molecule because the heme component is primarily iron.

Some heavy competition

Excesses of other heavy metals (such as lead) may compete for iron-binding sites and cause a lack of Hgb that may lead to iron deficiency. Iron-deficiency anemia is most common in the youngest and oldest children in the pediatric age range (infants, toddlers, and adolescents).

What causes it

Iron-deficiency anemia can be caused by inadequate intake of iron in the diet, malabsorption of iron through the GI tract, or chronic blood loss.

An in utero gift

In the last trimester of pregnancy, the fetus draws what iron it needs from the birthing parent. In the last month, it draws enough iron stores for approximately 6 to 12 months. If the birthing parent is deficient in iron or the neonate is more than 4 weeks premature, the infant may not have sufficient iron stores and, eventually, becomes anemic. This condition is usually evident by 9 to 12 months of life but can occur earlier if the child is more premature, especially less than 32 weeks' gestation.

How it happens

Anytime there is blood loss, there is loss of iron. Adolescents with heavy menses are at risk for iron-deficiency anemia because they lose blood during menstruation. If too little iron is consumed, over time, children can become iron deficient. Iron from food is absorbed into the bloodstream in the small intestine. An intestinal disorder, such as celiac disease, which affects the intestine's ability to absorb nutrients from digested food, can lead to iron-deficiency anemia. If part of the small intestine has been bypassed or removed surgically, it may affect the body's ability to absorb iron and other nutrients. In resource-limited countries, a leading cause of iron deficiency is infestation from parasitic worms (hookworms, whipworms, roundworms).

Got milk?

Cow's milk allergy, due to heat-labile protein in cow's milk, causes inflammation of the GI tract with chronic blood loss and decreased absorption. This allergy is a common source of iron-deficiency anemia. In adolescents, iron-deficiency anemia is commonly related to fad dieting and overconsumption of snack foods containing little or no iron.

You are what you eat

Adolescent females are at risk for iron-deficiency anemia during their growth spurt and at the beginning of menses, especially if periods are irregular. Adolescent males are at a lower risk, although any adolescent may have poor dietary habits or eat fad diet foods. Vegetarians and vegans are not at increased risk if they plan their diets with adequate sources of iron.

What to look for

Clinical symptoms may be mild until anemia is severe, causing a pale appearance and decreased activity. Toddlers may have a history of prematurity and poor weight gain. Other symptoms include:

- fatigue
- inability to concentrate
- palpitations
- dyspnea on exertion
- craving for nonnutritive substances such as ice, dirt, or starch (pica)
- tachycardia
- dry, brittle nails
- concave, or "spoon-shaped," fingernails.

What tests tell you

Hgb, hematocrit, red cell distribution width (RDW), and ferritin tests may be used in diagnosing iron-deficiency anemia. Lower than normal Hgb levels indicate anemia. The normal ranges for children vary depending on the child's age and sex. Hematocrit is the percentage of the blood volume made up by RBCs. Like Hgb, the hematocrit values differ according to the child's age. The RDW will show RBCs that are smaller and paler in color than normal cells in children with iron-deficiency anemia. Ferritin is a protein that helps the body store iron. A low level of ferritin usually indicates a low level of stored iron.

Bleached out bull's-eye

Iron-deficiency anemia is a microcytic, hypochromic anemia, meaning the RBCs are small and pale. RBCs with decreased iron appear bleached out, resembling a bull's-eye target. Because the cells are small, the mean corpuscular volume (MCV) and the mean corpuscular Hgb concentration are low. Serum iron levels are decreased.

Complications

Untreated iron-deficiency anemia can cause stress on all body tissue, with decreased oxygenation. Severe anemia poses the greatest risk to the respiratory and cardiovascular systems. Increasing evidence suggests that children with even mild iron deficiency have less ability to concentrate and greater difficulty in school. Overtreatment with replacement iron can occur when toxic levels of iron buildup, which may cause excessive iron deposits, affecting the liver, heart, pituitary glands, and joints. Pica may lead to eating lead-based paint and can result in lead poisoning.

How it's treated

The main treatment is correction of the underlying problem. If chronic blood loss or GI bleeding is suspected, appropriate intervention is needed.

In with the iron

If the problem is nutritional, the child's diet should be adjusted to increase iron intake. Good sources of dietary iron include red meat, organ meat, legumes (such as kidney and pinto beans), green leafy vegetables, raisins, and dried apricots as well as iron-fortified cereals and formula. Milk has little iron and may actually cause anemia by preventing the intake of other iron-rich foods if the child fills up on milk.

It's supplementary, my dear Watson!

In addition to dietary changes, the child may be placed on oral iron supplementation, although iron supplements aren't absorbed as well as iron from dietary sources. The American Academy of Pediatrics recommends that children with hematocrit below 34% (Hgb level less than 11.3 g/dL) be placed on supplemental iron. Ascorbic acid (vitamin C) helps with iron absorption. Breast milk has low levels of iron, but the iron that is present is extremely well absorbed and is adequate for most infants. If an infant is drinking formula, it should be iron fortified.

What to do

Nursing care focuses on educating the caregivers about diet and treatment regimens:

- Monitor the child's adherence with the prescribed iron supplement therapy.
- Teach the caregivers of infants the importance of using iron-fortified infant cereals or iron-fortified formula.
- Teach the caregivers or adolescents about good iron sources in the normal diet; if the child is a vegetarian, explain the importance of incorporating iron-rich vegetable sources into the diet.
- Caution the child and caregivers that taking iron supplements may result in dark green or black stool; supplements can also cause constipation, and this may need to be treated with prunes or a laxative.
- Make sure the caregivers understand the dosage and administration of oral iron supplements; stress the importance of storing the supplements safely because they are a major source of poisoning in children.
- Taking iron supplements with vitamin C sources (like orange juice) may help absorption. Discuss ways to mask the taste of iron, as this is often a major reason for nonadherence.

Leukemia

Leukemia is cancer of the body's blood-forming tissues, including the bone marrow and the lymphatic system. Leukemia usually starts in the WBCs with an abnormal, uncontrolled overproduction of WBCs by the stem cells in bone marrow. The nonfunctional, leukemic cells infiltrate the tissues of the body and replace normal cells. Children are most commonly diagnosed with B-cell acute lymphocytic leukemia (ALL), which involves the lymphocytic WBC cell line, or acute myelogenous leukemia (AML), which involves the granulocytic–myelocytic WBC cell line.

What causes it

The exact cause of leukemia is unknown. It seems to develop from a combination of genetic and environmental factors. There is an increased incidence of ALL in children with Down syndrome (trisomy 21). Other risk factors include exposure to large doses of ionizing radiation or drugs that suppress bone marrow. Certain viruses, such as human T-cell lymphotropic virus type I, are also associated with an increased risk for leukemia.

How it happens

Leukemia is thought to occur when some blood cells acquire mutations in their DNA. This causes a rapid production of WBCs, which results in the accumulation of immature, nonfunctional cells called *blast cells*. The blast cells multiply continuously, regardless of the body's needs. However, the proliferating blast cells do not attack and destroy normal cells. Rather, they crowd out other healthy, functional cells, robbing them of nutrition essential for metabolism, leading to *pancytopenia* (reduction in the number of blood cells being produced by all cell lines). Eventually, the bone marrow becomes packed with the malignant cells, and they spill out into the peripheral blood where they can be seen on microscopic slides.

What to look for

Signs and symptoms of ALL and AML are similar and are related to suppression of elements of the bone marrow:
- RBC and platelet levels are reduced as the stem cells are no longer producing them, which leads to anemia with decreased Hgb.
- A low platelet count leads to bruising, bleeding, and multiple nosebleeds; minor trauma, such as bumping into furniture, may cause large bruises.
- Because the WBCs are immature and nonfunctioning, the ability to fight infection is diminished, and the child may experience high fevers and show signs of sepsis.

What tests tell you

- Blood counts show thrombocytopenia and neutropenia. The WBC count in a CBC will be very high (usually over 25,000/mcL), and the differential determines cell type.
- Lumbar puncture is performed to detect meningeal involvement; cerebrospinal fluid analysis reveals abnormal WBC invasion of the CNS.
- Bone marrow aspiration and biopsy confirm the disease, showing blast cells present in large numbers. (These tests are also used to determine whether the leukemia is lymphocytic or myelogenous, which will help determine treatment and prognosis.)

Complications

Because leukemia and its treatment affect all blood cell lines and the immune system, complications vary and can be severe. Infections are of particular concern.

Fungus alert

Children on long-term immunosuppressive therapy may have overgrowth of fungal infections, such as candidiasis, or little resistance to severe fungal infections such as aspergillosis. Disruptions in the child's and family's routine may have major impacts on school and social development as well as cause stress and anxiety.

How it's treated

Both ALL and AML are treated with combinations of oral and IV chemotherapy drugs aimed at killing the malignant stem cells plus leukemia cells that may have migrated to other areas of the body. AML is more resistant to therapy; therefore, the treatment regimens are more severe, requiring more hospitalizations. Because IV chemotherapy can't penetrate the CNS and spinal fluid, treatment of the CNS involves intrathecal chemotherapy.

Treatment may also include:
- antibiotic, antifungal, and antiviral drugs
- colony-stimulating factors, such as filgrastim (Neupogen), are used in the treatment of AML
- transfusions of platelets to prevent bleeding and transfusions of RBCs to prevent anemia.

Transplant to the rescue

Bone marrow transplantation has become a standard treatment for some patients with leukemia because it can improve long-term survival.

What to do

Leukemia is a devastating diagnosis for the child and their family. The child must deal not only with the disease but also with the adverse effects of treatment. The child should be prepared for all tests and treatments, and emotional support should be offered to their family. Referral to additional support services may be needed.

In addition, follow these steps:

- Educate the child and their family about the disease and treatments (including treatment-related problems).
- Assess for bleeding, bruising, fatigue, and signs and symptoms of an impending infection.
- To control infection, place the patient in a private room with minimal interaction with those caring for patients with communicable illnesses.
- Provide guidelines for reducing adverse effects of chemotherapy such as nausea, vomiting, constipation, or diarrhea. Make sure the caregivers understand how to administer medications to treat these common effects.
- Make the caregivers aware that any fever is serious and may be life-threatening; a health care provider should immediately evaluate the child with a fever.
- Attempt to explain to families the need for flexibility because there are many events—including illness and appointments—that are unexpected. Cancer is a stressor for all family members.

Sickle cell anemia

Sickle cell anemia is an inherited, autosomal recessive genetic disease that affects the RBCs, which become acutely sickle shaped. They occlude small vessels, causing pain and decreased function. The two common variants of sickle cell anemia are hemoglobin SS (Hgb SS) and hemoglobin SC (Hgb SC) disease. Symptoms are usually severe with Hgb SS and moderate or undetectable in Hgb SC.

What causes it

The child must receive the autosomal recessive gene from both caregivers to have the condition. The defective hemoglobin (Hgb S) takes on the classic sickle shape with decreased oxygen-carrying capacity and inability to flow through capillaries. Carriers of sickle cell trait have few symptoms and only on rare occasions.

How it happens

Sickle cell anemia occurs as a result of a mutation in the gene that encodes the beta chain of Hgb. This mutation causes a structural change in Hgb. A single amino acid change from glutamic acid to valine occurs in the sixth position of the beta Hgb chain.

Hgb S is for sickle

When hypoxia (oxygen deficiency) occurs, the Hgb S in the RBCs becomes insoluble. As a result, the blood cells become rigid and rough, forming an elongated crescent, or sickle, shape. Sickling can cause hemolysis (cell destruction).

Capillary traffic jam

Sickle cells accumulate in capillaries and smaller blood vessels as they cannot pass through these areas, causing occlusions and increasing blood viscosity. This increased viscosity impairs normal circulation, causing pain, tissue infarctions (tissue death), swelling, and anoxic changes that lead to further sickling and obstruction.

Low on O_2

Sickle cell crisis occurs when a patient with sickle cell anemia experiences cellular oxygen deprivation from, for example, an infection, exposure to cold or high altitude, or overexertion. A chain of events then ensues. (See *Understanding sickle cell crisis.*)

What to look for

Infants are screened for sickle cell on the newborn screening test, so children with sickle cell disease and sickle cell trait should be identified early. Signs and symptoms of sickle cell anemia usually don't develop until after the age of 6 months because large amounts of fetal Hgb act in a protective manner. Fetal Hgb has a higher oxygen concentration and inhibits sickling. Swollen hands and feet (hand-foot syndrome) may be the first signs of sickle cell anemia in babies. The swelling is caused by sickle-shaped RBCs blocking blood flow out of their hands and feet. Periodic episodes of pain, called sickle cell crises, are a major symptom of sickle cell anemia. Pain develops when sickle-shaped RBCs block blood flow through tiny blood vessels to the chest, abdomen, and joints. Sickle cells can damage the spleen, an important organ in fighting infection—making children more vulnerable to infections. Children with sickle cell anemia usually receive prophylactic antibiotics until the age of 5 years to prevent potentially life-threatening bacterial infections. Children with sickle cell disease may have delayed growth and anemia because the sickle cells have a shortened lifespan compared to normal RBCs (20 days for sickle cells vs. 120 days for normal RBCs).

Understanding sickle cell crisis

Sickle cell crisis is triggered by infection, cold exposure, high altitudes, overexertion, dehydration, and other conditions that cause cellular oxygen deprivation. Here's what happens:

• Deoxygenated, sickle-shaped erythrocytes adhere to the capillary wall and to one another, blocking blood flow and causing cellular hypoxia.

• The crisis worsens as tissue hypoxia and acidic waste products cause more sickling and cell damage.

• With each new crisis, organs and tissues are destroyed and areas of tissue die slowly (especially in the spleen and kidneys).

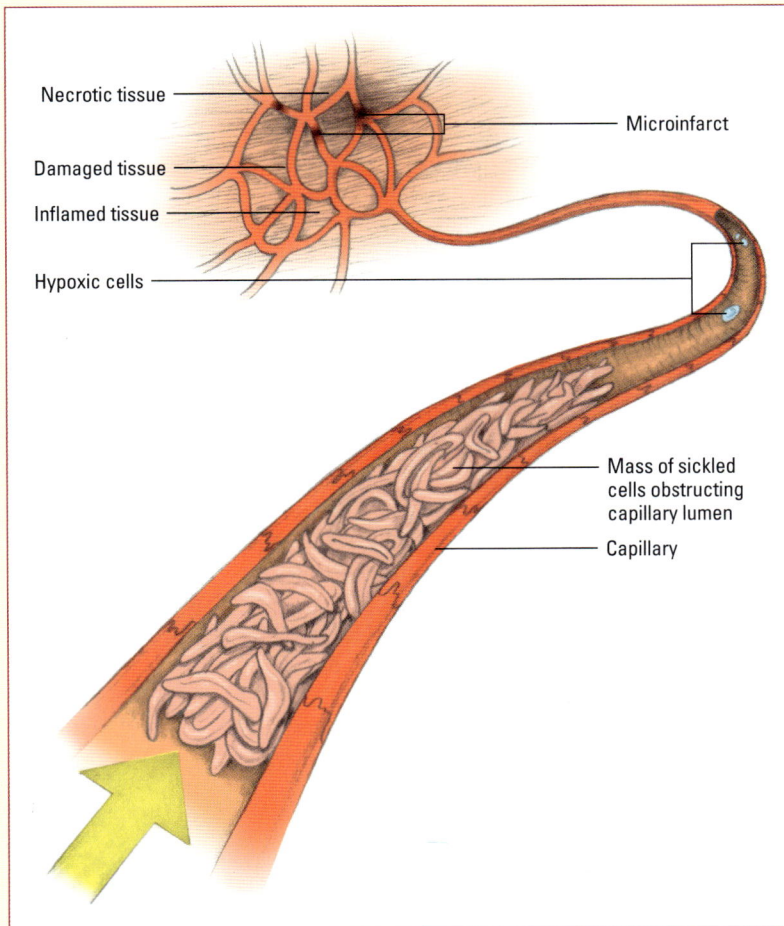

A telling history

The patient's history includes chronic fatigue (due to chronic anemia), unexplained dyspnea or dyspnea on exertion, joint swelling, aching bones, severe localized and generalized pain, leg ulcers (rare in children), and frequent infections. Inspection of the skin may reveal jaundice or pallor. A young child may appear small for their age. The spleen will usually be enlarged and palpable.

Sickle cell crisis

In sickle cell crisis, symptoms include severe pain; hematuria; lethargy; irritability; and pale lips, tongue, palms, and nail beds.

Isn't one enough?

Four different types of crisis can occur:

1. In *painful crisis*, patients report severe abdominal, thoracic, muscle, or bone pain and, possibly, increased jaundice, dark urine, or a low-grade fever.
2. *Aplastic crisis* results from bone marrow depression and is characterized by pallor, lethargy, sleepiness, dyspnea, markedly decreased bone marrow activity, RBC hemolysis, and possible coma.
3. *Acute sequestration crisis*, occurring in infants, may cause sudden, massive entrapment of RBCs in the spleen and liver; if untreated, lethargy and pallor progress to hypovolemic shock and death.
4. *Hemolytic crisis* results from complications of the disease rather than the disease itself; degenerative changes cause liver congestion and enlargement, and chronic jaundice develops and worsens. The spleen is often nonfunctioning from being infarcted by sickle cells.

What tests tell you

- Hgb levels will be low, and sickle cells will be seen on microscopic slide.
- Additional blood tests show low RBC counts, elevated WBC and platelet counts, a decreased ESR, increased serum iron levels, decreased RBC survival, and reticulocytosis.
- Genetic tests will help identify the status of the caregivers and can be used to assess sibling status. Because of the importance of early diagnosis, it has become standard for all neonates to be tested at birth for both carrier and disease states.

Complications

Clinical manifestations of sickle cell anemia vary, resulting in a wide range of complications related to occlusion of the blood vessels. Complications include stroke, acute chest syndrome, organ damage, retinal damage/blindness, and priapism. A stroke can occur if the sickle cells block blood flow to the brain. Acute chest syndrome is a life-threatening complication of sickle cell anemia that causes chest pain, fever, and difficulty breathing. Acute chest syndrome can be caused by a lung infection or by sickle cells blocking blood vessels in the lungs. It may require emergency medical treatment with antibiotics, oxygen, pain medications, and other treatments.

Sickle cells can block blood flow through blood vessels, immediately depriving an organ of blood and oxygen. Chronic deprivation of oxygen-rich blood can damage nerves and organs, including the kidneys, liver, and spleen. Organ damage can be fatal.

The blood vessels that supply the eyes can get blocked by sickle cells and, over time, can damage the retina and lead to blindness. Sickle cells can block the blood vessels in the penis. As a result, males with sickle cell anemia may experience painful, long-lasting erections—a condition called priapism. This can damage the penis and eventually lead to impotence.

How it's treated

Bone marrow transplant offers the only potential cure for sickle cell anemia. Transplants are recommended only for people who have significant symptoms and problems from sickle cell anemia. As a result, treatment for sickle cell anemia is usually aimed at avoiding crises, relieving symptoms, and preventing complications. Treatments may include medications to reduce pain and prevent complications, blood transfusions, and supplemental oxygen. To prevent life-threatening bacterial infections, children with sickle cell anemia may begin taking the antibiotic penicillin when they are about 2 months of age and continue taking it until they are 5 years old. To relieve pain during a sickle crisis, over-the-counter or prescription pain relievers may be recommended.

When taken daily, hydroxyurea reduces the frequency of painful crises and may reduce the need for blood transfusions. Hydroxyurea seems to work by stimulating production of fetalHgb—a type of Hgb found in newborns that helps prevent the formation of sickle cells. Long-term use of hydroxyurea may increase the risk of infection. In children with sickle cell anemia at high risk for stroke, regular blood transfusions can decrease their risk of stroke but may cause an excess amount of iron to build up in the body. Excess iron can damage the heart, liver, and other organs. Therefore, patients who undergo regular transfusions may need iron-chelating treatment with deferasirox (Exjade) to reduce iron levels. Because infections can be very serious in children with sickle cell anemia, children should be up to date on all of their immunizations.

What to do

A child who experiences the pain of a crisis will likely be fearful of future crises, as will their caregivers. This may have a significant impact on the child's life. They may be afraid to participate in normal activities for fear of bringing on a crisis, and their caregivers may become overprotective. Pain is often severe. Always believe the patient about their level of pain.

In pursuit of normal

Prevention and education are the keys to leading a normal life, and participation in a support group may be extremely helpful in this regard. To prevent sickle crisis, the goal is to maintain as high of a state of oxygenation as possible:

- Be aware that excessive exercise or activity may precipitate crisis.
- Avoid tight or restricting clothes such as elastic at the end of sleeves.
- Promote relaxation and stress-reducing activities because mental stress may play a role in crisis.
- Encourage the child to attend school and social functions while being aware that they may be more susceptible to infection.
- Explain the need to avoid flying in unpressurized aircrafts.
- Stress the importance of immediate evaluation of fever; children with sickle cell anemia are functionally asplenic and are at risk for pneumococcal sepsis.
- Impress upon the patient and family the importance of medication adherence and the possible consequences of nonadherence.
- Understand that sickle cell disease can cause great pain. Pain medications often include opioids. Treating pain appropriately (both with and without medications) and seeking emergency care during times of a pain crisis should be impressed upon patients and families.

Quick quiz

1. The main function of platelets is to:
    A. provide oxygen to tissue.
    B. fight viral infections and provide immunity.
    C. fight bacterial infections.
    D. form a blood clot.

Answer: D. Platelets adhere to one another and plug holes in vessels or tissues where there's bleeding.

2. Which type of cell induces cell-mediated immunity?
   A. T lymphocytes
   B. Monocytes
   C. Reticulocytes
   D. B lymphocytes

Answer: A. T lymphocytes and macrophages are the chief participants in cell-mediated immunity.

3. What causes ALL?
   A. RBCs are defective and can't fight infection.
   B. Bone marrow stem cells are defective and produce ineffective blast cells.
   C. WBCs mature into only one cell line and fight only one type of infection.
   D. Platelets can't form clots, leading to severe hemorrhaging.

Answer: B. Stem cells start to produce nonfunctional blast cells for no apparent reason. The blast cells compete with and deprive normal cells of their essential nutrients and gradually replace them.

4. An example of a type I hypersensitivity reaction is:
   A. anaphylaxis.
   B. transfusion reaction.
   C. autoimmune disorder.
   D. GVHD.

Answer: A. Examples of type I hypersensitivity reactions are anaphylaxis, hay fever (allergic rhinitis), and, in some people, asthma.

Scoring

⭐⭐⭐ If you answered all four items correctly, bravo! You're obviously immune to incorrect answers.

⭐⭐ If you answered three items correctly, great work! Your knowledge of hematologic and immunologic systems is coursing through your blood.

⭐ If you answered fewer than three items correctly, don't have an adverse reaction. There's only one more quiz to go!

Suggested References

Akrimi, S., Simiyu, V., Nchimba, L., & Ngongola, A. (2023). Children with sickle cell disease: Acute complications, acute pain and perioperative management. *Update in Anaesthesia, 37,* 28–33. https://doi.org/10.1029/WFSA-D-20-00010

Burnham, J., Cecere, L., Ukaigwe, J., Knight, A., Peterson, R., & Chang, J. (2021). Factors associated with variation in pediatric systemic lupus erythematosus care delivery. *ACR Open Rheumatology, 3,* 708–714.

Evangelista, T., Sosko, J., Weyant, D., & Schreiber, J. (2022). Integrative wellness program for pediatric oncology/bone marrow transplant patients. *Pediatric Nursing, 48,* 7–20.

Fyfe-Taylor, L., & Cockett, A. (2021). Addressing the psychosocial needs of young people with thalassaemia undergoing bone marrow transplantation. *Nursing Children & Young People, 33,* 19–24.

Gittus, A., & Roach, R. (2021). The human immunodeficiency virus in pediatrics. *International Journal of Child Health & Human Development, 14,* 265–279.

Gooch, M., & Jordan, K. (2023). Atopic dermatitis: A common pediatric diagnosis that is not just another rash. *Advanced Emergency Nursing Journal, 45,* 195–205.

Kato, M., & Manabe, A. (2018). Treatment and biology of pediatric acute lymphoblastic leukemia. *Pediatrics International, 60,* 4–12.

Khair, K. (2019). Management of haemophilia in children. *Paediatrics & Child Health, 29,* 334–338.

Lo, A. C., Dieckmann, K., Pelz, T., Gallop-Evans, E., Engenhart-Cabillic, R., Vordermark, D., Kelly, K. M., Schwartz, C. L., Constine, L. S., Roberts, K., & Hodgson, D. (2021). Pediatric classical Hodgkin lymphoma. *Pediatric Blood & Cancer, Supplement, 68*(S2), 1–10.

Mattiello, V., Schmugge, M., Hengartner, H., von der Weid, N., & Renella, R. (2020). Diagnosis and management of iron deficiency in children with or without anemia: Consensus recommendations of the SPOG Pediatric Hematology Working Group. *European Journal of Pediatrics, 179,* 527–545.

Tosca, M., Del Barba, P., Licari, A., & Ciprandi, G. (2020). The measurement of asthma and allergic rhinitis control in children and adolescents. *Children, 7,* 1–9.

Chapter 23

Dermatologic problems

Just the facts

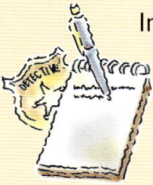

In this chapter, you'll learn:

◆ anatomy and physiology of the integumentary system

◆ tests used to diagnose dermatologic problems in children

◆ treatments and procedures for children with skin problems

◆ dermatologic disorders that may affect infants, children, and adolescents.

Anatomy and physiology

The integumentary system, which consists of the skin and its components, is the largest organ system in the body. At birth, the skin is only 1 mm thick; the dermal layer of the skin doubles in thickness at maturity.

The great protector

The skin protects most of the other organ systems by acting as a mechanical barrier. Other functions include sensory perception, temperature regulation, vitamin synthesis, and excretion of wastes through sweating.

Structures of the skin

The skin is composed of layers of tissue. Appendages of the skin include the hair and glands.

Skin layers

The skin consists of two layers and a sublayer, the hypodermis or sub-cutaneous tissue:

- The *epidermis*, or outermost covering, provides a protective barrier to external trauma and limits the loss of body contents to the environment; dermatologic problems are characteristically evident on the epidermis.
- The *dermis* consists of connective tissue that gives the skin strength and elasticity; it contains blood vessels, lymphatics, and nerves.
- The *hypodermis* lies below the dermis and is composed of loose connective tissue, or *adipose tissue*. It contains larger blood vessels, lymph channels, and nerve trunks. This layer attaches the skin to the underlying bones, acts as a cushion and temperature insulator, and determines the skin's contours. (See *Structure of the skin.*)

Structure of the skin

Major components of the skin include the epidermis, dermis, and epidermal appendages (hair and glands).

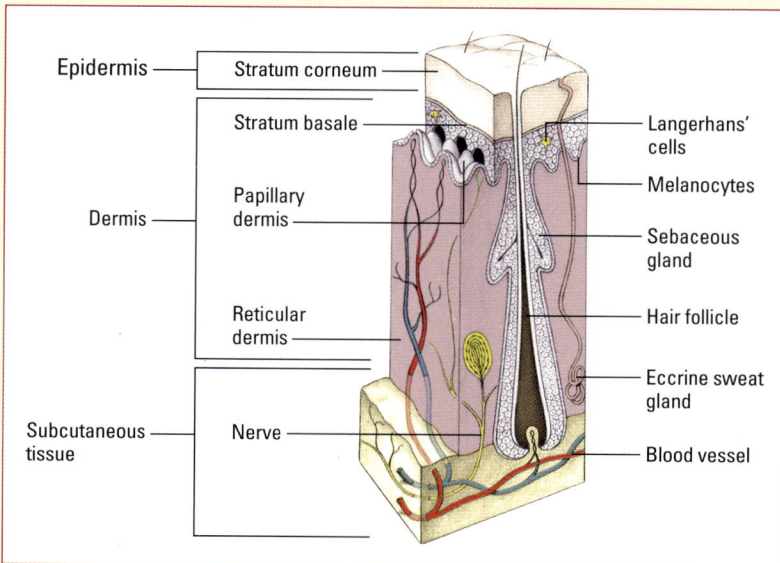

Epidermis — Stratum corneum —
Stratum basale —
— Langerhans' cells
— Melanocytes
Papillary dermis —
Dermis —
— Sebaceous gland
Reticular dermis —
— Hair follicle
— Eccrine sweat gland
Subcutaneous tissue — Nerve —
— Blood vessel

Thin-skinned

Skin layers act to prevent water loss, which varies with environmental temperature and humidity as well as the proportion of body surface exposed. Thus, fluid loss in the preterm neonate is greater than in an adult because the neonate's skin is thinner.

Hair

Hair changes markedly during the stages of development.

Fetal comb-over

Fine body hair, or *lanugo*, is found in utero over most of the fetus but decreases as the fetus approaches full term. The neonate's scalp hair varies greatly in amount and is usually lost before growth of permanent hair, which gradually thickens.

Growth spurt

Puberty causes additional growth of hair in the axilla and pubic regions of both genders; boys experience facial hair growth.

Glands

The main glands of the skin are:
- *sebaceous glands*, or sebum-producing glands, which contain the hair follicles and keep the skin supple by minimizing water loss. They are more prevalent on the scalp, forehead, nose, chin, and genitalia.
- *sweat glands*, which may be *eccrine* (function as the body's heat-regulating mechanism by producing sweat) or *apocrine* (mature at puberty and cause the unpleasant body odor associated with sweating).

Diagnostic tests

Various tests are used to help diagnose skin problems and related systemic diseases and to identify the causes of the disorder.

Potassium hydroxide preparation

Potassium hydroxide (KOH) preparation is an alkalinizing agent that is used to prepare clinical specimens for microscopic examination needed to help diagnose fungal disorders.

Fungus finder

A drop of 20% KOH is added to skin scrapings to dissolve debris before the scrapings are placed on a slide. When the slide is heated, the skin cells dissolve, leaving fungal elements visible on microscopic examination.

Nursing considerations

Explain the procedure to the caregivers and the child. Tell the child what to expect, including discomfort they may experience, and suggest coping strategies such as distraction techniques.

Skin biopsy

Skin biopsy is the removal of a section or an entire lesion for microscopic analysis to determine its cell structure and make a diagnosis. (See *Recognizing skin lesions.*) A skin biopsy specimen can be obtained by:

- shave biopsy
- punch biopsy
- excisional biopsy.

Recognizing skin lesions

These illustrations depict the most common primary and secondary skin lesions.

Macule

Flat, pigmented, circumscribed area less than 1 cm in diameter (freckle, rubella, petechiae)

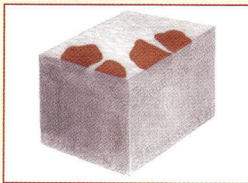

Plaque

Circumscribed, solid, elevated lesion more than 1 cm in diameter; elevation above skin surface occupies a larger surface area compared with height (psoriasis, mycosis fungoides).

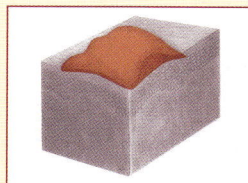

Papule

Firm, inflammatory, raised lesion up to 0.5 cm in diameter, may be the same color as skin or pigmented (acne papule, lichen planus, wart, basal cell carcinoma).

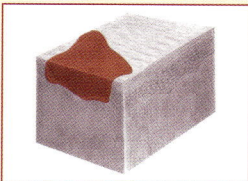

Patch

Flat, pigmented, circumscribed area more than 1 cm in diameter (herald patch [pityriasis rosea] and vitiligo)

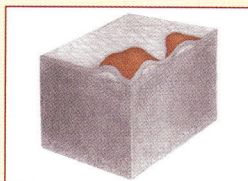

Recognizing skin lesions (*continued*)

Nodule

Firm, raised lesion; deeper than a papule, extending into the dermal layer; 0.5 to 2 cm in diameter (intradermal nevus, keloid, lipoma)

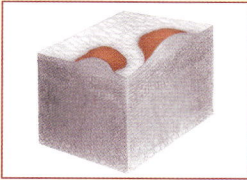

Tumor

Elevated, solid lesion more than 2 cm in diameter, extending into dermal and subcutaneous layers (dermatofibroma, hemangioma)

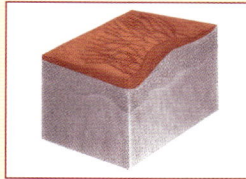

Wheal

Raised, firm lesion with intense localized skin edema, varying in size and shape; color ranging from pale pink to red, disappears in hours (hive [urticaria], insect bite)

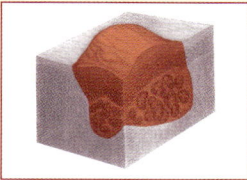

Comedone

Plugged pilosebaceous duct, exfoliative, formed from sebum and keratin (blackhead [open comedone], whitehead [closed comedone])

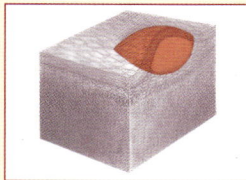

Cyst

Semisolid or fluid-filled encapsulated mass extending deep into the dermis (sebaceous cyst, cystic acne)

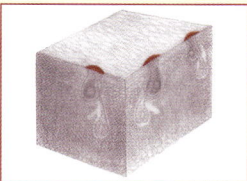

Vesicle

Raised, circumscribed, fluid-filled lesion less than 0.5 cm in diameter (chickenpox [varicella], herpes simplex)

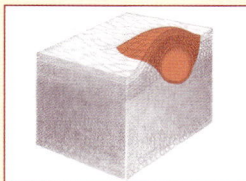

Pustule

Raised, circumscribed lesion usually less than 1 cm in diameter; containing purulent material that makes it a yellow-white color (acne pustule, impetigo, furuncle)

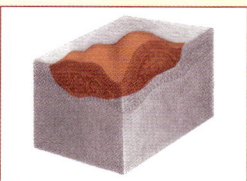

Bulla

Fluid-filled lesion more than 2 cm in diameter; also called a *blister* (severe poison oak or ivy dermatitis, bullous pemphigoid, second-degree burn)

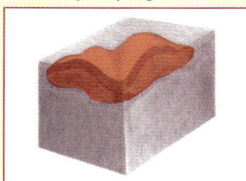

(*continued*)

Recognizing skin lesions (*continued*)

Atrophy
Thinning of skin surface at site of disorder (striae, aging skin)

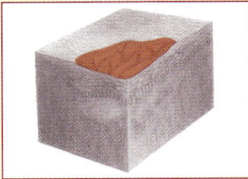

Erosion
Circumscribed lesion involving loss of superficial epidermis (rug burn, abrasion)

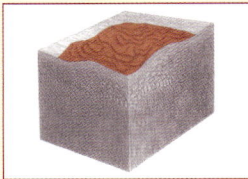

Ulcer
Epidermal and dermal destruction may extend into subcutaneous tissue; usually heals with scarring (pressure injury).

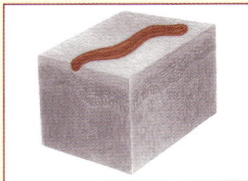

Scale
Thin, dry flakes of shedding skin (psoriasis, dry skin, newborn desquamation)

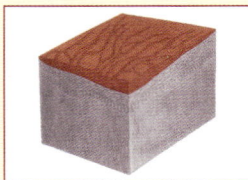

Crust
Dried sebum, serous, sanguineous, or purulent exudate overlying an erosion or weeping vesicle, bulla, or pustule (impetigo, secondarily infected dermatitis)

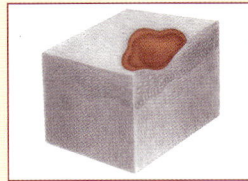

Excoriation
Linear scratched or abraded area, usually self-induced (abraded acne, eczema)

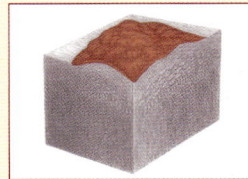

Fissure
Linear cracking of the skin extending into the dermal layer (hand dermatitis [chapped skin], interdigital tinea pedis)

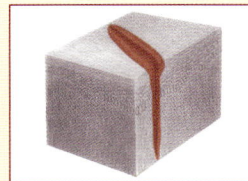

Lichenification
Thickened, prominent skin markings from constant rubbing (chronic atopic dermatitis)

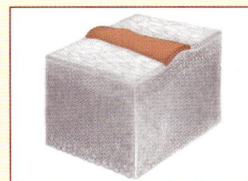

Recognizing skin lesions (*continued*)

Scar

Fibrous tissue caused by trauma, deep inflammation, or surgical incision; red and raised (recent), pink and flat (6 weeks), and depressed (old) (on a healed surgical incision)

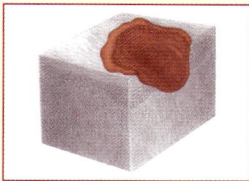

The closest shave

In a shave biopsy, the protruding portion of the growth is excised at skin level and the specimen is sent for microscopic examination.

Pulled and punched

In a punch biopsy, the skin surrounding the lesion is pulled taut, and the punch is introduced firmly into the lesion. The punch is then rotated to obtain a tissue specimen, or *plug*. The plug is lifted with forceps or a needle, and the surgeon severs as deeply as possible into the fat layer. The wound is then sutured closed.

Out, out, darn lesion

In an excisional biopsy, a scalpel is used to excise the lesion completely.

Nursing considerations

Explain the procedure to the caregivers and child. Tell the child what to expect, including discomfort they may experience, and suggest coping strategies such as distraction techniques.

Post punch, shave, and excise

After the procedure, follow these steps:
- Apply a pressure dressing to the site.
- Observe the site for bleeding.
- Administer analgesic agents for pain as ordered.

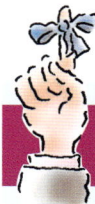

Memory jogger

Need help remembering what to assess when evaluating a skin lesion? Just think about your ABCDs.

Asymmetry
Border
Color and
    configuration
Diameter and
    drainage

Tzanck test

Tzanck test is a microscopic examination of cells taken from skin lesions to aid in the diagnosis of vesicular diseases. Cells are scraped from the base of a vesicle to obtain moist, cloudy debris, or *exudate*. The cells are then placed on a slide, air-dried, and stained with Wright or Giemsa stain. Multinucleated giant cells are indicative of either herpesvirus or varicella.

Nursing considerations

Explain the procedure to the caregivers and the child. Tell the child what to expect, including discomfort they may experience, and suggest coping strategies such as distraction techniques.

Treatments and procedures

Management of skin disorders may include a variety of therapeutic procedures, including laser surgery and skin grafting.

Laser surgery

Laser is the common term for light amplification by simulated emission of radiation. Lasers are used in surgery to divide adhesions or to treat lesions of the skin. The most common types of lasers used are the pulsed dye laser, the argon laser, and the carbon dioxide laser, each of which emits light at a different wavelength.

Complications

Complications associated with laser surgery include secondary infections, keloid or pyrogenic granuloma formation, localized dermatitis, and hyperpigmentation or hypopigmentation.

Nursing considerations

Explain the procedure to the caregivers and the child and prepare the child for discomfort they may experience. Make sure to prepare the child (and the caregivers) for the appearance of the treated area after laser surgery because it will probably look much worse (some laser treatments leave skin raw and oozing). Reassure the child that this is normal, and the area will heal quickly.

After the laser

After laser surgery, follow these steps:
- Apply dressings as ordered.
- Instruct the caregivers in care of the treated area.

- Stress to the child and caregivers the importance of avoiding trauma to the lesion or picking at the scab.

Skin grafting

During skin grafting, a section of skin is separated from its blood supply and implanted over an area where skin has been lost due to burns, injury, or surgical débridement of diseased tissue.

'Tis better to give than receive

The area from which the skin is removed is referred to as the *donor site*. For donor areas in which appearance or joint movement is important, the graft is transplanted intact. In flat areas where appearance is less critical, the graft may be meshed (fenestrated) to cover up to three times its original size. It is then placed on what is known as the *recipient site*.

A healthy loan

Skin from the patient's own healthy skin (autograft) may be used. If an autograft is not available, a *homograft* (cadaver skin) or *xenograft* (pigskin) may be surgically attached. Artificial skin may be used if there is not enough unburned skin surface. Artificial skin, which is composed of synthetic fibers, forms a new dermal layer, which dissolves as new skin replaces it.

Keys to success

The skin graft may be a *split-thickness graft* (involving the epidermis and superficial dermis) or a *full-thickness graft* (involving the epidermis and all layers of dermis). To be successful, grafts must have a sufficient blood supply, have contact with the recipient area, be free from infection and mechanical trauma, and have minimal bleeding or fluid accumulation.

Nursing considerations

Explain the procedure to the caregivers and the child. Prepare the child for the postgrafting appearance of the donor site and the recipient site. Reassure the child that the sites will heal, but tell them that this may take some time.

After graft

After grafting, follow these steps:
- Observe the donor and graft sites dressings for fluid drainage and odor; if these occur, notify the doctor.
- Observe the child for pain at the graft sites because this may indicate infection.

- Monitor the child's temperature every 4 hours because a rise in temperature may also indicate the presence of infection.
- Instruct the caregivers on care of the donor and recipient sites and include them in the child's care as much as possible (including dressing changes).
- Teach caregivers to recognize the signs of infection (such as pain, a rise in temperature, fluid drainage and odor) and instruct them to report these signs immediately.
- Stress to the caregivers and the child the importance of protecting the donor and recipient sites from trauma.
- Encourage the caregivers to hold and comfort the child despite the presence of the bulky dressings; reassure them that the dressings allow them to hold their child without hurting the child.

Dermatologic disorders

Dermatologic disorders that may affect children and adolescents include acne, burns, contact dermatitis, scabies, tinea capitis, and tinea corporis.

Acne

Acne is a chronic skin disorder of the *pilosebaceous unit*, which consists of sebaceous glands that produce sebum (an oily substance) and open onto the skin surface. Comedones, pustules, nodules, and nodular lesions characterize this inflammatory disease.

Facing up to acne

Acne is the most prevalent pediatric skin condition especially among adolescents and is typically observed on the face, chest, upper arms and back, and neck, where many sebaceous glands are located. It appears predominantly during middle to late adolescence often paralleling puberty and with a peak incidence at ages 14 to 17 years in females and ages 16 to 19 years in males. It is a common skin problem in all ethnic populations and affects males more severely than females. Neonatal acne takes approximately 1 month to resolve spontaneously.

Lasting legacy

Even though acne is self-limiting, the psychosocial impact and significance of acne on the quality of life of adolescents can have a negative effect on their self-esteem.

What causes it

Although the exact etiologic mechanism remains unknown, many factors affect the pathogenesis of the inflammatory response that is evident in acne:

- Androgynous hormones play a role in the development of acne; circulating androgens stimulate the production of sebum.
- Many adolescent females have an increased incidence of acne 2 to 7 days before their menstrual periods, also suggesting a hormonal link.
- Genetic factors seem to play a role because acne appears to run in families.
- Certain medications are known to aggravate acne, including corticosteroids, phenytoin, lithium, androgens, isoniazid, and hormonal contraceptives containing norethindrone and norgestrel.
- Adolescents commonly cite stress as a precipitating factor, but there is no evidence of a clear association.
- Ingestion of specific foods, such as chocolate, fried foods, and carbonated beverages, has not been found to be associated with the tendency to develop acne.

How it happens

Acne results from a combination of factors causing a keratin plug to develop within the follicular canal that opens onto the skin's surface.

During adolescence, androgens stimulate sebaceous gland growth and production of sebum, which is secreted into dilated hair follicles that contain bacteria. The resulting environment permits the overgrowth of gram-positive bacteria known as *Cutibacterium* (formerly *Propionibacterium*) *acnes* and *Staphylococcus epidermidis*, which thrive in the trapped secretions. Continued accumulation of follicular contents results in perforation of the follicular wall; the contents leak into surrounding tissue and cause an inflammatory reaction and the characteristic skin lesions of acne.

What to look for

Patients with acne usually exhibit two types of lesions:

1. *Noninflammatory* lesions consist of *closed comedones* (whiteheads) or *open comedones* (blackheads).
2. *Inflammatory* lesions consist of papules, pustules, and nodules or cysts that may result in permanent scarring of the skin.

In full view

Inspection reveals acne lesions, most commonly on the face, neck, shoulders, chest, and upper back. The area around the infected follicle may appear red and swollen. The rupture or leakage of an enlarged plug into the dermis produces inflammation and characteristic acne pustules, papules, or, in severe forms, acne cysts or abscesses. If the patient has previously picked or squeezed the lesions, scars may be visible.

Acne classifications

Classification of acne is based on the type of lesions observed. *Mild acne* involves primarily noninflammatory lesions with or without a limited number of inflammatory papules or pustules. *Moderate acne* involves noninflammatory lesions with more inflammatory papules and pustules present. Scarring is usually nonexistent or mild. *Severe acne* involves noninflammatory lesions along with numerous extensive inflammatory papules, pustules, and nodules. Scarring is more prevalent and usually dictates oral therapy.

What tests tell you

The diagnosis of acne is typically based solely on clinical appearance of the lesions. If a health condition such as polycystic ovarian syndrome is suspected, lab tests to diagnose that condition would be warranted.

Complications

Adolescents typically perceive acne as distressing and may need additional emotional support from the nurse as well as the family. In severe cases, the child may become withdrawn or depressed. Additional complications may occur:

- Permanent scarring can result from compulsive picking of acne lesions.
- Isotretinoin (Accutane), which is a retinoid or vitamin A compound, causes teratogenicity and cannot be taken if the adolescent is pregnant or lactating; two negative pregnancy test results must occur before initiating treatment and effective contraception must be used by the sexually active adolescent female starting at least 1 month before starting Accutane. Informed consent is necessary, and registration with the federally mandated iPLEDGE program requires routine laboratory studies (lipid levels and liver function tests) and office visits. Monitor for any indication of irritable bowel disease and depressive symptoms. Do not take with tetracycline, which may cause brain edema.
- Systemic antibiotics can interfere with the effectiveness of hormonal contraceptives; sexually active adolescent females using hormonal contraceptives should use a backup method of contraception for the first 2 weeks of systemic antibiotic therapy to prevent unwanted pregnancies.

- Sun exposure may cause excessive burning in a child taking certain medications (such as tetracycline and Accutane) and should be avoided. Encourage the use of protective clothing and noncomedonic sunscreen.

How it's treated

Various treatments are used and may be topical or systemic, depending on factors such as history, severity, types of lesions, psychological impact, cost-effectiveness, and benefit-risk assessment. Several treatments may be used simultaneously.

On the skin or in the mouth

Mild acne usually requires only topical therapy, such as retinoids and/ or benzoyl peroxide (available over the counter). Adolescents with persistent acne may need follow-up with a primary care provider or dermatologist for further treatment. Moderate acne generally requires a combination therapy including topical and oral medications. Female adolescents who experience premenstrual or menstrual acne flares may benefit from hormonal medications, such as oral contraceptives. Severe acne is treated initially with topical and oral medications, and isotretinoin (Accutane) is added if the acne fails to resolve. Acne lesions may be slow to resolve, with improvements typically taking up to 6 weeks. The patient should be taught to observe for adverse effects specific to these preparations, such as lethargy, insomnia, nausea, vomiting, and abdominal pain.

Skin care 101

The child can help ensure successful acne treatment by:
- developing health-promoting behaviors, such as getting adequate rest, participating in moderate exercise, eating a well-balanced diet, and reducing stress
- using good hygiene practices, including washing with mild soap and water twice per day, and avoiding abrasive and drying cleansers or aggressive measures (such as scrubbing)
- using noncomedogenic sunscreen, SPF of 30 or higher
- resisting the temptation to pick or squeeze blemishes
- avoiding the use of aggravating agents, such as oil-based cosmetics, face creams, and hair sprays and gels
- using noncomedogenic sensitive skin moisturizer if excessive dryness occurs.

A referral to a dermatologist may be necessary for further treatment. (See *Teaching about acne*.)

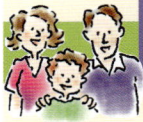

Teaching about acne

Be sure to include these points in your teaching plan for the child with acne:
- Myths about the causes of acne
- Predisposing factors
- How acne develops
- Stages of severity
- Medications (such as benzoyl peroxide, tretinoin, antibiotics, and isotretinoin)
- Other care measures, including hygiene and cosmetic use

Topical therapy

Lotions and creams tend to be less drying than topical medications in gels or solutions. There are three main categories of topical acne therapy:
1. Keratolytics include benzoyl peroxide (Benoxyl), azelaic acid (Azelex), salicylic acid (Propa pH), and sulfur (Novacet).
2. Retinoids include adapalene (Differin), tretinoin (Vesanoid), tazarotene (Tazorac), and trifarotene.
3. Topical antibiotics include erythromycin (Erygel), clindamycin (Cleocin), sodium sulfacetamide (Klaron), dapsone (Aczone), and minocycline (Minocin).

Systemic therapy

Adolescents who have moderate-to-severe inflammatory acne that is not successfully controlled with topical medications or those with widespread acne will generally require additional therapy with systemic oral medications. Antibiotic resistance may be minimized when used for short-term therapy or combined with topical agents rather than used as a monotherapy. All these medications, except isotretinoin, may be used along with the topical acne preparations.

The dope on drugs

Acne is treated systemically with antibiotics, such as tetracycline, erythromycin, co-trimoxazole (Bactrim), clindamycin, cephalexin (Keftab), doxycycline (Periostat), and minocycline (Dynacin). Instruct the adolescent that tetracycline and minocycline should be taken on an empty stomach, but if using doxycycline, it should be taken with food. (Tetracycline is contraindicated during pregnancy and in children younger than age 8 years because it discolors developing teeth; erythromycin is an alternative for these patients.) Antibiotics should be discontinued once the acne is under control.

Other systemic acne treatments include isotretinoin, hormonal contraceptives, and oral spironolactone. Oral contraceptives and spironolactone are used solely to treat female adolescents.

Intralesional therapy

Acne may also be treated with intralesional injections of corticosteroids to treat individual cysts and inflammatory papules. This procedure involves injection of a corticosteroid (usually triamcinolone [Kenalog]) into the acne cysts with a fine needle. This therapy reduces skin inflammation and may help prevent scarring.

What to do

Be prepared to discuss psychosocial concerns and self-esteem issues while reinforcing that acne is self-limiting and slow to resolve. Severe acne can lead to serious emotional problems. The child may endure teasing by their peers, leading to feelings of embarrassment or humiliation. They may become withdrawn and, in severe cases, clinically depressed. In these cases, referral to a psychologist, social worker, or other professional is indicated.

In addition, follow these steps:
- Encourage compliance with specific treatment regimens.
- Monitor the child for potential adverse effects associated with the prescribed drug therapy.
- Provide a written handout with specific instructions to improve adherence.
- Recommend additional reliable online educational resources.

A gentle touch

- Encourage the child to avoid vigorous scrubbing and picking at lesions and to eliminate mechanical irritation to lesions, such as headbands, shoulder pads, backpacks, or underwire bras.
- Help the child select safe, noncomedogenic, water-based skin care products, and hair pomades. Avoid oil-based cosmetics and hair products as well as astringents or abrasive cleansers.
- Educate about medication dosage, proper use and application of topical medications, expectations about the time needed for therapeutic response, side effects, and contraindications.
- Reinforce teaching about the adverse effects of isotretinoin, including increased cardiovascular risk, hepatotoxicity, and teratogenicity.
- Provide emotional support and refer to counseling if necessary for depression related to body image disturbances.
- Stress the need for follow-up care by a health care professional.

Myth busters

- Focus teaching on key aspects of good hygiene, information about specific medications and their adverse effects, and dispel myths about the causes of acne.
- Instruct the child not to take vitamin A supplements due to the risk of hepatotoxicity.
- Caution the child about a potential decrease in tolerance to wearing contact lenses.

Burns

Burns are not only caused by excessive heat but also related to exposure to cold, chemicals, electricity, or radiation. When the skin is burned, it loses its ability to perform its normal physiologic functions.

Educational efforts aimed at burn prevention have significantly decreased the number of burn injuries and deaths among children. However, fire and burn injuries remain a leading cause of unintentional, injury-related death in children younger than age 14 years. Burn injuries often cause extensive pain and may result in disfigurement.

What causes it

Burn injuries result from various causes and represent a severe trauma to the body. Exposure to thermal, chemical, electrical, and radioactive sources can cause burn injuries.

Thermal burns

Thermal burns, the most common type, are usually the result of residential fires, automobile accidents, children playing with matches, improperly stored gasoline, space heater or electrical malfunctions, or arson. Other causes include improper handling of firecrackers, scalding accidents, kitchen accidents (such as a child climbing on top of a stove), and access to dangerous items (such as a hot iron, hot curling iron, matches, and candles).

Chemical burns

Chemical burns result from contact, ingestion, inhalation, or injection of acids, alkalis, vesicants, or noxious agents commonly used in cleaning products.

Electrical burns

Electrical burns usually occur after contact with faulty electrical wiring or from inserting conductive objects into electrical outlets. Many infants and toddlers sustain electrical burns by chewing on electric cords.

Other burns

Burns also may occur from:
- skin being rubbed harshly against a coarse surface (called *friction* or *abrasion burns*)
- sun exposure (minor burns)
- child abuse (intentionally inflicted injuries from actions such as immersion in hot water and contact with hot objects such as cigarettes).

How it happens

Children, especially those younger than age 5 years, are at greater risk for burn injuries. Developmentally, children have a limited ability to act promptly and properly in a dangerous situation, such as a fire, an explosion, or when they are exposed to dangerous items (such as a pot on the stove and a hot iron).

Thermal and chemical burns disrupt the normal protective function of the skin, leading to various sequelae. In an electrical injury, the heat generated by the electricity passes through the body, causing injury to the tissues.

Two levels of response to the burn injury occur:
1. Local
2. Systemic

Local response

Local response represents local tissue damage to the skin:
- Edema results from increased capillary permeability and increased hydrostatic pressure forcing water, protein, and electrolytes into the interstitial spaces.
- Fluid loss from the burn-injured skin is a result of the inflammatory response.
- Significant circulatory alterations cause capillary stasis in the burned area.
- Thrombi develop, leading to tissue ischemia and necrosis, causing pain and edema.

Systemic response

Systemic response to burns may involve various body systems:
- Cardiovascular changes occur, such as burn shock caused by dramatic alterations in circulation; tachycardia and tachypnea occur to compensate for decreasing vascular volume and increased oxygen needs.

A tight squeeze

- Compartment syndrome, requiring surgical correction, may occur when severe edema causes a tourniquet-like effect that compromises circulation and entraps nerves.

- The respiratory system may be compromised by smoke inhalation; injuries can range from tissue edema of upper respiratory airways to impaired gas exchange in the alveoli.

Constricted and depressed

- Kidney changes occur, such as kidney vasoconstriction, reduced kidney plasma flow, and depressed glomerular filtration.
- Gastrointestinal (GI) ischemia may occur as perfusion to the GI tract and liver is decreased.
- Gastric ileus may occur, with digestion almost ceasing.
- Metabolism is greatly increased, which can lead to prolonged starvation and extensive energy needs.

Changing spaces

- Fluid shifts from the vasculature to the extravascular spaces and altered concentrations of potassium, sodium, chloride, and bicarbonate occur.
- Elevated body temperature occurs as a result of increased metabolism, even in the absence of infection.
- The neuroendocrine system attempts to restore equilibrium by secreting trophic hormones to stimulate various organs.

Fragile: handle with care

- Increased cell fragility and loss of circulatory red blood cells lead to anemia and the production of lactic acid.
- Growth and development are slowed with severe burn injuries due to growth hormone suppression.
- The patient is prone to infections, such as nosocomial infections, due to loss of skin and tissue integrity and an immature immune system.

What to look for

Assessment of the child with a burn injury should begin with a thorough history. A description of events surrounding the burn injury should include the cause and the duration the agent was in contact with the skin. The history also consists of how and when the injury occurred, treatment of the burn, and history of previous burns.

A matter of degree

Burns are assessed according to the degree (depth of damage), extent (percentage of body surface area), and specific body part involved. One goal of assessment is to determine the depth of skin and tissue damage:

1. In *first-degree burns*, (superficial) damage is limited to the epidermis, causing erythema and pain, usually healing within 4 to 5 days.

2. In *second-degree burns* (partial thickness), the epidermis and part of the dermis are damaged, producing blisters and mild-to-moderate edema and pain.
3. In *third-degree burns* (full thickness), the epidermis and the dermis are damaged; no blisters appear, but white, brown, or black leathery tissue and thrombosed vessels are visible.
4. *Fourth-degree burns* (full thickness) are rare, and damage extends through deeply charred subcutaneous tissue to muscle and bone. (See *Gauging burn depth*.)

Gauging burn depth

One method of assessing burns is determining their depth. As shown in this illustration, a partial-thickness burn damages the epidermis and part of the dermis, whereas a full-thickness burn damages the epidermis, dermis, subcutaneous tissue, and muscle. The burn depth determines the potential for healing and the need for surgical intervention.

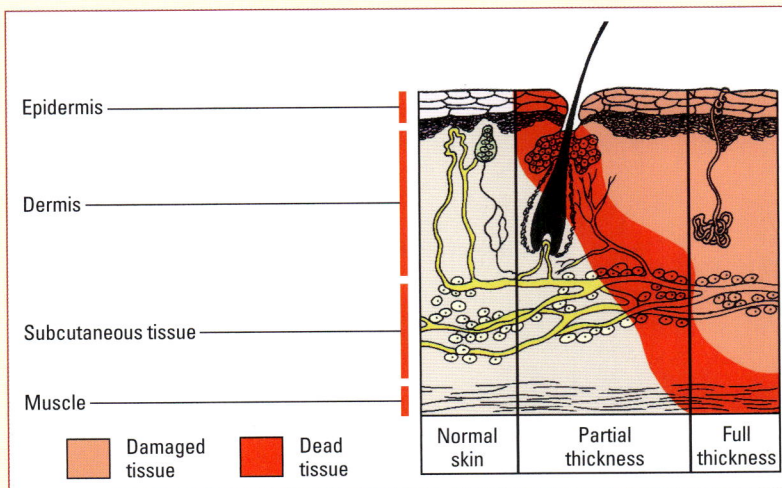

Total body surface area (TBSA) or not TBSA

Another assessment goal is to estimate the size of a burn, which is usually expressed as a percentage of the TBSA. The TBSA, together with the body part affected, determines morbidity, mortality, and management strategies.

10% of TBSA = a hospital stay

For children, burns that make up 10% or more of TBSA are considered critical and require hospitalization. In addition, significant burns on the hands, feet, face, ears, and genitalia also require immediate hospitalization. Children's larger body surface areas put them at high risk for fluid volume and heat loss, leading to dehydration. (See *Estimating the extent of a burn*.)

Estimating the extent of a burn

To estimate the extent of a burn in a pediatric patient, use the Lund and Browder chart. To use the chart:
• Mentally transfer your patient's burns to the body chart shown here.
• Then add up the corresponding percentages for each burned body section.

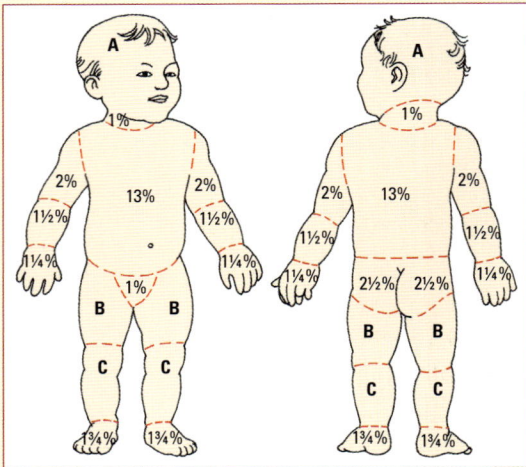

Relative percentages of areas affected by growth

At birth
0 to 1 year
2 to 4 years
5 to 9 years
10 to 15 years

A: Half of head
9½%
8½%
6½%
5½%
4½%

B: Half of thigh
2¾%
3¼%
4%
4¼%
4½%

C: Half of leg
2½%
2½%
2¾%
3%
3¼%

Inspect to detect

Inspection reveals other characteristics of the burn as well, including location, pattern, and extent. Assess for sensation and degree of pain and check for blanching and capillary refill of the nail beds.

- Lung auscultation may reveal respiratory compromise, tachypnea, or stridor.
- Assessment of the cardiovascular system may reveal tachycardia, narrow pulse pressure, and hypotension.
- The child may have decreased urine output.

Complications

Nursing care of a patient with burn is challenging because many organ systems are affected by the burn injury. Potential complications depend on the depth and severity of the burn as well as its specific cause. The most common complications and leading causes of death are respiratory complications and sepsis. Other possible complications include:

- burn shock
- fluid and electrolyte deficits
- hypothermia
- hypermetabolism
- hypovolemic shock
- infections
- scarring and disfigurement
- contractures
- multisystem organ failure.

How it's treated

Superficial first-degree burn injuries and partial-thickness burns heal spontaneously with reasonable care.

Minor burns

Management of minor burns includes removing burned clothing, cleaning with mild soap and tepid water, and leaving blisters intact. In addition, follow these steps:

- Nothing should be applied to the burn, except a clean cloth that is (usually) treated with antimicrobial ointment or cream until reepitheliazation occurs.
- Tetanus prophylaxis is necessary if no history of immunization is available, if more than 5 years have passed since the last immunization, or if the child has not completed the full vaccine series.
- A mild analgesic or moist soaks may be administered to relieve pain.
- Use sun protection.

Moderate or severe burns

If the burn involves a large area of the body surface or critical body parts, it represents severe trauma and usually requires treatment at a specialized burn center. Emergency management of major burns begins with stopping the burning process and placing the child in a horizontal position. In addition, follow these steps:

- Establish and maintain a patent airway, initiating cardiopulmonary resuscitation if necessary.
- Remove burned clothing and jewelry while keeping the child warm.
- Cover the burn to prevent contamination.
- Until transported to a medical facility or burn center, do not allow the patient to eat or drink anything; intravenous (IV) fluids with lactated Ringer or normal saline solution should be started and oxygen therapy provided at 100%.
- Keep the child warm to prevent the risk of hypothermia.

In the unit

Initial management of the major burn in the burn unit includes maintenance of an adequate airway. IV fluid replacement should be started as soon as possible. Intubation and mechanical ventilation may be necessary. In addition, follow these steps:

- A pulse oximeter, a cardiac/apnea monitor, and a chest radiography to evaluate pulmonary status may be ordered.
- A urinary catheter is inserted to adequately measure urine output.
- A nasogastric tube may be necessary to decompress the stomach; later, it may be used to administer a high-protein, high-calorie diet or total parenteral nutrition (which may be necessary if the GI tract is dysfunctional).
- Baseline laboratory studies are performed which may include electrolytes and complete blood count (CBC).
- IV pain medication is administered.
- Topical wound cleaning is begun to prevent infections.
- Tetanus prophylaxis is administered if required.

In general

General wound management includes wound débridement, hydrotherapy for dressing removal and débridement, topical antimicrobial therapy, nutritional therapy, physiotherapy focusing on range of motion and contracture prevention, and skin grafting.

What to do

Burns are one of the most painful injuries a child can sustain. Severe burns are life threatening. The child and their caregivers will need a great deal of emotional support and reassurance.

Every effort should be made to make the child as comfortable as possible during painful procedures such as débridement. Depending on the child's age, it may be difficult for them to understand why doctors and nurses are inflicting pain during such procedures. The reasons for these treatments should be explained repeatedly, and the child should be encouraged to express their feelings, which may include fear and anger.

Referral to a therapist and a support group may be needed to help the child and caregivers deal with the traumatic injury and any altered body image because such traumas can have long-lasting psychological effects. Similar referrals are needed if severe scarring or disfigurement is anticipated.

In the heat of the moment

During the acute phase—the first 24 to 48 hours after the burn occurs—nursing care includes:

- treating burn shock
- monitoring respiratory status
- maintaining a patent airway
- monitoring vital signs and fluid status every hour
- maintaining adequate fluid and electrolyte balance
- caring for the burn wound
- managing pain
- providing emotional support.

When the fire dies down

Ongoing management and rehabilitation should include preventing wound infections and complications (such as heat loss and contractures), promoting wound healing, managing the child's pain, promoting comfort, adequate nutrition, and providing psychosocial support for the child and their family. The child and their caregivers should be educated about long-term needs and follow-up care. Education about safety issues, including prevention of future burns, should be conducted in a nonjudgmental manner with genuine interest and concern, making appropriate referrals as needed. Summer camps are available for children with burns. These camps provide a supportive space for children who have experienced a burn injury where they can build relationships with other burn survivors.

Contact dermatitis

Contact dermatitis occurs as an acute or chronic inflammatory response due to a hypersensitivity reaction to a natural or synthetic chemical substance, resulting in a localized flare. The irritating substance can be a primary irritant or a sensitizing agent or allergen.

What causes it

Irritant dermatitis is caused by the toxic effect of the substance directly on the skin. The extent of the rash and itching depends on the length of exposure and the concentration of the irritant. Common irritants include:

- detergents, harsh soaps, fabric softeners, bubble bath, baby wipes, and hydrocarbons (crude petroleum lubricating oils)
- bathing too frequently
- saliva, urine, and feces. (*Diaper dermatitis*, the most common form of irritant dermatitis, is a reaction to urine and byproducts of feces.)

Allergic annoyances

Allergic dermatitis (a delayed hypersensitive response) occurs with exposure to substances that cause an immunologic response triggered by an allergen to which the child has become sensitized. Sensitizing reactions occur with repeated or prolonged exposure to substances such as:

- plant oils (poison ivy, oak, and sumac)
- nickel-containing jewelry, buckles, eyeglasses, buttons, snaps, and zippers
- clothing with woolen or rough textures
- topical medications, such as neomycin and lanolin
- perfumed soaps or cosmetics
- latex.

How it happens

In primary irritant dermatitis, the toxic substance causes damage to the stratum corneum and the skin's lipid film, impairing the protective barrier mechanism of the skin. The toxic substance is then absorbed into the skin, resulting in vasodilatation, edema of the upper dermis, inflammatory infiltrates, and breakdown of epidermal cells. Vesicles or bullae that rupture ooze and crust may develop as a result of the fluid accumulating between the epidermal cells that act as a sponge.

Not immune to an immune response

Allergic dermatitis is due to an immune response caused by the sensitizing chemical entering the dermis and combining with epidermal proteins to form a new molecule that acts as an antigen. This antigen enters the local cutaneous lymphoid tissue, causing an inflammatory reaction.

What to look for

A thorough history should elicit information about:

- exposure to new or unusual substances
- repeated exposure to a substance

- history of diarrhea or infrequent diaper changes
- location and distribution of the rash related to specific areas of the body
- treatments or forms of at-home management.

Oozing, scaling, and itching

Mild irritants and allergens produce erythema and small vesicles that ooze, scale, and itch. Strong irritants may also cause blisters and ulcerations.

It's a classic

A classic allergic response produces clearly defined lesions with straight lines following the points of contact. A severe allergic reaction also produces marked edema of the affected area.

What tests tell you

Tests should be reserved for a time when the child is not experiencing acute, active dermatitis. There are two methods used to determine allergy:

- The *patch test* identifies specific allergens. The suspected substance is applied to a patch left in place on the child's skin for a specified period. If the area under the patch is red and swollen when the patch is removed, the test is positive and the child is considered allergic to the offending substance.
- In *skin testing*, the suspected allergen is introduced intradermally on the child's back or upper arm. A wheal response demonstrates an allergic response to the allergen. Emergency equipment should be available in the event of rare anaphylaxis.

Complications

Complications of contact dermatitis include secondary infections and trauma from scratching. The child may have serious concerns about their appearance and body image.

How it's treated

The keys to successful treatment are identification and removal or elimination of the causative agent and appropriate skin care and management. Topical treatment may include cool compresses and topical corticosteroids. Resolution of contact dermatitis typically takes 2 to 3 weeks. More severe cases may require systemic steroids.

How offensive!

When the offending substance has been identified and eliminated from the child's environment, management consists primarily of treating and preventing worsening of symptoms:

- For diaper dermatitis, change diapers frequently, use air-drying if possible, and avoid rubber pants. Barrier ointments containing vitamins A, D, and E or zinc oxide may provide protection and comfort.

- Hydrocortisone 1% cream should be used sparingly for no more than 5 days.
- Use an emollient/moisturizer if needed to minimize dry skin, apply after bathing.
- Antifungal agents may be necessary if secondary infection develops.

A soak in the tub

- Burow solution soaks, Aveeno or oatmeal baths, and cool saline compresses may soothe itching and vesicular rashes.
- Petroleum-based or combination of lanolin- and petroleum-based emollients may be applied to dry and chaffed skin but must be avoided if the skin is inflamed.

Ditch the itch!

- Topical corticosteroids (clobetasol [Temovate] or betamethasone [Diprolene]) may be administered two times per day; oral antihistamines (hydroxyzine [Atarax] or diphenhydramine [Benadryl]) are commonly prescribed for itching.
- Referral to a dermatologist for patch testing may be necessary.

What to do

Management requires problem-solving to determine the cause of the skin reaction and to find a mutually agreeable solution:

- Educate the child and caregivers about hygiene practices to prevent infections.
- Teach the caregivers about antipruritic agents and their proper use to relieve discomfort and itching.

Replace; don't recycle

- Discuss proper use and regular replacement of skin care and makeup products.
- Educate the caregivers and the child about ways to prevent future exposures, such as wearing protective clothing and using blocking agents such as Ivy Block for the prevention of plant oil contact dermatitis.

Don't judge

- Establish a professional rapport with the child and caregivers and provide education in a nonjudgmental manner; caregivers may become defensive and are less likely to listen when they feel they are being judged or their caregiver skills are being questioned.
- Encourage the child to express concerns about their appearance and body image.

Scabies

Scabies, a highly transmissible parasitic skin infestation, is characterized by burrows, pruritus, and excoriations with secondary infections. It characteristically spreads by skin-to-skin contact to family members, intimate contacts, and among schoolchildren. Prolonged contact is needed to become infected.

What causes it

Scabies is a contagious disease caused by the scabies mite, *Sarcoptes scabiei*, which burrows into the stratum corneum of the epidermis and deposits eggs and feces. (See *Scabies: cause and effect*.)

Scabies: cause and effect

Infestation with *S. scabiei*—the itch mite—causes scabies. The top illustration shows the mite (enlarged); it has a hard shell and measures a microscopic 0.1 mm. The bottom illustration depicts the erythematous nodules with excoriation that appear in patients with scabies.

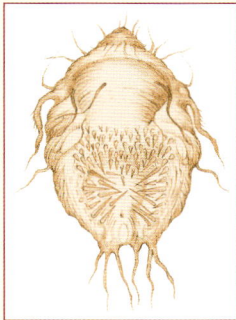

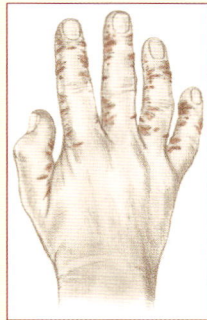

How it happens

Transmission occurs when the child is exposed by direct contact with infected people or fomite (such as infected bedding or clothing). The female scabies mite burrows under the skin and forms a small tunnel that is evident as a fine, wavy, dark line with a black dot at the end. The mite extends the burrow, laying up to three eggs per day as they travel. The eggs hatch in about 2 weeks, thus continuing the process.

What to look for

- The lesions initially produce no symptoms, but sensitization to the mites occurs in about 3 weeks. At that time, intense itching occurs, becoming more severe at night.

Loads of lesions

- Infants have dozens of lesions, whereas older children commonly have fewer than 10. Children younger than age 2 years usually have lesions on the feet and ankles; in older children, most lesions are found on the hands and wrists.
- Inspection reveals characteristic gray-brown burrows, which may appear as erythematous nodules when excoriated; secondary excoriation and bacterial infections commonly obscure the burrows and papules.
- Papules of various sizes may exist simultaneously and are typically distributed in areas such as the finger webs, flexor surfaces of the wrist, elbows, and axillary folds, along the belt line, and on the lower buttocks.

What tests tell you

- Microscopic examination reveals the characteristic eight-legged scabies mite, eggs, or feces. (Scrapings from an unscratched burrow should be placed in saline or mineral oil. The scrapings should not be placed in KOH because it can dissolve the mites, eggs, or feces.)
- The burrow ink test reveals the presence of burrows. This test involves applying a drop of ink or a blue or black felt–tipped pen to a suspected burrow, wiping off the excess ink with an alcohol pad, and examining the area with a magnifying glass for an ink-stained burrow.

Complications

A secondary bacterial infection from scratching is one possible complication of scabies. Postscabetic syndrome may occur, characterized by lesions and itching that commonly persist for days to weeks following treatment.

How it's treated

Pharmacologic treatment with a thin layer of scabicide (applied after a soap and water bath) to the entire body (except the eyes) is usually recommended:

- Be especially careful to gently massage the cream into the fingernails, scalp, behind the ears, all folds and creases, and the feet and hands; in 7 days, reapply the cream to the child and all symptomatic contacts.

- Permethrin 5% cream (Elimite) is the treatment of choice and is safe for infants as young as age 2 months; the cream should be left on for 8 to 12 hours and then removed with bathing and shampooing. Repeat application in 7 days may be advised. The use of mitts for the hands and socks to cover the feet may reduce the chance of the young child sucking and ingesting the scabicide during the time that the cream is on the skin.
- Antimicrobial agents may be ordered if a secondary infection has developed.

What to do

All caregivers, friends, and school and day care contacts should undergo treatment simultaneously with the infected individual, even if they are asymptomatic. Caregivers should be educated about the course of the disease and told that the rash and itching commonly persist for up to 3 weeks. Oral antihistamines may be necessary if itching is pronounced. Children are no longer infectious 24 hours after treatment has started and may return to school or day care.

Instruct the caregivers to:

- wash all bed linens and clothing with hot water 140°F (60°C) and then dry for 40 minutes in a hot dryer—the day after treatment and again in 1 week.

Hoover Whole House

- Vacuum the entire house and upholstery discarding the vacuum bags immediately.
- Store nonwashable items in sealed plastic bags for 2 weeks.
- Use meticulous handwashing and good hygiene to avoid secondary infections.
- Trim the child's fingernails short to avoid excoriation from scratching.
- Use soothing lotions and bathe with Aveeno or a similar product to control itching.

Tinea capitis (ringworm of the scalp)

Tinea capitis is a superficial cutaneous fungal infection of the scalp and hair. It characteristically spreads through direct and indirect contact with infected humans and animals, such as dogs and cats, and sharing of personal items, such as hats, combs, and brushes, in addition to close contact with infected fomites such as bedding, couches, and soft stuffed toys. It occurs more frequently in hot, humid climates and among individuals living in overcrowded conditions and in disadvantaged areas. It is important to allay the child's misperception that tinea capitis is caused by worms. Fungi are commonly found in the environment.

What causes it

Tinea capitis is the most common contagious fungal infection in children younger than 12 years old. It is caused predominately by the dermatophyte *Trichophyton tonsurans* and involves both the scalp and hair shaft.

How it happens

Dermatophytes attach to the epidermis skin layer of the scalp and may invade the hair shaft, often resulting in hair breakage and temporary alopecia. An exaggerated cell-mediated response occurs and results in severe inflammation, leading to varying degrees of itching, scaling, pustules, and papules.

What to look for

- Erythema and scaling of the scalp
- Pustules, papules, and often yellow honeycomb crusts
- Varying degrees of pruritus
- Broken hairs at the scalp level resembling a dotted black stubbled appearance or patchy hair loss (sometimes called "black dot alopecia")
- Adenopathy that may occur

What tests tell you

Microscopic examination of hair and scalp scrapings using KOH wet mount can detect and immediately confirm the dermatophytes. The use of a fungal culture is more sensitive but does take additional time to obtain the results.

Complications

In severe cases of tinea capitis, permanent alopecia may result. If symptoms do not improve, refer to a dermatologist. Hair regrowth may take 3 to 12 months.

How it's treated

- Oral antifungal medication such as griseofulvin is given for 4 to 8 weeks. Medication absorption is enhanced if given with whole milk or other foods high in fat. Topical antifungals are ineffective against tinea capitis and thus are not recommended.
- Selenium sulfide shampoo is recommended as an adjunctive therapy. It is applied two to three times weekly, leaving it on the scalp for 10 minutes before rinsing to eradicate the scalp spores and reduce transmission. This adjunctive therapy should be used for 2 to 4 weeks.

What to do

- Use shampoo with selenium sulfide for all family members for several weeks to prevent infection.
- Clean all potentially contaminated objects that came into contact with the infected child's head. Wash sheets and clothes in hot water to decrease the potential spread to others.
- Avoid sharing personal items, such as hats, combs, brushes, towels, and bedding, or anything that may have had close physical contact with the infected child's head.
- Discourage scratching or touching of scalp and hair.

Tinea corporis (ringworm of the body)

Tinea corporis is a superficial dermatophyte fungal skin infection commonly known as *ringworm* because of the characteristic pattern of annular (ring-shaped), scaling, erythematous plaques with sharply defined borders. It is found on the trunk and limbs, excluding hands, feet, head, and groin.

What causes it

Tinea corporis is most prevalent during the preadolescent years. It is caused by *Trichophyton rubrum*, *Trichophyton mentagrophytes*, *Microsporum canis*, and *Epidermophyton floccosum*. Contact with these dermatophytes occurs typically with infected humans, infected animals, fomites (such as wrestling mats and towels), and, less frequently, from the soil or from infection on other anatomic locations on the same person, such as tinea pedis (athlete's foot).

How it happens

Dermatophytes that are transmitted from infected people, animal, or fomite attach to the superficial epidermis skin layer and release keratinases that invade and multiply within the stratum corneum. About 1 to 3 weeks later, the dermatophytes invade the epidermis peripherally and increase the proliferation of the basal cell layer. This results in epidermal thickening, and the lesion begins to appear as a ring-shaped lesion with an erythematous, scaly border with a healthy center.

What to look for

- There are slightly raised ring-shaped lesions with pink borders ranging in size from 0.5 to 3 cm.
- Lesions may be singular or multiple but usually not very numerous.
- Lesions are more commonly found on exposed areas of the body.
- Mild pruritus or burning sensation may be present.

What tests tell you

KOH scraping of the lesion's border can confirm the dermatophyte's branching hyphae and spores but cannot identify the specific species of dermatophyte involved. Dermatophyte test medium (DTM) is used for selective recognition of the dermatophytic fungus, which is the causative agent in ringworm. A fungal culture is more sensitive but takes more time to obtain results.

How it's treated

- Treat with topical antifungal medications (creams) such as clotrimazole, miconazole, econazole, terbinafine, tolnaftate, naftifine, ciclopirox, or ketoconazole for up to 8 weeks or until the lesions resolve. Apply cream once or twice daily as prescribed.
- Do not use topical corticosteroids or combination antifungal/corticosteroid preparations, which can cause infections to persist or recur.
- Use oral antifungal agents if unresponsive to topical therapy or the ringworm recurs or is extensive. Griseofulvin is often the drug of choice.

What to do

- Avoid sharing of personal items to prevent the spread of the lesions.
- Wash hands before and after applying the cream to the lesions.
- Avoid touching or scratching the lesions.
- Wash clothing that comes in contact with affected areas once removed.
- Clean wrestling mats after use.
- Discourage athletes from practice until at least 72 hours after treatment begins, and lesions should be covered before resumption of any contact sport.

Quick quiz

1. Which statement about the integumentary system and its components is true?
   A. It's the largest organ in the body and serves primarily as an insulator.
   B. It can only protect the body from trauma that's mechanical in nature.
   C. It consists of just the dermis and epidermis.
   D. Its main function is to act as an organ of excretion.

Answer: A. The integumentary system, which consists of the skin and its components, is the largest organ system in the body. It functions to shelter most of the other organ systems, protecting them while acting as a mechanical barrier.

2. The glands that are primarily responsible for the odor associated with sweating are known as the:
    A. endocrine sweat glands.
    B. eccrine sweat glands.
    C. cutaneous sweat glands.
    D. apocrine sweat glands.

Answer: D. The sweat glands consist of the eccrine sweat glands, which function as the body's heat-regulating mechanism by producing sweat, and the apocrine sweat glands, which mature at puberty and cause the unpleasant body odor associated with sweating.

3. The proportion of a child's body that's burned is typically estimated according to:
    A. rule of nines.
    B. TBSA.
    C. depth of injury.
    D. three-dimensional analysis.

Answer: B. One goal in assessing burns is to estimate its size, which is usually expressed as a percentage of TBSA. The TBSA and body part affected determine morbidity, mortality, and management strategies.

4. When assessing a child with a rash consistent with irritant dermatitis, which question should the nurse ask?
    A. "Has your child been playing with children who may have chickenpox?"
    B. "Has your child been ill lately?"
    C. "Has your child been exposed to new or unusual substance?"
    D. "Has your child visited mountainous regions?"

Answer: C. Irritant dermatitis is caused by the toxic effect of the substance directly on the skin. Common irritants include detergents, harsh soaps, bubble bath, baby wipes, saliva, urine or feces, or overbathing.

5. Pruritus caused by contact dermatitis can usually be treated at home with:
    A. oatmeal or Aveeno baths.
    B. soothing scented bath oils.
    C. ice and heat alternately.
    D. patch skin applications.

Answer: A. Burow solution soaks, Aveeno or oatmeal baths, and cool compresses may soothe itching and vesicular rashes.

Scoring

☆☆☆ If you answered all five items correctly, hooray! Your knowledge of dermatologic problems is more than skin deep.

☆☆ If you answered three to four items correctly, congratulations! The material in this chapter has gotten under your skin.

☆ If you answered fewer than three items correctly, take an oatmeal bath, relax, and then reread the chapter! This is the last quick quiz to irritate you.

Suggested References

American Academy of Dermatology Association. (2023). *Acne clinical guideline.* https://www.aad.org/member/clinical-quality/guidelines/acne

Bland, T. (2022). Dermatologic disorders. In D. Garzon-Maaks, N. Starr, M. Brady, N. Gaylord, M. Driessnack, & K. Duderstadt (Eds.), *Burns' pediatric primary care* (pp. 567–615). Elsevier.

Bolognia, J. L., Schaffer, J. V., Duncan, K. O., & Lo, C. J. (2022). *Dermatology essentials* (2nd ed.). Elsevier.

Centers for Disease Control and Prevention. (2024). *Treatment of Scabies.* https://www.cdc.gov/scabies/treatment/

Habeshian, K. A., & Cohen, B. A. (2020). Current issues in the treatment of acne vulgaris. *Pediatrics, 145*(S2), S225–S230. https://doi.org/10.1542/peds.2019-2056L

Heath, C., & Usatine, R. (2022). Tinea capitis. *Journal of Family Practice, 71,* 370–371. https://doi.org/10.12788/cutis.0630

Kyle, T., & Carmen, S. (2021). *Essentials of pediatric nursing* (4th ed.). Wolters Kluwer.

Linnard-Palmer, L. (2019). Skin integrity. In L. Linnard-Palmer (Ed.), *Pediatric nursing care: A concept-based approach* (pp. 232–246). Jones & Bartlett Learning.

Mancini, A. J., & Krowchuk, D. P. (Eds.). (2021). *Pediatric dermatology* (4th ed.). American Academy of Pediatrics.

Seth, D., Poowuttikul, P., Kamat, D., & Pansare, M. (2021). Contact dermatitis in children. *Pediatric Annals, 50,* e198–e205. https://doi.org/10.3928/19382359-20210418-01

Silbert-Flagg. J. (2023). *Maternal & child health nursing: Care of the childbearing & childrearing family* (9th ed.). Wolters Kluwer.

Index

A

AAP. *See* American Academy of Pediatrics (AAP)
Abdomen
  assessment tips, 695
  liver, 688
  neonatal assessment, 331–332
  small intestine, 687
  stomach, 686
Abdominal breathing, 584
Abdominal discomfort, 143
Abducens nerve (CN VI), 486
Abduction, joint movement, 650
Abruptio placentae. *See* Placental abruption
Abrysvo. *See* RSV vaccine (Abrysvo)
ACC. *See* American College of Cardiology (ACC)
Accessory glands/organs, 688–689
  biliary duct system, 688
  liver, 688
  pancreas, 688–689
Accessory reproductive glands, 13
Accommodate growth, loop of catheter in peritoneum to, 512
Accutane. *See* Isotretinoin (Accutane)
Acini of lobule, 21
Acne, 434, 794–800
  classification of, 796
  complications, 796–797
  diagnosis of, 796
  gentle touch, 799
  intralesional therapy, 799
  myth busters, 800
  skin care 101, 797
  skin/mouth, 797
  systemic therapy, 798–799
  topical therapy, 798
Acoustic nerve (CN VIII), 486
Acquired immunodeficiency syndrome (AIDS), 631
Acrocyanosis, 313
Acrosome, 25
Acupressure, for labor pain, 237
Acupuncture, for labor pain, 237

Acute asthma, 593
Acute laryngotracheobronchitis, 601
Acute lymphocytic leukemia (ALL), 775, 776
Acute myelogenous leukemia (AML), 775, 776
Acute poststreptococcal glomerulonephritis, 625–628
Acute slipped capital femoral epiphysis, 674
Acute stage, infection, 452
Aczone. *See* Dapsone (Aczone)
Adapalene (Differin), 798
Additives, and pregnancy, 132
Adduction, joint movement, 650
Adenohypophysis. *See* Anterior pituitary
Adenoid, 581
Adenovirus, 609
Adipose tissue, 21
Adrenal glands, 712, 714
  changes during pregnancy, 87
Adventitious breath sounds, 585–586
Aerosol therapy, 589–590
Afferent arteriole, 615
AFP testing, 129
Aganglionic position, 700
AHA. *See* American Heart Association (AHA)
AIDS. *See* Acquired immunodeficiency syndrome (AIDS)
Air/barium enema, 689
Airway resistance, 583
Albuterol (Proair, Proventil), 596
Alcohol
  misuse, 151, 438–442
  and pregnancy, 132
Alcohol misuse disorder, 438
Aldomet. *See* Methyldopa (Aldomet)
ALL. *See* Acute lymphocytic leukemia (ALL)
Allergic dermatitis, 808
Allergic rhinitis, 763–766
Allergic shiners, 764
Allergy shots, 596

Allergy skin testing, 758
  nursing considerations, 758
  radioallergosorbent test to rescue, 758
Alternative feeding methods, 692–693
Alveoli, 580, 583
Amenorrhea, 76
American Academy of Pediatrics (AAP), 261, 385, 389
American College of Cardiology (ACC), 158
American Heart Association (AHA), 158
AML. *See* Acute myelogenous leukemia (AML)
Amnion, 33, 34, 36
Amniotic sac/fluid, 34–35
Amniotomy, 211
Amoxicillin (Amoxil), 467
Amoxil. *See* Amoxicillin (Amoxil)
Amphidiarthrodial joints, 650
Ampicillin, 353
Ampulla, 12, 20
Anemia, 771–774
Anencephaly, 516–517
ANS. *See* Autonomic nervous system (ANS)
Anterior pituitary, 23, 713
Antibody screening tests, 127–128
  hepatitis B test, 128
  indirect Coombs test, 128
  Rubella titer test, 128
Antiinflammatory agents, 595–596
Antivert. *See* Meclizine (Antivert)
Anus, 10, 16, 17
Aorta, 91, 542, 546, 550, 553, 557, 559, 564, 567
Aortic arch, 527
Aortic semilunar valve, 527
Aortic valve atresia/stenosis, 561
Aortic valves, 528
Apgar score, 311–313
Appendicitis, 695–697
Apresoline. *See* Hydralazine (Apresoline)
Aqueduct of Sylvius, 509

Arachnoid membrane, 483, 484
Arachnoid villi, 484, 509
Arcuate artery and vein, 615
Areola, 21, 260
Arnold–Chiari malformation, 511
Arteries, 528
Articular cartilage, 648
Articulate, 649
Artificial sweeteners, and
        pregnancy, 132
Artificially acquired active
        immunity, 453
Artificially acquired passive
        immunity, 454
Ascending loop of Henle, 615
ASD. *See* Atrial septal defect (ASD)
Aseptic meningitis, 500
Aspiration pneumonia, 609
Association of Women's Health,
        Obstetric and Neonatal Nurses
        (AWHONN), 225
Asthma, 579, 591–598
Astrocytoma, 502
Atarax. *See* Hydroxyzine (Atarax)
Ataxia/uncoordinated gait, 503
Ataxic cerebral palsy, 506
Athetoid cerebral palsy, 506
Atopic dermatitis, 766–768
        infant with, 767
Atrial septal defect (ASD), 542–545, 564
Atrial septum, 526
Atrioventricular (AV) bundle, 529
Atrioventricular (AV) node, 529
Atrioventricular (AV) valves, 528
Autoimmune thyroid disease, 697
Autonomic nervous system (ANS), 487
AWHONN. *See* Association of
        Women's Health, Obstetric and
        Neonatal Nurses (AWHONN)
Axons, 483
Azelaic acid (Azelex), 798
Azelex. *See* Azelaic acid (Azelex)
Azotemia, 638

B

B cells/B lymphocytes, 754–755
Baby blues, 247–248, 285
        vs. depression, 248

Bacteria, 464–470
        classification, 466
        Lyme disease, 466–468
        pertussis, 468–470
Bacteria blocker, 84
Bacteriuria without symptoms, 123
Bactrim. *See*
        Trimethoprimsulfamethoxazole
        (Bactrim)
Ballard gestational age assessment
        tool, 314–319
Ballottement, 79
Barium swallow, 690
Barium/diatrizoate meglumine
        (Gastrografin), 690
Bartholin duct opening, 16
Basal body temperature (BBT) method,
        contraception, 44–45
Basophils, 751
BBT method. *See* Basal body
        temperature (BBT) method
Benadryl. *See* Diphenhydramine
        (Benadryl)
Benoxyl. *See* Benzoyl peroxide
        (Benoxyl)
Benzoyl peroxide (Benoxyl), 798
Betamethasone (Diprolene), 810
Beyfortus. *See* Nirsevimab (Beyfortus)
Bidirectional Glenn procedure, 563
Biphasic oral contraceptives, 48
Birth, cardiac adaptations at, 530–531
Bishop score, 209–210
Bladder, 17, 70, 628–631
Bladder catheterization, 621–623
Blast cells, 748, 775
Bleeding, 280
        uterine, 83
Blood components, 749–752
Blood culture, 353
Blood formation, 748–749
Blood glucose test, 720
Blood pressure
        low, 283
        pregnancy, 118
Blood transfusion, 760–761
Blood urea nitrogen (BUN), 618–619
Body, GI, 686

Body piercings/tattoos, 434
Bone marrow aspiration/biopsy,
        758–759
Bone marrow transplantation, 761–763
Bones, 645–649
Bordetella pertussis, 468, 469
Bottle-feeding with breast milk,
        268–270
        breast milk storage, 270
        breast pumping, 268
                battery-powered/electric, 269
                manual, 269
Bottle-feeding with formula, 270–273
        burping, 272–273
        commercial formulas, 270–271
        elemental formulas, 271
        feeding steps, 272
        milk-based formulas, 270
        soy-based formulas, 271
Bowman capsule, 615
Brain, 481–485
Brain stem glioma, 502
Brain tumors, 501–504
Branches of left pulmonary artery, 527
Branches of right pulmonary artery, 527
Braxton Hicks contractions, 79, 143
Breast
        changes during pregnancy, 76, 84
        lactation preparation, 85
        nonpregnant *vs.* pregnant, 85
Breast care, 273–274
        for breastfeeding patients, 274
        for non-breastfeeding patients, 274
Breast milk
        bottle-feeding with, 268–270
                breast pumping, 268–269
        composition, 260–261
        storage, 270
Breast stimulation, 210–211
Breastfeeding, 261–268, 366, 385–387
        advantages, 262–263
        assistance and instruction, 263–264
        contraindications, 261–262
        feeding/hunger cues, 266
        hydration, 263
        infant latch, 265–266
        manual breast milk expression,
                267–268

and maternal nutrition, 263
positions, 264–265
   biologic/laid-back, 265
   cradle, 264
   cross-body, 264
   football, 265
   side-lying, 265
Breathing techniques, for labor
   pain, 236
Breech presentation, 203–204, 205–206
Brethine. *See* Terbutaline (Brethine)
Bronchioles, 580, 582–583
Bronchiolitis, 598–601
Bronchodilators, 596
Bronchopneumonia, 609
Brow cephalic presentation, 203, 205
Brudzinski sign, 498
Budesonide (Pulmicort), 595
BUN. *See* Blood urea nitrogen (BUN)
Burns, 800–807
   chemical burns, 800
   complications, 805
   electrical burns, 800
   estimate the extent of, 804
   first 24 to 48 hours, 807
   in general, 806
   inspect to detect, 805
   local response, 801
   matter of degree, 802
   minor burns, 805
   moderate/severe burns, 806
   other burns, 801
   systemic response, 801–802
      changing spaces, 802
      constricted and depressed, 802
      fragile, 802
      tight squeeze, 801–802
   thermal burns, 800
   things to do, 806–807
   total body surface area (TBSA)/not
      TBSA, 803–804
   treatment, 805–806
Burping, 272–273

C

C-reactive protein (CRP), 353
Caffeine, and pregnancy, 132
Calcium, 135, 433

Calories, 133
Cancellous bone, 648
Cancer, 631
Candida infection, 84
Capillary, 779
Caput succedaneum, 327
Carbon dioxide, 70
Cardiac catheterization, 536–537, 551,
   558, 560
Cardiac disease, for pregnant patient,
   156–160
Cardiac output, 529
Cardiac physiology, 529
Cardiac screening, 350–351
Cardiac surgery, 538–540
Cardiac transplantation, 540–541
Cardinal movements of labor, 220
Cardiovascular system, 380–381, 639
   anatomy and physiology, 526–532
      birth, cardiac adaptations at,
         530–531
      cardiac physiology, 529
      circulation, 528
      conduction system, 529
      heart, structures of, 526–528
      murmurs, 531–532
   congenital heart defects that
      decrease pulmonary blood
      flow, 566–569
      tetralogy of Fallot, 566–569
   congenital heart defects that
      increase pulmonary blood
      flow, 541–552
      atrial septal defect, 542–545
      patent ductus arteriosus,
         545–549
      ventricular septal defect,
         549–552
   congenital obstructive defects,
      553–560
      coarctation of the aorta,
         553–556
      pulmonic stenosis, 559–560
      stenosis, aortic, 556–558
   diagnostic tests, 532–534
      echocardiography, 532–533
      electrocardiography, 533
      exercise testing, 534

      magnetic resonance imaging,
         533
   disorders, 569–576
      endocarditis, 569–574
      Kawasaki disease, 574–576
   mixed congenital heart defects,
      560–566
      hypoplastic left heart syndrome,
         561–563
      transposition of the great
         arteries, 563–566
   during pregnancy, 89–93
      anatomic changes, 89–90
      auscultatory changes, 90
      hemodynamic changes, 90–93
      rhythm disturbances, 90
   treatments and procedures,
      534–541
      cardiac catheterization, 536–537
      cardiac surgery, 538–540
      cardiac transplantation, 540–541
      teach expectations, 534–536
Carina, 580
Cartilage, 648
Cast care, 655
Casting/splints, 652–656
CAT (computerized axial tomography)
   scan. *See* Computed
   tomography (CT) scan
Catheter in enlarged ventricle, 512
Cavities, 647
CBC. *See* Complete blood count (CBC)
CDC. *See* Centers for Disease Control
   and Prevention (CDC)
Cecum, 703
Ceftin. *See* Cefuroxime (Ceftin)
Cefuroxime (Ceftin), 467
Celiac disease, 697–699
Centers for Disease Control and
   Prevention (CDC), 4, 434
Central command, 480
Central nervous system (CNS), 381,
   480–485, 639
   brain, 481–485
   central command, 480
   spinal cord, 485
Cephalexin (Keftab), 798

Cephalic fetal presentation, 202–203, 205
  brow, 203, 205
  face, 205
  mentum, 203, 205
  vertex, 202, 205
Cephalocaudal development, 489
Cephalohematoma, 327
Cerebellar astrocytoma, 502
Cerebellum, 482
Cerebral palsy (CP), 505–508
Cerebrospinal fluid (CSF), 353, 484
  circulation, 509
Cerebrum, 481–482
Cervical canal, 17, 232
Cervical cap, 63–64
  advantages of, 64
  disadvantages of, 64
  insertion, 63
Cervical effacement and dilation, labor, 232
Cervical mucus (Billings) method, contraception, 45–46
Cervix, 17, 19–20, 33
Cervix, changes during pregnancy, 83
Cetirizine (Zyrtec), 765
CF. *See* Cystic fibrosis (CF)
CFTR. *See* Cystic fibrosis transmembrane conductance regulator (CFTR)
Chadwick sign, 79
Chain of infection, 451–452
CHDs. *See* Congenital heart defects (CHDs)
Chemical burns, 800
Chemotherapy, 642
Chest, 579–580
Chest, neonatal assessment, 330
Chest x-ray, 544, 547, 551, 558, 560, 561, 565, 568, 586–587
Chickenpox. *See* Varicella
Child maltreatment, 410–414
Child sexual abuse, 410–411
Childhood mortality rates, 4
Children
  bacterial infections, 464–470
    Lyme disease, 466–468

    pertussis, 468–470
  brain tumors in, 502
  cardiovascular disorders, 569–576
    endocarditis, 569–574
    Kawasaki disease, 574–576
  cast types for, 653
  common fractures in, 669
  dermatologic disorders, 794–816
    acne, 794–800
    burns, 800–807
    contact dermatitis, 807–810
    scabies, 811–813
    tinea capitis, 813–815
    tinea corporis, 815–816
  endocrine and metabolic disorders, 729–744
    congenital hypothyroidism, 729–732
    diabetes, 732–739
    Graves disease, 739–742
    phenylketonuria, 742–744
  gastrointestinal (GI) disorders, 694–708
    appendicitis, 695–697
    celiac disease, 697–699
    Hirschsprung disease, 699–702
    intussusception, 702–705
    pyloric stenosis, 706–708
  hematologic and immunologic disorders, 763–782
    allergic rhinitis, 763–766
    atopic dermatitis, 766–768
    hemophilia, 769–771
    iron-deficiency anemia, 771–774
    leukemia, 775–777
    sickle cell anemia, 777–782
  immunization schedule, 455–464
  musculoskeletal disorders, 658–680
    congenital clubfoot, 659–662
    developmental dysplasia of the hip, 662–668
    fractures, 668–673
    Osgood-Schlatter disease, 675–676
    scoliosis, 677–680
    slipped capital femoral epiphysis, 673–675

  neurologic disorders, 496–523
    bacterial meningitis, 496–501
    brain tumors, 501–504
    cerebral palsy, 505–508
    hydrocephalus, 508–513
    neural tube defects, 513–519
    seizure disorders, 519–523
  respiratory disorders, 591–612
    asthma, 591–598
    bronchiolitis, 598–601
    croup, 601–604
    cystic fibrosis, 605–608
    pneumonia, 608–612
  T_3 levels, 726
  T_4 levels, 725
  urine output in, 616
  urinary disorders, 625–642
    acute poststreptococcal glomerulonephritis, 625–628
    congenital anomalies of the ureter/bladder/urethra, 628–631
    hemolytic uremic syndrome, 631–634
    kidney failure, acute, 637–640
    nephrotic syndrome, 634–637
    Wilms tumor, 641–642
  viral infections, 470–477
    COVID-19, 477
    fifth disease, 471–472
    not so rash, 471
    rash of rashes, 470
    roseola infantum, 472–473
    rubeola, 473–475
    varicella, 476–477
Chlamydia, 572
Choana, 580
Choking hazards, 685
Cholecystokinin, 687
Chordae tendineae, 527, 528
Chorion, 34
Chorion frondosum, 34
Chorion laeve, 34
Chorionic vesicle, 33
Chorionic villi, 30
Choroid plexus, 484, 509
Chronic SCFE, 674

Chyme, 686
CICU. *See* Coronary intensive care unit (CICU)
Cigarette smoking, 434–435
Circulation, 528
Circumduction, joint movement, 650
Claritin. *See* Loratadine (Claritin)
Clavicle, 21
Clavicular, 585
Cleocin. *See* Clindamycin (Cleocin)
Climacteric years, 24
Clindamycin (Cleocin), 798
Clindamycin, 798
Clitoris, 16, 17
Clobetasol (Temovate), 810
Clubfoot (talipes), 659
CMV. *See* Cytomegalovirus (CMV)
CN V. *See* Trigeminal nerve (CN V)
CNS. *See* Central nervous system (CNS)
Co-trimoxazole (Bactrim), 798
Coarctation of the aorta, 553–556
Cognitive development, 385
Coitus interruptus, contraception, 47
Collecting and main ducts, 21
Collecting tubule, 615
Colonoscopy, 690
Colostrum, 250, 260
Commercial formulas, bottle-feeding, 270–271
Communicating hydrocephalus, 509
Compact bone, 648
Compact bone replacing cartilage, 648
Compartment syndrome, 801
Complete blood count (CBC), 353, 759–760, 765, 767
Computed tomography (CT) scan, 489–490, 548
Conception/fetal development
  female reproductive system, 16–25
    external genitalia, 16–19
    hormonal function/menstrual cycle, 22–25
    internal genitalia, 19–20
    mammary glands, 21–22
  fertilization, 25–28
    disperse and penetrate, 27–28

help along the way, 27
survival of the fittest, 27
timing is everything, 27
  male reproductive system, 9–15
    accessory reproductive glands, 13
    duct system, 12–13
    hormonal control/sexual development, 14–15
    making introductions, 10
    penis, 11
    scrotum, 11–12
    spermatogenesis, 13–14
    testes, 12
  pregnancy, 28–37
    making predictions, 28
    ovaries and uterus, structural changes in, 32–37
    stages of fetal development, 28–32
Conduction system, 529
Confluence of venous sinuses, 509
Congenital anomalies of the ureter, 628–631
Congenital clubfoot, 659–662
Congenital heart defects (CHDs), 350
Congenital hypothyroidism, 729–732
Congenital neonatal infections, 351–354
  bacterial sepsis, 351–354
Congenital obstructive defects, 553–560
  coarctation of the aorta, 553–556
  pulmonic stenosis, 559–560
  stenosis, aortic, 556–558
Constipation, 142
Contact dermatitis, 807–810
Contraception, 40–42
  abstinence, 42–43
  barrier methods, 59–67
    cervical cap, 63–64
    diaphragm, 60–63
    female condom, 65–67
    male condom, 64–65
    spermicides, 59–60
  combined oral contraceptives, 48–51

    advantages of, 50
    biphasic, 48
    disadvantages of, 50–51
    monophasic, 48
    pills, 48
    tips on, 49
    triphasic, 48
    21- or 28-day packs, 49
  complications, 41
  factor in partner, 41
  implantable methods, 58–59
    advantages of, 58
    disadvantages of, 59
  implementation, 41–42
  injections, 54–55
    advantages of, 54
    disadvantages of, 54–55
  intrauterine device (IUD), 55–58
    advantages of, 57
    copper interference, 56
    disadvantages of, 57
    insertion, 55–56
    progesterone reserve, 56–57
  intravaginal method, 52–53
    advantages of, 52
    disadvantages of, 52–53
  morning-after pill, 51–52
    advantages of, 51
    disadvantages of, 52
  natural family planning methods, 43–47
    basal body temperature (BBT) method, 44–45
    cervical mucus (Billings) method, 45–46
    coitus interruptus, 47
    ovulation awareness (cycle beads), 46–47
    rhythm (calendar) method, 43
    symptothermal method, 46
  patient history, 41
  tips on, 42
  transdermal contraceptive patch, 53–54
    advantages of, 53
    disadvantages of, 53–54
Contraction, without relaxation, 227

Convalescent stage, 452
Coronary intensive care unit (CICU), 541
Corpus, 20
Corpus callosum, 481
Corpus cavernosum, 10
Corpus of uterus, 17
Corpus spongiosum, 10
Corpus uterus, 17
Corticosteroids, 604
Coumadin. *See* Warfarin (Coumadin)
Counterpressure, for labor pain, 237
COVID-19 pandemic, 3, 5, 477, 609
    vaccine, 455, 456
CP. *See* Cerebral palsy (CP)
Cranial abnormalities, types of, 327
Cranial nerves, 486
Creatinine, 618–619
Croup, 601–604
CRP. *See* C-reactive protein (CRP)
CSF. *See* Cerebrospinal fluid (CSF)
CT. *See* Computed tomography
    (CT) scan
Cutaneous, 639
Cutibacterium acnes, 795
Cyanosis/crying, 543, 568
Cystic fibrosis (CF), 579, 600, 605–608
Cystic fibrosis transmembrane
    conductance regulator
    (CFTR), 605
Cytomegalovirus (CMV), 355, 356

D
Damaged tissue, 779
Dapsone (Aczone), 798
DDAVP. *See* Desmopressin acetate
    (DDAVP)
DDH. *See* Developmental dysplasia of
    the hip (DDH)
Decadron. *See* Dexamethasone
    (Decadron)
Decidua, 32–33
Decidua basalis, 33, 34
Decidua capsularis, 33
Decidua parietalis, 33
Deep vein thrombosis (DVT), 298–305
    femoral *vs.* pelvic, 300
    and pulmonary embolism, 304–305

Deformity, 660
Demerol. *See* Meperidine (Demerol)
Dendrites, 483
Denis Browne boots/splint, 661
Dennie sign, 764
Dense tissue, 586
Dermatitis herpetiformis, 697
Dermatologic problems
    anatomy and physiology, 785–787
        great protector, 785
        structures of skin, 785–787
    diagnostic tests, 787–792
        potassium hydroxide
            preparation, 787–788
        skin biopsy, 788–791
        tzanck test, 792
    disorders, 794–816
        acne, 794–800
        burns, 800–807
        contact dermatitis, 807–810
        scabies, 811–813
        tinea capitis, 813–815
        tinea corporis, 815–816
    treatments and procedures,
        792–794
        laser surgery, 792–793
        skin grafting, 793–794
Dermatophyte test medium
    (DTM), 816
Dermis, 786, 803
Descending aorta, 527
Descending loop of Henle, 615
Desmopressin acetate (DDAVP), 770
Detoxification, 441
Developmental dysplasia of the hip
    (DDH), 662–668
Dexamethasone (Decadron),
    499, 604
DHA. *See* Docosahexaenoic acid
    (DHA)
Diabetes, 732–739
    gestational, 160
    for pregnant patient, 160–166
        classifications, 160
        losing balance, 160–161
    type 1, 160, 732–733, 735
    type 2, 160, 732–733, 735

Diabetic ketoacidosis (DKA), 735
Diaper dermatitis, 808
Diaphragm, 60–63
    advantages of, 62
    disadvantages of, 62–63
    insertion, 61–62
Diaphysis, 647
Diarthrodial joints, 650
Differentiation, 748
Differin. *See* Adapalene (Differin)
DiGeorge syndrome, 567
Digestion, 684–688
Digoxin (Lanoxin), 158, 558, 560
Diminutive/absent left ventricle, 561
Diphenhydramine (Benadryl), 176,
    768, 810
Diphtheria and tetanus toxoids and
    acellular pertussis (DTaP)
    vaccine, 459
Diprolene. *See* Betamethasone
    (Diprolene)
Dislocation, 663, 664
Dispersed granulosa cells, 26
Distal convoluted tubule, 615
Distended sigmoid colon, 700
DKA. *See* Diabetic ketoacidosis (DKA)
Docosahexaenoic acid (DHA), 263
Doppler ultrasound stethoscope, 121
Dornase alfa (Pulmozyme), 607
Double-footling breech, 206
Doula, 236
Down Syndrome, 28, 543, 697
Doxycycline (Periostat), 798
DTaP vaccine. *See* Diphtheria and
    tetanus toxoids and acellular
    pertussis (DTaP) vaccine
DTM. *See* Dermatophyte test medium
    (DTM)
Duct system, 12–13
Ductus arteriosus, 530
Ductus venosus, 530, 531
Duodenum, 693
Dura mater/"hard mother," 239, 483
DVT. *See* Deep vein thrombosis (DVT)
Dynacin. *See* Minocycline (Dynacin)
Dysplasia, 663
Dyspnea, 143

E

E-cigarettes, 434–435
Early adolescence, 430
Early blastocyst, 29
Early pregnancy loss (spontaneous abortion), 193–196
  types of, 193
Ears, neonatal assessment, 329–330
EC. *See* Emergency contraception (EC)
ECG. *See* Electrocardiography (ECG)
Echocardiogram, 350
Echocardiography, 532–533, 544, 547, 551, 561, 568
Eclampsia, 118, 167
Ectoderm, 30
Eculizumab (Soliris), 633
Eczema. *See* Atopic dermatitis
Edinburgh postnatal depression scale, 288
EEG. *See* Electroencephalogram (EEG)
Efferent arteriole, 615
Ejaculatory duct, 10
Electrical burns, 800
Electrocardiography (ECG), 533, 544, 547, 551, 558, 560, 565
Electroencephalogram (EEG), 490–491
Elemental formulas, bottle-feeding, 271
Embryo, 21–22
  to fetus, 31
Embryonic disk, 30
Emergency contraception (EC), 51
  advantages of, 51
  disadvantages of, 52
Encephalocele, 516–517
Endocarditis, 569–574
Endocrine and metabolic system
  anatomy and physiology, 711–719
    endocrine system components, 712
    glands, 711–715
    hormones, 715–719
    too little, too much, 711
  changes during pregnancy, 86–88
    adrenal gland, 87
    pancreas, 88
    parathyroid gland, 87
    pituitary gland, 86–87

placenta, 86
prostaglandins, 86
relaxin, 86
thyroid gland, 87
congenital hypothyroidism, 729–732
diabetes, 732–739
diagnostic tests, 720–727
  GH, human, 721–722
  GH, suppression, 722–723
  glucose, fasting plasma, 720–721
  neonatal T4/TSH blood-spot test, 723–725
  T_3 test (serum), 726–727
  T_4 test, 725–726
Graves disease, 739–742
phenylketonuria, 742–744
treatments and procedures, 727–729
  ^{131}I therapy, 727–728
  thyroidectomy, 728–729
Endoderm, 30
Endometrium, 17, 20
Endoscopy, 690–691
Engorgement, 250
Enlarged cartilage cells, 647
Enterobacter aerogenes, 867
Eosinophils, 751
Epidermis, 786, 803
Epidermophyton floccosum, 815
Epididymis, 10, 12
Epidural space, 239, 484
Epiglottis, 580
Epilepsy, 519
Epileptogenic focus, 520
Epiphyseal line, 648
Epiphyseal plate, 647, 648
Epiphysis, 646, 647
Epstein pearls, 328–329
Erygel. *See* Erythromycin (Erygel)
Erythema migrans, 466–467
Erythromycin (Erygel), 798
Erythromycin, 798
Erythropoietin. *See* Red blood cells (RBCs)
Escherichia coli, 497, 631, 634, 867
Esophagogastroduodenoscopy, 690

Esophagus, 580
Etonogestrel implant (Nexplanon), 58
Excretory urography, 619–620
Exercise-induced asthma, 592
Exercise testing, 534
Extension, joint movement, 650
External genitalia, 16–19
  adjacent structures, 18
  clitoris, 18
  featuring glands, 18–19
  labia majora, 18
  labia minora, 18
  mons pubis, 18
  not too simple, 19
External inguinal ring, 10
External os, 19, 232
External rotation, joint movement, 650
Extremities, neonatal assessment, 332
Extrinsic cascade, 752
Eyes, neonatal assessment, 327–328

F

Face cephalic presentation, 205
Facial nerve (CN VII), 486
Fallopian tube, 17, 29, 70
Fallopian tubes, 20
Family-centered care, 1–2
  benefits of, 2
Family planning, 40
  natural methods, 43–47
    basal body temperature (BBT) method, 44–45
    cervical mucus (Billings) method, 45–46
    coitus interruptus, 47
    ovulation awareness (cycle beads), 46–47
    rhythm (calendar) method, 43
    symptothermal method, 46
  surgical methods, 67–70
    sterilization, 67
    tubal sterilization, 69–70
    vasectomy, 67–69
Family types, 2–3
Fascia, 649
Fatigue, and pregnancy, 76
Fats, 134

FDA. *See* U.S. Food and Drug
    Administration (FDA)
Female condom, 65–67
    advantages of, 66
    disadvantages of, 67
    insertion, 65–66
Female reproductive system, 16–25
    external genitalia, 16–19
    hormonal function/menstrual cycle,
        22–25
    internal genitalia, 19–20
    mammary glands, 21–22
    structures of, 16–17
Females, sexual maturity in, 424–427
Femoral DVT *vs.* pelvic DVT, 300
Ferritin, 773
Fertilization, 25–28, 29
    disperse and penetrate, 27–28
    help along the way, 27
    survival of the fittest, 27
    timing is everything, 27
Fetal engagement, 207–208
Fetal heart rate, 120–121
    baseline, 230
    classifications of, 230–231
    Doppler ultrasound stethoscope, 121
    episodic or periodic, 230
    evaluation of, 121
    fetoscope, 121
    heart to heart, 120
    variability, 230
Fetal presentation, labor and birth,
        199–208
    engagement, 207–208
    fetal attitude, 200
    fetal lie, 200, 202
    fetal position, 200–201
    types of, 202–207
        breech presentation, 203–204,
            205–206
        cephalic presentation, 202–203,
            205
        shoulder presentation, 206–207
Fetal strip evaluation, 228–231
Fetoscope, 121
Fibrinogen, 93
Fibrous septa, 21

Fifth disease, 471–472
Fimbria, 17
Fimbriae, 20
Finnegan Neonatal Abstinence Scoring
    Tool (FNAST), 365
Firearms, 435
First-degree burns, 802
First mitotic division, 29
First trimester
    ambivalence, 101–102
    pregnancy discomforts, 138–140
        fatigue, 140
        nausea and vomiting, 139
        queasiness cause, 139
    psychosocial challenge, 101–102
Flexion, joint movement, 650
Flovent. *See* Fluticasone (Flovent)
Fluticasone (Flovent), 595
FNAST. *See* Finnegan Neonatal
    Abstinence Scoring Tool
    (FNAST)
Foley catheter. *See* Indwelling catheter
Follicle-stimulating hormone (FSH), 15,
    429–430
Fontanels, 326–327
Footling breech, 206
Foramen of Luschka, 509
Foramen of Magendie, 509
Foramen of Monro, 509
Foramen ovale, 530, 531
Formula feeding, 387
Fourth-degree burns, 803
Fourth ventricle, 509
Fractures, 668–673
Frontal lobe, 482
Frontal sinus, 580
FSH. *See* Follicle-stimulating hormone
    (FSH)
Fundal height throughout pregnancy, 82
Fundal palpation, complications of, 252
Fundus, 20, 252
    GI, 686
    of uterus, 17

G
Galactosemia, 361–362
Galeazzi sign, 664

Gamma-globulin, 454
Gastrografin. *See* Barium/diatrizoate
    meglumine (Gastrografin)
Gastrointestinal (GI) system
    anatomy and physiology, 683–689
        accessory glands and organs,
            688–689
        digestion, 684–688
        structures of, 683
    diagnostic tests, 689–691
        air/barium enema, 689
        barium swallow, 690
        endoscopy, 690–691
        stool specimen, 691
    disorders, 694–708
        appendicitis, 695–697
        celiac disease, 697–699
        Hirschsprung disease, 699–702
        intussusception, 702–705
        pyloric stenosis, 706–708
    during pregnancy, 96–98
        anatomic changes, 96–98
        functional changes, 98
    treatments and procedures,
        691–694
        alternative feeding methods,
            692–693
        GI intubation, 693–694
Gastrostomy feedings, 693
Gauging burn depth, 803
GCS. *See* Glasgow Coma Scale (GCS)
Genitalia, neonatal assessment, 332
Gentamicin, 353
Gestation, 28
Gestational age (AGA), 347
Gestational diabetes, 160
Gestational hypertension, 118
    for pregnant patient, 167–172
        administering magnesium
            sulfate safely, 171–172
        emergency interventions for,
            171
GH. *See* Growth hormone (GH)
GI. *See* Gastrointestinal (GI) system
Glands, 711–715
    adrenal glands, 714
    gonads, 715

pancreas, 714–715
parathyroid glands, 714
pituitary gland, 713
thyroid gland, 713
Glandular lobe, 21
Glans penis, 10
Glasgow Coma Scale (GCS), 487–488
Glomerulus, 615
Glossopharyngeal nerve (CN IX), 486
Glucose challenge values, in
pregnancy, 163
Glucose, fasting plasma, 720–721
Glucose tolerance testing, 129
Goiter, 740
Gonads, 715
Goodell sign, 79
Graft-versushost disease (GVHD),
762, 763
Granular leukocytes, 750–751
Graves disease, 739–742
Growing cartilage, 647, 648
Growing hyaline cartilage, 647
Growth hormone (GH)
human, 721–722
suppression, 722–723
tests, 720
GVHD. See Graft-versushost disease
(GVHD)

H

Haemophilus influenzae, 601
Haemophilus influenzae type B (Hib)
vaccine, 460, 496
Hard palate, 581
hCG. See Human chorionic
gonadotropin (hCG)
HDN. See Hemorrhagic disease of the
newborn (HDN)
Head, neonatal assessment, 326
Head-to-toe assessment, prenatal
care, 116–119
back, 119
breasts, 117
ears, 117
extremities and skin, 119
eyes, 116
general appearance, 116

head and scalp, 116
heart, 117–118
lungs, 118
mouth, 117
neck, 117
nose, 117
rectum, 119
Health problems
alcohol and drug misuse, 438–442
sexually transmitted infections,
442–445
suicide and attempted suicide,
446–448
Healthy People 2030, 3
social determinants of health, 5–6
Heart, 526–528
heart chambers, 526–527
atria, 526
ventricles, 526–527
heart valves, 527
aortic/pulmonic valves, 528
tricuspid/mitral valves, 528
neonatal assessment, 331
Heart rate, neonate, 322
Heart to heart, fetal heart rate, 120
Heartburn, 141
Heat and cold application, for labor
pain, 236–237
Heat loss prevention, in neonate,
337–338
conduction, 337
convection, 337
evaporation, 338
radiation, 338
Hegar sign, 79
HELLP. See Hemolysis, elevated liver
enzymes, and low platelets
(HELLP) syndrome
Hematocrit, 773
Hematologic/immunologic systems
anatomy and physiology, 747–752
blood components, 749–752
blood formation, 748–749
hemostasis, 752
complement system, 756
diagnostic tests, 757–760
allergy skin testing, 758

bone marrow aspiration/biopsy,
758–759
CBC with differential, 759–760
disorders, 763–782
allergic rhinitis, 763–766
atopic dermatitis, 766–768
hemophilia, 769–771
iron-deficiency anemia,
771–774
leukemia, 775–777
sickle cell anemia, 777–782
hypersensitivity, 756–757
immune system cells, 754–756
immune system organs, 753–754
treatments and procedures,
760–763
blood transfusion, 760–761
bone marrow transplantation,
761–763
Hematopoiesis, 748
Hemi-Fontan. See Bidirectional Glenn
procedure
Hemodialysis, 623
Hemoglobin (Hgb), 750, 773, 778
Hemoglobin SC (Hgb SC) disease, 777
Hemoglobin SS (Hgb SS) disease, 777
Hemolysis, elevated liver enzymes, and
low platelets (HELLP) syndrome,
118, 173–174
temporary, 173
Hemolytic uremic syndrome (HUS),
631–634
Hemophilia, 769–771
Hemorrhage, postpartum, 277–285
Hemorrhagic disease of the newborn
(HDN), 688
Hemorrhoids, 141–142
Hemostasis, 752
Hepatitis A vaccine, 456–458
Hepatitis B test, 128
Hepatitis B vaccine, 458–459
Hereditary bleeding disorder, 769
Herpes simplex virus (HSV), 355, 356
Heterotopic procedure, 540
Hgb. See Hemoglobin (Hgb)
Hgb SC. See Hemoglobin SC (Hgb SC)
disease

Hgb SS. *See* Hemoglobin SS (Hgb SS) disease
HIE. *See* Hypoxic–ischemic encephalopathy (HIE)
High-risk neonate
  birth weight classification, 347–350
    large for gestational age, 347–348
    small for gestational age, 348–350
  cardiac screening, 350–351
  congenital neonatal infections, 351–354
    bacterial sepsis, 351–354
  hyperbilirubinemia, 357–360
  metabolism, inborn errors of, 360–362
    galactosemia, 361–362
    phenylketonuria, 360–361
  neurologic issues, 362–366
    neonatal abstinence syndrome, 364–366
    seizures, 362–364
  prematurity, 366–369
  respiratory problems, 369–375
    meconium aspiration syndrome, 373–374
    pneumothorax, 374–375
    respiratory distress syndrome, 371–373
    transient tachypnea of the newborn, 369–371
  at risk for impaired parenting, 346–347
  syphilis, 354–355
  viral infections, 355–357
High-risk pregnancy
  age, 147–148
  cardiac disease, 156–160
  current obstetric status, 148
  diabetes, 160–166
  early pregnancy loss (spontaneous abortion), 193–196
    types of, 193
  family history, 152
  gestational hypertension, 167–172
    administering magnesium sulfate safely, 171–172
  emergency interventions for, 171
  gravida aggravations, 150
  gynecologic history, 148–149
  HELLP syndrome, 173–174
    temporary, 173
  hyperemesis gravidarum, 174–177
  insulin influx, 150
  isoimmunization, 177–181
    RhoGAM, 179–180
  lifestyle, 150–151
  medical history, 149–150
  nutrition, 151
  obstetric history, 148–149
  placenta previa, 181–185
    types of, 182
  placental abruption (abruptio placentae), 152–156
  premature labor, 185–189
  premature rupture of membranes (PROM), 189–193
  substance misuse, 151
Hilum, 580
Hirschsprung disease, 699–702
Hirsutism, 100
HIV testing, 128–129
HLA. *See* Human leukocyte antigen (HLA)
Home pregnancy tests, 78
Homograft/xenograft, 793
Hormonal control/sexual development, 14–15
Hormonal function/menstrual cycle, 22–25
Hormones, 715–719
  adrenal hormones, 718
  hormonal action, 719
  hormonal regulation, 719
  hormone release and transport, 718–719
  pancreatic hormones, 718
  pituitary hormones, 715–718
  TH hormones, 718
HPL. *See* Human placental lactogen (HPL)
HPV vaccine. *See* Human papillomavirus (HPV) vaccine
HSV. *See* Herpes simplex virus (HSV)
Human blood cell development, 749
Human chorionic gonadotropin (hCG), 32–33, 78
Human chorionic somatomammotropin. *See* human placental lactogen
Human leukocyte antigen (HLA), 762
Human papillomavirus (HPV) vaccine, 460
Human placental lactogen (HPL), 37
HUS. *See* Hemolytic uremic syndrome (HUS)
Hydralazine (Apresoline), 170
Hydrocephalus, 508–513
Hydroxyzine (Atarax), 768, 810
Hyperbilirubinemia, 357–360
Hyperemesis gravidarum, 174–177
Hyperimmune/convalescent serum globulin, 454
Hypersensitivity, 756–757
  atopy/anaphylaxis, 756
  cell-mediated hypersensitivity, 757
  cytotoxic response, 756–757
  immune complex, 757
Hyperthyroidism. *See* Graves disease
Hypertrophy of right ventricle, 567
Hypodermis/subcutaneous tissue, 786
Hypoglossal nerve (CN XII), 486
Hypoglycemia, 735
Hypophysis/master gland. *See* Pituitary gland
Hypoplastic ascending aorta, 561
Hypoplastic left heart syndrome, 561–563
Hypotension, supine, 91
Hypothyroidism, 674
Hypoxia, 363
Hypoxic cells, 779
Hypoxic–ischemic encephalopathy (HIE), 363
Hysterical scoliosis, 677

I

Ibuprofen (Motrin/Advil), 676
ICP monitoring, 493–495
Idiopathic scoliosis, 678
IgA. *See* Immunoglobulin A (IgA)

IgD. *See* Immunoglobulin D (IgD)
IgE. *See* Immunoglobulin E (IgE)
IgG. *See* Immunoglobulin G (IgG)
IgM. *See* Immunoglobulin M (IgM)
Igs. *See* Immunoglobulins (Igs)
Immature immunity, 452
Immune protection, 452–464
    immunization schedule, 455–464
    methods of, 453–454
        artificially acquired active
            immunity, 453
        artificially acquired passive
            immunity, 454
        natural (innate) immunity, 453
        naturally acquired active
            immunity, 453
        naturally acquired passive
            immunity, 453
    types of immunizations, 454–455
        inactivated/killed vaccines,
            454–455
        live, attenuated vaccines, 454
        other vaccines, 455
    vaccine administration,
        contraindications to, 464
Immune system, 381, 752–757
    changes during pregnancy, 101
    complement system, 756
    hypersensitivity, 756–757
        atopy or anaphylaxis, 756
        cell-mediated
            hypersensitivity, 757
        cytotoxic response, 756–757
        immune complex, 757
    immune system cells, 754–756
        B cells, 754–755
        phagocytes, 755
        T cells, 755–756
    immune system organs, 753–754
        lymph nodes, 753
        spleen, 754
        thymus, 753
        tonsils, 754
Immunization schedule, 455–464
    COVID-19 vaccine, 456
    DTaP vaccine, 459
    hepatitis A vaccine, 456–458

    hepatitis B vaccine, 458–459
    Hib vaccine, 460
    human papillomavirus vaccine, 460
    influenza vaccine, 463–464
    IPV, 461
    meningococcal vaccine, 461–462
    MMR vaccine, 461
    pneumococcal 15- or 20-valent
        conjugate vaccine, 462
    rotavirus vaccine, 462
    varicella virus vaccine, 463–464
Immunoglobulin A (IgA), 754–755
Immunoglobulin D (IgD), 755
Immunoglobulin E (IgE), 755, 756,
    764, 767
Immunoglobulin G (IgG), 755, 756
Immunoglobulin M (IgM), 755, 756
Immunoglobulins (Igs), 754
Implantable methods, contraception,
    58–59
    advantages of, 58
    disadvantages of, 59
Inactivated poliovirus vaccine (IPV)
    vaccine, 461
Inactivated vaccines, 454–455
Incubation stage, 452
Incubator, 336, 338
Indigestion, 140
Indirect Coombs test, 128
Indocin. *See* Indomethacin (Indocin)
Indomethacin (Indocin), 187, 548
Indwelling catheter, 622
Infancy and early childhood, 380–385
    child maltreatment, 410–414
    growth and development, principles
        of, 379–380
        stages of, 379
        teach your children well, 379–380
    injury prevention, 391–392, 400–401,
        407–410
        aspiration, 391, 400–401
        burns, 401, 407
        child passenger safety, 391
        childproofing, 392
        drowning, 407–408
        falls, 392, 401, 408
        inadvertent ingestions, 392

        motor vehicle and bicycle
            injuries, 408–409
        poisoning, 409–410
        suffocation, 410
    maintaining health, 385–391
        dental hygiene, 390–391
        nutritional guidelines, 385–388
        sleep and rest guidelines,
            389–390
    physical development, 381–382
        fine motor development, 382
        gross motor development, 382
        head circumference, 382
        height, 381
        infant reflexes, 382, 383
        normal infant reflexes, 382
        teeth, 382
        weight, 381–382
    preschool, 402–407
        coping with concerns, 406–407
        keys to health, 404–406
        physical development, 402
        psychological development,
            403–404
    psychological development, 382–385
        cognitive development, 385
        language development/
            socialization, 383–385
    sleep requirements, 390
    system development, 380–381
        cardiovascular/respiratory
            systems, 380–381
        immune system, 381
        neurologic system, 380
    toddlerhood, 393–400
        keys to health, 396–400
        psychological development,
            394–396
        toddlerhood, 393–394
Infant mortality rates, 4
Infections
    bacteria, 464–470
        a class by any other class, 466
        Lyme disease, 466–468
        pertussis, 468–470
    chain of infection, 451–452
        immature immunity, 452

Infections (*continued*)
  immune protection, 452–464
    immunization schedule, 455–464
    methods of, 453–454
    types of immunizations, 454–455
    vaccine administration,
      contraindications to, 464
  stages of, 452
  viruses, 470–477
    COVID-19, 477
    fifth disease, 471–472
    not so rash, 471
    rash of rashes, 470
    roseola infantum, 472–473
    rubeola, 473–475
    varicella, 476–477
Infective or bacterial endocarditis.
  See Endocarditis
Inferior nasal concha, 580
Inferior vena cava, 527
Inflamed laryngeal area, 602
Inflamed subglottic tissue, 602
Inflamed tissue, 779
Influenza, 609
Influenza vaccine, 463–464
Infratentorial ependymoma, 502
Injections, contraceptive, 54–55
  advantages of, 54
  disadvantages of, 54–55
Injury prevention, 391–392, 400–401,
  407–410
  aspiration, 391, 400–401
  burns, 401, 407
  child passenger safety, 391
  childproofing, 392
  drowning, 407–408
  falls, 392, 401, 408
  firearms, 435
  inadvertent ingestions, 392
  motor vehicle accidents,
    435–436
  motor vehicle and bicycle injuries,
    408–409
  poisoning, 409–410
  risk-taking behaviors, 436–437
  sports injuries, 437
  suffocation, 410

Innate immunity, 453
Inspiration/expiration, 584–586
  adventitious breath sounds, 585–586
  muscles to stabilize/muscles to
    breathe, 584–585
Insulin, 735–737
Integumentary system, 785
  changes during pregnancy, 99–100
    bubbled gums, 100
    pigmentation, 100
    pink-handed, 100
    striae gravidarum, 99–100
    vascular markings, 100
Intentional physical abuse, 410
Intercostal, 585
Interlobular artery and vein, 615
Internal genitalia, 19–20
  cervix, 19–20
  fallopian tubes, 20
  ovaries, 20
  uterus, 20
  vagina, 19
Internal inguinal ring, 10
Internal os, 19, 232
Internal os of cervix, 17
Internal rotation, joint movement, 650
Interstitial cell–stimulating hormone, 15
Interstitial pneumonia, 609
Interventricular septum, 526, 527
Intrarenal failure, 638
Intrauterine device (IUD), 55–58
  advantages of, 57
  copper interference, 56
  disadvantages of, 57
  insertion, 55–56
  progesterone reserve, 56–57
Intravaginal contraceptive method,
  52–53
  advantages of, 52
  disadvantages of, 52–53
Intrinsic cascade system, 752
Intrinsic or parenchymal kidney failure.
  See Intrarenal failure
Intussusception, 702–705
Invaginated bowel, 703
Invisible bone, 651–652
Involution, 245

Iodine, 135
IPV vaccine. *See* Inactivated poliovirus
  vaccine (IPV) vaccine
Iron, 135–136, 688
Iron deficiencies, 92–93, 771–774
Irritant dermatitis, 808
Ischemia, 363
Islet cells/islets of Langerhans, 715
Isoimmunization, 177–181
  RhoGAM, 179–180
Isotretinoin (Accutane), 796, 797
Isthmus, 713
IUD. *See* Intrauterine device (IUD)

J

JCIH. *See* Joint Committee on Infant
  Hearing (JCIH)
Jejunostomy feedings, 693
Jejunum gavage, 693
Joint Committee on Infant Hearing
  (JCIH), 329
Joints, 649–650

K

Kangaroo care, 337
Kawasaki disease (KD), 574–576
Kayexalate, 640
KD. *See* Kawasaki disease (KD)
Keftab. *See* Cephalexin (Keftab)
Kernig sign, 498
Kidney, 614–615
  biopsy, 621
  failure, acute, 637–640
  nephron, 614–615
  transplantation, 624
Kidneys, ureters, and bladder (KUB)
  radiography, 619
Klaron. *See* Sodium sulfacetamide
  (Klaron)
KOH. *See* Potassium hydroxide (KOH)
  preparation
KUB. *See* Kidneys, ureters, and bladder
  (KUB) radiography
Kyphosis, 677

L

Labia majora, 16
Labia minora, 16

Labor and birth
  cardinal movements, 220
  fetal presentation, 199–208
    engagement, 207–208
    fetal attitude, 200
    fetal lie, 200, 202
    fetal position, 200–201
    types of, 202–207
  labor stimulation, 208–212
    Bishop score, 209–210
    conditions for, 208–210
    methods, 210–212
  nursing interventions, 241
  nursing procedures, 225–233
    cervical examination, 231–233
    continuous external electronic
      monitoring, 227
    continuous internal electronic
      monitoring, 228
    fetal strip evaluation, 228–231
    intermittent monitoring of fetal
      status, 226–227
  onset of labor, 212–215
    preliminary signs and
      symptoms, 213–214
    true labor signs, 214–215
  pain
    local anesthesia, 240–241
    lumbar epidural anesthesia,
      238–240
    nonpharmacologic methods,
      235–237
    perception, 234–235
    pharmacologic methods,
      237–241
    sources of, 233–234
    spinal anesthesia, 240
  stages of labor, 215–225
    first, 216–218
    fourth, 224–225
    second, 218–223
    third, 223–224
Lactation, 259–261
  breast milk composition, 260–261
  and menstrual cycle, 261
  physiology of, 259
Lactiferous duct, 21, 260

Lactiferous duct orifice, 21
Lactiferous sinus, 21, 260
Lanoxin. *See* Digoxin (Lanoxin)
Laparoscope, 70
Large for gestational age (LGA), 347–348
Large intestine, GI, 687–688
Laryngopharynx, 580
Larynx, 582
Laser surgery, 792–793
  complications, 792
  nursing considerations, 792–793
Lasix/mannitol (Osmitrol), 640
Late adolescence, 431
Late blastocyst, 29
Left atrium, 527, 542
Left primary (mainstem) bronchus, 580
Left pulmonary veins, 527
Left secondary (lobar) bronchus, 580
Left ventricle, 527, 550, 557, 564
Leukemia, 775–777
Leukotriene modifiers, 596
Levalbuterol (Xopenex), 596
LGA. *See* Large for gestational age
  (LGA)
LH. *See* Luteinizing hormone (LH)
Ligaments, 649
  pain around round, 143–144
Ligamentum arteriosus, 531
Ligamentum teres, 531
Lightheadedness, 142–143
Linea nigra, 77
Listeria monocytogenes, 497
Live, attenuated vaccines, 454
Lobar pneumonia, 609
Lobe, 260
Lochia, 253–255
  types of, 253
Long bones, 645–646
Loose connective tissue/adipose
  tissue, 786
Lordosis, 677
Low blood pressure, 283
Lower GI series. *See* Air/barium enema
Lower respiratory tract, 580, 582–583
  alveoli, 583
  bronchi, 582–583
  trachea, 582

Lumbar epidural anesthesia, 238–240
Lumbar puncture, 491–492
Lumbar vertebra, 91
Lungs, 579–580
Lungs, neonatal assessment,
  330–331
Luteinizing hormone (LH), 15, 429–430
Lyme disease, 466–468
Lymph nodes, 753
Lymphocytes, 752
Lymphokines, 757

M

Magnetic resonance imaging (MRI),
  492–493, 533, 544, 547, 551,
  565, 568
Maintaining health, 385–391
  dental hygiene, 390–391
  nutritional guidelines, 385–388
    breastfeeding, 385–387
    formula feeding, 387
    introducing solid foods, 388
  sleep and rest guidelines, 389–390
Male condom, 64–65
  advantages of, 64
  disadvantages of, 65
Male reproductive system, 9–15
  accessory reproductive glands, 13
  duct system, 12–13
  hormonal control/sexual
    development, 14–15
  making introductions, 10
  penis, 11
  scrotum, 11–12
  spermatogenesis, 13–14
  testes, 12
Males, sexual maturity in, 428–429
Mammary glands, 21–22
Manual breast milk expression,
  267–268
MAS. *See* Meconium aspiration
  syndrome (MAS)
Mass of sickled cells obstructing
  capillary lumen, 779
Mastitis, 295–298
Maternal morbidity, 4–5
Maternal mortality, 3–4

Maternal serum AFP (MSAFP) test.
    See AFP testing
Maternity/pediatric nursing
    family-centered care, 1–2
    infant and childhood mortality, 4
    maternal and childhood morbidity,
        4–5
    maternal mortality, 3–4
    role of nurse in, 1
    social determinants of health
        (SDOH), 5–6
        family's health-related beliefs
            and practices, 6
        health-related beliefs and
            practices, 6
MDIs. *See* Metered-dose inhalers
    (MDIs)
Measles. *See* Rubeola
Measles, mumps, and rubella (MMR)
    vaccine vaccine, 461
Meclizine (Antivert), 176
Meconium, 260
Meconium aspiration syndrome (MAS),
    373–374
Mediastinum, 579, 580
Medulla oblongata, 483
Medullary cavity, 647, 648
Medulloblastoma, 502
Meninges, 483–484
Meningitis, 496–501
Meningocele, 514–517
Meningococcal B vaccine, 461–462
Meningococcal serogroup A, C, W, and
    Y vaccine, 461–462
Meningococcal vaccines (MenACWY/
    MenB), 496
Menopause, 24
Mentum cephalic presentation,
    203, 205
Meperidine (Demerol), 238
Mesoderm, 30
Messenger RNA (mRNA) vaccine, 455
Metabolism, inborn errors of, 360–362
    galactosemia, 361–362
    phenylketonuria, 360–361
Metered-dose inhalers (MDIs), 589–590
Metformin, 735

Methimazole (Tapazole), 741
Methyldopa (Aldomet), 170
Microinfarct, 779
Microscopic colitis, 697
Microsporum canis, 815
Midbrain, 483
Middle adolescence, 430–431
Middle childhood/adolescence
    coping with concerns, 423, 434–435
    health problems, 437–448
        alcohol and drug misuse,
            438–442
        sexually transmitted infections,
            442–445
        suicide and attempted suicide,
            446–448
    injury prevention, 435–437
        firearms, 435
        motor vehicle accidents,
            435–436
        risk-taking behaviors, 436–437
        sports injuries, 437
    keys to health, 420–422, 432–433
    physical development, 417–418,
        423–430
    psychological development,
        419–420, 430–432
Middle nasal concha, 580
Mild acne, 796, 797
Milk-based formulas, bottle-feeding,
    270
Mini assessment, 487
Minocin. *See* Minocycline (Minocin)
Minocycline (Dynacin), 798
Minocycline (Minocin), 798
Mitral valve, 527, 528
Mitral valve atresia/stenosis, 561
Mixed congenital heart defects,
    560–566
    hypoplastic left heart syndrome,
        561–563
    transposition of the great arteries,
        563–566
MMR. *See* Measles, mumps, and
    rubella (MMR) vaccine vaccine
Moderate acne, 796, 797
Moderna, 456

Modified Fontan procedure, 563
Molding, 327
Moles. *See* Nevi
Monocytes, 752
Monophasic oral contraceptives, 48
Mons pubis, 16
Montelukast (Singulair), 596
Montgomery tubercle, 21
Morbidity, 4–5
Morning-after pill, 51–52
    advantages of, 51
    disadvantages of, 52
Morning sickness, 139
Morula, 29
Motor function, 489
Motor vehicle accidents, 435–436
Motrin/Advil. *See* Ibuprofen (Motrin/
    Advil)
Mouth and pharynx, neonatal
    assessment, 328–329
Mouth/oropharynx, 581
MRI. *See* Magnetic resonance imaging
    (MRI)
mRNA. *See* Messenger RNA (mRNA)
    vaccine
Mucocutaneous lymph node
    syndrome. *See* Kawasaki
    disease (KD)
Multigravida, 112
Multipara, 112
Murmurs, 531–532
Muscle, 649, 803
    bone marrow biopsy, 651
Musculoskeletal system
    anatomy and physiology, 645–650
        bones, 645–649
        joints, 649–650
        muscles, 649
    changes during pregnancy, 98–99
        muscles, 99
        nerves, 99
        skeleton, 99
    diagnostic tests, 650–652
        muscle/bone marrow
            biopsy, 651
        x-rays, 651–652
    disorders, 658–680

congenital clubfoot, 659–662
developmental dysplasia of the
hip, 662–668
fractures, 668–673
Osgood-Schlatter disease,
675–676
scoliosis, 677–680
slipped capital femoral
epiphysis, 673–675
treatments and procedures,
652–658
casting/splints, 652–656
prevent/restore, 652
traction, 656–658
Mycoplasma, 572
Mycoplasma pneumoniae, 601
Myelinization, 381
Myelomeningocele, 514–517
Myocardium, 527
Myometrium, 17, 20

N

Nägele rule, 28
Naprosyn/Aleve. *See* Naproxen
(Naprosyn/Aleve)
Naproxen (Naprosyn/Aleve), 676
Naris, 580
Narrowed trachea, 602
NAS. *See* Neonatal abstinence
syndrome (NAS)
Nasogastric (NG) gavage, 692–693
Nasopharynx, 580
National Institute of Child Health and
Human Development (NICHD),
211
Natural family planning methods,
43–47
basal body temperature (BBT)
method, 44–45
cervical mucus (Billings) method,
45–46
coitus interruptus, 47
ovulation awareness (cycle beads),
46–47
rhythm (calendar) method, 43
symptothermal method, 46
Naturally acquired active immunity, 453

Naturally acquired passive immunity,
453
Nausea and vomiting
during pregnancy, 76
reducing, 139–140
Nebulized racemic epinephrine, 603
Nebulizer therapy, 589
Neck, neonatal assessment, 330
Necrotic tissue, 779
Negativism, 398
Neisseria meningitidis, 496
Neonatal abstinence syndrome (NAS),
364–366
Neonatal intensive care unit (NICU),
347, 353, 360, 368
Neonatal screening, 720
Neonatal T4/TSH blood-spot test,
723–725
Neonatal thyrotropin test, 723
Neonatal TSH interference, 724
Neonate
adapting to extrauterine life, 309
care
eye prophylaxis, 334–335
oxygen administration, 339–344
physical, 334
thermoregulation, 335–339
head-to-toe assessment, 325–333
abdomen, 331–332
chest, 330
ears, 329–330
extremities, 332
eyes, 327–328
genitalia, 332
head, 326
heart, 331
lungs, 330–331
mouth and pharynx, 328–329
neck, 330
nose, 328
respiratory distress, 328
skin, 325–326
spine, 333
initial assessment, 311–320
Apgar score, 311–313
Ballard gestational age
assessment tool, 314–319

birth weight, 320
large-for-gestational-age infant,
caring for, 321
neurologic assessment, 333
physical assessment, 320
physiology of, 309–310
preterm, caring for, 320
size assessment, 324–325
chest circumference, 324
head circumference, 324
head-to-heel length, 324–325
vital signs, 321–323
axillary temperature, 322–323
blood pressure, 323
heart rate, 322
rectal temperature, 322
respiratory rate, 321–322
weight assessment, 324–325
Nephroblastoma. *See* Wilms tumor
Nephron, 614–615
Nephrotic syndrome, 634–637
Neural tube defects (NTDs), 513–519
anencephaly, 516
encephalocele, 516
spina bifida, 513–515
Neurohypophysis, 713
Neurologic issues, 362–366
neonatal abstinence syndrome,
364–366
seizures, 362–364
Neurologic system, 380
anatomy and physiology, 480–487
autonomic nervous system, 487
central nervous system, 480–485
peripheral nervous system,
485–487
assessment, 487–489
Glasgow Coma Scale, 487–488
mini assessment, 487
motor function, 489
pupillary response, 489
changes during pregnancy, 101
diagnostic tests, 489–493
computed tomography scan,
489–490
electroencephalogram, 490–491
lumbar puncture, 491–492

Neurologic system (*continued*)
    magnetic resonance imaging, 492–493
  disorders, 496–523
    bacterial meningitis, 496–501
    brain tumors, 501–504
    cerebral palsy, 505–508
    hydrocephalus, 508–513
    neural tube defects, 513–519
    seizure disorders, 519–523
  procedures and treatments, 493–496
    ICP monitoring, 493–495
    ventriculoperitoneal shunt insertion, 495–496
Neurons, 483
Neutrophils, 751
Nevi, 100
New trabeculae, 648
Newborns, 351, 353, 355, 362, 366, 369, 374
  common clinical signs of sepsis in, 352
NG. *See* Nasogastric (NG) gavage
NICHD. *See* National Institute of Child Health and Human Development (NICHD)
NICU. *See* Neonatal intensive care unit (NICU)
Nipple, 21, 260
Nirsevimab (Beyfortus), 600
Noncommunicating hydrocephalus, 509
Nongranular leukocytes, 751
Nonparent families, 3
Nonsteroidal antiinflammatory drugs (NSAIDs), 752
Normal pediatric respiratory rates, 584
Normally closed ductus arteriosus, 553
Norwood procedure, 562–563
Nose, neonatal assessment, 328
Nosebleeds (epistaxis), 765
Nose/nasal passages, 580–581
Not so rash, 471
Novacet. *See* Sulfur (Novacet)
NSAIDs. *See* Nonsteroidal antiinflammatory drugs (NSAIDs)
NTDs. *See* Neural tube defects (NTDs)
Nulligravida, 112

Nursing procedures, labor, 225–233
  cervical examination, 231–233
  continuous external electronic monitoring, 227
  continuous internal electronic monitoring, 228
  fetal strip evaluation, 228–231
  intermittent monitoring of fetal status, 226–227
Nutrition, 421, 432–433

O

Occipital lobe, 482
Oculomotor nerve (CN III), 486
OG. *See* Orogastric (OG) gavage
Olfactory nerve (CN I), 486
$131_{I\ therapy}$, 727–728
Optic nerve (CN II), 486
Oral cavity, 580
Orogastric (OG) gavage, 692–693
Oropharynx, 580
Orthotopic procedure, 540
Osgood-Schlatter disease, 675–676
Osmitrol. *See* Lasix/mannitol (Osmitrol)
Ossification, 646
Ossifying cartilage, 648
Osteoblasts creating bone, 647
Osteoclasts, 649
Osteocytes, 649
Ostium primum defect, 543
Ostium secundum defect, 542
Ovary, 17, 20, 29, 70
  changes during pregnancy, 81
Ovulation awareness (cycle beads), contraception, 46–47
Ovum, 25, 29
Oxygen, 596
Oxygen deficiency, 778
Oxygen therapy, 590–591
  hazards of, 343
Oxytocin, 211–212

P

Pacemaker of the heart. *See* Sinoatrial node
Pain, labor and birth
  nonpharmacologic methods, 235–237
    acupressure, 237

    acupuncture, 237
    breathing techniques, 236
    counterpressure, 237
    doula, 236
    heat and cold application, 236–237
    relaxation techniques, 236
    transcutaneous electrical nerve stimulation, 237
    yoga, 237
  perception, 234–235
  sources of, 233–234
Palivizumab (Synagis), 600
Pancreas, 712, 714–715
  changes during pregnancy, 88
Pancytopenia, 775
Papillary muscle, 527
Papilledema, 502
Parainfluenza, 601, 609
Parasympathetic nervous system, 487
Parathyroid glands, 714
  changes during pregnancy, 87
Parathyroid hormone (PTH), 714
Parietal lobe, 482
Partially implanted blastocyst, 29
Patent ductus arteriosus (PDA), 531, 545–549, 564
Patient-family-centered care. *See* Family-centered care
Pavlik harness, 666–667
PDA. *See* Patent ductus arteriosus (PDA)
PDSS. *See* Postpartum Depression Screening Scale (PDSS)
Pediatric coma scale, 488
Pelvic DVT *vs.* femoral DVT, 300
Pelvic examination, prenatal care, 119–120
Pelvic inflammatory disease (PID), 57–58
  signs of, 58
Penetration of zona pellucida, 26
Penis, 11
Pericardium, 526
Perineal nerves, 241
Perineum, 16
Period of communicability, 452
Periostat. *See* Doxycycline (Periostat)

Periosteum, 646
Peripheral nervous system, 485–487
  cranial nerves, 486
  somatic nervous system, 487
  spinal nerves, 485
Peritoneal dialysis, 624–625
Peritubular capillaries, 615
Pertussis, 468–470
Pfizer-BioNTech, 456
PFTs. *See* Pulmonary function
  tests (PFTs)
Phagocytes, 755
Pharynx, 581
Phenylalaninemia/phenylpyruvic
  oligophrenia. *See*
  Phenylketonuria (PKU)
Phenylketonuria (PKU), 360–361,
  742–744
Phosphorus, 135
Phototherapy, 359
Pia mater/"tender mother," 483, 484
PID. *See* Pelvic inflammatory
  disease (PID)
Pineal gland, 712
Pituitary gland, 712, 713
Pituitary gland, changes during
  pregnancy, 86–87
PKU. *See* Phenylketonuria (PKU)
Placenta, 35–37
  changes during pregnancy, 86
Placenta previa, 181–185
Placental abruption, 152–156
Platelets, 748, 752
Pluripotential stem cell, 747
Pneumococcal 15- or 20-valent
  conjugate vaccine (PCV15/
  PCV20), 462
Pneumococcal conjugate vaccine
  (PCV20), 611
Pneumococcal polysaccharide
  vaccine (PPSV/PPV23), 611
Pneumococcal vaccine (PCV7/
  PCV20), 496
Pneumonia, 608–612
Pneumothorax, 374–375
Pons, 483
Posterior fornix of vagina, 17
Posterior pituitary, 713

Postpartum blues. *See* Baby blues
Postpartum complications
  deep vein thrombosis (DVT),
    298–305
  hemorrhage, 277–285
  mastitis, 295–298
  psychiatric disorders, 285–291
    baby blues, 285
    postpartum depression, 285–289
    postpartum psychosis, 289–291
  puerperal infection, 291–295
Postpartum depression, 285–289
Postpartum Depression Screening
  Scale (PDSS), 290
Postpartum period
  care, 256–258
    bowel movement, 257
    catheterization, 257
    maternal self-care, 257–258
    patient education, 257
  lactation, 259–261
    breast milk composition,
      260–261
    and menstrual cycle, 261
    physiology of, 259
  neonatal nutrition, 261–274
    bottle-feeding with breast milk,
      268–270
    bottle-feeding with formula,
      270–273
    breast care, 273–274
    breastfeeding, 261–268
  patient history, 249
  phases of, 246
  physical examination, 249–256
    breasts, 250–251
    fundus, 252
    lochia, 253–255
    sitz bath, 256
    uterus, 251–253
  physiologic changes, 244–246
  psychological changes, 246–248
Postpartum psychosis, 289–291
Postrenal failure, 638
Potassium hydroxide (KOH)
  preparation, 787–788
  fungus finder, 787
  nursing considerations, 788

Pre-embryonic development, 29
Preeclampsia, 118, 167
Pregnancy, 28–37. *See also* High-risk
  pregnancy
  classification system, 112
  diabetes, 150
    classifications, 160
    losing balance, 160–161
  discomforts, 137–138
    first trimester, 138–140
    second and third trimesters,
      140–144
  foods to avoid during, 132
  fundal height throughout, 82
  glucose challenge values in, 163
  making predictions, 28
  obstetric history, 133
  ovaries and uterus, structural
    changes in, 32–37
  physiologic changes in body
    systems, 80–101
    cardiovascular system, 89–93
    endocrine system, 86–88
    gastrointestinal (GI) system,
      96–98
    immune system, 101
    integumentary system,
      99–100
    musculoskeletal system,
      98–99
    neurologic system, 101
    reproductive system, 80–85
    respiratory system, 88–89
    urinary system, 93–95
  physiologic signs of, 73
  positive signs of, 79–80
    fetal heart rate, 80
    fetal movement, 80
    ultrasonography, 79–80
  presumptive signs of, 75–80
    amenorrhea, 76
    breast changes, 76
    fatigue, 76
    nausea and vomiting, 76
    quickening, 77
    skin changes, 77
    urinary frequency, 76
    uterine enlargement, 76

Pregnancy (*continued*)
  probable signs of, 78–79
    ballottement, 79
    Braxton Hicks contractions, 79
    Chadwick sign, 79
    Goodell sign, 79
    hCG test, 78
    Hegar sign, 79
    home pregnancy tests, 78
    laboratory tests, 78
    ultrasonography, 79
  psychosocial changes, 101–104
    first trimester, 101–102
    second trimester, 102–103
    third trimester, 103–104
  signs of, 74–75
  stages of fetal development, 28–32
Pregnancy-induced hypertension. *See*
  Gestational hypertension
Premature labor, 185–189
Premature menopause, 24
Premature rupture of membranes
  (PROM), 189–193
Prematurity, 366–369
Prenatal care
  amniocentesis, 124–125
  assessment, 108
  biographic data, 109–111
    age, 109
    education, 110
    family history, 111
    medical history, 110
    nutritional status, 110
    obstacle course, 111
    occupation, 110
    previous and current medical
      problems, 110
    race, ethnicity, and religion, 109
    relationship status, 109
  biophysical profile, 126–127
  blood studies, 127–130
    AFP testing, 129
    antibody screening tests, 127–128
    blood typing, 127
    glucose tolerance testing, 129
    HIV testing, 128–129
    quadruple screen, 130
    serologic tests, 129

chorionic villi sampling, 125–126
  complications, 126
  transcervical or transabdominal
    approach, 125
contraction stress test, 131
fetal activity determination, 123
fetal heart rate, 120–121
  Doppler ultrasound
    stethoscope, 121
  evaluation of, 121
  fetoscope, 121
  heart to heart, 120
fetoscopy, 126
foods to avoid during
  pregnancy, 132
gynecologic history, 111
  contraceptive history, 111
  menarche, 111
  menstrual history, 111
health history, 108–109
interview tips, 108
maternal serum assays, 123–124
  fetal fibronectin (fFN),
    123–124
  human chorionic
    gonadotropin, 124
  human placental lactogen, 124
maternal urinalysis, 123
minimizing discomforts of
  pregnancy, 136–144
  first trimester, 138–140
  second and third trimesters,
    140–144
nonstress testing, 130
nutritional care, 132
  calcium, 135
  calories, 133
  fats, 134
  fluid, 136
  iodine, 135
  iron, 135–136
  phosphorus, 135
  protein, 133–134
  sodium, 136
  vitamins, 134–135
  zinc, 136
obstetric history, 112–114
  gravid, 114

GTPAL classification
  system, 114
GTPALM classification
  system, 114
para, 114
patient education, 107
percutaneous umbilical blood
  sampling, 126
physical assessment, 115–120
  head-to-toe assessment,
    116–119
  monitoring vital signs, 115
  pelvic examination, 119–120
  scheduled surveillance, 115
prenatal testing, 120
traditional elements of, 107
ultrasonography, 121–122
Prepuce, 10
Prepuce of clitoris, 16
Preschool, 402–407
  coping with concerns, 406–407
  keys to health, 404–406
  physical development, 402
  psychological development,
    403–404
Preslip SCFE, 674
Preterm labor. *See* Premature labor
Prevent/restore, 652
Primigravida, 112
Primipara, 112
Proair, Proventil. *See* Albuterol (Proair,
  Proventil)
Proctosigmoidoscopy, 690
Prodromal stage, 452
PROM. *See* Premature rupture of
  membranes (PROM)
Propa pH. *See* Salicylic acid
  (Propa pH)
Propylthiouracil (PTU), 741
Prostaglandins, changes during
  pregnancy, 86
Prostate gland, 10
Protein, 133–134
Proximal convoluted tubule, 615
Proximodistal development, 489
Psychoactive substance misuse/
  dependence, 438
PTH. *See* Parathyroid hormone (PTH)

PTU. *See* Propylthiouracil (PTU)
Pubarche, 18
Puerperal infection, 291–295
Puerperium. *See* Postpartum period
Pulmicort. *See* Budesonide (Pulmicort)
Pulmonary artery, 528, 542, 546, 550, 553, 557, 559, 564
Pulmonary circulation, 583–584
Pulmonary embolism, 304–305
Pulmonary function tests (PFTs), 587–588, 595
Pulmonary stenosis, 559
Pulmonic semilunar valve, 527
Pulmonic stenosis, 559–560
Pulmonic valves, 528
Pulmozyme, 607. *See* Dornase alfa (Pulmozyme)
Pulse oximetry, 588–589
Pupillary response, 489
Purkinje fibers, 529
Pyloric stenosis, 706–708
Pylorus, GI, 686

Q

Quadruple screen, 130
Quickening, 123
    during pregnancy, 77

R

Radiant warmer, 336
Radioallergosorbent test (RAST), 758
Radiography, 651
Radioimmunoassay, 720
Rash of rashes, 470
RAST. *See* Radioallergosorbent test (RAST)
Loratadine (Claritin), 765
RBCs. *See* Red blood cells (RBCs)
RDS. *See* Respiratory distress syndrome (RDS)
RDW. *See* Red cell distribution width (RDW)
Rectum, 10, 17, 700
Red blood cells (RBCs), 92, 748, 749–750, 761, 773, 777, 778
Red cell distribution width (RDW), 773
Relaxation techniques, for labor pain, 236

Relaxin, 86
Released enzymes, 26
Renal cortex, 614
Renal medulla, 614
Reproductive system, changes during pregnancy, 80–85
    bacteria blocker, 84
    breasts, 84–85
    cervix, 83
    ovaries, 81
    uterus, 81–83
    vagina, 84
    vascular growth, 83
Resolution stage, 452
Resorption, 649
Respiratory, 639
Respiratory distress syndrome (RDS), 371–373
    neonate, 328
Respiratory problems, 369–375
    meconium aspiration syndrome, 373–374
    pneumothorax, 374–375
    respiratory distress syndrome, 371–373
    transient tachypnea of the newborn, 369–371
Respiratory syncytial virus (RSV), 598, 600, 601, 609
Respiratory system, 380–381, 802
    anatomy and physiology, 579–586
        airway resistance, 583
        chest and lungs, 579–580
        inspiration and expiration, 584–586
        lower respiratory tract, 582–583
        pulmonary circulation, 583–584
        upper respiratory tract, 580–582
    changes during pregnancy, 88–89
    diagnostic tests and monitoring techniques, 586–589
        chest x-ray, 586–587
        pulmonary function tests, 587–588
        pulse oximetry, 588–589
    disorders, 591–612
        asthma, 591–598
        bronchiolitis, 598–601

croup, 601–604
cystic fibrosis, 605–608
pneumonia, 608–612
        treatments and procedures, 589–591
            aerosol therapy, 589–590
            oxygen administration, 590–591
Rh incompatibility. *See* Isoimmunization
Rh isoimmunization, pathogenesis of, 178
Rh sensitization, 128
Rhinovirus, 609
RhoGAM, 179–180
Rhythm (calendar) method, contraception, 43
Right atrium, 527, 542, 559
Right pulmonary veins, 527
Right upper quadrant (RUQ), 688
Right ventricle, 527, 550, 559, 564
Risk-taking behaviors, 436–437
Roseola infantum, 472–473
Rotarix, 462
RotaTeq, 462
Rotavirus vaccine, 462
RSV. *See* Respiratory syncytial virus (RSV)
RSV vaccine (Abrysvo), 600
Rubella titer test, 128
Rubeola, 473–475
RUQ. *See* Right upper quadrant (RUQ)

S

Salicylic acid (Propa pH), 798
Salmonella, 631
Salter-Harris classification system, 670–672
Same-sex cliques, 419
Sarcoptes scabiei, 811
Scabies, 811–813
SCFE. *See* Slipped capital femoral epiphysis (SCFE)
School phobias, 423
School refusal/school avoidance. *See* School phobias
Scoliosis, 677–680
Scrotum, 10, 11–12

SDOH. *See* Social determinants of health (SDOH)

Sebaceous glands/sebum-producing glands, 787

Second-degree burns, 803

Second trimester, pregnancy discomforts, 140–144
  abdominal discomfort, 143
  Braxton Hicks contractions, 143
  constipation, 142
  dyspnea (shortness of breath), 143
  heartburn, 141
  hemorrhoids, 141–142
  indigestion, 140
  lightheadedness, 142–143
  pain around round ligaments, 143–144
  psychosocial challenge, 102–103
  varicose veins, 141

Secretin, 687

Seizures, 362–364
  disorders, 519–523

Semen, 13

Semilunar valves, 528

Seminal vesicle, 10

Serologic tests, 129

Setting-sun sign, 510

Severe acne, 796, 797

Severe acute respiratory syndrome coronavirus 2019 (SARS-COVID-19). *See* COVID-19 pandemic

Severe maternal morbidity (SMM), 4

Severe preeclampsia, 118

Sexually transmitted infections (STIs), 442–445

SGA. *See* Small for gestational age (SGA)

Shigella, 631

Shigella dysenteriae, 633

Short bones, 645–646

Shortness of breath. *See* Dyspnea

Shoulder presentation, 203, 206–207

Sickle cell anemia, 777–782

Sickle cell crisis, 778, 779

SIDS. *See* Sudden infant death syndrome (SIDS)

Single-footling breech, 206

Single-parent family, 3

Singulair. *See* Montelukast (Singulair)

Sinoatrial node, 528

Sinus venosus defect, 542

Sitz bath, 256

Sjögren syndrome, 697

Skeletal traction, 657
  types of, 657

Skene duct opening, 16

Skin, 239
  biopsy, 788–791
    closest shave, 791
    nursing considerations, 791
    out, out, darn lesion, 791
    pulled and punched, 791
    recognizing skin lesions, 788–791
  changes during pregnancy, 77
  grafting, 793–794
    better to give than receive, 793
    healthy loan, 793
    keys to success, 793
    nursing considerations, 793–794
  as great protector, 785
  neonatal assessment, 325–326
  structures of, 785–787
    hair, 787
    sebaceous glands/sebum-producing glands, 787
    skin layers, 786–787
    sweat glands, 787
  traction, 656
    types of, 656–657

Slipped capital femoral epiphysis (SCFE), 673–675

Small for gestational age (SGA), 348–350

Small intestine, GI, 687

SMM. *See* Severe maternal morbidity (SMM)

Smoking, 598

Smooth/involuntary muscles, 649

Social determinants of health (SDOH), 5–6
  family's health-related beliefs and practices, 6
  health-related beliefs and practices, 6

Sodium, 136

Sodium sulfacetamide (Klaron), 798

Soft palate, 580, 581

Solid foods, 388

Soliris. *See* Eculizumab (Soliris)

Somatic nervous system, 487

Soy-based formulas, bottle-feeding, 271

Spastic cerebral palsy, 506

Spermatoblasts, 14

Spermatogenesis, 13–14

Spermatogonia, 14

Spermatozoon, 25

Spermatozoon nucleus released into the ovum, 26

Spermicides, 59–60
  advantages of, 60
  disadvantages of, 60

Sphenoid sinus, 580

Spica cast, 667

Spina bifida, 513–515

Spina bifida cystica, 514

Spina bifida occulta, 514, 516

Spinal accessory nerve (CN XI), 486

Spinal cord, 485

Spinal nerves, 485

Spine, neonatal assessment, 333

Spinous process, 239

Spleen, 754

Sports injuries, 437

Staphylococcus aureus, 570, 571

Staphylococcus epidermidis, 795

Steeple sign, 603

Stenosis, aortic, 556–558

Stenosis of pulmonary artery, 567

Stepfamily, 2

STIs. *See* Sexually transmitted infections (STIs)

Stomach, GI, 686

Stool specimen, 691

Streptococcus mutans, 390, 391

Streptococcus pneumoniae, 462, 496, 497, 754

Streptococcus viridans, 570

Stress, 766

Striae gravidarum, 77

Striated/skeletal muscles, 649

Stroke volume, 529

Subaortic stenosis, 557

Subarachnoid space, 484, 509

Subcostal, 585
Subcutaneous catheter, 512
Subcutaneous tissue, 803
Subdural space, 484
Subgaleal hemorrhage, 327
Subluxated/dislocated hip, 663, 664
Substance use disorder, 438
Substernal, 585
Subtotal thyroidectomy, 728
Sudden infant death syndrome
      (SIDS), 389
Sudden unexpected infant deaths
      (SUIDs), 389
Suicide/attempted suicide,
      446–448
SUIDs. *See* Sudden unexpected infant
      deaths (SUIDs)
Sulfur (Novacet), 798
Superior nasal concha, 580
Superior sagittal venous sinus, 509
Superior vena cava, 527
Supine hypotension, 91
Suprasternal, 585
Supratentorial ependymoma, 502
Surgical correction, 667
Sutures, 326
Sweat glands, 787
Sympathetic nervous system, 487
Symphysis pubis, 10, 17, 252
Symptothermal method,
      contraception, 46
Synagis. *See* Palivizumab (Synagis)
Synarthrodial joints, 650
Synovial joints, 650
Syphilis, 354–355

T
T cells/T lymphocytes, 755–756
T_3 test (serum), 726–727
T_4 test, 725–726
Tanner stages, 430
Tapazole. *See* Methimazole (Tapazole)
Tazarotene (Tazorac), 798
Tazorac. *See* Tazarotene (Tazorac)
TBSA. *See* Total body surface area
      (TBSA)
Teach expectations, 534–536
TEE. *See* Transesophageal
      echocardiography (TEE)

Temovate. *See* Clobetasol (Temovate)
Temporal lobe, 482
Tendons, 649
Terbutaline (Brethine), 187, 188
Testis, 10
Testosterone, 14
Tetracycline, 798
Tetralogy of Fallot, 566–569
Thermal burns, 800
Thermoregulation, neonatal care,
      335–339
Thermoregulators, 336
Third-degree burns, 803
Third trimester, pregnancy discomforts,
      140–144
   abdominal discomfort, 143
   Braxton Hicks contractions, 143
   constipation, 142
   dyspnea (shortness of breath), 143
   heartburn, 141
   hemorrhoids, 141–142
   indigestion, 140
   lightheadedness, 142–143
   pain around round ligaments,
      143–144
   psychosocial challenge, 103–104
   varicose veins, 141
Third ventricle, 509
Thymus, 712, 753
Thyroid cartilage, 580
Thyroid function test, 720
Thyroid gland, 712, 713
   changes during pregnancy, 87
Thyroidectomy, 728–729
Tinea capitis, 813–815
Tinea corporis, 815–816
To left lung, 550
To right lung, 550
Toddlerhood, 393–400
   keys to health, 396–400
   psychological development,
      394–396
   toddlerhood, 393–394
Tonsils/adenoids, 581, 754
Total body surface area (TBSA), 803–804
Toxoid, 454–455
Trabeculae, 647
Trachea, 580, 581, 582
Traction, 656–658

Transcutaneous electrical nerve
      stimulation, 237
Transdermal contraceptive patch,
      53–54
   advantages of, 53
   disadvantages of, 53–54
Transesophageal echocardiography
      (TEE), 532–533
Transient tachypnea of the newborn
      (TTN), 369–371
Transposition defect, 564
Transposition of the great arteries,
      563–566
Trendelenburg gait, 665
Trendelenburg test, 665
Treponema pallidum, 354
Tretinoin (Vesanoid), 798
Trichophyton mentagrophytes, 815
Trichophyton rubrum, 815
Trichophyton tonsurans, 814
Tricuspid valves, 527, 528
Trifarotene, 798
Trigeminal nerve (CN V), 486
Trimethoprimsulfamethoxazole
      (Bactrim), 469
Triphasic oral contraceptives, 48
Trochlear nerve (CN IV), 486
True labor signs, 214–215
TTN. *See* Transient tachypnea of the
      newborn (TTN)
Tubal sterilization, 69–70
   advantages of, 70
   disadvantages of, 70
   procedure, 70
Tunica albuginea, 12
Tunica vaginalis, 12
Turner syndrome, 697
21- or 28-day packs, contraceptives, 49
Two-cell stage, 29
Two-parent families, 2
Type 1 diabetes, 160, 732–733, 735
Type 2 diabetes, 160, 732–733, 735
Tzanck test, 792

U
Ultrasonography, pregnancy, 79
Umbilical arteries, 530
Umbilical cord, 36
Umbilical vein, 530

Umbilical vessels, 36
United Network for Organ Sharing (UNOS) list, 540
Universal neonatal hearing screening, 329
UNOS. *See* United Network for Organ Sharing (UNOS) list
Upper airway, 602
Upper GI series. *See* Barium swallow
Upper respiratory tract, 580–582
  larynx, 582
  mouth and oropharynx, 581
  nose and nasal passages, 580–581
  pharynx, 581
Urethra, 10, 17, 628–631
Urethral meatus, 10, 16
Urinalysis/urine culture, 617–618
Urinary bladder, 10
Urinary frequency, and pregnancy, 76
Urinary system
  anatomy and physiology, 614–616
    kidneys, 614–615
    urinary tract, 616
  diagnostic tests, 617–621
    BUN and creatinine, 618–619
    excretory urography, 619–620
    kidney biopsy, 621
    KUB radiography, 619
    urinalysis and urine culture, 617–618
    voiding cystourethrogram, 620–621
  disorders, 625–642
    acute poststreptococcal glomerulonephritis, 625–628
    congenital anomalies of the ureter/bladder/urethra, 628–631
    hemolytic uremic syndrome, 631–634
    kidney failure, acute, 637–640
    nephrotic syndrome, 634–637
    Wilms tumor, 641–642
  during pregnancy, 93–95
    anatomic changes, 93–94
    functional changes, 94–95
    posture of elimination, 95

treatments and procedures, 621–625
  bladder catheterization, 621–623
  hemodialysis, 623
  kidney transplantation, 624
  peritoneal dialysis, 624–625
Urinary tract, 616
U.S. Food and Drug Administration (FDA), 735–736
Uterine atony, 279
  risk factors for, 279
Uterine bleeding, 83
Uterine cavity, 29
Uterine contraction, 245
Uterine enlargement, during pregnancy, 76
Uterine stabilizing instrument, 70
Uterine wall, 29
Uterus, 20, 70, 91, 232
  changes during pregnancy, 81–83
Uvula, 581

V

Vagina, 17, 19, 33, 232
  changes during pregnancy, 84
Vaginal orifice, 16
Vagus nerve (CN X), 486
Varicella, 476–477
Varicella virus vaccine, 463–464
Varicose veins, 141
Vas deferens, 10, 68
Vascular growth, changes during pregnancy, 83
Vasectomy, 67–69
  advantages of, 69
  disadvantages of, 69
  procedure, 68
VATS. *See* Video-assisted thoracoscopic surgery (VATS)
VCUG. *See* Voiding cystourethrogram (VCUG)
Vena cava, 91, 542, 550, 553
Ventricles, 485
Ventricular septal defect (VSD), 549–552, 567
Ventriculoperitoneal (VP) shunt, 495–496
Vertex cephalic presentation, 202, 205
Vesanoid. *See* Tretinoin (Vesanoid)

Video-assisted thoracoscopic surgery (VATS), 548
Viral infections, 355–357
Viruses, 470–477
  COVID-19, 477
  fifth disease, 471–472
  not so rash, 471
  rash of rashes, 470
  roseola infantum, 472–473
  rubeola, 473–475
  varicella, 476–477
Vitamin B_{12}, 688
Vitamin D, 433, 688
Vitamin K, 687–688
Vitamins, 134–135
Voiding cystourethrogram (VCUG), 620–621
von Willebrand disease, 770
VP. *See* Ventriculoperitoneal (VP) shunt
VSD. *See* Ventricular septal defect (VSD)

W

Warfarin (Coumadin), 158
WBCs. *See* White blood cells (WBCs)
White blood cells (WBCs), 93, 748, 750–752, 775
WHO. *See* World Health Organization (WHO)
Whooping cough. *See* Pertussis
Wilms tumor, 641–642
World Health Organization (WHO), 4

X

X chromosome, 14
X-rays, 651–652
Xopenex. *See* Levalbuterol (Xopenex)

Y

Y chromosome, 14
Yersinia/Campylobacter, 631
Yoga, for labor pain, 237
Yolk sac, 33, 34, 35

Z

Zinc, 136
Zona fasciculata, 714
Zona glomerulosa, 714
Zona reticularis, 714
Zygote, 9, 21–22, 27, 29
Zyrtec. *See* Cetirizine (Zyrtec)